Hirschsprung's Disease and Allied Disorders

Prem Puri
Editor

Hirschsprung's Disease and Allied Disorders

Fourth Edition

Springer

Editor
Prem Puri
National Children's Research Centre
Our Lady's Childrens Hospital, University College Dublin
Dublin
Ireland

Originally published by Hippokrates Verlag GmbH, Thieme-Stratton Inc., New York, 1982

ISBN 978-3-030-15646-6   ISBN 978-3-030-15647-3 (eBook)
https://doi.org/10.1007/978-3-030-15647-3

This Springer imprint is published by the registered company Springer Nature Switzerland AG
The registered company address is: Gewerbestrasse 11, 6330 Cham, Switzerland

To the ever patient Veena, for her love and inspiration

Foreword

Harald Hirschsprung (1830–1916) was born in Copenhagen in 1830. His father was a tobacco merchant and founder of the tobacco factory A. M. Hirschsprung & Sønner. He was the younger son and was expected to take over the family business, but he refused. However, the father gave in to his son's wish which was to become a physician. He was attracted to gastroenterology, and his doctoral thesis was on the topic of atresia of the oesophagus and small bowel. His interest in rare paediatric surgical conditions, especially of the gut, continued throughout his life and produced a steady stream of publications in this field. In 1870, he became the first paediatrician in Denmark. In 1886, at the Congress of the Gesellschaft für Kinderheilkunde in Berlin, he gave a lecture titled "Stuhlträgheit Neugeborener in Folge von Dilatation und Hypertrophie des Colons" (Bowel Inertia following Dilatation and Hypertrophy of the Colon). In this lecture, which was published the following year, he described the problem of two infants who had died from the disease that was to bear his name: constipation associated with dilatation and hypertrophy of the colon. He concluded his account by commenting "it appears unquestionable that the condition is caused in utero, either as a developmental abnormality or as a disease process". Fifteen years later, in 1901, K. Tittel reported the first histological study of the intrinsic plexus myentericus of the colon and described its absence in the colon of a patient. Bretano made a similar observation in 1904, and the nature of the basic abnormality was eventually confirmed in 1949 by Bodian et al. who reviewed a large number of autopsy specimens at The Hospital for Sick Children, London. Since the end of the nineteenth century, the congenital disease, based on the absence of ganglion cells in the colon, has been called "Hirschsprung's disease". Its first logical and most effective therapy, the introduction of the rectosigmoidectomy, was performed by Swenson and Bill in 1948. Orvar Swenson (1909–2012) was Professor of Pediatric Surgery at this time at Harvard Medical School in Boston.

The first book on "Hirschsprung's disease" was edited in 1970 by Theodor Ehrenpreis (1918–1999), Professor of Pediatric Surgery at the Karolinska Institute in Stockholm. His books started with a small chapter on the "Basic Facts" of the disease; the rest were clinical generalities and results. The book was a famous part of a series called "Surgical Conditions in Infancy and Childhood" published by the Year Book Medical Publishers Inc., Chicago. In the following years, the knowledge about A- and dysganglionosis in the colon developed fundamentally and rapidly, increasing "like a little snowball anticipated in a big avalanche" as Theodor Ehrenpreis wrote in the Preface of the next, my own first book, on "Hirschsprung's Disease".

After Ehrenpreis's retirement, I got the permission from him to edit this book, which was published in 1982 by Hippokrates-Thieme-Stratton Inc. Publishers, Stuttgart-New York. Orvar Swenson himself gave me the honour of adding two chapters to this new book: a historical review of the disease and details of the surgical treatment of his own, very effective surgical technique. The neuronal colonic development and its physiology were described by Marvin Schuster, Baltimore, and the pathophysiology of Hirschsprung's congenital disease by Alois Schärli, Luzern. He had been trained by Marvin Schuster in the new diagnostic technique of anorectal manometrical studies in patients with imperforate anus and had published this experience in his first book *Die Angeborenen Mißbildungen des Rectums und Anus, Verlag Hans Huber Bern, Stuttgart, Wien, 1971*. I learned this new diagnostic procedure from him and used it effectively for patients with chronic constipation, dysganglionosis or Hirschsprung's disease. Apart from this new diagnostic experience and new histochemical studies of biopsies of the bowel wall, chapters on "Particular Forms of Hirschsprung's Disease" like IND (Intestinal Neuronal Dysplasia) and Anal Sphincter Achalasia were also described for the first time in this book. Additionally, new surgical techniques like Duhamel's (France) "Retro rectal and transanal pull through", Soave's (Italy) "Extra mucosal colorectal pull-through procedure" and Rehbein's (Germany) "Deep anterior resection" were described in detail and their different steps explained by the paediatric surgeons themselves, who had invented these techniques.

In the following 18 years, the scientific knowledge about this disease increased very much again. According to Th. Ehrenpreis, its "curtain was suddenly raised". In the second edition of my book, which I had the great honour to publish together with Prem Puri at Harwood Academic Publishers in 2000, our international contributors increased the quality of the book very much. For the first time, the developmental genetics of the enteric nervous system were mentioned by J.H.C. Meyers, D.T. Cass, I. Ceccherini, G. Martucciello and others. Very important too was the detailed description of the "Functional Anatomy of the Nervous System" with "A Developmental Perspective relevant to the Pathogenesis of Hirschsprung's Disease". Its author, Michael Gershon, Professor of Pathology and Cell Biology, at the Columbia University, New York, has been called the "Father of Neurogastroenterology" and later on wrote his famous, popular book *The Second Brain*, a groundbreaking new understanding of nervous disorders of the gastrointestinal tract. Besides, many new aspects concerning different visceral myo- and neuropathies mimicking Hirschsprung's disease were described. For the first time, intestinal neuronal dysplasia was described by its discoverer, William Meier-Ruge, and "Newer Neuronal markers for the Investigation of Enteric Plexus Disorders" were analysed by Prem Puri. In addition, a new surgical laparoscopic technique for pull-through procedures was introduced by Keith E. Georgeson, Birmingham, Alabama. Therefore, this second edition was not anymore called "Hirschsprung's Disease" but

Hirschsprung's Disease and Allied Disorders. It was Alberto Pena who gave us the honour to write the foreword of this book.

The following edition of this book was published 8 years later, again by Springer Publisher, Berlin-Heidelberg, in 2008. In this short interval of 8 years, not very much of our knowledge had changed, but it was no longer possible to get further copies of the excellent edition from Harwood Academic Publishers. Therefore, Prem Puri and I myself started the third edition of the book with special regard to some new aspects. A chapter on "Animal Models of Aganglionosis" by A.M. Alzahem and D.T. Cass was introduced, and "Molecular Genetics" and "Genetic Associations in Hirschsprung's Disease" became more important chapters of this new edition. Enterocolitis, as a difficult complication of Hirschsprung's disease, was described for the first time in a separate chapter. Prem Puri and his co-workers added for the first time new chapters on "NADPH-Diaphorase Histochemistry" and "Immunohistochemical Studies". In addition, T. Wedel and H.J. Krammer published for the first time new aspects on "Electron Microscopic Studies of Hirschsprung's Disease". Concerning "Allied Disorders", the "Megacystis-Microcolon-Intestinal Hypoperistalsis Syndrome", the "Degenerative Hollow Visceral Myopathy mimicking Hirschsprung's Disease", the "Adynamic Bowel Syndrome" and the "Ultrashort Hirschsprung's Disease" were added to this further edition.

Now, 11 years have passed since the last publication, and I am very happy that Prem Puri has now edited the fourth edition of our book. It is very well known that medical knowledge outdates approximately every 7–8 years. If we want to help our patients, we have to continue with the publication of the newest and most important results of newer scientific studies. In my eyes, these days, Prem Puri is one of the most important paediatric surgeons in the world. He is Clinical Research Professor at the UCD School of Medicine and Medical Science and President of the National Children's Research Centre at Our Lady's Children's Hospital in Dublin. He has a vast experience in scientific studies and was my coeditor of the last two editions of our book. In his institute, he has performed many further clinical and experimental studies in this interesting disease. I am sure that Harald Hirschsprung would be proud of him. I congratulate Prem on his professional expertise in bringing to fruition this fifth book on "Hirschsprung's Diseases" and this fourth edition of *Hirschsprung's Disease and Allied Disorders*.

Alexander Holschneider

Preface to the Fourth Edition

It is 11 years since the third edition of this book was published in 2008. During the past decade, major advances have occurred both in the understanding and in the treatment of "Hirschsprung's disease and allied disorders". The fourth edition of *Hirschsprung's Disease and Allied Disorders* has been thoroughly updated either in the form of entirely new or substantially revised chapters. The new edition contains 32 chapters by 71 contributors from various parts of the world. This edition contains 14 new chapters on important topics including familial Hirschsprung's disease, stem cell therapy for enteric neuropathies, association between Hirschsprung's disease and multiple endocrine neoplasia type 2a, manometric diagnosis of Hirschsprung's disease, rectal biopsy for the diagnosis of Hirschsprung's disease, total colonic aganglionosis, Hirschsprung's disease in adolescents and adults, variant Hirschsprung's disease, redo surgery for Hirschsprung's disease, morphological basis of persistent bowel problems following a properly performed pull-through operation for Hirschsprung's disease, bowel management for the treatment of chronic constipation in patients operated on for Hirschsprung's disease, inflammatory bowel disease in patients with Hirschsprung's disease, intestinal transplantation for total intestinal aganglionosis and urological and sexual outcome in patients with Hirschsprung's disease. Each chapter has been written by expert contributors with a significant experience in their respective fields of interest.

The fourth edition of this book provides an authoritative, comprehensive and complete account of the enteric neuronal disorders of the lower gastrointestinal tract. I hope that the trainees as well as established paediatric surgeons, paediatricians, neonatologists and paediatric gastroenterologists will find this textbook useful as a guide when dealing with Hirschsprung's disease and allied disorders in infants and children.

I wish to thank most sincerely all the contributors for their outstanding work in producing this innovative textbook. I also wish to express my gratitude to Dr. Anne Marie O'Donnell and Dr. Hiroki Nakamura for all their help in the preparation of this book. I wish to thank the editorial staff of Springer Nature, particularly Ms. Evgenia Koutsouki and Mr. Prakash Jagannathan, for all their help during the preparation and publication of this book.

Dublin, Ireland Prem Puri

Contents

Contributors

Eleni Athanasakos Department of Paediatric Surgery, The Royal London Hospital, Barts Health, Whitechapel, London, UK

Andrea Bischoff International Center for Colorectal and Urogenital Care, Children's Hospital Colorado, Aurora, CO, USA

Julia Brendel Department of Pediatric Surgery, Hannover Medical School, Hannover, Germany

Robin Brown Division of Paediatric Surgery, Red Cross War Memorial Children's Hospital, Cape Town, South Africa

Faculty of Health Sciences, University of Cape Town, Cape Town, South Africa

Alan J. Burns Stem Cells and Regenerative Medicine, UCL Great Ormond Street Institute of Child Health, London, UK

Department of Clinical Genetics, Erasmus University Medical Centre, Rotterdam, The Netherlands

Takeda Pharmaceuticals International, Cambridge, MA, USA

Stephanie Chen Division of Pediatric Surgery, Department of Surgery, Cedars-Sinai Medical Center, Los Angeles, CA, USA

James Christensen Department of Internal Medicine, University of Iowa Carver College of Medicine, Iowa City, IA, USA

Stewart Cleeve Department of Paediatric Surgery, The Royal London Hospital, Barts Health, Whitechapel, London, UK

Arnold G. Coran Pediatric Surgery, University of Michigan, Ann Arbor, MI, USA

David Coyle Temple Street Children's University Hospital, Dublin, Ireland

Jie-xiong Feng Department of Pediatric Surgery, Tongji Hospital, Tongji Medical College, Huazhong University of Science and Technology, Wuhan, China

Florian Friedmacher Department of Pediatric Surgery, The Royal London Hospital, Whitechapel, London, UK

National Children's Research Centre, Our Lady's Children's Hospital, Crumlin, Dublin, Ireland

Philip K. Frykman Division of Pediatric Surgery, Department of Surgery, Cedars-Sinai Medical Center, Los Angeles, CA, USA

Maria-Mercè Garcia-Barceló Department of Surgery, Li Ka Shing Faculty of Medicine, The University of Hong Kong, Hong Kong SAR China, Hong Kong SAR

Michael D. Gershon Department of Anatomy and Cell Biology, Columbia University, College of Physicians and Surgeons, New York, NY, USA

Allan M. Goldstein Department of Pediatric Surgery, Massachusetts General Hospital, Harvard Medical School, Boston, MA, USA

Ankush Gosain Division of Pediatric Surgery, Department of Surgery, University of Tennessee Health Science Center, Memphis, TN, USA

Children's Foundation Research Institute, Le Bonheur Children's Hospital, Memphis, TN, USA

Anna Löf Granström Division of Pediatric Surgery, Department of Women's and Children's Health, Karolinska Institutet, Stockholm, Sweden

Pediatric Surgery, Karolinska University Hospital, Stockholm, Sweden

J. L. Grosfeld University Clinic of Paediatric and Adolescent Surgery, Medical University of Graz, Graz, Austria

Devendra K. Gupta Department of Pediatric Surgery, All India Institute of Medical Sciences, New Delhi, India

Roisin Hayes Department of Radiology, Our Ladys Childrens Hospital, Crumlin, Dublin, Ireland

Robert M. W. Hofstra Department of Clinical Genetics, Erasmus University Medical Centre, Rotterdam, The Netherlands

M. E. Höllwarth University Clinic of Paediatric and Adolescent Surgery, Medical University of Graz, Graz, Austria

Ryo Hotta Department of Pediatric Surgery, Massachusetts General Hospital, Harvard Medical School, Boston, MA, USA

Kishore Iyer Recanati/Miller Transplantation Institute, Mount Sinai Medical Center, New York, NY, USA

Raj P. Kapur Department of Pathology, Seattle Children's Hospital and University of Washington, Seattle, WA, USA

Jerry Kelleher Department of Radiology, Our Ladys Childrens Hospital, Crumlin, Dublin, Ireland

Kristiina Kyrklund Section of Pediatric Surgery, Pediatric Liver and Gut Research Group, Pediatric Research Center, Children's Hospital, University of Helsinki and Helsinki University Hospital, Helsinki, Finland

Joanne Lai Icahn School of Medicine at Mount Sinai, New York, NY, USA

Ning Li Department of Pediatric Surgery, Tongji Hospital, Tongji Medical College, Huazhong University of Science and Technology, Wuhan, China

Ting Li Department of Pediatric Surgery, Tongji Hospital, Tongji Medical College, Huazhong University of Science and Technology, Wuhan, China

Conor J. McCann Stem Cells and Regenerative Medicine, UCL Great Ormond Street Institute of Child Health, London, UK

Sandra Montedonico National Children's Research Centre, Our Lady's Children's Hospital, Crumlin, Dublin, Ireland

Hospital Carlos Van Buren, Escuela de Medicina, Universidad de Valparaíso, Valparaíso, Chile

Samuel William Moore Division of Pediatric Surgery, Faculty of Medicine and Health Sciences, University of Stellenbosch, Stellenbosch, South Africa

Annika Mutanen Section of Pediatric Surgery, Hospital for Children and Adolescents, University of Helsinki, Helsinki, Finland

Hiroki Nakamura National Children's Research Centre, Our Lady's Children's Hospital, Crumlin, Dublin, Ireland

Alp Numanoglu Division of Paediatric Surgery, Red Cross War Memorial Children's Hospital, Cape Town, South Africa

Faculty of Health Sciences, University of Cape Town, Cape Town, South Africa

Anne Marie O'Donnell National Children's Research Centre, Our Lady's Children's Hospital, Crumlin, Dublin, Ireland

Mikko P. Pakarinen Section of Pediatric Surgery, Pediatric Liver and Gut Research Group, Pediatric Research Center, Children's Hospital, University of Helsinki and Helsinki University Hospital, Helsinki, Finland

Section of Pediatric Surgery, Hospital for Children and Adolescents, University of Helsinki, Helsinki, Finland

Deven C. Patel Division of Pediatric Surgery, Department of Surgery, Cedars-Sinai Medical Center, Los Angeles, CA, USA

Alberto Peña International Center for Colorectal and Urogenital Care, Children's Hospital Colorado, Aurora, CO, USA

Prem Puri National Children's Research Centre, Our Lady's Childrens Hospital, University College Dublin, Dublin, Ireland

School of Medicine and Medical Science and Conway Institute of Biomedical Research, University College Dublin, Dublin, Ireland

Matthew W. Ralls Pediatric Surgery, University of Michigan, Ann Arbor, MI, USA

Rebecca M. Rentea Department of Surgery, Children's Mercy Hospital, Kansas City, MI, USA

Risto J. Rintala Section of Pediatric Surgery, Hospital for Children and Adolescents, University of Helsinki, Helsinki, Finland

Heinz Rode Division of Paediatric Surgery, Red Cross War Memorial Children's Hospital, Cape Town, South Africa

Faculty of Health Sciences, University of Cape Town, Cape Town, South Africa

Udo Rolle Department of Paediatric Surgery and Paediatric Urology, Goethe-University Frankfurt/M., Frankfurt/M, Germany

Shilpa Sharma Department of Pediatric Surgery, All India Institute of Medical Sciences, New Delhi, India

Charles L. Snyder Department of Surgery, Children's Mercy Hospital, Kansas City, MI, USA

Masahiro Takeda Department of Pediatric Surgery, Juntendo University School of Medicine, Tokyo, Japan

Paul K. H. Tam Department of Surgery, Li Ka Shing Faculty of Medicine, The University of Hong Kong, Hong Kong SAR China, Hong Kong SAR

Clara S. M. Tang Department of Surgery, Li Ka Shing Faculty of Medicine, The University of Hong Kong, Hong Kong SAR China, Hong Kong SAR

Nikhil Thapar Stem Cells and Regenerative Medicine, UCL Great Ormond Street Institute of Child Health, London, UK

Laura V. Veras Division of Pediatric Surgery, Department of Surgery, University of Tennessee Health Science Center, Memphis, TN, USA

Dirk von Delft Division of Paediatric Surgery, Red Cross War Memorial Children's Hospital, Cape Town, South Africa

Faculty of Health Sciences, University of Cape Town, Cape Town, South Africa

Tomas Wester Division of Pediatric Surgery, Department of Women's and Children's Health, Karolinska Institutet, Stockholm, Sweden

Pediatric Surgery, Karolinska University Hospital, Stockholm, Sweden

Atsuyuki Yamataka Department of Pediatric Surgery, Juntendo University School of Medicine, Tokyo, Japan

Yuta Yazaki Department of Pediatric Surgery, Juntendo University School of Medicine, Tokyo, Japan

Hirschsprung's Disease: A Historical Perspective – 1691–2018

1

M. E. Höllwarth and J. L. Grosfeld*

Contents

Hirschsprung's disease (HSCR) is a rare cause of neonatal intestinal obstruction that is of great interest to pediatric surgeons throughout the world. The prevalence shows some geographic heterogeneity with an incidence of 1.09/10,000 births in Europe and 1.0/5343 in Japan [7, 168].

The first prehistoric experience of Hindu doctors can be found in the Sushruta Samhita which is an ancient monograph of Ayurvedic surgery compiled by Sushruta (circa 1200–600 BC). It described a pathology called "Baddha Gudodaram" which is clinically very similar to HSCR characterized by abdominal distension due to blockage of the rectum. The distal colon of the affected patients is stuffed with feces, fecaliths, and undigested fibers [137]. Prior reports from the Western world ascribe the initial description of this condition to Fredericus Ruysch, a Dutch anatomist in Amsterdam in 1691 [99, 149]. He described a 5-year-old girl with abdominal pain who did not respond to the "usual treatment of the day to relieve pain, pass wind and kill worms." She eventually died. The information regarding the patient was incomplete in regard to the events that occurred at the time of her birth; the autopsy findings were not clearly described apart from enormous dilatation of the colon. Although this may have represented a case of HSCR, there was inadequate evidence to be sure of the actual diagnosis [38]. Similarly, in 1800, Domenico Battini in Italy described very carefully the clinical history of a child whom he followed up for 10 years with severe constipation who eventually died and demonstrated severe rectal and colonic dilatation at autopsy consistent with megacolon. A number of characteristic features including familiarity – both parents suffered from constipation and tedious abdominal hardness, and similar complaints could be traced back to the maternal grandmother and one uncle – and the selective involvement of "neural layers" at autopsy of the bowel were postulated by Battini [44, 156]. Further case reports of clinical observations were published in the nineteenth century by Monterossi (1819), Parry (1825), Billard (1829), von Ammon (1842), Oulmont (1843), Banks (1846), Favalli (1846), Porro (1871), Vulpian (1877), and Chapmann (1878) [44]. In 1869, Jacobi was the first to describe two newborn infants with intestinal obstruction that may have been attributable to congenital megacolon. One recovered after the administration of enemas; the other required a

* Deceased

M. E. Höllwarth (✉) · J. L. Grosfeld
University Clinic of Paediatric and Adolescent Surgery, Medical University of Graz, Graz, Austria
e-mail: michael.hoellwarth@medunigraz.at

P. Puri (ed.), *Hirschsprung's Disease and Allied Disorders*,
https://doi.org/10.1007/978-3-030-15647-3_1

colostomy which completely resolved the symptoms but died of subsequent peritonitis [79]. No obstruction was found at autopsy, and the colonic dilatation had disappeared.

Scattered reports concerning the autopsy findings in anecdotal cases of constipation in older children and adults that started at birth or early youth and progressed to intestinal obstruction appeared in the literature during the following 15 years [21, 38]. In 1884, Gee (as reported by Cass [21]) considered it possible, based on the findings of an autopsy of a 4-year-old child, that the condition was related to the presence of "spasm" of the sigmoid colon since the rectum was not involved in the typical dilatation and hypertrophy noted in his patient. In 1885, Bristowe described the course of an 8-year-old girl who died of intestinal obstruction after longstanding constipation. Her autopsy demonstrated dilatation of the colon and upper rectum that ceased abruptly 2 inches from the anus. No anal stricture or stenosis was observed [15]. This may have represented an instance of low-segment HSCR.

Dr. Harald Hirschsprung, a Danish pediatrician from Queen Louise Children's Hospital, Copenhagen, presented the most telling and concise description of the "congenital megacolon" at the Society of Pediatrics in Berlin in 1886. His treatise was entitled "Constipation in newborns due to dilatation and hypertrophy of the colon" [38, 63]. At the time, he was unaware of the previous reports concerning the subject [38]. He presented the pathologic colon specimens and case reports of two infant boys who had symptoms of constipation soon after birth and who eventually died at 11 months and 8 months old. The first patient failed to pass stool at birth and required repeated enemas to relieve his obstruction. Constipation continued in the ensuing months despite breast feeding and was managed by laxatives. He was hospitalized for a 2-month period when he was 8 months old. Spontaneous bowel motions never occurred, and the boy's abdomen was enormously distended. After a bowel motion was provoked, the distension decreased. Following discharge from the hospital he developed abdominal distension and frequent loose stools. He experienced rapid weight loss and was readmitted to the hospital and died the same day at 11 months of age. At autopsy, the sigmoid and transverse colon was enormously dilated, and the muscle wall of the bowel was hypertrophied. The rectum was described as not being dilated and there was no site of narrowing. The second patient basically had the same presenting history of constipation from birth. He died at 8 months of age following the onset of severe abdominal distension and diarrhea (probably enterocolitis). At autopsy, the colon appeared similar to that of the first patient, but the appearance of the rectum was not described, although it was noted that the rectum was empty on digital examination. Hirschsprung's presentation was published in 1888 [56]. He neither offered a method of treatment nor proposed an etiology for this condition.

In 1898, Treves described a patient with idiopathic dilatation of the colon. He treated the patient with colon irrigation and performed a rectosigmoid resection and colostomy [186]. He documented the presence of a "narrow distal rectum" and presumed that this was the cause of the obstruction (a fact that went unrecognized for many years) [186]. A year later (1899), Grith published a collective review of 55 similar cases in the literature [55]. In 1900, Fenwick attributed the findings in infants with hypertrophy and dilatation of the colon to "spasm of the anal sphincters" [43]. The same year, Lennander was the first to suggest a neurogenic origin for this condition. He observed megasigmoid in the absence of mechanical obstruction in a 4-year-old boy and interpreted the findings as due to "deficient innervation" and treated the boy successfully with faradic (electric) enemas [100]. In 1901, Tittel in Austria is credited with the first histologic study suggestive of Hirschsprung's disease noting the absence and/or sparse development of plexuses in the colon but normal findings in the ileum [184]. Brentano corroborated these findings in a patient 3 years later [14].

In 1904, Hirschsprung described his personal experience with ten patients with this condition that he now referred to as "congenital dilatation of the colon." Nine of the ten patients were boys, and at the time of his report, five had died between 2 and 11 months of age. The other patients continued to have significant problems with constipation. The bowel was dilated and hypertrophied in each of the patients autopsied. There was no evidence of mechanical obstruction. The mucosa of the colon showed morphological changes and ulceration that Harold Hirschsprung interpreted as the result of fecal retention. While he now considered the condition to be congenital in nature, he continued his fixation on the abnormally dilated and hypertrophied colon and still did not speculate on the etiology nor offer specific treatment. Hirschsprung's observations were published in 1904 as the first textbook chapter devoted to congenital dilatation of the colon in "Traite des maladies de l'enfance" (2nd edition) edited by Grancher and Comby. The year 2016 is a noteworthy centenary anniversary, because Dr. Harald Hirschsprung born in 1930 died in 1916 at 86 years of age.

Ehrenpreis indicated that Mya had actually invented the term "megacolon congenita" in 1894, and some years later the term Hirschsprung's disease was brought into use to describe the condition that Harald Hirschsprung so carefully described and brought into focus [38]. Although Hirschsprung was not a pediatric surgeon, in addition to his acclaim regarding congenital megacolon, he made other important contributions to the field of pediatric surgery in the areas of esophageal and intestinal atresia, pyloric stenosis, and the non-operative management of intussusception [64, 65, 135, 185]. Interested readers are referred to additional publications concerning this unusual personality [13, 21, 45, 81, 101, 135, 145, 185].

With the world now more aware of this common condition, additional reports describing similar clinical findings began to appear in the literature. Many of these reports concerned adult patients with a short history of constipation and atypical or inadequate autopsy studies that likely had other diagnoses. In regard to surgical interventions, Perthes described transanal resection of the rectal folds and valves in 1905, and Finney in 1908 and Barington-Ward in 1915 reported "temporary success" following resection of the dilated bowel [6, 21, 38]. Patients continued to do poorly and the etiology of this condition remained elusive. In 1920, Dalla Valla shed new light on the subject when he reported the absence of ganglion cells in the sigmoid colon in two brothers who had normal ganglion cells in the proximal colon [27]. These observations were corroborated by Cameron 8 years later [16]. In 1923, Ishikawa noted the absence of parasympathetic nerves in the pelvic colon in a 4-year-old girl and he and others induced experimental megacolon in laboratory animals by resecting the parasympathetic nerves to the distal colon [1, 38, 76]. In 1927, Wade and Royle performed a lumbar sympathectomy to reduce sympathetic tone in the affected bowel in a patient who relapsed after a sigmoid resection [192]. Other reports appeared documenting the use of sympathectomy for this condition [2, 82, 136]. In the 1930s, spinal anesthesia was also employed to treat the sympathetic hyperfunction that was presumed to be the cause of symptoms in patients with megacolon with some improvement noted [60]. In 1931, Irwin provided a careful description of Auerbach's plexus [75]. In the late 1930s and early 1940s clinical reports described some improvement in symptoms after administration of parasympathomimetic drugs to patients with megacolon [86]. In 1940, Tiffin and associates described local absence of ganglion cells in the myenteric plexus in a patient with congenital megacolon with ganglia present above and below the area in question [183].

Despite these observations, many authors including Ehrenpreis, refuted the evidence regarding sympathetic hyperfunction, and for that matter any neurogenic disturbance, as the cause of the disease [1, 37]. In 1945, Grimson and colleagues similarly recommended a one-stage resection for "obstinate megacolon and ileosigmoidostomy" [56]. Ehrenpreis considered the loss of ganglion cells reported by others as a secondary event resulting from persistent colonic dilatation and stasis and in 1946, he defined HSCR as "a dysfunction of evacuation of the colon of as yet unknown origin, occurring in the absence of morphological and mechanical causations giving rise secondarily to a characteristic dilatation of the colon" [37, 38]. In 1948, Whitehouse et al. investigated histologic specimens, not only from HSCR patients but also from patients with constipation [198]. They found in controls that dilatation of the colon created only a wider separation of the ganglia and inflammatory diseases had little effect on the plexus at all, concluding that aganglionosis is a congenital anomaly.

Following the end of World War II in 1945, further light was shed on the subject that would dramatically change the course for children with HSCR. In 1948, Drs. Swenson, Neuhauser (a radiologist) and Pickett in Boston using a barium enema and fluoroscopy, recognized an area of spasm in the rectum or rectosigmoid that defined the site of obstruction in patients with congenital megacolon [170]. This established the barium enema as a useful diagnostic tool in HSCR. In six patients, Swenson and Bill performed a lifesaving proximal colostomy that relieved obstructive symptoms. This improvement following colostomy was similar to the observations made by Jacobi in 1869 and Treves in 1898 [79, 169, 173, 186]. Closure of the colostomy in three of the infants resulted in recurrence of obstructive symptoms. These astute clinical observations led to the decision to resect the colon from a point proximal to the abnormal area of obstruction identified on the barium studies and the narrow distal rectum (now recognized as the site of physiologic obstruction), and perform a coloanal anastomosis above the dentate line to preserve continence. This was a historic landmark event, the first successful operative procedure for HSCR – the Swenson procedure [169]. The procedure was initially developed in the experimental surgical laboratory at Boston Children's Hospital and then applied in the clinical setting. The operation was undertaken based on careful clinical observations and thoughtful deduction ignoring the controversy at the time regarding the influence of bowel innervation and the presence or absence of ganglion cells in this disorder [170, 173, 174].

That same year, Zuelzer and Wilson described the autopsy findings in 11 infants who died of HSCR [208]. No mechanical cause of obstruction was noted. All 11 had an absence of ganglion cells in the distal segment with six having a recognizable definitive level of obstruction. They suggested that HSCR was a functional intestinal obstruction that had a congenital neurogenic basis and that an enterostomy should be considered [208]. Also in 1948, Whitehouse and Kernohan described the autopsy findings in 11 children who died of megacolon [199]. None had ganglion cells present, and nonmyelinated nerve trunks between the longitudinal and circular muscle layers were identified in the distal bowel. They noted variations in the length of the transition zone between the aganglionic distal rectum and when normal ganglion cells were noted proximally [199].

In 1949, Bodian et al. reviewed 73 patients who presented with findings consistent with congenital megacolon [8]. In 39 patients, he confirmed the diagnosis of HSCR by recognizing the presence of a spastic segment in the rectosigmoid and noting absence of ganglion cells in the spastic distal segment. The 34 patients who did not fit these criteria were labeled as "idiopathic cases" [8]. These findings may explain the controversy noted in early reports concerning the presence or absence of ganglion cells, and finally separated patients with HSCR from those with other motility disturbances and causes of colonic dilatation. In1951, Bodian reported the first instance of aganglionosis affecting the entire bowel from the duodenum to the rectum [9]. All of these studies reaffirmed the importance of Dalla Valla's original report in 1920 describing an absence of ganglion cells [27]. In 1951, Hiatt performed manometric studies in patients with HSCR and confirmed that the abnormal distal segment was the area of obstruction. The rectum lacked peristaltic activity but showed mass contraction and there was a loss of anorectal relaxation of the internal anal sphincter [62].

Although Swenson's operation now provided surgeons with a satisfactory method to treat HSCR, some considered this a tedious operation and the results were not quite as good in other people's hands. Alternative procedures were sought. In 1952, State (Minneapolis, Minnesota) described the use of a low anterior resection to manage this condition [165]. The operation left considerable residual aganglionic tissue in place frequently causing recurrence of symptoms and was ultimately abandoned. In 1953, Sandegard in Sweden reported the first successful operation in a patient with total colonic aganglionosis (TCA) by performing a total colectomy and an ileoanal anastomosis [150]. In 1956, Bernard Duhamel of St Denis, France, described the retrorectal transanal pull-though procedure for the treatment of HSCR [35]. This concept was developed to preserve the nerves to the bladder and nervi erigente and left the aganglionic rectum in place. The normal proximal bowel was brought down to the perineum through an incision 1.0 cm above the dentate line in the posterior rectal wall. Since that time, numerous modifications have been employed to alter the location of the anal incision to preserve part of the internal anal sphincter to avoid incontinence and to ablate the residual blind aganglionic rectal pouch to avoid the development of an obstructing fecaloma.

In 1960, Grob in Zurich, Switzerland, used a different location for the posterior incision. He made the incision 2.0–2.5 cm above the pectinate line, but this resulted in constipation [57]. Pagès in Paris made the rectal incision1.5 cm above the pectinate line to avoid incontinence and constipation [125]. A variety of clamps and subsequently stapling devices were employed to divide the colorectal spur comprising the posterior wall of the aganglionic rectal stump and the anterior wall of the normally innervated pull-through segment by Martin, Ikeda, Soper and Miller and Steichen et al. [74, 108, 109, 163, 166]. In 1958, Rehbein of Bremen, Germany, reported his experience with low anterior resection using multiple stay sutures in order to elevate the pelvic floor, thereby allowing the colorectal anastomosis 2–3 cm above the pectinate line [139]. This procedure is still used in some German-speaking countries.

In 1963, Soave of Genoa, Italy, described the endorectal pull-through procedure bringing the innervated bowel down to the perineum through a muscular sleeve of the aganglionic rectum [162]. Performing the mucosal stripping dissection within the muscle wall reduced the risk of injury to the nerves to the bladder and nervi erigentes. The original Soave procedure left the pulled through bowel segment extending from the anal opening. After a period to allow adherence of the bowel to the anal tissues, the protruding segment was resected [162]. The preservation of the muscular sleeve was not an original technique as it had been described by Hochenegg in Austria in 1898, and was used by Ravitch in an adult patient with a benign colonic condition in 1948 [66, 138]. Similarly, Kiesewetter used the concept during repair of high anorectal malformations [84]. Pellerin in France (1962) and Cutait in Brazil (1965) modified the endorectal technique by performing a delayed anastomosis, and in 1964 Boley (New York) further modified the procedure by performing a primary anastomosis at the time of the pull-through procedure [11, 26, 128].

Recognizing that the barium enema was not always diagnostic, particularly in the neonate, in 1959, Swenson et al. described the full-thickness rectal biopsy to obtain material for a tissue diagnosis [171]. Shandling reported his experience with a simple punch biopsy to obtain tissue in 1960 [157]. That same year, Gherardi noted that the level of aganglionosis was similar in the submucosal and myenteric plexuses [51]. Bodian was the first to use a submucosal biopsy for the diagnosis of HSCR [10]. In 1965, Dobbins and Bill employed a suction rectal biopsy instrument to obtain tissue for diagnosis [33]. This was successfully employed by Campbell and Noblett in 1969, and was modified by Noblett later that year using a special suction biopsy tube [17, 123]. In 1968, Meier-Ruge confirmed the effective use of submucosal rectal biopsy in Europe [111]. In the current era, suction rectal biopsy remains the preferred technique used to diagnose HSCR, particularly in neonates and infants [180]. A rapid acetylcholinesterase staining test was proposed by Kobayashi in 1994 allowing intraoperative diagnosis within 10 minutes [87].

During the same period, other investigators evaluated the diagnostic efficacy of anorectal manometrics in infants with HSCR [98, 153, 154]. The technique measures resting anal canal pressures and determines if the normal anorectal tone resulting in relaxation of the sphincter is present when the rectum is distended by a balloon. Loss of the anorectal response is interpreted as being consistent with HSCR [122]. These studies were inconsistent in premature infants and some neonates because of perceived immaturity of the anorectal response and limitations in equipment sensitivity in this age group [69, 77, 102]. However, additional studies using advanced semiconductor technology and miniature probes have demonstrated a normal anorectal pressure in premature and full-term neonates [177].

Despite the ability of clinicians to histologically diagnose HSCR by confirming the absence of ganglion cells on rectal biopsy, there remained a significant number of children with conditions that resembled aganglionic megacolon but who had ganglion cells present on their specimens. This was the condition that Bodian referred to as "idiopathic megacolon" in his observations on the histology of HSCR in 1949 and in more detail described by Puri since [8, 46].

In 1971, Meier-Ruge in Switzerland published his classic article describing colonic neuronal dysplasia [111, 112]. The following year he described the benefit of acetylcholinesterase staining of the hypertrophied nerve fibers in the lamina propria and muscularis in the diagnosis of HSCR [113]. Special staining techniques that were employed to identify instances of hypoganglionosis, immaturity of the submucosal and myenteric plexuses and anorectal achalasia became commonplace in evaluating conditions that mimicked HSCR [152, 153].

Over the next three decades, numerous articles appeared in the literature regarding intestinal neuronal dysplasia (IND). The condition seemed to be common in Europe, but was a rare entity on the North American continent. Puri and associates and Scharli were advocates of Meier-Ruge's observations regarding IND and reported a series of cases with this condition and other variants of HSCR [131, 133, 134]. IND is divided into two subtypes, A and B, with the former being quite rare and the latter far more common, and can be treated conservatively in most cases. Puri and colleagues noted that IND can coexist with HSCR and might be responsible for the persistence of motility disturbances seen in some patients following pull-through operations [131]. Controversy surrounds this condition regarding whether it is a distinct primary entity or a secondary phenomenon resulting from stasis or obstruction.

Meier-Ruge and colleagues have reported follow-up studies in patients with IND-B [114]. IND–B was identified in 6% of their patients with HSCR and 2.3% of other children evaluated for chronic constipation. The criteria for diagnosis were a rectal biopsy obtained 8–10 cm above the pectinate line in which 15–20% of the ganglia were giant-sized, and more than eight nerve cells in 30 sections of the same biopsy [114]. He considered the findings consistent with delayed maturation of the ENS and recommended conservative management up to 4 years of age. The authors suggested that children with hypoganglionosis required surgical intervention [114]. The precise management of IND in association with HSCR remains unclear, but conservative treatments with laxatives and enema are usually sufficient [132].

In regard to anal achalasia, in 1934, Hurst considered that this was related to parasympathetic underactivity [71]. Others suggested this was a manifestation of very low segment HSCR. Doodnath and Puri [34] described the anal sphincter achalasia as a clinical condition similar to HSCR, but with normal ganglia within the rectal mucosa and absence of the recto-anal relaxation reflex during manometry. According to these authors, the pathogenesis is multifactorial characterized by the absence of nitrergic innervation and an altered distribution of the interstitial cells of Cajal. Currently, the diagnosis of anal achalasia requires both a rectal biopsy showing the presence of ganglion cells and absence of anorectal reflex relaxation on manometric studies [180]. Thomas [181] and Holschneider et al. [69] performed a posterior sphincterotomy, and Thomas [182] and Lynn and van Heerdon [103] recommended a transanal posterior rectal myectomy for those with low-segment disease [69, 103, 181, 182]. In 1990, Neilson and Yazbeck described five children with "ultra-short segment Hirschsprung's disease" [119]. Each of the children had a loss of anorectal reflex relaxation on manometry but ganglion cells were found on rectal biopsy. They responded to posterior sphincterotomy [119]. In 1994, Krebs and Acuna noted that internal sphincter pressures initially are reduced following sphincter myotomy, but with time they return to above normal levels [89]. Prato and associates have reported the benefit of myectomy in anal achalasia using a posterior sagittal approach [130]. Long-term follow-up showed that the majority of patients have normal bowel control following internal sphincter myotomy [34].

As experience was obtained, it became clear that HSCR is more common in boys and in 80–85% of patients, aganglionosis is limited to the rectum and rectosigmoid. However, in 10% of patients aganglionosis extends to more proximal areas of the colon, and in 5–8% TCA is noted with proximal extension of the aganglionic segment to various levels of the small intestine. A Japanese nationwide survey showed an incidence of 10–11% of all HSCR cases or 1:58,000 neonatal births [73]. As noted above, Bodian documented the first instance of aganglionosis of the entire bowel in 1951 [10]. Talwalker's review on the subject in 1976 identified 11 patients [175]. Sporadic reports have documented even more rare extensions of aganglionosis to the stomach and esophagus [193]. In 1985, Caniano et al. described one patient and noted that no intestinal distension, evidence of bowel obstruction or transition zone could be detected at laparotomy. In addition, a review of similar patients in the literature indicated that 33% pass meconium at birth and 25% do not demonstrate hypertrophied nerve fibers on histologic study [19]. In 1986, Rudin et al. described three neonates with absence of the entire ENS and described 13 additional patients from the literature [147].

As noted above, Sandegard performed the first successful operative repair of TCA with colon resection and ileoanal anastomosis in 1953 [150]. The morbidity and mortality with TCA was greater than in those with the typical rectosigmoid involvement [66, 74, 167]. In an effort to improve the absorptive capacity of the colon, in 1968, Martin described a modification of the Duhamel procedure utilizing a side-to-side anastomosis to the aganglionic colon up to the level of the splenic flexure [106]. In 1981, Kimura used an aganglionic right colon patch inserted in the anti-mesenteric surface of the ileum to slow transit and improve absorption following ileostomy. The patch was left in place at the time of the pull-through procedure [85]. Boley used the left colon as a patch in 1984 [12]. In 1982, Martin further revised his procedure for TCA by using the entire aganglionic colon [107]. This latter procedure was associated with severe enterocolitis and has subsequently been abandoned by most pediatric surgeons [41, 42, 180, 202]. Most recent reports suggest that reasonably good results can be achieved in TCA affecting the distal ileum up to the mid-small bowel using a standard modification of the Duhamel procedure, endorectal pull-through or a Swenson operation [42, 120, 167, 174, 180, 202]. Rintala and Lindahl and Lal et al. have suggested that an ileoanal J pouch or S pouch may also be of benefit in these patients [92, 144].

The outlook for extension of aganglionosis into the more proximal small bowel remains guarded. These children essentially have short bowel syndrome and frequently require long-term support with total parenteral nutrition (TPN). Escobar et al. [42], Kimura [85], Kottmeier et al. [88], and Nishijima et al. [121] have found the aganglionic patch procedure beneficial in this subset of patients; however, iron deficiency anemia is a late complication. In 1987, Ziegler described the concept of myotomy/myectomy of aganglionic bowel for patients with near total aganglionosis (NTAG) with less than 40 cm of normally innervated small bowel [206]. The concept of myotomy in HSCR was first described by Martin-Burden in 1927 [38], using the procedure in the rectosigmoid, and by Kasai et al. in 1971 [83] who performed myotomy of the intact aganglionic rectal segment following proximal colon resection. In 1993, Ziegler et al. reported the outcomes of 16 myotomy/myectomies for NTAG that had been performed at multiple centers [207]. They suggested that myectomized aganglionic bowel has the capacity to adapt and absorb nutrients, and that the procedure may be viewed as a bridge to intestinal transplantation [207]. In 2000, Saxton et al. described their experience with seven patients with NTAG of the bowel. Only two of the seven survived despite the use of myectomy and aganglionic patch procedures. These adjunctive procedures were associated with a high complication rate [151]. A meta-analysis published by Ruttenstock and Puri reported the findings from 68 cases of total intestinal aganglionosis – 6 up to the stomach, 19 up to the duodenum, and 43 up to 20 cm below the duodenojejunal flexure. Forty-five patients died either pre- or postoperatively at ages ranging from 1 day to 8 years.

Twelve patients received either intestinal or liver-intestinal transplantation. Twenty-three patients were alive; the longest survivor was 10 years old after a liver-intestinal transplantation [148]. A recent single center study of 21 patients with total colonic aganglionosis showed that restorative proctocolectomy for aganglionosis extending up to the small bowel had promising results [70].

In the 1990s, intestinal transplantation became an option in the management of patients with NTAG of the small intestine. Instances complicated by total parenteral nutrition (TPN)-induced liver failure are candidates for combined liver and bowel transplantation. In 1995, Tzakis et al., from Dr. Starzl's group in Pittsburgh, described a 16-month-old girl with extensive aganglionosis who had a successful combined liver/bowel transplantation and a Soave endorectal pull-through using donor descending colon [187]. In 1998, Reyes et al. found that 4 of 55 children undergoing small bowel transplantation had HSCR [142]. In 1999, Goulet et al. described preliminary experience with small-bowel transplantation at the Enfants Malades Hospital in Paris. Four of 20 patients had HSCR with aganglionosis extending to the proximal jejunum [54]. In 2003, Revillon et al., from the same institution, reported an improved quality of life in three children with extensive aganglionosis who underwent successful combined liver-bowel transplantation and a subsequent pull-through procedure (two had a Duhamel procedure; one a Swenson procedure) [141]. Also in 2003, Sharif et al., from Birmingham, UK, reported a successful outcome in four of five infants with extensive aganglionosis (between 10 and 50 cm of normal jejunum remaining) and TPN-related liver failure following combined liver/bowel transplantation in four and an isolated small-bowel graft in one [158]. The authors stressed preservation of the aganglionic bowel and avoidance of extensive enterectomy to preserve the size of the abdomen for subsequent graft insertion. At present, this group is recommending transplantation in patients with NTAG and severe TPN-related liver disease [158]. Seven percent of 814 children with intestinal failure needed transplantation for HSCR. Their 5-year survival rate is with 56% in the same range as the overall survival rate [97]. Nakamura et al. recently reviewed the outcome of intestinal transplantation in patients with NTAG. Of the 63 patients who had intestinal transplantation for NTAG, 37% of patients had isolated intestinal transplantation and 63% had liver and intestinal transplantation. Mean follow up was 40 months. Overall survival rate was 60%, the longest survivor was 12.8 years after transplantation [118].

One of the major complications observed in children with HSCR, both prior to and after a pull-through operation, is Hirschsprung-associated enterocolitis (HAEC). This was probably the cause of the demise of both of the infants described by Hirschsprung in his original report in 1886, and continued to be a problematic cause of morbidity and mortality over the next century. Swenson was the first to key in on the significance of this complication in babies with HSCR [172]. Enterocolitis is likely the result of functional obstruction and stasis. The reported incidence of HAEC varies widely, ranging from 6% to 60% prior to definitive surgery and from 25% to 37% after surgery depending on the diagnostic criteria used [60, 178]. Enterocolitis is associated with explosive diarrhea (70%), vomiting (50%), fever (34%), and lethargy (27%) [178]. The diarrhea is often associated with abdominal distension suggesting an obstructive cause. Acute inflammatory infiltrates have been noted in the anal crypts and colon mucosa that may lead to crypt abscesses and mucosal ulceration. The exact etiology is still unknown, but impaired mucosal defense mechanisms have been implicated with deficiency in secretory IgA, absence of mucin precursors and the muc-2 gene [4, 178, 203]. Recent studies have shown a close relationship with the disturbance of the intestinal microbiota elucidating significant differences between "normal" HSCR patients – prevalence of Bacteroidetes – and HAEC patients – prevalence of Proteobacteria.

Although enterocolitis has been observed after all of the procedures used to treat HSCR, the incidence is higher after a Soave pull-through, long-segment aganglionosis, prior HAEC, and any kind of causes of anal obstructions (presumably because of a tight anastomosis or snug aganglionic muscular cuff), in patients with TCA (especially after a long Martin modification of the Duhamel procedure), and in infants with Down syndrome probably related to immunologic factors. [18, 53, 178, 180]. These observations led to further operative modifications such as division of the posterior muscular cuff in the Soave procedure and abandoning the long Martin modification of the Duhamel procedure. A systematic review and meta-analysis of HAEC after one-stage transanal pull-through procedures showed an overall incidence of 10.2% with recurrent episodes in 2% [148]. Recently, guidelines have been published for the diagnosis and management of HAEC by the Hirschsprung's Disease Group of the APSA [53].

Aside from the availability of intestinal transplantation as a treatment option, the 1990s and the first few years of the twenty-first century have been the era of continued technical modifications with a trend toward one-stage procedures earlier in life using advances in minimally invasive technology, employing the transanal approach and managing treatment failures. In addition, this has been a time characterized by significant advances in understanding the ENS in general and the genetic basis of HSCR; in particular due to a veritable explosion of new information especially following the elucidation of the human genome.

In 1981, So and colleagues were the first to report a one-stage pull-through procedure in neonates with HSCR without a preliminary colostomy [161]. In 1982, Carcassone and associates from Marseilles similarly described a favorable experience with a one-stage procedure in the first 3 months of life [20]. These reports refuted Swenson's contention that a definitive procedure in early infancy is associated with an increased morbidity and mortality. The one-stage approach became increasingly popular in the 1990s [59, 95, 179]. Georgeson et al. described a laparoscopically assisted Soave endorectal pull-through procedure avoiding an open laparotomy [48]. He adapted this to a primary procedure in 1999 [49]. Successful application of the laparoscopic technique has also been reported by pediatric surgeons performing the Swenson procedure [25, 67, 90] and modified Duhamel operation [28, 52, 160, 188]. In 1993, Rinatala and Lindahl of Helsinki described a predominantly transanal pull-through operation but performed a laparotomy to mobilize the proximal colon [143]. In 1998, de la Torre-Mondregon and Ortega-Salgado of Mexico were the first to perform a one-stage totally transanal pull-through procedure [30]. Results with the transanal endorectal pull-through were favorable when compared to the open procedure [31]. Since then, the transanal operation has been used extensively in the neonatal period by Langer et al. [93], Albanese et al. [3], and Teitelbaum et al. [179]. Three multicenter studies in Europe [68], North America [96] and Egypt [39] have supported the use of this approach.

The Swenson, modified Duhamel, and Soave endorectal pull-through procedures all give satisfactory results, and each has its advocates and detractors [35, 41, 96, 125, 140, 162, 169, 173, 174, 180, 190]. Each of the procedures has required modification since their inception in attempts to deal with subsequent postoperative complications [11, 61, 85, 108, 109, 172, 180, 181, 191, 194, 206]. Although most patients do well over time, aside from the previously mentioned instances of enterocolitis and IND, there are a subset of patients who have other recurring problems [41, 180, 189]. These include instances of "acquired" aganglionosis following a pull-through performed with normally innervated proximal bowel. These problems are likely related to ischemia of the pull-through segment and respond to a second pull-through procedure [22, 32, 197]. Similarly, occasional poor outcomes related to persistent postoperative stricture or severe obstipation also require a re-do pull-through procedure [90, 94, 189, 196, 200]. According to a recent meta-analysis, the Duhamel pull-through seems to be associated with a lower incidence of anastomotic strictures compared to transanalendorectal pull-throughs [155]. In all transanal procedures, the preservation of the complete anal canal is crucial to have postoperative fecal control. However, long aganglionic segments may be associated with Hirschsprung-associated enterocolitis (HAEC)

[29]. Persistent constipation problems have been treated with partial internal sphincterotomy, rectal myotomy/myectomy, botulinum toxin injections, and topical nitric oxide [41, 115, 116, 172, 201]. In a series of 348 patients, 9.1% needed a myotomy or myectomy later on [201].

While the exact etiology of HSCR is still unknown, the last two decades have provided new insights into the complexities of this condition and its variants. HSCR has been observed to coexist with anorectal malformations, ileal atresia, colon atresia, achalasia of the esophagus, and the Currarino syndrome [5, 47, 72, 80, 84, 159, 195]. A better understanding of the enteric nervous system (ENS) and the molecular genetic basis of this disorder has provided a wealth of new information. Since the early studies of Okamoto and Ueda [124] on the embryogenesis and cranio-caudal migration of the neuroblast along the gastrointestinal tract in 1967, many investigators have focused on uncovering the mysteries surrounding the ENS through genomic analysis of the ENS and neural crest development and migration and colonization of enteric neurons. The association of HSCR with other neurocristopathies is linked to various genetic disturbances. These include instances of Ondine's curse (Congenital central hypoventilation syndrome; PHOX-2B), Waardenburg-Shah syndrome (SOX-10), Mowat-Wilson syndrome (ZFHX1B), Goldberg-Shprintzen syndrome, Smith-Lemli-Opitz syndrome, MEN-2A and B, neuroblastoma, and ganglio-neuromatosis of the bowel [23, 24, 105, 117, 129, 133, 176, 180, 205].

While early studies by Passarge [127] and Engum and Grosfeld [40] identified familial instances of HSCR, it was the elucidation of the human genome that opened the door to the genetic basis of the disease. Collaboration between basic scientists, medical geneticists, and pediatric surgeons led the way to these discoveries. In 1992, Martucciello et al. of Genoa reported the association of TCA with interstitial deletion of the long arm of chromosome 10 [110]. This was confirmed in 1993 by Angrist et al. [104] and Yin et al. [204] who described the close linkage of the RET protooncogene in autosomal dominant HSCR and by Pasini et al. in 1995 [126]. Mutations were identified in 50% of the patients from families with HSCR. In 1994, Romeo et al. identified point mutations affecting the tyrosine kinase domain of the RET proto-oncogene [146]. In the same year, Edery et al. [36] reported that loss of function of the RET protooncogene led to HSCR, whereas gain of RET function led to MEN-2B. Additional studies have uncovered genetic linkages involved in the development of the ENS. Most belong to the RET and endothelin signaling pathways. In 1995, Gershon demonstrated that endothelin and the endothelin-B receptor are necessary for the development of the ENS in the colon [50]. In 1997, Kusafuka et al. identified mutations in endothelin-B and endothelin-B receptor in isolated cases of HSCR [91]. Iwashita et al. noted that the glial cell line-derived neurotropic factor receptor (GDNF) RET is necessary for neural crest stem cell migration in the gut [78]. Gene expression profiling, reverse genetics and analysis of stem cell function have implicated neural crest stem cell function as the likely cause of HSCR [78]. These studies suggest that HSCR is a genetically complex and heterogeneous inborn error of neural crest cell development that may involve a number of mutations affecting different genes and signaling pathways and other biologic and molecular factors yet to be determined. Recent advances in genetic technologies including next-generation sequencing provide more insights into the development and complexity of the human ENS and reveal new HSCR genes [58].

1.1 Conclusion and Future Directions

Since the clinical presentations by Harald Hirschsprung in Berlin in 1886, the condition that bears his name has had a rich history. The seminal events that influenced progress in the understanding and management of this complex congenital disorder have been briefly covered in this historical review. More than 100 years ago, the condition was considered incurable and uniformly fatal over time [21, 38]. Mortality rates continued to be high in the 1940s (70%) and remained high even in the 1970s (25%). By the 1990s, more than 90% of patients survived [140].

Currently, the survival in most advanced medical environments is greater than 95% [180], excluding cases with chromosomal disorders or advanced comorbidities. While mortality has improved, there remains much to be learned. Why some patients with HSCR do poorly following operative repair remains an enigma. Similarly, the proper management of many patients with variants of HSCR needs to be more clearly elucidated. Continuing studies of the ENS and the molecular genetics of these conditions may shed further light on these issues and provide a better understanding of the choice of management in the future for affected children. Recent studies have transplanted human enteric neural progenitors into the mouse colon and shown engraftment [164]. Currently, researchers are working to develop novel stem cell therapies, whereby stem cells could be transplanted into the aganglionic segment of bowel to replace the missing ENS.

References

1. Adamson WAD, Aird I. Megacolon: evidence in favor of a neurogenic origin. Br J Surg. 1932;20:220–3.
2. Adson A. Hirschsprung's disease: indications for and results obtained by sympathectomy. Surgery. 1937;1:859–77.
3. Albanese CT, Jennings RW, Smith B, Bratton B, Harrison MR. Perineal one-stage pull-through for Hirschsprung's disease. J Pediatr Surg. 1999;34:377–80.
4. Aslam A, Spicer RD, Corfield AP. Turnover of radioactive mucin precursors in the colon of patients with Hirschsprung's disease correlates with the development of enterocolitis. J Pediatr Surg. 1998;33:103–5.
5. Baltogiannis N, Mavridis G, Soutis M, Keramidas D. Currarino syndrome associated with Hirschsprung's disease. J Pediatr Surg. 2003;38:1086–9.
6. Barington-Ward LE. Colectomy for Hirschsprung's disease. Br J Surg. 1915;2:655.
7. Best KE, Addor MC, Arriola L, et al. Hirschsprung's disease prevalence in Europe; a register based study. Birth Defects Res A Clin Mol Teratol. 2014;100:695–702.
8. Bodian M, et al. Hirschsprung's disease and idiopathic megacolon. Lancet. 1949;1:6–11.
9. Bodian M, et al. Hirschsprung's disease. Lancet. 1951;1:32.
10. Bodian M. Pathological aids in the diagnosis and management of Hirschsprung's disease. In: Recent advances in clinical pathology. London: Churchill Livingstone; 1960.
11. Boley SJ. New modification of the surgical treatment of Hirschsprung's disease. Surgery. 1964;56:1015–7.
12. Boley SJ. A new operative approach to total colonic aganglionosis. Surg Gynecol Obstet. 1984;159:481–4.
13. Breathnach CS. Biographical sketches. Hirschsprung. Ir Med J. 1987;80:437.
14. Brentano A. Uber einen Fall von HirschsprungscherKrankheit. Verh Dtsch Ges Chir. 1904;1:265–8.
15. Bristowe JS. The consequences of long continued constipation. BMJ. 1885;1:1085–8.
16. Cameron JAM. On the etiology of Hirschsprung's disease. Arch Dis Child. 1928;3:210–1.
17. Campbell PE, Noblett HR. Experience with rectal suction biopsy in the diagnosis of Hirschsprung's disease. J Pediatr Surg. 1969;4:410–5.
18. Caneiro P, Brereton R, Drake D, et al. Enterocolitis in Hirschsprung's disease. Pediatr Surg Int. 1992;7:356–60.
19. Caniano D, Ormsbee HS 3rd, Polito W, Sun CC, Barone FC, Hill JL. Total intestinal aganglionosis. J Pediatr Surg. 1985;20:456–60.
20. Carcassonne M, Morisson-Lacombe G, Letourneau JN. Primary corrective operation without decompression in infants less than three months of age with Hirschsprung's disease. J Pediatr Surg. 1982;17:241–3.
21. Cass D. Hirschsprung's disease: an historical review. Prog Pediatr Surg. 1986;20:199–214.
22. Cohen MSW, Neveling U, Kaschula RO. Acquired Hirschsprung's disease: a report of five cases during a 33 year experience with pull through procedures. Histopathology. 1993;22:163–8.
23. Coyle D, Friedmacher F, Puri P. The association between Hirschsprung's disease and multiple endocrine neoplasia type 2a: a systematic review. Pediatr Surg Int. 2014;30:751–6.
24. Coyle D, Puri P. Hirschsprung's disease in children with Mowat-Wilson syndrome. Pediatr Surg Int. 2015;31:711–7.
25. Curran TJ, Raffensperger JG. Laparoscopic Swenson pull-through: a comparison with the open procedure. J Pediatr Surg. 1996;31:1155–6.
26. Cutait DE. Technique of rectosigmoidectomy for megacolon. Dis Colon Rectum. 1965;151:107–14.
27. Dalla Valla A. Richerche istologiche su di un caso di megacolon congenito. Pediatria. 1920;28:740–52.
28. De Lagausie P, Berrebi D, Geib G, Sebag G, Aigrain Y. Laparoscopic Duhamel procedure: management of 30 cases. Surg Endosc. 1999;13:972–4.
29. De La Torre L, Cogley K, Santos K, et al. The anal canal is the fine line between "fecal incontinence and colitis" after a pull-through for Hirschsprung disease. J Pediatr Surg. 2017;52:2011–7.
30. De la Torre-Mondregon L, Ortega-Salgado JA. Transanal endorectal pull-through for Hirschsprung's disease. J Pediatr Surg. 1998;33:1283–6.
31. De la Torre-Mondregon L, Ortega-Salgado JA. Transanal vs. open endorectal colon pull-through for Hirschsprung's disease. J Pediatr Surg. 2000;35:1630–2.

32. Dimler M. Acquired Hirschsprung's disease. J Pediatr Surg. 1981;16:844–5.
33. Dobbins WO, Bill AH. Diagnosis of Hirschsprung's disease excluded by rectal suction biopsy. New Engl J Med. 1965;272:990–3.
34. Doodnath R, Puri P. A systematic review and meta-analysis of Hirschsprung's disease presenting after childhood. Pediatr Surg Int. 2010;26:1107–10.
35. Duhamel B. Une nouvelle operation pan le megacolon congenital l'abaisement retrorectal et transanal du colon of san application possible au traitement de quelques autres malformation. Presse Med. 1956;64:2249–50.
36. Edery P, Lyonnet S, Mulligan LM, Pelet A, Dow E, Abel L, Holder S, Nihoul-Fekete C, Ponder BA, Munnich A. Mutations of the RET proto-oncogene in Hirschsprung's disease. Nature. 1994;367:378–80.
37. Ehrenpreis T. Megacolon in the newborn. A clinical and roentgenological study with special regard to the pathogenesis. Acta Chir Scand Suppl. 1946;94:112.
38. Ehrenpreis T. Hirschsprung's disease. Chicago: Year Book Medical Publishers; 1970.
39. Elhalaby EA, Hashish A, Elbarbary MM, Soliman HA, Wishahy MK, Elkholy A, Abdelhay S, Elbehery M, Halawa N, Gobran T, Shehata S, Elkhouly N, Hamza AF. Transanal one-stage endorectal pullthrough for Hirschsprung's disease: a multicenter study. J Pediatr Surg. 2004;39:345–51.
40. Engum SA, Grosfeld JL. Long-term results of treatment of Hirschsprung's disease. Semin Pediatr Surg. 2004;13:273–85.
41. Engum SA, Petrites M, Rescorla FJ, Grosfeld JL, Morrison AM, Engles D. Familial Hirschsprung's disease: 20 cases in 12 kindreds. J Pediatr Surg. 1993;28:1286–90.
42. Escobar MA, Grosfeld JL, West KW, Scherer LR, Rouse TM, Engum SA, Rescorla FJ. Long-term outcomes in total colonic aganglionosis: a 32-year experience. J Pediatr Surg. 2005;40:955–61.
43. Fenwick W. Hypertrophy and dilatation of the colon in infants. BMJ. 1900;2:564–7.
44. Fiori MG. Domenico Battini and his description of congenital megacolon: a detailed case report one century before Hirschsprung. J Peripher Nerv Syst. 1998;3:197–206.
45. Frenckner B. The man behind the syndrome: Harald Hirschsprung. A pioneer in pediatric research – a popular clinician but less valued lecturer. Lakartidningen. 1983;80:4664–5.
46. Friedmacher F, Puri P. Classification and diagnostic criteria of variants of Hirschsprung's disease. Pediatr Surg Int. 2013;29:855–72.
47. Gauderer MW, Rothstein FC, Izant RJ Jr. Ileal atresia with long segment Hirschsprung disease in a neonate. J Pediatr Surg. 1984;19:15–7.
48. Georgeson KE, Fuenfer MM, Hardin WD. Primary laparoscopic pullthrough for Hirschsprung's disease in infants and children. J Pediatr Surg. 1995;30:1017–22.
49. Georgeson KE, Cohen RD, Hebra A, Jona JZ, Powell DM, Rothenberg SS, Tagge EP. Primary laparoscopic-assisted endorectal colon pull through for Hirschsprung's disease: a new gold standard. Ann Surg. 1999;229:678–82.
50. Gershon M. Neural crest development: do developing enteric neurons need endothelin? Curr Biol. 1995;1:601–4.
51. Gherardi GJ. Pathology of the ganglionic-aganglionic junction in congenital megacolon. Arch Pathol. 1960;69:520–3.
52. Goh DW, Ford WD, Little KE. Primary neonatal Duhamel procedure using the ENDO GIA stapler. Aust N Z J Surg. 1995;65:120–1.
53. Gosain A, Frykman PK, Cowles RA, et al. Guidelines for the diagnosis and management of Hirschsprung-associated enterocolitis. Pediatr Surg Int. 2017;33:517–21.
54. Goulet O, Jan D, Lacaille F, Colomb V, Michel JL, Damotte D, Jouvet P, Brousse N, Faure C, Cezard JP, Sarnacki S, Peuchmaur M, Hubert P, Ricour C, Revillon Y. Intestinal transplantation in children: preliminary experience in Paris. JPEN J Parenter Enteral Nutr. 1999;23(5 Suppl):S121–5.
55. Grffith C. Congenital idiopathic dilatation of the colon. Am J Med Sci. 1899;118:283.
56. Grimson KS, Vandergrift L, Datz HM. Surgery in obstinate megacolon: one stage resection and ileosigmoidostomy. Surg Gynecol Obstet. 1945;80:164.
57. Grob M. Intestinal obstruction in the newborn infant. Arch Dis Child. 1960;35:40–50.
58. Gui H, Schriemer D, Cheng WW, et al. Whole exome sequencing coupled with unbiased functional analysis reveals new Hirschsprung disease genes. Genome Biol. 2017;18:48.
59. Hackam DJ, Superina RA, Pearl RH. Single stage repair of Hirschsprung's disease: a comparison of 109 patients over five years. J Pediatr Surg. 1997;32:1028–31.
60. Hawksley M. Spinal anaesthesia in the treatment of Hirschsprung's disease. With reports of 12 cases. Br J Surg. 1943/1944;31:245–53.
61. Hedlund H. Posterior sagittal resection for rectal aganglionosis: preliminary results of a new approach. J Pediatr Surg. 1997;32:1717–20.
62. Hiatt RB. The pathological physiology of congenital megacolon. Ann Surg. 1951;133:313–20.
63. Hirschsprung H. Struhltragheit Neugeborener in folge von Dilatation and Hypertrophie des colons. Jahrbuch Kinderheilkunde. 1888;27:1–7.
64. Hirschsprung H. Tilfaelde af medfodt Tillukning af Spiseroret. Hospitalstidende. 1895;38:1037–41.
65. Hirschsprung H. Stenosis pylori congenital. Hospitalstidende. 1901;44:1169–75.
66. Hochenegg J. Beitrage zur Chirurgie des rectum und der Beckenorgane. Wien Klin Wochenschr. 1898;2:515.
67. Hoffmann K, Schier F, Waldschmidt J. Laparoscopic Swenson's procedure in children. Eur J Pediatr Surg. 1996;6:15–7.

68. Hollwarth ME, Rivosecchi M, Schleef J, Deluggi S, Fasching G, Ceriati E, Ciprandi G, DePeppo F. The role of transanal endorectal pull through in the treatment of Hirschsprung's disease: a multicenter study. Pediatr Surg Int. 2002;18:344–6.
69. Holschneider AM, Kellner E, Streibl P, Sippell WG. The development of anorectal continence and its significance in the diagnosis of Hirschsprung's disease. J Pediatr Surg. 1976a;11:151–6.
70. Hukkinen M, Koivusalo A, Merras-Salmio L, et al. Postoperative outcome and survival in relation to small intestinal involvement of total colonic aganglionosis. J Pediatr Surg. 2015;50:1859–64.
71. Hurst AF. Anal achalasia and megacolon. Hirschsprung's disease: idiopathic dilatation of the colon. Guys Hosp Rep. 1934;84:317–50.
72. Hyde G Jr, de Lorimier AA. Colon atresia and Hirschsprung's disease. Surgery. 1968;64:976–8.
73. Ieiri S, Suita S, Nakatsuji T, et al. Total colonic aganglionosis with or without small bowel involvement: a 30-year retrospective nationwide survey in Japan. J Pediatr Surg. 2008;43:2226–30.
74. Ikeda K, Goto S. Total colonic aganglionosis with or without small bowel involvement: an analysis of 137 patients. J Pediatr Surg. 1986;21:319–22.
75. Irwin DA. The anatomy of Auerbach's plexus. Am J Anat. 1931;49:141.
76. Ishikawa N. Experimentelle und klinische Untersuchungen uber die Pathogenese und das Wesen des megaco- lons. Mitt med Fak kaiserl, Kyushu Univ. 1923;7:339.
77. Ito Y, Donahoe PK, Hendren WH. Maturation of the rectoanal response in premature and perinatal infants. J Pediatr Surg. 1977;12:477–81.
78. Iwashita T, Kruger GM, Pardal R, Kiel MJ, Morrison SJ. Hirschsprung disease is linked to defects in neural crest stem cell function. Science. 2003;301:972–6.
79. Jacobi A. On some important causes of constipation in infants. Am J Obstet. 1869;2:96.
80. Janik JP, Wayne ER, Janik JS, Price MR. Ileal atresia with total colonic aganglionosis. J Pediatr Surg. 1997;32:1502–3.
81. Jay V. The legacy of Harald Hirschsprung. Pediatr Dev Pathol. 2001;4:203–4.
82. Judd ES, Adson AW. Lumbar sympathetic ganglionectomy and ramisection for congenital idiopathic dilatation of the colon. Ann Surg. 1928;88:479–98.
83. Kasai M, Suzuki H, Watanabe K. Rectal myotomy with colectomy: a new radical operation for Hirschsprung's disease. J Pediatr Surg. 1971;6:36–41.
84. Kiesewetter WB, Sukarochana K, Sieber WK. The frequency of aganglionosis in association with imperforate anus. Surgery. 1965;58:877–80.
85. Kimura K. A new surgical approach to extensive aganglionosis. J Pediatr Surg. 1981;16:840–9.
86. Klingmann W. The treatment of neurogenic megacolon with selective drugs. J Pediatr. 1938;13:805.
87. Kobayashi H, O'Briain DS, Hirakawa H, et al. A rapid technique of acetylcholinesterase staining. Arch Pathol Lab Med. 1994;118:1127–9.
88. Kottmeier PK, Jongco B, Velcek FT, Friedman A, Klotz DH. Absorptive function of the aganglionic ileum. J Pediatr Surg. 1981;16:275–8.
89. Krebs C, Acuna R. Transanal internal sphincter myomectomy: indications, operative procedure and results. Eur J Pediatr Surg. 1994;4:151–7.
90. Kumar R, Mackay A, Borzi P. Laparoscopic Swenson procedure—an optimal approach for both primary and secondary pull through for Hirschsprung's disease. J Pediatr Surg. 2003;38:1440–3.
91. Kusafuka T, Wang Y, Puri P. Mutation analysis of the RET, the endothelin-B receptor, and the endothelin-3 genes in sporadic cases of Hirschsprung's disease. J Pediatr Surg. 1997;32:501–4.
92. Lal DR, Nichol PF, Harms BA, Go LL, Lund DP. Ileoanal S-pouch reconstruction in patients with total colonic aganglionosis after failed pull-through procedure. J Pediatr Surg. 2004;39:e7–9.
93. Langer JC. Repeat pull-through surgery for complicated Hirschsprung's disease: indications, technique and results. J Pediatr Surg. 1999;34:1136–41.
94. Langer JC, Fitzgerald PG, Winthrop AL, Srinathan SK, Foglia RP, Skinner MA, Ternberg JL, Lau GY. One-stage versus two-stage Soave pull-through for Hirschsprung's disease in the first year of life. J Pediatr Surg. 1996;31:33–6.
95. Langer JC, Minkes RK, Mazziotti MV, Skinner MA, Winthrop AL. Transanal one-stage Soave procedure for infants with Hirschsprung's disease. J Pediatr Surg. 1999;34:148–51.
96. Langer JC, Durrant AC, de la Torre L, Teitelbaum DH, Minkes RK, Caty MG, Wildhaber BE, Ortega SJ, Hirose S, Albanese CT. One-stage transanal Soave pull- through for Hirschsprung's disease: a multicenter experience with 141 cases. Ann Surg. 2003;238:569–76.
97. Lao OB, Healey PJ, Perkins JD, et al. Outcomes in children after intestinal transplant. Pediatrics. 2010;125:e550–8.
98. Lawson JON, Nixon HH. Anal canal pressures in the diagnosis of Hirschsprung disease. J Pediatr Surg. 1967;2:544–52.
99. Leenders E, Sieber WK. Congenital megacolon, observation by Frederici Ruysch 1691. J Pediatr Surg. 1970;5:1–3.
100. Lennander KG. Fall av medfodd (?) dilatation och hypertro av exura simoides hos ett barn (malade de Hirschsprung?). Nord Med Ark. 1900;11:1.
101. Lister J. Hirschsprung: the man and the disease. J R Coll Surg Edinb. 1977;22:377–84.
102. Loening-Bauke VA. Anorectal manometry: experience with strain gauge pressure transducers for the diagnosis of Hirschsprung's disease. J Pediatr Surg. 1983;18:595–600.
103. Lynn H, van Heerdon J. Rectal myectomy in Hirschsprung's disease: a decade of experience. Arch Surg. 1975;110:991–4.
104. Lyonnet S, Bolino A, Pelet A, et al. A gene for Hirschsprung's disease maps to the proximal long arm of chromosome 10. Nat Genet. 1993;4:346–50.

105. Maris JM, Chatten J, Meadows AT, Biegel JA, Brodeur GM. Familial neuroblastoma: a three-generation pedigree and a further association with Hirschsprung disease. Med Pediatr Oncol. 1997;28:1–5.
106. Martin LW. Surgical management of Hirschsprung's disease involving the small intestine. Arch Surg. 1968;97:183–9.
107. Martin LW. Total colonic aganglionosis preservation and utilization of entire colon. J Pediatr Surg. 1982;17:635–7.
108. Martin LW, Altemeier WA. Clinical experience with a new operation (modified Duhamel procedure) for Hirschsprung's disease. Ann Surg. 1962;156:678–81.
109. Martin LW, Caudill DR. A method of elimination of the blind rectal pouch in the Duhamel operation for Hirschsprung's disease. Surgery. 1967;62:951.
110. Martucciello G, Biocchi M, Dodero P, et al. Total colonic aganglionosis associated with interstitial deletion of the long arm of chromosome 10. Pediatr Surg Int. 1992;7:308–10.
111. Meier-Ruge W. Causistic of colon disorder with symptoms of Hirschsprung's disease. Verh Dtsch Ges Pathol. 1971;35:506–10.
112. Meier-Ruge W, Morger R. Neve Gesichtspunkle zur pathogenese und klinik des morbus Hirschsprung. Schweitz Med Wochenschr. 1968;98:209.
113. Meier-Ruge W, Lutterbeck PM, Herzog B, Morger R, Moser R, Scharli A. Acetylcholinesterase activity in suction biopsies of the rectum in the diagnosis of Hirschsprung's disease. J Pediatr Surg. 1972;7:11–7.
114. Meier-Ruge WA, Ammann K, Bruder E, Holschneider AM, Scharli AF, Schmittenbecher PP, Stoss F. Updated results on intestinal neuronal dysplasia (IND B). Eur J Pediatr Surg. 2004;14:384–91.
115. Millar AJ, Steinberg RM, Raad J, Rode H. Anal achalasia after pull-through operations for Hirschsprung's disease – preliminary experience with topical nitric oxide. Eur J Pediatr Surg. 2002;12:207–11.
116. Minkes RK, Langer JC. A prospective study of botulinum toxin for internal anal sphincter hypertonicity in children with Hirschsprung's disease. J Pediatr Surg. 2000;35:1733–6.
117. Mowat DR, Wilson MJ, Goossens M. Mowat-Wilson syndrome. J Med Genet. 2003;40:305–10.
118. Nakamura H, et al. A meta-analysis of clinical outcome of intestinal transplantation in patients with total intestinal aganglionosis. Pediatr Surg Int. 2017;33:837–41.
119. Neilson M, Yazbeck S. Ultrashort Hirschsprung's disease: myth or reality. J Pediatr Surg. 1990;25:1135–8.
120. N-Fekete C, Ricour C, Martelli H, Jacob SL, Pellerin D. Total colonic aganglionosis (with or without ileal involvement): a review of 27 cases. J Pediatr Surg. 1986;21:251–4.
121. Nishijima E, Kimura K, Tsugawa C, Muraji T. The colon patch graft procedure for extensive aganglionosis: long-term follow-up. J Pediatr Surg. 1998;33:215–9.
122. Nixon HH. Problems in the diagnosis of Hirschsprung's disease. Paediatr Paedol [Suppl]. 1972;2:21.
123. Noblett H. A rectal suction biopsy tube for use in the diagnosis of Hirschsprung's disease. J Pediatr Surg. 1969;4:406–9.
124. Okamoto E, Ueda T. Embryogenesis of the intra-neural ganglia of the gut and its relation to Hirschsprung's disease. J Pediatr Surg. 1967;2:437–43.
125. Pagès R. Maladie Hirschsprung. In: Patel J, Leger L, editors. Nouveau traite de technique chirurgicale. Paris: Maison etcie; 1969. p. 636–52.
126. Pasini B, Borrello MG, Greco A, Bongarzone I, Luo Y, Mondellini P, Alberti L, Miranda C, Arighi E, Bocciardi R, et al. Loss of function effect of RET mutations causing Hirschsprung disease. Nat Genet. 1995;10:35–40.
127. Passarge E. The genetics of Hirschsprung's disease — evidence for heterogeneous etiology and a study of 63 families. N Engl J Med. 1967;276:138–43.
128. Pellerin D. The surgical treatment of Hirschsprung's disease by resection and exterior anastomosis. J Int Coll Surg. 1962;37:591–3.
129. Pingault V, Bondurand N, Kuhlbrodt K, Goerich DE, Prehu MO, Puliti A, Herbarth B, Hermans-Borgmeyer I, Legius E, Matthijs G, Amiel J, Lyonnet S, Ceccherini I, Romeo G, Smith JC, Read AP, Wegner M, Goossens M. SOX10 mutations in patients with Waardenburg-Hirschsprung disease. Nat Genet. 1998;18:171–3.
130. Pini Prato A, Martucciello G, Torre M, Jasonni V. Feasibility of perineal sagittal approaches in patients without anorectal malformations. Pediatr Surg Int. 2004;20:762–7.
131. Puri P. Intestinal neuronal dysplasia. Semin Pediatr Surg. 2003;12:259–64.
132. Puri P, Gosemann JH. Variants of Hirschsprung disease. Semin Pediatr Surg. 2013;21:310–8.
133. Puri P, Rolle U. Variant Hirschsprung's disease. Semin Pediatr Surg. 2004;13:293–9.
134. Puri P, Lake BD, Nixon HH, Mishalany H, Claireaux AE. Neuronal colonic dysplasia: an unusual association of Hirschsprung's disease. J Pediatr Surg. 1977;12:681–5.
135. Raffensperger JG. Hirschsprung's disease: an historical review. Bull Soc Sci Med Grand Duche Luxemb. 1987;124(Spec):31–6.
136. Rankin FW, Learmouth JR. Section of sympathetic nerves of the distal part of the colon and rectum in the treatment of Hirschsprung's disease and certain types of constipation. Ann Surg. 1930;92:710.
137. Raveenthiran V. Knowledge of ancient Hindu surgeons on Hirschsprung disease: evidence from Sushruta Samhita of circa 1200–600 BC. J Pediatr Surg. 2011;46:2204–8.

138. Ravitch MM. Anal ileostomy with sphincter preservation in patients requiring total colectomy for benign conditions. Surgery. 1948;24:170.
139. Rehbein F. Intraabdominalle Resektion oder rectosigmoidektomie (Swenson) bei der Hirschsprungschen Krankheit? Chirurg. 1958;29:366–9.
140. Rescorla FJ, Morrison AM, Engles D, West KW, Grosfeld JL. Hirschsprung's disease: evaluation of mortality and long-term function in 260 cases. Arch Surg. 1992;127:934–41.
141. Revillon Y, Yves A, Dominique J, THierry Y, Olivier G, Florence L. Improved quality of life by combined transplantation in Hirschsprung's disease with a very long aganglionic segment. J Pediatr Surg. 2003;38:422–4.
142. Reyes J, Bueno J, Kocoshis S, Green M, Abu-Elmagd K, Furukawa H, Barksdale EM, Strom S, Fung JJ, Todo S, Irish W, Starzl TE. Current status of intestinal transplantation in children. J Pediatr Surg. 1998;33:243–54.
143. Rintala R, Lindahl H. Transanal endorectal coloanal anastomosis for Hirschsprung's disease. Pediatr Surg Int. 1993;8:128–31.
144. Rintala RJ, Lindahl HG. Proctocolectomy and J-pouch ileo-anal anastomosis in children. J Pediatr Surg. 2002;37:66–70.
145. Roed-Peterson K, Erichsen G. The Danish pediatrician Harald Hirschsprung. Surg Gynecol Obstet. 1988;166:181–5.
146. Romeo G, Ronchetto P, Luo Y, Barone V, Seri M, Ceccherini I, Pasini B, Bocciardi R, Lerone M, Kaariainen H, et al. Point mutations a ecting tyrosine kinase do- main of the RET proto-oncogene in Hirschsprung patients. Nature. 1994;367:377–8.
147. Rudin C, Jenny P, Ohnacker H, Heitz PU. Absence of the ENS in the newborn: presentation of three patients and review of the literature. J Pediatr Surg. 1986;21:313–8.
148. Ruttenstock E, Puri P. A meta-analysis of clinical outcome in patients with total intestinal aganglionosis. Pediatr Surg Int. 2009;25:833–9.
149. Ruysch F (1691) Observationum anatomico-chirurgi- carum centuria. Amstelodami.
150. Sandegard E. Hirschsprung's disease with ganglion cell aplasia of the colon and terminal ileum. Report of a case treated with total colectomy and ileoanostomy. Acta Surg Scand. 1953;106:367–76.
151. Saxton ML, Ein SH, Hoehner J, Kim PC. Near-total intestinal aganglionosis: long-term follow-up of a morbid condition. J Pediatr Surg. 2000;35:669–72.
152. Scharli AF, Sossai R. Hypoganglionosis. Semin Pediatr Surg. 1998;7:187–91.
153. Schnaufer L, Talbert JL, Haller JA, Reid NC, Tobon F, Schuster MM. Differential sphincteric studies in the diagnosis of ano-rectal disorders of childhood. J Pediatr Surg. 1967;2:538–43.
154. Schuster MM, Hendrix TR, Mendelo AI. The internal anal sphincter response: manometric studies on its normal physiology, neural pathways, and alteration in bowel disorders. J Clin Invest. 1963;42:196–207.
155. Seo S, Miyake H, Hock A, et al. Duhamel and transanal endorectal pull-throughs for Hirschsprung's disease: a systematic review and meta-analysis. Eur J Pediatr Surg. 2018;28:81–8.
156. Sergi C. Hischsprung's disease: historical notes and pathological diagnosis on the occasion of the 100(th) anniversary of Dr. Harald Hirschsprung's death. World J Clin Pediatr. 2015;8:120–5.
157. Shandling B. New technique in the diagnosis of Hirschsprung's disease. Can J Surg. 1961;4:298–305.
158. Sharif K, Beath SV, Kelly DA, McKiernan P, van Mourik I, Mirza D, Mayer AD, Buckels JA, de Ville de Goyet J. New perspective for the management of near total or total intestinal aganglionosis in infants. J Pediatr Surg. 2003;38:25–8.
159. Siu KL, Kwok WK, Lee WY, Lee WH. A male newborn with colon atresia and total colonic aganglionosis. Pediatr Surg Int. 1999;15:141–2.
160. Smith BM, Steiner RB, Lobe TE. Laparoscopic Duhamel pullthrough procedure for Hirschsprung's disease in childhood. J Laparoendosc Surg. 1994;4:273–6.
161. So HB, Schwartz DL, Becker JM, Daum F, Schneider KM. Endorectal pull-through without preliminary colostomy in neonates with Hirschsprung's disease. J Pediatr Surg. 1980;15:470–1.
162. Soave F. A new surgical technique for treatment of Hirschsprung's disease. Surgery. 1964;56:1007–14.
163. Soper RT, Miller FE. Modification of the Duhamel procedure: elimination of rectal pouch and colorectal septum. J Pediatr Surg. 1968;3:376–85.
164. Stamp LA, Young HM. Recent advances in regenerative medicine to treat enteric neuropathies: use of human cells. Neurogastroenterol Motil. 2017;29 https://doi.org/10.1111/nmo.12993.
165. State D. Surgical treatment for idiopathic congenital megacolon (Hirschsprung's disease). Surg Gynecol Obstet. 1952;95:201–12.
166. Steichen FM, Talbert JL, Ravitch MM. Primary side-to-side colorectal anastomosis in the Duhamel operation for Hirschsprung's disease. Surgery. 1968;64:475–83.
167. Suita S, Taguchi T, Kamimura T, Yanai K. Total colonic aganglionosis with or without small bowel involvement: a changing profile. J Pediatr Surg. 1997;32:1537–44.
168. Suita S, Taguchi T, Ieiri S, et al. Hirschsprung's disease in Japan: analysis of 3852 patients based on a nationwide survey in 30 years. J Pediatr Surg. 2005;40:197–201.
169. Swenson O. Partial internal sphincterectomy in the treatment of Hirschsprung's disease. Ann Surg. 1964;160:540–50.
170. Swenson O. How the cause and cure of Hirschsprung's disease was discovered. J Pediatr Surg. 1999;34:1580–1.
171. Swenson O. Hirschsprung's disease — a complicated therapeutic problem: some thoughts and solutions based on data and personal experience over 56 years. J Pediatr Surg. 2004;39:1449–53.

172. Swenson O, Bill AH. Resection of rectum and rectosigmoid with preservation of the sphincter for benign spastic lesions producing megacolon. Surgery. 1948;24:212–20.
173. Swenson O, Neuhauser EBD, Pickett LK. New concepts of etiology, diagnosis, and treatment of congenital megacolon (Hirschsprung's disease). Pediatrics. 1949;4:201–9.
174. Swenson O, Fisher JH, MacMahon HE. Rectal biopsy as an aid in the diagnosis of Hirschsprung's disease. N Engl J Med. 1959;253:632–5.
175. Talwalker VC. Aganglionosis of the entire bowel. J Pediatr Surg. 1976;11:213–6.
176. Tam PK, Garcia-Barcelo M. Molecular genetics of Hirschsprung's disease. Semin Pediatr Surg. 2004;13:236–48.
177. Tamate S, Shiokawa C, Yamada C, Takeuchi S, Nakahira M, Kadowaki H. Manometric diagnosis of Hirschsprung's disease in the neonatal period. J Pediatr Surg. 1984;19:285–8.
178. Teitelbaum DH, Coran AG. Enterocolitis. Semin Pediatr Surg. 1998;7:162–9.
179. Teitelbaum DH, Coran AG. Hirschsprung disease and related conditions. In: Grosfeld JL, O'Neill JA, Fonkalsrud EW, Coran AG, Caldamone A, editors. Pediatric surgery. 6th ed. Philadelphia: Elsevier; 2005.
180. Teitelbaum DH, Cilley RE, Sherman NJ, Bliss D, Uitvlugt ND, Renaud EJ, Kirstioglu I, Bengston T, Coran AG. A decade of experience with the primary pull-through for Hirschsprung disease in the newborn period: a multicenter analysis of outcomes. Ann Surg. 2000;232:372–80.
181. Thomas CG Jr. Posterior sphincterotomy in Hirschsprung's disease. Surg Gynecol Obstet. 1967;124:365–6.
182. Thomas CG Jr, Bream CA, DeConnick P. Posterior sphincterotomy and rectal myotomy in the management of Hirschsprung's disease. Ann Surg. 1970;171:796–810.
183. Tiffin ME, Chandler LR, Faber HK. Localized absence of ganglion cells of the myenteric plexus in congenital megacolon. Am J Dis Child. 1940;59:1071–82.
184. Tittel K. Uber eine angeborene Missbildung des Dickdarmes. Wien Klin Wochenschr. 1901;14:903–7.
185. Touloukian RJ. Pediatric surgery between 1860 and 1900. J Pediatr Surg. 1995;30:911–6.
186. Treves F. Idiopathic dilatation of the colon. Lancet. 1898;1:276–9.
187. Tzakis AG, Nour B, Reyes J, Abu-Elmagd K, Furukawa H, Todo S, Starzl TE. Endorectal pull-through of transplanted colon as part of intestinal transplantation. Surgery. 1995;117:451–3.
188. van der Zee DC, Bax NM. Duhamel-Martin procedure for Hirschsprung's disease in neonates and infants: one stage operation. J Pediatr Surg. 1996;31:901–2.
189. van Leeuwen K, Teitelbaum DH, Elhalaby EA, Coran AG. Long term follow up of re-do pull-through procedures for Hirschsprung's disease: efficacy of the endorectal pull-through. J Pediatr Surg. 2000;35:829–33.
190. Vrsansky P, Bourdelat D, Pages R. Early history of the therapy of Hirschsprung's disease: facts and personal observations over 50 years. J Pediatr Surg. 1997;32:935–6.
191. Vrsansky P, Bourdelat D, Pages R. Principal modifications of the Duhamel procedure in the treatment of Hirschsprung's disease. Analysis based on results of an international retrospective study of 2,430 patients. Pediatr Surg Int. 1998;13:125–32.
192. Wade RB, Royle ND. Preoperative treatment of Hirschsprung's disease: a new method. Med J Aust. 1927;14:137–41.
193. Walker AW, Kempson RL, Ternberg JL. Aganglionosis of the small intestine. Surgery. 1966;60:449–57.
194. Wang G, Sun XY, Wei MF, Weng YZ. Heart shaped anastomosis for Hirschsprung's disease: operative technique and long term follow up. World J Gastroenterol. 2005;11:296–8.
195. Watanatittan S, Suwatanaviroj A, Limprutithum T, Rattanasuwan T. Association of Hirschsprung's disease and anorectal malformation. J Pediatr Surg. 1991;26:192–5.
196. Weber TR, Fortuna RS, Silen ML, Dillon PA. Re-operation for Hirschsprung's disease. J Pediatr Surg. 1999;34:153–6.
197. West KW, Grosfeld JL, Rescorla FJ, Vane DW. Acquired aganglionosis: a rare occurrence following pull-through procedures for Hirschsprung's disease. J Pediatr Surg. 1990;25:104–9.
198. Whitehouse FR, Kernohan JW. Myenteric plexus in congenital megacolon. Arch Intern Med. 1948;82:75–111.
199. Whitehouse F, et al. Congenital megacolon: favorable end results of treatment by resection. Gastroenterology. 1943;1:922–37.
200. Wilcox DT, Kiely EM. Repeat pull-through for Hirschsprung's disease. J Pediatr Surg. 1998;35:1507–9.
201. Wildhaber BE, Pakarinen M, Rintala RJ, Coran AG, Teitelbaum DH. Posterior myotomy/myectomy for persistent stooling problems in Hirschsprung's disease. J Pediatr Surg. 2004;39:920–6.
202. Wildhaber BE, Teitelbaum DH, Coran AG. Total colonic Hirschsprung's disease a 28 year experience. J Pediatr Surg. 2005;40:203–7.
203. Wilson-Storey G, Scobie WG. Impaired gastrointestinal mucosal defense in Hirschsprung's disease: a clue to the pathogenesis of enterocolitis? J Pediatr Surg. 1989;24:462–4.
204. Yin L, Ceccherini I, Pasini B, Matera I, Bicocchi MP, Barone V, Bocciardi R, Kääriäinen H, Weber D, Devoto M, Romeo G. Close linkage with the RET protooncogene and boundaries of deletion mutations in autosomal dominant Hirschsprung disease. Hum Mol Genet. 1993;2:1803–8.
205. Yomo A, Taira T, Kondo I. Goldberg-Shprintzen syndrome: Hirschsprung disease, hypotonia, and ptosis in sibs. Am J Med Genet. 1991;41:188–91.

206. Ziegler MM, Ross AJ 3rd, Bishop HC. Total colonic aganglionosis: a new technique for prolonged survival. J Pediatr Surg. 1987;22:82–3.
207. Ziegler MM, Royal RE, Brandt J, Drasnin J, Martin LW. Extended myotomy-myectomy: a therapeutic alternative for total intestinal aganglionosis. Ann Surg. 1993;218:504–9.
208. Zuelzer WW, Wilson JL. Functional intestinal obstruction on a congenital neurogenic basis in infancy. Am J Dis Child. 1948;75:40–64.

Development of the Enteric Nervous System

2

Udo Rolle and Prem Puri

Contents

U. Rolle (✉)
Department of Paediatric Surgery and Paediatric Urology, Goethe-University Frankfurt/M., Frankfurt/M., Germany
e-mail: udo.rolle@kgu.de

P. Puri
National Children's Research Centre, Our Lady's Children's Hospital, Crumlin, Dublin, Ireland

2.1 Introduction

The enteric nervous system (ENS) is the largest and the most complex division of the peripheral nervous system and comprises enteric neurons and glial cells, which are organized in two concentric ganglionated plexuses [1, 2]. The ENS contains more neurons than the spinal cord and is capable of mediating reflex activity in the absence of the central nervous system. About 80–100 million enteric neurons can be classified into functional distinct subpopulations, including intrinsic primary neurons, interneurons, motor neurons, secretomotory and vasomotor neurons [3, 4]. The ENS plays a crucial role in normal gastrointestinal motility. Therefore, insights into the development of the gastrointestinal tract and the ENS are relevant for the understanding of the pathophysiology and treatment of infants and children with motility disorders.

2.2 Embryonic Origin of ENS

There are two major steps in the development of the gastrointestinal tract: (1) formation of the gut tube and (2) formation of individual organs, each with their specialized cell types (Table 2.1) [5].

Gastrulation is an early step in the development of all multicellular organisms. During gastrulation, the axes of the embryo are determined, and the development of the gastrointestinal tract starts. Gastrulation gives rise to three germ layers, endo-

P. Puri (ed.), *Hirschsprung's Disease and Allied Disorders*,
https://doi.org/10.1007/978-3-030-15647-3_2

Table 2.1 Developmental milestones of the human gastrointestinal tract [5]

Developmental stage	Gestation
Gastrulation	Week 3
Gut tube largely closed	Week 4
Liver and pancreas buds	Week 4
Growth of intestines into cord	Week 7
Intestinal villus formation	Week 8
Retraction of intestines into abdominal cavity	Week 10
Organ formation complete	Week 12
Parietal cells detectable, pancreatic islets appear, bile secretion, intestinal enzymes detectable	Week 12
Swallowing detectable	Weeks 16 and 17
Mature motility	Week 36

derm, mesoderm and ectoderm. The mammalian gastrointestinal system originates from all three embryonic germ layers [5]. The epithelial lining of the gastrointestinal tube and the parenchymal cells of the liver and pancreas are formed by the endoderm. The mesoderm provides mesenchymal elements including smooth muscle and stromal cells. The neurons of the ENS which regulate gastrointestinal motility are derived from ectoderm.

The ectoderm divides into three types of cells: outer ectoderm, neural tube and neural crest. The neural crest arises from the dorsal region of the neural tube. Melanocytes, the adrenal medulla, the dentine of teeth, the sympathetic and parasympathetic arms of the peripheral nervous system, and the neurons of the ENS are derived from the neural crest. These tissues and cell types originate from different regions of the neural crest, which means that the cells need to migrate to the site of the mature organs. The gene mutations that result in disrupted neural crest cell migration to one region also cause altered migration of other neural crest-derived tissues [6].

2.3 Origin and Development of Neural Crest-Derived Cells

The neural crest (NC) is located along the entire length of the body axis. Two groups of undifferentiated cells, derived from neural crests, colonize the gut wall and migrate in craniocaudal and caudocranial directions.

The embryonic NC arises in the neural tube, originating with the central nervous system, but neural crest cells (NCCs) detach from this tissue via reduction of cell-cell and cell-matrix adhesion. The epithelio-mesenchymal transformation allows NCC to migrate along pathways of defined routes to various tissues, where they stop moving and differentiate into various cell types. Pathway selection is most likely achieved by balanced combinations of molecules that promote and reduce adhesions [7, 8]. NCCs give rise to neuronal, endocrine and paraendocrine, craniofacial, conotruncal heart and pigmentary tissues. Neurocristopathies encompass tumours, malformations and single or multiple abnormalities of tissues, mentioned above in various combinations [9].

In the human foetus, NCCs first appear in the developing oesophagus at the third week of gestation and then migrate down to the anal canal in a craniocaudal direction during the fourth week and the seventh week of gestation (Table 2.2) [2]. The NCCs first form the myenteric plexus just outside the circular muscle layer. The mesenchymally derived longitudinal muscle layer then forms, sandwiching the myenteric plexus after it has been formed in the 12th week of gestation. In addition, after the craniocaudal migration has ended, the submucous plexus is formed by the neuroblasts, which migrate from the myenteric plexus across the circular muscle layer and into the submucosal; this progresses in a craniocaudal direction during the 12th to 16th week of gestation [7]. The absence of ganglion cells in Hirschsprung's disease has been attributed to a failure of migration

Table 2.2 Time of vagal ENCC arrival at designated sites [2]

	Proximal foregut	Stomach	Caecal region	Distal end of hindgut
Zebrafish	32 hpf			66 hpf
Quail	E2.5	E4	E5	E7
Chick	E2.5	E4.5	E5.5	E8
Mouse	E9.5	E10.5	E11.5	E14.5
Human	Week 3	Week 4	Week 6	Week 7

of NCC. The earlier the arrest of migration, the longer the aganglionic segment is.

It is generally accepted that the enteric ganglion cells are derived primarily from the NCC [10–13]. Studies in the avian system provide strong evidence for the contribution of the sacral NC to the hindgut ENS [14–16]. Whether the sacral NC contributes to the ENS in the mammalian hindgut still remains unknown. Failure of the vagal-derived NCC to colonize the hindgut results in failure of hindgut ENS development, suggesting that interaction between sacral and vagal enteric NCC may be necessary for sacral NCC contribution to the ENS [17].

Furthermore, it has been shown that the major difference between vagal- and sacral-derived enteric NCC is the higher invasiveness of the vagal cells. If the vagal tube replaces the sacral tube, vagal-derived NCCs colonize the distal bowel much faster and with higher numbers [18].

In more detail, Yntema and Hammond first performed neural crest ablations in chick embryos and identified the vagal neural crest (somites 1–7) as the source of the ENS stem cells [13].

Le Douarin and Teillet showed an additional source of neural crest stem cells originating from the lumbosacral region to colonize the gut [14]. Later, the lumbosacral-derived crest cells were found principally in the myenteric plexus, with very few in the submucous plexus. The number of these cells declines rostrally. Cells derived from the lumbosacral neural crest were never observed in any gut region above the umbilicus [16].

The colonization of the gut by sacral neural crest-derived cells and the contribution of the cells to the development of the ENS are controversial [19]. The dual origin of enteric neurons has been negated by studies on chick embryos as well as human embryos. Allen and Newgreen [20] isolated bowel segments from fowl embryos at various stages of development and grew these segments on chorioallantoic membrane and found that enteric neurons appeared in a craniocaudal sequence, showing a vagal source.

Meijers et al. [21] transected the chicken bowel in ovo at an early stage, before the passage of NCC had occurred, preventing craniocaudal migration of vagal NCC. They found that the hindgut remained aganglionic, showing that there was no colonization by sacral NCC.

Some studies showed that sacral NCCs migrate from the neural plate early in development and extraenteric pelvic ganglia. Later, these cells are able to colonize the gut and contribute to the ENS, coincident with the migration of vagal NCC [16, 22–24]. In contrast, other studies suggest that sacral NCCs invade the hindgut mesenchyme several days before the colonization of the hindgut by vagal NCC and contribute to the development of ENS [15, 25–27].

The current concept in human gut development is that the ENS is derived primarily from cells of the vagal segment of the neural crest [3, 14]. Fujimoto et al. [28] studied NCC migration in the developing gut in the human embryo using anti-neurofilament protein triplet antibody and found that enteric ganglia originated from a single vagal neural crest source.

The vast majority of studies have revealed that vagal NCCs provide the main source of enteric neurons and the sacral neural crest innervates the distal bowel in addition [14–16, 29–31].

Recently, some alternative pathways of neuronal cell population in the gut have been described, as transmesenteric migration of a crest cell subpopulation or the migration of Schwann cells precursors along extrinsic nerves [32]. In particular, transmesenteric migration comprises an alternative pathway for enteric nervous precursor cells to reach the hindgut [33].

The final requirement for the development and maturation of the ENS is the formation of ganglia. Several days after NCCs have colonized the gut, these cells are evenly distributed, with no indication of cell clustering, except the caecum. As the gut increases later in length and diameter, the cells start forming ganglionic groups [34]. One previous study has shown that cells forming a ganglion do not arise from a single precursor cell [35]. Human foetal intestine has been used to investigate nitrergic neurons in the developing myenteric plexus. The distribution of nitrergic neurons was found to change markedly between 14 and 22 weeks of gestation. Nitrergic neurons were randomly distributed at week 14 and were later aggregated in the plexus and within individual ganglia at week 19 [36]. How cells are induced to cluster into ganglia is as yet unknown.

2.4 Functional Development of ENS

The complexity of the mature ENS is exemplified by many different functional types of neurons containing various neurotransmitters occurring in various combinations. Types of neurotransmitters vary according to the time of their appearance [34, 37]. The development of the human ENS is characterized by the early appearance (between 9 and 12 weeks' gestation) of adrenergic and cholinergic nerves. Strong evidence has emerged that the ENS is not only composed of adrenergic and cholinergic nerves but also non-adrenergic, non-cholinergic (NANC) autonomic nerves, which contain different peptides. These peptides act as neurotransmitters, or neuromodulators, or both. These nerves have been termed peptidergic nerves. The development of peptidergic innervation occurs much later.

In recent years, pharmacologic and physiologic studies have provided evidence that nitric oxide (NO) is the most important mediator in non-adrenergic, non-cholinergic relaxation of the gastrointestinal tract. By 12 weeks' gestation, nitrergic neurons appear in the myenteric ganglia, at all levels of the gut, and begin plexus formation. Nitrergic innervation in the submucous plexus becomes evident after 14 weeks. As gestational age increases, nitrergic innervation becomes richer and more organized. Increasing numbers of nitrergic nerve fibres are seen in the circular muscle; some of these fibres project from the myenteric plexus. Thus, the onset and pace of development of nitrergic innervation are similar to adrenergic and cholinergic innervation and occur before peptidergic innervation [38].

Serotonin (5-HT) together with glucagon, insulin, peptide XY, gastrin and somatostatin are the earliest neurohumoral substances to be expressed at about 8 weeks of gestation. By 24 weeks of gestation, most of the known gastrointestinal neurohumoral substances have been identified.

Further contacts between enteric nerves and effectors are developed at 26 weeks and first signs of motility are detected at 25 weeks of gestation [5].

2.5 Development of Intestinal Motility

The innervation of the gastrointestinal tract in utero is accompanied by functional activity of increasing complexity. The first studies to measure intestinal transit in humans used amniography; aboral transport of contrast did not occur in the intestinal tract of foetuses younger than 30 weeks of gestation [39]. With increasing gestational age, increasing aboral transit and rate of propagation develops. Subsequent studies of gastrointestinal motility in premature infants have been performed using intraluminal catheters [40]. The data from these studies reveal no regular periodicity or rhythmicity at 25 weeks of gestation. Further development occurs during the next 15 weeks, so that by term, mature motor patterns of the gastrointestinal tract are well established. Responses to feeding vary considerably among preterm infants; in general, intestinal motility studies can predict feeding intolerance [41].

Enteric nerve cells continue to differentiate throughout the first couple of years of life, which means that the infant's nervous system is plastic and developing [42]. There is clear evidence that the development of the ENS continues after birth. In rats, nitric oxide synthase-expressing neurons are already present at birth but increase in number and location postnatally during the first 3 weeks of life [37]. Normal ganglion cell distribution is present at 24 weeks of gestation in humans. These ganglia continue to mature on into childhood. Previous studies on human bowel specimens have revealed that the density of NADPH-diaphorase-positive ganglion cells decreases in the submucous plexus of the human distal colon and the myenteric plexus of human small bowel, colon and rectum [43, 44].

2.6 Genes Involved in ENS Development

Normal development of ENS is related to migration, proliferation, differentiation and survival of NCC [45]. Several genes and signalling molecules have been identified that control morphogenesis and differentiation of the ENS. These genes, when mutated or deleted, interfere with ENS development (Table 2.3) [9, 46–48]. A short description of the main functions of these genes is provided in Table 2.4 [49].

2.6.1 RET/GDNF/GFRα1 Signalling System

This signalling pathway is of importance for subpopulations of both peripheral and central neurons, having been shown by in vitro and in vivo assays to promote survival of neurons, mitosis of neuronal progenitor cells, differentiation of neurons and neurite extension [30, 50]. The RET receptor is the signalling component of receptor complexes with four ligands, glial-derived neurotropic factor (GDNF), neurturin (NTN), artemin (ATM) and persephin (PSP) [50, 51]. The complete receptor complex includes the RET receptor tyrosine kinase and a glycosylphosphatidylinositol-anchored binding component (GFRα1, GFRα2, GFRα3 and GFRα4) [51–53]. In vivo, the absence of GDNF/GFRα1-mediated signalling leads to the failure of ENS development, whereas absence of NTN/GFRα2-mediated signalling leads to more subtle abnormalities in ENS development [51]. RET has its role in promoting migration, but also proliferation and survival of enteric NCC [54–59]. The importance of RET in mammalian organogenesis has been further illustrated by the generation of RET knockout mice [60]. These RET-deficient mice exhibit apoptosis of enteric NCC in the foregut [57] leading to intestinal aganglionosis, which has been shown in mice deficient in RET, GDNF and GFR [61–65]. Sufficient proliferation and survival of enteric NCC is required to colonize the entire gut. Insufficient numbers of progenitor cells

Table 2.3 Genes involved in the morphogenesis and differentiation of the ENS [9, 46–48]

Genes	Chromosomal assignment	Function
RET	10q11.2	Tyrosine kinase receptor
GDNF NTN GFRα	5p12–13.1 19q13.3 10q26	Glial cell-derived neurotropic factor Neurturin, RET ligand GDNF family receptor alpha 1
EDNRB	13q22	Endothelin B receptor
EDN-3	20q13.2–13.3	Endothelin B
ECE-1	1p36.1	Endothelin-converting enzyme
SOX 10 Phox2b	22q13.1 4p12	Sry/HMG box transcription factor Paired-like homeobox 2b
Pax3 SIP1	2q35 2q22	Paired box gene 3 Siah-interacting protein

Table 2.4 Role of selected genes in ENS development [49]

Gene	Role in ENS development	Protein function/ comments
RET	Supports ENS precursor survival, proliferation, migration, neuronal differentiation, neurite growth and axon patterning	Transmembrane tyrosine kinase receptor Most commonly inactivated gene in patients with HD
GDNF	RET-activating ligand	Neurotrophic factor Rarely mutated in patients with HD
EDNRB	Prevents premature differentiation of enteric NCCs	G-protein-coupled receptor Mutated in 5% of people with HD Also causes hearing loss and pigmentation defects (Waardenburg-Shah, WS4)
EDN3	EDNRB-activating ligand	Peptide Rarely mutated in patients with HD
SOX 10	Required for bowel colonization by enteric NCCs Activates RET expression	Transcription factor Mutations cause HD plus hearing loss and pigmentation defects (WS4)
PHOX2B	Required for bowel colonization by enteric NCCs Activates RET expression	Transcription factor Mutations cause HD plus congenital central hypoventilation (Haddad syndrome)

lead to intestinal aganglionosis, as observed in Hirschsprung's disease. The RET proto-oncogene has been demonstrated to be a major gene causing Hirschsprung's disease [66–70]. Mutations of RET account for 50% of familial and 15%–20% of sporadic cases of Hirschsprung's disease [70, 71].

Interestingly, there is evidence that the effect of RET on the proliferation and survival of enteric NCC are dose dependent. RET-deficient homozygous mice develop near-total aganglionosis, whereas heterozygous mice present with a normal ENS [61]. The level of RET expression influences the length of aganglionosis, since colorectal aganglionosis occurs if RET is expressed at one-third of normal expression levels [72]. RET signalling is also important for neuron survival and ENS maturation after full colonization [72].

The development of the ENS is dependent upon the actions of GDNF, which stimulates the proliferation and survival of NC-derived precursor cells in the embryonic gut [73–76]. It has been reported that GDNF is the ligand of RET [77]. GDNF acts as a chemoattractive agent and promotes the migration of enteric NCC [78]. Mice carrying the homozygous null mutation in GDNF have been generated, and these mice demonstrate the lack of kidneys and ENS, confirming the crucial role of GDNF in the development of the ENS [79, 80].

The role of GDNF-Ret signalling pathway on differentiation of enteric neuronal precursor cells is controversially reported, which reflects the complexity of this pathway.

Although a causative role for GDNF mutations in some patients with Hirschsprung's disease has been suggested, the occurrence of such cases is uncommon, and it is more likely that the GDNF mutations are involved in modulation of Hirschsprung's disease phenotype via its interaction with other susceptibility loci such as RET [7, 63].

2.6.2 Endothelin Signalling Pathway

The endothelins (EDN1, EDN2 and EDN3) are intercellular local messengers that act via cell surface receptors, EDNRA and EDNRB [51]. EDN is initially produced as an inactive prepro-endothelin that undergoes two proteolytic steps to produce an active peptide. The first cleavage produces inactive big endothelins, and these are finally cleaved by a specific protease, endothelin-converting enzyme (ECE) to produce biologically active EDN [9, 81].

EDN3 and EDNRB have a role in the migration and development of the ENS [82–84]. Endothelin-3 (ET3) is the ligand of EDNRB. Deletions of the genes or ECE lead to colorectal aganglionosis [82, 84]. In mice, in which the EDN3 or EDNRB gene was disrupted, intestinal aganglionosis was demonstrated experimentally. Several reports suggest that the downregulation of EDN3 expression may play a role in the pathogenesis of Hirschsprung's disease in the sporadic cases [85–91]. ECE1 knockout mice show craniofacial and cardiac abnormalities in addition to colonic aganglionosis [92]. Besides its role for the proliferation of enteric NCC, EDNRB also inhibits the differentiation of the neuronal precursor cells. Disturbance of this function results in precursor cell populations which cannot further divide or migrate leading to a failure of full colonization of the gut [93].

2.6.3 SOX10

SOX10 (sex determining region Y-box) gene is expressed in NCCs that contribute to the formation of the peripheral nervous system during embryogenesis [94, 95]. SOX10 is required for survival of enteric NCC as well as for maintaining enteric NCC in an undifferentiated and proliferative state [96–99]. The latter function is similar to EDNRB [100]. The involvement of SOX10 in the development of enteric neurons was demonstrated in the Dom (dominant megacolon) mouse model of Hirschsprung's disease which exhibit distal intestinal aganglionosis [94]. Mutations in SOX10 have been identified as a cause of the dominant megacolon mouse and Waardenburg-Shah syndrome in human, both of which include defects in the ENS and pigmentation abnormalities [100, 101].

2.6.4 PHOX2B

The Phox2B gene is a homeodomain-containing transcription factor that is involved in neurogenesis and regulates RET expression in mice, in which disruption of the Phox2B gene results in a Hirschsprung's disease-like phenotype [78, 102]. Enteric Phox2B expression begins in vagal and truncal NCC as they invade the foregut mesenchyme and is contained in the adult submucosal and myenteric plexus [78]. Phox2B is involved in the formation of enteric ganglia by promotion of enteric NCC proliferation and survival [78].

2.6.5 HOX11L1

Hox11L1 is a homebox gene involved in peripheral nervous system development and is reported to play a role in the proliferation or differentiation of NC cell lines. Two different Hox11L1 knockout mouse models have been generated [103, 104]. In both cases, homozygous mutant mice were viable but developed megacolon at the age of 3–5 weeks. Histological and immunohistochemical analysis showed hyperplasia of myenteric ganglia, a phenotype similar to that observed in human intestinal neuronal dysplasia.

2.7 Other Non-genetic Factors Implicated in the Control of ENS Development

Several studies have implicated the importance of the gut microenvironment during development of the ENS. It has been shown that factors such as laminin [105], fibronectin [106], vitronectin [107] and collagen type I [108] support enteric NCC migration, whereas collagen type VI [109] inhibits migration. Mice lacking EDN-3 showed increased expression of laminin, one of extracellular matrix (ECM) proteins, which lead to the conclusion that EDN-3 also affects the environment through which the NCCs migrate [110]. Altered ECM proteins such as tenascin, fibronectin and nidogen have been shown in patients with Hirschsprung's disease, suggesting the importance of ECM molecules during development of ENS [111, 112].

2.8 Interstitial Cells of Cajal

Kit, another receptor with tyrosine kinase activity, is involved in the development of interstitial cells of Cajal (ICC) [113]. These are nonneuronal cells that serve as pacemaker cells and are responsible for the spontaneous, rhythmic, electrical excitatory activity of gastrointestinal smooth muscle. Recent studies have found that the c-kit receptor is essential for the development of ICC. Mesenchymal ICC precursors that carry the c-kit receptor require the kit ligand, which can be provided by neuronal cells or smooth muscle cells. According to the influence of the kit ligand from either neuronal or smooth muscle cells, the ICCs develop as either myenteric ICC or muscular ICC [114]. These cells are also important in modulating communications between nerve and muscle. Mice with mutations in the KIT gene lack ICC and have changes in skin pigment and abnormal intestinal motility [115]. No such mutations have been reported in humans so far, but several studies reported disturbed expression of ICC in patients with motility disorders [116–120].

2.9 Summary

The development of the ENS requires the complex interaction of genes encoding transcription factors, signalling molecules and their receptors. Normal ENS development is based on survival of NCC and their coordinated proliferation, movement and differentiation into neurons and glia. These processes are influenced by the microenvironment of the developing gut. Alterations in gene function, defects in NCC or changes in the gut microenvironment may result in abnormal development of the ENS.

References

1. Gershon MD, Jerde SM. The nervous system of the gut. Gastroenterology. 1981;80:1571–94.
2. Nagy N, Goldstein AM. Enteric nervous system development: a crest cell's journey from neural tube to colon. Semin Cell Dev Biol. 2017;66:94–106.
3. Furness JB, Clere N, Vogalis F, Stebbing MJ. The enteric nervous system and its extrinsic connections. In: Yamada T, Alpers DH, editors. Textbook of gastroenterology. Philadelphia: Lippincott Williams; 2003. p. 13–34.
4. Furness JB. Types of neurons in the enteric nervous system. J Auton Nerv Syst. 2000;81(1–3):87–96.
5. Montgomery RK, Mulberg AE, Grand RJ. Development of the human gastrointestinal tract: twenty years of progress. Gastroenterology. 1999;116:702–31.
6. Bates MD. Development of the enteric nervous system. Clin Perinatol. 2002;29:97–114.
7. Rolle U, Nemeth L, Puri P. Nitrergic innervation of the normal gut and in motility disorders of childhood. J Pediatr Surg. 2002;36:551–67.
8. Puri P, Ohsiro K, Wester T. Hirschsprung's disease: a search for etiology. Semin Pediatr Surg. 1998;7:140–7.
9. Amiel J, Lyonnet S. Hirschsprung disease, associated syndromes and genetics: a review. J Med Genet. 2001;38:729–39.
10. Gershon MD, Chalazonitis A, Rothman TP. From neural crest to bowel: development of the enteric nervous system. J Neurobiol. 1993;24:199–214.
11. Goyal RK, Hirano I. The enteric nervous system. N Engl J Med. 1996;334:1106–15.
12. Gershon MD. The enteric nervous system: a second brain. Hosp Pact. 1999;34:31–2, 35–8, 41–2
13. Yntema CL, Hammond WS. The origin of intrinsic ganglia of trunk viscera from vagal neural crest in the chick embryo. J Comp Neurol. 1954;101:515–41.
14. Le Douarin NM, Teillet MA. The migration of neural crest cells to the wall of the digestive tract in avian embryo. J Embryol Exp Morphol. 1973;30:31–48.
15. Pomeranz HD, Gershon MD. Colonization of the avian hindgut by cells derived from the sacral neural crest. Dev Biol. 1990;137:378–94.
16. Burns AJ, Le Duoarin NM. The sacral neural crest contributes neurons and glia to the post-umbilical gut: spatiotemporal analysis of the development of the enteric nervous system. Development. 1998;125:4335–47.
17. Caniano DA, Ormsbee HS III, Polito W. Total intestinal aganglionosis. J Pediatr Surg. 1985;20:456–60.
18. Burns AJ, Delalande JM, Le Douarin NM. In ovo transplantation of enteric nervous system precursors from vagal to sacral neural crest results in extensive hindgut colonisation. Development. 2002;129(12):2785–96.
19. Gariepy CE. Developmental disorders of the enteric nervous system: genetic and molecular bases. J Pediatr Gastroenterol Nutr. 2004;39:5–11.
20. Allan IJ, Newgreen DF. The origin and differentiation of enteric neurons of the intestine of the fowl embryo. Am J Anat. 1980;157(157):137–54.
21. Meijers JHC, Tibboel D, Van der Kamp AWM. A model for aganglionosis in the chicken embryo. J Pediatr Surg. 1989;24:557–61.
22. Kapur RP. Colonization of the murine hindgut by sacral crest-derived neural precursors: experimental support for an evolutionarily conserved model. Dev Biol. 2000;227:146–55.
23. Burns AJ, Champeval D, le Douarin NM. Sacral neural crest cells colonise aganglionic hindgut in vivo but fail to compensate for lack of enteric ganglia. Dev Biol. 2000;219:30–43.
24. Young HM, Hearn CJ, Ciampoli D, Southwell BR, Brunet JF, Newgreen DF. A single rostrocaudal colonization of the rodent intestine by enteric precursors is revealed by the expression of Phox2b, Ret, and p75 and by explants grown under the kidney capsule in organ culture. Dev Biol. 1998;202:67–84.
25. Erickson CA, Goins TL. Sacral neural crest cell migration to the gut is dependent upon migratory environment and not cell-autonomous migratory properties. Dev Biol. 2000;219:79–97.
26. Serbedzija GN, Burgan S, Fraser SE, Bronner-Fraser M. Vital dye labelling demonstrates a sacral neural crest contribution to the enteric nervous system of chick and mouse embryos. Development. 1991;111:857–66.
27. Pomeranz HD, Rothman TP, Gershon MD. Colonization of the post-umbilical bowel by cells derived from the sacral neural crest: direct tracing of cell migration using an intercalating probe and replication-deficient retrovirus. Development. 1991;111:647–55.
28. Fujimoto T, Hata J, Yokoyama S, Mitomi T. A study of the extracellular matrix protein as the migration pathway of neural crest cells in the gut: Analysis in human embryos with special reference to the pathogenesis of Hirschsprung's disease. J Pediatr Surg. 1989;24:550–6.
29. Le Douarin NM, Dupin E, Ziller C. Genetic and epigenetic controls in neural crest development. Curr Opin Genet Dev. 1994;4:685–95.
30. Taraviras S, Pachnis V. Development of the mammalian enteric nervous system. Curr Opin Genet Dev. 1999;9:321–7.
31. Young HM, Hearn CJ, Newgreen DF. Embryology and development of enteric nervous system. Gut. 2000;47:iv12–4.
32. Uesaka T, Nagashimada M, Enomoto H. Neuronal differentiation in Schwann cell lineage underlies postnatal neurogenesis in the enteric nervous system. J Neurosci. 2015;35:9879–88.
33. Nishiyama C, Uesaka T, Manabe T, Yonekura Y, Nagasawa T, Newgreen DF, Young HM, Enomoto H. Trans-mesenteric neural crest cells are the principal source of the colonic enteric nervous system. Nat Neurosci. 2016;15:1211–8.

34. Young HM, Newgreen DF. Enteric neural crest-derived cells: origin, identification, migration, and differentiation. Anat Rec. 2001;262:1–15.
35. Rothman TP, Le Douarin NM, Fontaine-Perus JC, Gershon MD. Colonization of the bowel by neural crest-derived cells migrating from foregut backtransplanted to vagal or sacral regions of host embryos. Dev Dyn. 1993;196:217–33.
36. Roman V, Bagyanszki M, Krecsmarik M, Horvath A, Resch BA, Fekete E. Spatial pattern analysis of nitrergic neurons in the developing myenteric plexus of the human fetal intestine. Cytometry A. 2004;57A:108–12.
37. Matini P, Mayer B, Faussone-Pellegrini MS. Neurochemical differentiation of rat enteric neurons during pre- and postnatal life. Cell Tissue Res. 1997;288:11–23.
38. Brandt CT, Tam PKH, Gould SJ. Nitrergic innervation of the human during early foetal development. J Pediatr Surg. 1996;31:661–4.
39. Grand RJ, Watkins JB, Torti FM. Development of the human gastrointestinal tract. A review. Gastroenterology. 1976;70:790–810.
40. Dumont RC, Rudolph CD. Development of gastrointestinal motility in the infant and child. Gastroenterol Clin North Am. 1994;23:655–71.
41. Berseth CL, Nordyke CK. Manometry can predict feeding readiness in preterm infants. Gastroenterology. 1992;103:1523–8.
42. Gershon MDV. Genes, lineages, and tissue interactions in the development of the enteric nervous system. Am J Physiol. 1998;275:G869–73.
43. Wester T, O'Briain S, Puri P. Morphometric aspects of the submucous plexus in whole-mount preparations of normal human distal colon. J Pediatr Surg. 1998;33(4):619–22.
44. Wester T, O'Briain S, Puri P. Notable postnatal alterations in the myenteric plexus of normal human bowel. Gut. 1999;44:666–74.
45. Wallace AS, Burns AJ. Development of the enteric nervous system, smooth muscle and interstitial cells of Cajal in the human gastrointestinal tract. Cell Tissue Res. 2005;319:367–382, 2005.
46. Gariepy CE. Intestinal motility disorders and development of the enteric nervous system. Pediatr Res. 2000;49:605–13.
47. Parisi MA, Kapur RP. Genetics of Hirschsprung's disease. Curr Opin Pediatr. 2000;12:610–7.
48. Passarge E. Dissecting Hirschsprung's disease. Nat Genet. 2002;31:11–2.
49. Heuckeroth RO, Schäfer KH. Gene-environment interactions and the enteric nervous system: neural plasticity and Hirschsprung disease prevention. Dev Biol. 2016;417:188–97.
50. Newgreen D, Young HM. Enteric nervous system: development and developmental disturbances part 1. Pediatr Dev Pathol. 2002;5:224–47.
51. Newgreen D, Young HM. Enteric nervous system: development and developmental disturbances part 2. Pediatr Dev Pathol. 2002;5:329–49.
52. Jing S, Wen D, Yu Y, Holst PJ, Fang M, Tamir R, et al. GDNF-induced activation of the ret protein tyrosine kinase is mediated by GDNFR-α, a novel receptor for GDNF. Cell. 1996;85:1113–24.
53. Jing S, Yu Y, Fang M, Hu Z, Holst PL, Boone T, et al. GFRα-2 and GFRα-3 are two new receptors for ligands of the GDNF family. J Biol Chem. 1997;272:33111–7.
54. Chalazonitis A, Rothman TP, Chen J, Gershon MD. Age-dependent differences in the effects of GDNF and NT-3 on the development of neurons and glia from neural crest-derived precursors immunoselected from the fetal rat gut: expression of GFRalpha-1 in vitro and in vivo. Dev Biol. 1998;204:385–406.
55. Hearn CJ, Murphy M, Newgreen D. GDNF and ET-3 differentially modulate the numbers of avian enteric neural crest cells and enteric neurons in vitro. Dev Biol. 1998;197:93–105.
56. Heuckeroth RO, Lampe PA, Johnson EM, Milbrandt J. Neurturin and GDNF promote proliferation and survival of enteric neuron and glial progenitors in vitro. Dev Biol. 1998;200:116–29.
57. Taraviras S, Marcos-Gutierrez CV, Durbec P, Jani H, Grigoriou M, Sukumaran M, Wang LC, Hynes M, Raisman G, Pachnis V. Signalling by the RET receptor tyrosine kinase and its role in the development of the mammalian enteric nervous system. Development. 1999;126:2785–97.
58. Barlow A, de Graaff E, Pachnis V. Enteric nervous system progenitors are coordinately controlled by the G protein-coupled receptor EDNRB and the receptor tyrosine kinase RET. Neuron. 2003;40:905–16.
59. Mwizerwa O, Das P, Nagy N, Akbareian SE, Mably JD, Goldstein AM. Gdnf is mitogenic, neurotrophic, and chemoattractive to enteric neural crest cells in the embryonic colon. Dev Dyn. 2011;240:1402–11.
60. Schuchardt A, D'Agati V, Larsson-Blumberg L, Constantini F, Pachnis V. Defects in the kidney and enteric nervous system of mice lacking the tyrosine kinase receptor Ret. Nature. 1994;367:380–3.
61. Pichel JG, Shen L, Sheng HZ, Granholm AC, Drago J, Grinberg A, Lee EJ, Huang EP, Saarma M, Hoffer BJ, Sariola H, Westphal H. Defects in enteric innervation and kidney development in mice lacking GDNF. Nature. 1996;382:73–6.
62. Moore MW, Klein RD, Farinas I, Sauer H, Armanini M, Phillips H, Reichardt LF, Ryan AM, Carver-Moore K, Rosenthal A. Renal and neuronal abnormalities in mice lacking GDNF. Nature. 1996;382:76–9.
63. Sanchez MP, Silos-Santiago I, Frisen J, He B, Lira SA, Barbacid M. Renal agenesis and the absence of enteric neurons in mice lacking GDNF. Nature. 1996;382:10–73.
64. Enomoto H, Araki T, Jackman A, Heuckeroth RO, Snider WD, Johnson EM Jr, Milbrandt J. GFR alpha1-deficient mice have deficits in the enteric nervous system and kidneys. Neuron. 1998;21:317–24.
65. Luo Y, Cecchernin I, Pasini B, Matera I, Bicochi MP, Barone V, et al. Close linkage with the RET proto-

oncogene and boundaries of deletion mutations in autosomal dominant Hirschsprung's disease. Hum Mol Genet. 1993;2:1803–8.
66. Romeo G, Ronchetto P, Luo Y, Barone V, Seti M, Ceccherini I, et al. Point mutations affecting the tyrosine kinase domain of the RET proto-oncogene in Hirschsprung's disease. Nature. 1994;367:377–87.
67. Edery P, Lyonnet S, Mulligan LM, Pelet A, Dow E, Abel L, et al. Mutations of the RET proto-oncogene in Hirschsprung's disease. Nature. 1994;367:378–80.
68. Kusafuka T, Puri P. Altered RET gene mRNA expression in Hirschsprung's disease. J Pediatr Surg. 1997;32:600–4.
69. Kusafuka T, Puri P. The RET proto-oncogene: a challenge to understanding of disease pathogenesis. Pediatr Surg Int. 1997;12:11–8.
70. Martucciello G, Ceccherini I, Lerone M, Jasonni V. Pathogenesis of Hirschsprung's disease. J Pediatr Surg. 2000;35:1017–25.
71. Uesaka T, Nagashimada M, Yonemura S, Enomoto H. Diminished Ret expression compromises neuronal survival in the colon and causes intestinal aganglionosis in mice. J Clin Investig. 2008;118:1890–8.
72. Uesaka T, Jain S, Yonemura S, Uchiyama Y, Milbrandt J, Enomoto H. Conditional ablation of GFRalpha1 in postmigratory enteric neurons triggers unconventional neuronal death in the colon and causes a Hirschsprung's disease phenotype. Development. 2007;134:2171–81.
73. Hellmich HL, Kos L, Cho ES, Mahon KA, Zimmer A. Embryonic expression of glial-line derived neurotrophic factor (GDNF) suggests multiple developmental roles in neural differentiation and epithelial-mesenchymal interactions. Mech Dev. 1996;54:95–105.
74. Worley DS, Pisano JM, Choi ED, Walus L, Hession CA, Cate RL, et al. Developmental regulation of GDNF response and receptor expression in the enteric nervous system. Development. 2000;127:4383–93.
75. Fock PJ, Schiltz CA, Jones SE. Enteric neuroblasts require the phosphatidylinositol 3-kinase pathway for GDNF-stimulated proliferation. J Neurobiol. 2001;47:306–17.
76. Young HM, Hearn CJ, Farlie PG, Canty AJ, Thomas PQ, Newgreen DF. GDNF is a chemoattractant for enteric cells. Dev Biol. 2001;229:503–16.
77. Durbec P, Marcos-Guitierrez CV, Klikenny C, Grigoriou M, Wartiowaara K, Suvanto P, et al. GDNF signaling through the ret receptor tyrosine kinase. Nature. 1996;381:789–93.
78. Pattyn A, Morin X, Cremer H, Goridis C, Brunet JF. The homeobox gene Phox2b is essential for the development of autonomic neural crest derivates. Nature. 1999;399:366–77.
79. Sanchez M, Silos-Santiago I, Frisen J, He B, Lira SA, Barbacid M. Renal agenesis and the absence of enteric neurons in mice lacking GDNF. Nature. 1996;382:70–3.
80. Pichel JG, Shen L, Sheng HZ, Granholm AC, Drago J, Grinberg A, et al. Defects in enteric innervation and kidney development in mice lacking GDNF. Nature. 1996;382:73–6.
81. Angrist M, Bolk S, Thiel B, Puffenberger EG, Hofstra RM, Buys CH, et al. Mutations analysis of the RET receptor tyrosine kinase in Hirschsprung's disease. Hum Mol Genet. 1995;4:821–80.
82. Baynash AG, Hosoda K, Giaid A, Richardson JA, Emoto N, Hammer RE, et al. Interaction of endothelin-3 with endothelin-B receptor is essential for development of epidermal melanocytes and enteric neurons. Cell. 1994;79:1277–85.
83. Leibl MA, Ota T, Woodward MN, Kenny SE, Lloyd DA, Vaillant CR, et al. Expression of endothelin-3 by mesenchymal cells of embryonic mouse caecum. Gut. 1999;44:246–52.
84. Hosoda K, Hammer RE, Richardson JA, Baynash AG, Cheung JC, Giaid A, et al. Targeted and natural (piebald-lethal) mutations of endothelin-B receptor gene produce megacolon associated with spotted coat color in mice. Cell. 1994;79:1267–76.
85. Kusafuka T, Wang Y, Puri P. Mutation analysis of the RET, endothelin-B receptor, and the endothelin-3 genes in sporadic cases of Hirschsprung's disease. J Pediatr Surg. 1997;32:501–4.
86. Kusafuka T, Wang Y, Puri P. Novel mutations of the endothelin-B receptor gene in isolated patients with Hirschsprung's disease. Hum Mol Genet. 1996;5:347–9.
87. Kusafuka T, Puri P. Mutations of the endothelin-B receptor and endothelin-3 genes in Hirschsprung's disease. Pediatr Surg Int. 1997;12:19–23.
88. Bidaud C, Salomon R, Pelet A, van Camp G, Attie T, Eng C, et al. Endothelin-3 gene in isolated and syndromic Hirschsprung's disease. Eur J Hum Genet. 1997;5:247–51.
89. Amiel J, Attie T, Jan D, Pelet A, Edery P, Bidaud C, et al. Heterozygous endothelin receptor B (EDNRB) mutations in isolated Hirschsprung's disease. Hum Mol Genet. 1996;5:355–7.
90. Oue T, Puri P. Altered endothelin-3 and endothelin-B receptor mRNA expression in Hirschsprung's disease. J Pediatr Surg. 1999;34:1257–60.
91. Abe Y, Sakurai T, Yamada T, Nakamura T, Yanagisawa M, Goto K. Functional analysis of five endothelin-B receptor mutations found in human Hirschsprung's disease patients. Biochem Biophys Res Commun. 2000;275:524–31.
92. Yanagisawa H, Yanagisawa M, Kapur RP, Richardson JA, Williams SC, Clouthier DE, et al. Dual genetic pathways of endothelin-mediated intercellular signalling revealed by targeted disruption of endothelin converting enzyme-1 gene. Development. 1998;125:825–36.
93. Gershon MD. Endothelin and the development of the enteric nervous system. Clin Exp Pharmacol Physiol. 1999;26:1161–73.
94. Southard-Smith EM, Kos L, Pavan WJ. Sox10 mutations disrupts neural crest development in

Dom Hirschsprung mouse model. Nat Genet. 1998;18:60–4.
95. Kuhlbrodt K, Herbarth B, Sock E, Enderich J, Hermans-Borgmeyer I, Wegner M. Sox10, a novel transcriptional modulator in glial cells. J Neurosci. 1998;18:237–50.
96. Kapur RP. Early death of neural crest cells is responsible for total enteric aganglionosis in Sox10 (Dom)/ Sox10 (Dom) mouse embryos. Pediatr Dev Pathol. 1999;2:559–69.
97. Paratore C, Eichenberger C, Suter U, Sommer L. Sox10 haploinsufficiency affects maintenance of progenitor cells in a mouse model of Hirschsprung disease. Hum Mol Genet. 2002;11:3075–85.
98. Bondurand N, Natarajan D, Barlow A, Thapar N, Pachnis V. Maintenance of mammalian enteric nervous system progenitors by Sox10 and endothelin 3 signalling. Development. 2006;133:2075–86.
99. Nagashimada M, Ohta H, Li C, Nakao K, Uesaka T, Brunet JF, Amiel J, Trochet T, Wakayama T, Enomoto H. Autonomic neurocristopathy-associated mutations in PHOX2B dysregulate Sox10 expression. J Clin Invest. 2016;122:3135–58.
100. Pingault V, Bondurand N, Kuhlbrodt K, Goerich DE, Prehu MO, Puliti A, et al. SOX 10 mutations in patients with Waardenburg-Hirschsprung's disease. Nat Genet. 1998;18:171–3.
101. Kuhlbrodt M, Schmidt C, Sock E, Pingault V, Bondurand N, Goosssens M, et al. Functional analysis of Sox 10 mutations found in human Waardenburg-Hirschsprung's disease. J Biol Chem. 1998;273:23033–8.
102. Pattyn A, Morin X, Cremer H, Goridis C, Brunet JF. Expression and interactions of the two closely related homebox genes Phox2a and Phox2b during neurogenesis. Development. 1997;124:4065–75.
103. Hatano M, Aoki T, Dezawa M, Yusa S, Iitsuka Y, Koseki H, et al. A novel pathogenesis of megacolon in NCX/HOX11L1 deficient mice. J Clin Invest. 1997;100:795–801.
104. Shirasawa S, Yunker AMR, Roth KA, Brown GA, Horning S, et al. ENX (HOX11L1) deficient mice develop myenteric neuronal hyperplasia and megacolon. Nat Med. 1997;3:646–50.
105. Nagy N, Mwizerwa O, Yaniv K, Carmel L, Pieretti-Vanmarcke R, Weinstein BM, Goldstein AM. Endothelial cells promote migration and proliferation of enteric neural crest cells via beta 1 integrin signaling. Dev Biol. 2009;330:263–72.
106. Akbareian SE, Nagy N, Steiger CE, Mably JD, Miller SA, Hotto R, Molnar D, Goldstein AM. Enteric neural crest-derived cells promote their migration by modifying their microenvironment through tenascin-C production. Dev Biol. 2013;125:4483–96.
107. Breau MA, Dahmani A, Broders-Bondon F, Thiery JP, Dufour S. Beta 1 integrins are required for the invasion of the caecum and proximal hindgut by enteric neural crest cells. Development. 2009;136:2791–801.
108. Nagy N, Goldstein AM. Endothelin-3 regulates neural crest cell proliferation and differentiation in the hindgut enteric nervous system. Dev Biol. 2006;293:203–17.
109. Soret R, Mennetrey M, Bergeron KF, Dariel A, Neinlist M, Grunder F, Faure C, Silverside DW, Pilon N. A collagen VI-dependent pathogenic mechanism for Hirschsprung's disease. J Clin Invest. 2017;125:4483–96.
110. Rothman TP, Chen J, Howard MJ, Costantini F, Schuchardt A, Pachnis V, et al. Increased expression of laminin-1 and collagen (IV) subunits in the aganglionic bowel of ls/ls, but not c-ret−/− mice. Dev Biol. 1996;178:498–513.
111. Parikh DH, Tam PK, Van Velzen D, Edgar D. The extracellular matrix components, tenascin and fibronectin, in Hirschsprung's disease: an immunohistochemical study. J Pediatr Surg. 1994;29: 1302–6.
112. Parikh DH, Leibl M, Tam PK, Edgar D. Abnormal expression and distribution of nidogen in Hirschsprung's disease. J Pediatr Surg. 1995;30:1687–93.
113. Huizinga JD, Thuneberg L, Kluppel M, Malysz J, Mikkelsen HB, Bernstein A. W/kit gene required for interstitial cells of Cajal and for intestinal pacemaker activity. Nature. 1995;373:347–9.
114. Wu JJ, Rothman TP, Gershon MD. Development of the interstitial cell of Cajal: origin, kit dependence and neuronal and nonneuronal sources of kit ligand. J Neurosci Res. 2000;59:384–401.
115. Maeda H, Yamagata A, Nishikawa S, Yoshinaga K, Kobayashi S, Nishi K, et al. Requirement of c-kit for development of intestinal pacemaker system. Development. 1992;116:369–75.
116. Feldstein AE, Miller SM, El-Youssef M, Rodeberg D, Lindor NM, Burgart LJ, et al. Chronic intestinal pseudoobstruction associated with altered interstitial cells of Cajal networks. J Pediatr Gastroenterol Nutr. 2003;36:492–7.
117. Hagger R, Finlayson C, Kahn F, De Oliveira R, Chimelli L, Kumar D. A deficiency of interstitial cells of Cajal in Chagasic megacolon. J Auton Nerv Syst. 2000;80:108–11.
118. Kenny S, Connell MG, Rintala RJ, Vaillant C, Edgar DH, Lloyd DA. Abnormal colonic interstitial cells of Cajal in children with anorectal malformations. J Pediatr Surg. 1998;33:130–2.
119. Rolle U, Piotrowska AP, Nemeth L, Puri P. Altered distribution of interstitial cells of Cajal in Hirschsprung's disease. Arch Pathol Lab Med. 2002;126:928–33.
120. Tong WD, Liu BH, Zhang LY, Zhang SB, Lei Y. Decreased interstitial cells of Cajal in the sigmoid colon of patients with slow transit constipation. Int J Colorectal Dis. 2004;19:467–73.

Functional Anatomy of the Enteric Nervous System

3

Michael D. Gershon and Hiroki Nakamura

Contents

M. D. Gershon (✉)
Department of Anatomy and Cell Biology, Columbia University, College of Physicians and Surgeons, New York, NY, USA
e-mail: mdg4@columbia.edu

H. Nakamura
The National Children's Research Centre, Our Lady's Children's Hospital, Crumlin, Dublin, Ireland

P. Puri (ed.), *Hirschsprung's Disease and Allied Disorders*,
https://doi.org/10.1007/978-3-030-15647-3_3

3.1 Introduction

Congenital birth defects, of which Hirschsprung disease is an example, are among the most difficult of illnesses to study in the human patients who suffer from them. By the time the condition is identified in an affected individual, the process that brought it about is over and done with. It is thus impossible to study the ontogeny of birth defects, such as Hirschsprung disease, in the fetus in which the problems develop. An investigator seeking to uncover the pathogenesis of such a condition must search, like a detective, for clues left behind by the perpetrator who has fled the scene of a crime. Even the identification of genes that may have mutated, important an achievement as that is, does not, by itself, explain why the defect develops. Human life, moreover, is so precious that human subjects are terrible laboratory animals. As a result, more can often be learned about the origins of human illness by studying animal models than by investigating the patients themselves. Invasive research, which is only possible on animals, can be used to develop a conceptual framework to devise hypotheses that can subsequently be tested for applicability to human patients. Experiments, based on these hypotheses, can be targeted to what can be confirmed or denied by diagnostic tests or by analyzing the restricted materials available from human subjects. Studies of animal biology can thus make investigations of human biology possible.

The importance of animal models in learning why developmental defects occur and what can be done to prevent them cannot be emphasized too strongly. Recent research, facilitated by the use of rodents, avians, and zebrafish as model systems, has greatly advanced our understanding of the factors that govern the development of the enteric nervous system (ENS). Clearly, comprehension of the pathogenesis of the neuromuscular defects of the bowel, including Hirschsprung disease, requires a detailed understanding of the processes that govern normal enteric neuronal and glial ontogeny. This research has already provided enough insight to systematize current thinking about the origin of Hirschsprung disease. This review is concentrated on the important progress made in the developmental biology of the ENS (provided mainly by research on animals) that now provides a logical basis for explaining the origin of the human disease.

Hirschsprung disease is a well-defined clinical entity. It is a congenital absence of neurons in the terminal portion of the gut. The length of the aganglionic region varies, and short- and long-segment varieties have been distinguished, although these entities represent the extremes of a continuum. In fact, classical Hirschsprung disease, in which a segment of the bowel is totally aganglionic, is itself only one of a series of conditions that encompass a variety of allied disorders that include hypoganglionosis, neuronal intestinal dysplasias (hyperganglionosis), immaturity of ganglion cells, and dysganglionoses that have yet to be thoroughly classified. Most often, Hirschsprung disease is limited to the colon, although occasionally greater lengths of bowel may be involved. The gut is hypoganglionic in the region immediately rostral to the aganglionic segment and, in some patients, the junction between the abnormal hypoganglionic tissue and the normal bowel may not be obvious. The aganglionic segment is invariably narrowed in comparison to the bowel rostral to it, which often becomes massively dilated, so that another name for Hirschsprung disease is congenital megacolon. The aganglionic portion of the gut evidently functions as an obstruction causing the ganglionated bowel orad to the aganglionic segment to dilate.

Although various investigators have proposed a number of hypotheses to explain why the aganglionic tissue should be a functional obstruction, including denervation hypersensitivity of the smooth muscle and a selective deficiency of fibers able to relax the bowel [1, 2], a more general explanation is that the ENS is essential for normal propulsive intestinal motility [3]. Given the absence of the ENS from the aganglionic zone, a failure of propulsive reflexes and thus a functional obstruction are to be expected. Aside from propulsion, moreover, the net effect on intestinal muscle of the ENS is relaxant [4]; therefore, contraction and narrowing would be the predicted behavior of gut that lacks ganglia.

In thinking about the physiology of the colon in a patient with Hirschsprung disease, it is important to emphasize the difference between aganglionosis and denervation. Although the terminal bowel is aganglionic in Hirschsprung disease, it is not denervated [1, 2, 5–7]. Actually, many investigators have reported that the aganglionic gut may be hyperinnervated, especially by catecholaminergic and cholinergic nerve fibers [2, 8]. What is missing in the diseased bowel are the cell bodies of intrinsic enteric neurons, which are essential for the mediation of reflexes, not nerve fibers. Certain types of intrinsic axon are also selectively lost, including those which contain serotonin (5-HT) [9] or nitric oxide synthase (NOS) [10, 11]; however, the apparent selectivity of these deficiencies may be attributable to the fact that these are transmitters of intrinsic neurons. Given the lack of intrinsic neurons, one might expect that the transmitter of virtually any type of intrinsic neuron would be diminished. The confirmation that what is expected actually occurs is thus of limited value in understanding the pathogenesis of the disease, although a loss of relaxant fibers (such as those which contain NOS) is often invoked to explain the narrowing of the aganglionic segment as a contracted region. To understand why a loss of nerve cell bodies, despite an abundance of axons should be so devastating, it is important to consider the nature of the ENS.

3.2 The Normal Enteric Nervous System

The gastrointestinal tract is responsible for performing complex functions that are essential for host survival including (1) transport of food and waste; (2) digestion and absorption of nutrients; (3) secretion of water, electrolytes, mucus, signaling molecules, and antimicrobial substances; (4) preservation of intestinal barrier function;, (5) maintenance of healthy microbiota; and (6) protection from ingested pathogens, allergens, and toxins [12]. The regulation of these critical processes is under the control of the ENS. The mature ENS is absolutely unique and different from any other region of the peripheral nervous system (PNS). First, the ENS is independent and can function in the absence of input from the brain or spinal cord [13]. Second, in contrast to the remainder of the PNS, the ENS can mediate reflexes, even when it is isolated from the central nervous system (CNS). This ability of the ENS is often overlooked, even though it has long been known to be true. As the nineteenth century turned to the twentieth century, Bayliss and Starling reported that enteric reflexes could be mediated by "the local nervous mechanism" of the gut [14, 15]. These investigators described what they called the "law of the intestine" (now known as the peristaltic reflex) in extrinsically denervated loops of dog intestine. This is a reflex, evoked by increased intraluminal pressure, that consists of a wave of oral excitation and anal relaxation that descends in the bowel and is propulsive. Essentially, the same reflex can also be elicited in vitro in preparations of guinea pig intestine [16]. The fact that reflex activity can be manifested by segments of gut in vitro, which have clearly lost all connection to dorsal root or cranial nerve ganglia, the brain, and the spinal cord, indicates that every neural element of the peristaltic reflex arc (sensory receptors, primary interneurons, motor neurons, and effectors) must be intrinsic components of the wall of the gut.

These observations were known to J.N. Langley who first defined the autonomic nervous system [17]. Together with Langley's own idea that most enteric neurons receive no direct input from the CNS, the independence of the ENS caused Langley to classify the ENS as a third component of the autonomic nervous system. The sympathetic division was defined as that with a thoracic and lumbar outflow of preganglionic axons from the CNS, while the parasympathetic was the division with a cranial and sacral outflow. The ENS, which mainly lacks either outflow, had to be classified as a separate division, since it met the criteria of neither of the other two. Anatomical observations have more recently confirmed the distinct nature of the enteric innervation. The internal ultrastructure of the ENS is more similar to that of the CNS than to any other region of the PNS [6–11, 18–23]. The ENS lacks internal collagen, and its neurons receive support from enteric glia; although enteric glia resemble astrocytes and Schwann cells, they are a distinct and unique cell type [24, 25]. Phenotypic diversity of peripheral neurons peaks in the ENS, and every class of neurotransmitter known to be present in the CNS is also represented in the ENS. Intrinsic neuronal reflexes evoke secretion as well as motility [26]; furthermore, most enteric neurons not only lack connection to the CNS, but some actually project centripetally, beyond the confines of the gut, to innervate extra-enteric targets [27]. These outside-the-bowel projections of enteric neurons make it possible for the ENS to affect directly the function of prevertebral sympathetic ganglia [28–30], the gallbladder [31], and the endocrine and exocrine pancreas [32, 33].

3.3 Organization of Enteric Neurons

The ENS of most adult mammals is comprised of two major interconnected ganglionated plexuses, the myenteric and the submucosal [3, 27, 34]. The myenteric plexus lies between the circular and longitudinal muscle layers of the gut. It manifests integrated neuronal activity and provides motor innervation to the circular and longitudinal muscle layers of the muscularis externa. The submucosal plexus is the smaller of the two major neural plexuses. The submucosal plexus is located between the mucosa and circular muscle of the gut within the dense irregularly arranged connective tissue of the submucosa, innervating secretory cells, endocrine cells, and blood vessels in the mucosa and submucosa. The two enteric plexuses also project to each other. In larger animals, including humans, the submucosal plexus can be divided into separate plexuses of Schabadasch (external) and Meissner (internal) [35]; however, these plexuses interconnect extensively and clear functional distinctions are not yet known. The submucosal plexus is thus usually treated as a single entity, although this practice will probably have to be changed in the future as new information accumulates that suggests a significant segregation of function to the subplexuses of Schabadasch and Meissner [36]. Submucosal neurons project to one another, to the mucosa, and to the myenteric plexus. The neurons that project to the mucosa include intrinsic sensory [37, 38] and secretomotor neurons [26, 39, 40]. Some submucosal neurons are bipolar or pseudounipolar in shape and also project to the myenteric plexus; these have been postulated to be primary afferent in function [37]. A subset of submucosal neurons, which evoke vasomotor responses when activated by mucosal stimuli, project both to the mucosa and to blood vessels [27, 41]. These cells may actually function as a unicellular reflex arc, which if true would be a structure that, in vertebrates, is unique to the bowel.

Both the submucosal and the myenteric plexuses contain many interneurons involved in interganglionic projections and the formation of complex microcircuits that are just beginning to be mapped. Motor neurons that excite or relax the muscularis externa are located exclusively in the myenteric plexus. The myenteric like the submucosal plexus [38] also contains intrinsic sensory neurons that project to the mucosa [27, 42–44]. Some myenteric neurons project centripetally out of the gut [27]. Projections that leave the bowel have been called "enterofugal" to distinguish them from the "centrifugal" extrinsic innervation, derived ultimately from the CNS, which enters the gut. Depending on the level of the bowel, targets of "enterofugal" neurons include prevertebral sympathetic ganglia (small and large intestine), the trachea (from esophagus), pancreas (from duodenum and stomach), gall bladder (from stomach), brain stem (from stomach), and sacral cord (from colon). The extreme complexity of the ENS, the behaviors of the gut that it regulates, and the multitude of neurological disorders to which it contributes have only recently been appreciated [45]. Certainly, the ENS is not, as once was thought, a system of "relay ganglia" interposed between the brain and effectors in the bowel [46]. Because the ENS is so different from the other components of the PNS, it stands to reason that the factors and/or processes that dictate the development of the ENS are likely to be different from those of other peripheral ganglia [12, 34, 47].

3.4 The ENS Is Derived from the Neural Crest

The first clear demonstration that the ENS is derived from the neural crest was made by Yntema and Hammond who noted that enteric ganglia fail to appear when the "anterior" neural crest is deleted in chick embryos [48]. Their work was confirmed, and levels of the crest that contribute to the ENS were more precisely identified by Le Douarin and her colleagues [49]. These investigators took advantage of the distinctive nucleolar-associated heterochromatin of quail cells, which allows these cells to be readily identified following their transplantation into embryos of other species. Le Douarin and her co-workers replaced segments of the chick neural crest with those of quail (or the reverse) and traced the migration of crest-derived cells in the resulting interspecies chimeras by identifying cells of the donor (chick or quail, depending on the particular experiment). These studies suggested that the ENS is derived from both the vagal (somites 1–7) and the sacral (caudal to somite 28) crest. The vagal crest colonizes the entire bowel, while the sacral crest colonizes only the postumbilical gut. The conclusion that there are two sites of origin of enteric neuronal precursors was soon challenged, because other investigators could recognize only a single proximodistal progression of cells thought to be "neuroblasts" in the avian gut [50]. This progression was believed to imply that neuronal precursors in the bowel only descend, as would be expected of vagal progenitors. No ascent, of the kind predicted for precursors from the sacral crest, could be found. These observations led to the suggestion that the data derived from experiments with interspecies chimeras could have been obtained if crest-derived cells were to be more invasive in a foreign embryo than they are when they migrate in embryos of their own species. If so, then quail cells might reach ectopic destinations in a chick embryo and chick cells might behave in a similarly abnormal manner in a quail embryo. There are, however, reasons why only a single proximodistal progression of cells that can be recognized as belonging to a neuronal lineage can be detected, even though multiple levels of the crest contribute precursors to the bowel. Neuronal progenitors colonize various levels of the gut before they actually give rise to progeny that express recognizable neural properties [51]; thus, neurons develop in vitro in segments of gut that appear to be aneuronal at the time of explantation, thereby demonstrating that otherwise unrecognizable neural precursor cells were present in the explants. The delay, however short it might be, between the arrival of progenitors and their differentiation into neurons provides an opportunity for crest-derived precursors to interact with, and be influenced by, the enteric microenvironment. In fact, the enteric microenvironment plays a critical role in the development of enteric neurons and glia [34, 47, 52–54]. The observed proximodistal progression of perceived "neuroblasts," therefore, may be due to a proximodistal gradient in the maturation of the enteric microenvironment, rather than to the timing of the descent of the neuronal precursors. Subsequent studies, in which endogenous crest cells were traced by labeling them with a vital dye or a replication-deficient retrovirus, confirmed that both the avian and murine gut are each colonized by cells from both vagal and sacral levels of the neural crest [55, 56]. Most recently, studies involving lineage tracing in mice have confirmed that the ENS is derived from vagal and sacral levels of the crest [12] and, further, have shown the distal gut is colonized by additional precursors that arrive in the bowel with the extrinsic innervation [57–59]. These latter precursors enter the gut as cells that appear to be in the Schwann lineage, but within the enteric microenvironment, they give rise to neurons. The avian and human bowel, like that of mice, thus appears to be colonized, not only by sacral and vagal crest cells but also by the Schwann cells of the extrinsic innervation [12, 60, 61]. In the mouse, studies with labeled crest-derived cells have also revealed that truncal crest contributes to the rostral-most foregut (esophagus and adjacent stomach) [62]. Retroviral and lineage tracing in avian embryos has suggested that vagal crest that contributes to the formation of the ENS is complex [12]. Crest-derived cells from somite levels 1–2 appear to give rise to neurons only in the esophagus, while those from levels 3–5 colonize the bowel from the stomach to the hindgut [12, 63]. Cells from levels 6–7 are more controversial and may go only to the hindgut [64], although labeling studies tracing cells in fetal mice with a lipophilic dye have suggested that crest-derived cells from somite levels 6–7 colonize the esophagus rather than the hindgut [62]. Crest-derived cells from somite level 3 seem to be the most invasive portion of the vagal crest and can compensate for the ablation of the remainder of the vagal crest [65].

The specificity of vagal and sacral regions as sources of enteric neuronal progenitors is well illustrated by back-transplantation experiments. Back-transplantation consists of grafting a developing organ or piece of tissue from an older to a younger host embryo. It is a technique that provides insight into whether cells in the older tissue retain and can manifest, in a suitably permissive environment, properties associated with earlier stages of development. Crest-derived cells that have colonized the bowel will leave segments of gut that are back-grafted into a younger embryo and re-migrate in their new host [66]. These cells will only reach the bowel of their host if the graft is situated so as to replace the host's vagal or sacral crest [67]. A subset of the vagal crest-derived cells that colonize the gut can be visually identified in transgenic mice directed to express *lacZ* by the promoter for dopamine β-hydroxylase (DBH) [68]. The *DBH-lacZ* transgene is permanently expressed in these mice by neurons that are not catecholaminergic in the adult gut. The colonization of the bowel by the transgenically labeled cells has been studied in detail in both normal mice and in murine models of Hirschsprung disease [69, 70]; however, it is important to note that the *DBH-lacZ* transgene probably demonstrates only a subset of vagal crest-derived cells and does not reveal those of sacral origin. Some enteric neurons develop from precursors that are transiently catecholaminergic (TC) [71–74]. DBH is one of the enzymes that participate in the formation of norepinephrine (NE), and thus its presence is a component of the catecholaminergic phenotype. Even in normal mice, and especially in rats, the genes encoding DBH are not completely repressed in the non-catecholaminergic neurons that develop from TC cell progenitors. Neurons derived from TC cells continue to express DBH, although they inactivate other elements of the catecholaminergic phenotype [72]. It is likely that the cells that are marked by the expression of the *DBH-lacZ* transgene are members of this lineage, that is, they are cells that originate from transiently catecholaminergic progenitors. Unfortunately, not every enteric neuron originates from a TC cell precursor. In fact, the subset of neurons that arises from progenitors that never exhibit catecholaminergic properties is larger than that which is TC cell-derived [74]. As a result, many enteric neuronal precursors are not subject to surveillance by the *DBH-lacZ* transgene-tracing technique. However cells are traced, it is now apparent that in both fetal mice and in avian embryos, the ENS arises from multiple regions of the neural crest, not just one [12]. Although the number of sources of enteric neurons in the neural crest is limited, it is necessary to take account of this multiplicity in attempting to explain the abnormal colonization of the gut that arises in Hirschsprung disease and other dysganglionoses.

Recent genetic studies have suggested that much of what has traditionally been considered vagal crest may not be [57]. Properties of the vagal crest are transitional between cranial and truncal [75]. Crest-derived cells next to somites 1–2 have been reported to give rise to Schwann cells that migrate to the esophagus and stomach along descending vagus nerve fibers and give rise to the ENS in these regions [57]. These Schwann cell/neuronal precursors would literally have to be considered vagal-crest-derived, because they migrate as components of the vagus nerves. In contrast, crest-derived cells from somite levels 3–7 have been suggested to be analogous to the more distal truncal crest-derived cells and actually to be contributors to sympathetic chains; moreover, their ventral migration provides precursors, not only for sympathetic chain ganglia, but also for the ganglia of the entire GI tract. These data might account for the abnormalities that occur both in enteric and sympathetic ganglia when the gene encoding the receptor tyrosine kinase, ERBB3, is deleted [57, 76, 77]. The atrophy in half of the esophageal ganglia when the nerve-associated form of the ERBB3 ligand, neuregulin 1 (considered essential for parasympathetic neuronal development), is deleted may also be evidence that esophageal neurons are parasympathetic. As a result of these recent observations, the ENS has been postulated to have four origins: (i) crest-derived cells from levels 1–2 of the neuraxis, which reach the esophagus and stomach as Schwann cells in the descending vagus nerves; (ii) a "sympatho-enteric" component from levels 3–7 of the neuraxis, which colonize the entire remainder of the bowel; (iii) crest-derived cells from the sacral level of the neuraxis (caudal to somite 28) that contribute to the post-umbilical gut; (iv) Schwann cells that migrate into the bowel late with extrinsic nerves to the ileum and colon [59]. Further studies, perhaps including some carried out by means of live imaging of genetically labeled cell populations and new genetic tracers, are needed to verify whether this interesting new hypothesis is correct.

3.5 The Crest-Derived Cells that Colonize the Gut Are Originally Multipotent and Migrate to the Bowel Along Defined Pathways in the Embryo

The restriction of the levels of the premigratory crest that contribute precursors to the ENS raises the possibility that cells in the pre-migratory crest of these regions might be predetermined to migrate to the bowel and give rise to enteric neurons and/or glia. Such a predestination, however, is not supported by experimental evidence, which indicates instead that premigratory crest cells are multipotent. For example, when levels of the crest are interchanged so as to replace a region that normally colonizes the gut with one that does not, the heterotopic crest cells still migrate to the bowel and there give rise to neurons the phenotypes of which are ENS-appropriate, not level of origin-appropriate [78, 79]. An analogous process, moreover, is seen when the interchange of crest cells is reversed. Vagal and sacral crest cells give rise to non-enteric neurons in ectopic locations, such as sympathetic ganglia, when they are grafted so as to replace crest cells at other axial levels. Clones derived from single crest cells, furthermore, give rise, both in vitro [80–84] and in vivo [85–87], to progeny that may express many different phenotypes. A single cell that gives rise to a clone containing many phenotypes has to be multipotent.

The crest-derived cells that colonize the gut remain multipotent with respect to their ability to give rise to neurons and glia, even after they have completed their migration to the bowel. This potency is well demonstrated by back-transplantation experiments (similar to those described above). Again, back-transplantation involves the transplantation of tissues or organs into younger embryos. When already colonized segments of gut are back-transplanted into a neural crest migration pathway of a younger embryo at a truncal level, donor crest-derived cells leave the graft, but they do not migrate to the host's gut. Instead, they migrate to the host's sympathetic ganglia, adrenal gland, and peripheral nerves which are the classical targets of the truncal crest; moreover, despite their previous migration to and residence in the bowel, the donor crest cells now form catecholaminergic neurons in the ganglia, chromaffin cells in the adrenals, and Schwann cells in the nerves of the host embryos [66]. Analogous results have been obtained from in vitro studies of cells developing from cloned crest-derived cells of enteric origin. The progeny found in these clones express a variety of different phenotypes, including some that are not present in the normal

ENS [88]. Despite their multipotent nature, however, the developmental potential of enteric crest-derived cells in vivo [66] and in clonal culture is not as great as that of their progenitors in the premigratory crest [88, 89]. The pluripotency of the crest-derived cells that colonize the gut, revealed by studies of clones and the behavior of cells emigrating from back-transplants [67], indicates that the bowel does not become colonized by precursors from restricted regions of the neural crest because these regions are the only ones that contain crest cells endowed with homing information that programs them to migrate to the gut. Instead, these regions are the only levels of the crest from which there are defined migratory pathways that lead to the bowel.

The pathway from the vagal crest (taking the latest definition as "vagal" and including the critical axial level of the third somite) conveys the largest cohort of crest-derived emigres to the gut. In avian embryos, this migration pathway leads crest-derived cells to the entire bowel between the proventriculus and the cloaca. In mammals, the equivalent region would extend from the corpus of the stomach to the rectum. The cohort of crest-derived cells that follows the sacral pathway is much smaller and leads crest-derived emigres only into the portion of the bowel that is distal to the umbilicus. The cohort of crest-derived cells that follow the pathway that leads to the presumptive esophagus and the most rostral portion of the stomach is the smallest. The origin of this pathway is controversial; it may be rostral crest [57, 90] or truncal crest [62]. The possibility that crest-derived cells of different origins are intrinsically different has some experimental support. It is also conceivable that the crest-derived emigres from different levels interact with one another during the formation of the ENS.

The molecular nature of the migratory pathways and the nature of the mechanisms that guide progenitors to their correct destinations within the gut itself have yet to be fully understood. Chemoattractant or repellent molecules for growing axons have been identified in the vertebrate CNS [88]. These molecules include netrins [88, 91–93], semaphorins [94–96], and slit proteins [97]. The directional growth of migrating crest-derived cells is a property also shown by pathfinding axonal growth cones [98, 99]. Netrins are expressed in the developing bowel [91] and mice with a targeted mutation in netrin-1 die at birth with a bloated bowel and no milk in their stomach (Tessier-Lavigne, personal communication). Netrins play a role in the formation of the submucosal plexus [100]. There are radial secondary migrations of crest-derived cells, perpendicular to the longitudinal axis of the gut, that lead these cells out of the distal-directed stream of migration toward the enteric mucosa and the pancreas. These secondary migrations give rise, respectively, to submucosal and pancreatic ganglia. Netrins help to guide these secondary migrations. Netrin-1 and netrin-3 in mice and netrin-2 in chicks are expressed by the epithelia of fetal mucosa and pancreas. Crest-derived cells express the netrin receptors, deleted in colorectal cancer (DCC), neogenin, and adenosine A2b. Of these receptors, DCC, which is developmentally regulated, seems to be most important. Crest-derived cells migrate out of explants of gut in vitro toward co-cultured cells that express netrin-1. Enteric crest-derived cells also migrate in vitro toward co-cultured explants of pancreas and, in rings of cultured gut, inwardly toward the mucosa. Antibodies to DCC and inhibitors of protein kinase A, which interfere with DCC signaling, specifically block these migrations of crest-derived cells in the direction of the mucosa or pancreas. Mice that lack DCC also lack submucosal and pancreatic ganglia. Netrins, moreover, promote the survival/development of enteric crest-derived cells in addition to guiding their migration. These data strongly support the idea that netrins and DCC participate in the formation of submucosal and pancreatic ganglia. An important question, not answered by these data, is why crest-derived cells migrating toward the netrin that mucosal epithelial cells secrete stop migrating in the submucosa and fail to invade the mucosa itself. Part of the answer is that laminin, which is abundant in the fetal enteric mucosa, converts the netrin/DCC effect from attraction to repulsion [101]. Mucosal laminin repels advancing crest-derived cells. More recently, netrins have been found to be expressed within neurons of the ENS and to attract vagal axons [102]. The sensory vagal innervation of the gut, moreover, appears to depend on the presence of intrinsic neurons within the bowel; sensory vagal axons grow away from explants of aganglionic ret-/- gut but toward explants of wild-type gut. It is thus possible that enteric neurons help to guide vagal sensory axons to the bowel. Such a role would help to explain the known termination of vagal sensory axons within the ganglia of the ENS.

New mouse genetic tools have formally confirmed that crest-derived precursors of neurons migrate from the myenteric to the submucosal plexus [103]. The *Confetti* transgene was used to map the fates in adult small intestines of individual crest-derived precursors that express Sox10 at E12.5 [103]. Most of the cells that were clonally related formed columns along the radial axis of the gut. Individual *Sox10*-expressing precursors differentiated into clones of neurons, glia, or both (called NG clones). Each type of clone participated in forming the myenteric plexus; however, but only glial and NG clones added to the submucosal plexus. Observations suggest that the cells that migrate from the myenteric to the submucosal plexus are bipotent. In the adult gut, moreover, neurons that were clonally related tended to display synchronous Ca^{2+} responses when stimulated with single electrical pulses, suggesting that developmental relationships are preserved in the functional wiring of the ENS [103]. Enteric neuronal subtypes are born in a reproducible phenotypic order [104], and subsets of neurons with similar birthdates may be more likely than cells with dissimilar birthdates to connect to one another. At least one additional factor is critical in the radial migration, at least of enteric glia. These cells respond to the presence of the enteric microbiota and are attracted toward the lumen as they migrate from their origin in the layer of the presumptive myenteric plexus [105, 106]. The extent to which lineage relationships and timing of phenotypic determination contribute to enteric circuit formation has not yet been explored.

Vagal crest-derived cells are clearly different from the sacral crest-derived cells that migrate to the bowel. Crest-derived cells from somites 8 and below express roundabout (ROBO) receptors; SLIT2, however, is expressed in the proximal gut [107, 108]. Slit proteins are repellent ligands for ROBO receptors. This distribution would allow vagal crest-derived cells, which fail to express ROBO to colonize the entire bowel (as they do) but would prevent the ascending stream of sacral crest-derived cells from entering the SLIT2-expressing rostral portion of the gut.

3.6 Differentiation of Crest-Derived Precursors Within the Enteric Microenvironment

No matter where in the crest enteric neuronal/glia precursors originate, after they colonize the bowel, the cells have to continue to proliferate to maintain an adequately sized precursor pool while at the same time giving rise to neurons. Because neurons are post-mitotic, their very formation necessarily diminishes the size of the proliferating precursor pool. The pool thus has to maintain itself even while engaged in an activity, neuronal differentiation, that threatens to deplete it. This paradoxical task, moreover, has to be solved as the crest-derived precursors move along the long routes of migration that lead from the rostral to the distal gut, into the pancreatic buds, and from the myenteric to the submucosal plexus. Proliferation at the colonizing wavefront is critical to keeping the mass of migrating cells sufficiently large to allow the population to keep on migrating [65, 109, 110]. If crest-derived precursors differentiate too quickly or prematurely into neurons, the distal bowel will not be adequately colonized [111–113].

Crest-derived cells encounter many molecules that influence their differentiation as they travel to their final destinations, and the cells must be endowed with receptors that enable them to respond to the molecules they encounter. Louis Pasteur said that "chance favours the prepared mind," and in an analogous fashion, signaling molecules favor the receptor-bearing crest-derived cell. Profiles of transcripts that cells *Sox10* marks at two times during murine ENS ontogeny have identified over 150 signaling molecules and receptors that developing enteric crest-derived precursors and the surrounding mesenchyme express [114]. Pathways that influence the development of the ENS are thus complex and have abundant molecular constituents; nevertheless, enteric crest-derived precursors express three regulatory molecules that are of central importance in preparing them to be enteric neurons or glia. These are the homeodomain paired-like homeobox 2B (PHOX2B) transcription factor, the Sry-related HMg-Box gene 10 (SOX10) transcription factor, and rearranged during transfection (RET) receptor tyrosine kinase.

When PHOX2B is deleted, vagal crest-derived precursors enter the foregut appropriately but fail to give rise to an ENS; expression of PHOX2B thus appears to be necessary for the subsequent expression of all other molecules critical for ENS development including RET and the transcription factors SOX10 and achaete-scute homologue 1 (ASCL1) [115, 116]. Loss-of-function mutations in human *PHOX2B* are not embryonically lethal but cause congenital central hypoventilation syndrome (CCHS), which in 16% of affected individuals is associated with Hirschsprung disease (HSCR) [117, 118]. PHOX2B is thus so important that even its haploinsufficiency can disturb ENS development. The risks for HSCR and neuroblastoma (a neural crest-derived tumor) are especially great in patients with CCHS who harbor a nonpolyalanine repeat expansion mutation in PHOX2B [116]. When a nonpolyalanine repeat expansion mutation of the PHOX2B was introduced into the mouse Phox2b locus, the clinical features of the association of CCHS with HSCR and neuroblastoma were recapitulated. Enteric and sympathetic ganglion precursors demonstrated sustained expression of Sox10. Proliferation of crest-derived precursors was impaired and their differentiation was biased against neurons and toward glia. Phox2B transactivation of target genes was affected in a dominant-negative fashion and the transcriptional effect of PHOX2B on a Sox10 enhancer was converted from repression to transactivation. The nonpolyalanine repeat expansion mutation of PHOX2B thus acts both as a dominant-negative and gain-of-function mutation. The ability of PHOX2B to regulate SOX10 is thus critical in development of the ENS and other autonomic ganglia.

SOX10, which is expressed by virtually every crest-derived cell as it delaminates from the neural tube, is nearly as fundamental to ENS development as PHOX2B. The initial expression of SOX10 is independent of PHOX2B. Once in the bowel, precursors need to express SOX10 in order to survive and maintain their multipotency. One of the first manifestations of the importance of SOX10 to the developing ENS to be realized came from the study of a naturally occurring autosomal dominant mutation in mice (*Dom*) that caused a pronounced hypoplasia of myenteric neurons, terminal bowel aganglionosis, and congenital megacolon [119]. *Dom* was subsequently found to be located in the *Sox10* locus [120, 121]. Even the haploinsufficiency of *Sox10* is enough to lead, in mice, to a hypoganglionic colon and megacolon [122]. *SOX10* haploinsufficiency in humans is associated with the HSCR-like aganglionosis of Waardenburg-Shah syndrome [123].

SOX10-expressing cells colonize the bowel and must maintain SOX10 expression. That allows them to survive and remain multipotent as they initiate their expression of PHOX2B and another gene important to a subset of enteric neurons, ASCL1 [124, 125]. Interestingly, as crest-derived precursors lose potency and differentiate, SOX10 expression is retained as the precursors generate glia; SOX10 expression thus becomes a glial marker in the adult ENS [122, 124]. Downregulation of SOX10 expression appears to be important in enteric neurogenesis [125]. Genetic lineage tracing has recently been employed to investigate enteric crest-derived cells in *Sox10*$^{Dom/+}$ mice [126]. Varying lengths of distal aganglionosis was found in the colons of *Sox10*$^{Dom/+}$ mice; nevertheless, the ENS of the small intestines of the *Sox10*$^{Dom/+}$ animals contained normal numbers of neurons and glia [126]. There were, however, abnormalities in the types of neurons generated in *Sox10*$^{Dom/+}$ mice and associated deficits in gastrointestinal motility [126]. It is possible that the extreme sensitivity of the terminal colon to SOX10 haploinsufficiency is due to the role that SOX10 plays in maintaining survival and multipotency of the colonizing stem cells. Premature depletion of the stem population (due to precocious differentiation) in the absence of adequate SOX10 leads to a failure to colonize the last (most distal) portion of the bowel. Surprisingly, however, SOX10 evidently also plays a role in specifying small intestinal neuronal subtypes. It is interesting to speculate that defects in the types of cells that populate enteric ganglia may occur as a result of diminished activity of SOX10 or developmentally active factors and give rise to an unsuspected dysmotility of the bowel. Alternatively, these defects of the proximal ganglionated bowel might be the cause of residual dysmotility of the gut that is frequently seen after the surgical correction of HSCR.

The *Ret* protooncogene is a gene upon which most enteric neurons are critically dependent for survival [62, 127, 128]. This gene encodes the third member of the trio of crucial regulators of ENS development, RET, a receptor tyrosine kinase, for which glial cell line-derived growth factor (GDNF) is a functional ligand [129–131]. GDNF was first identified as a factor, produced by a glial cell line (B49) that promotes the survival of midbrain dopaminergic neurons [132]. GDNF was later observed to enhance the survival of spinal motor neurons [133]. GDNF is a distant relative of transforming growth factor-β (TGF-β). It is a homodimer, consisting of two peptide chains of 134 amino acids linked by a disulfide bridge. A larger precursor of 211 amino acids is synthesized first. This big molecule is proteolytically cleaved intracellularly to produce mature GDNF, which is secreted. During development, GDNF is not restricted to the brain, but rather is very highly expressed in the gut and other peripheral organs [133, 134]. In keeping with its peripheral distribution, GDNF is not just a survival factor for central CNS neurons [130], but also enhances the in vitro survival of peripheral sensory and sympathetic neurons, and also promotes their extension of neurites [133]. The observation that GDNF affects sympathetic neurons suggests that it should also affect at least some neurons of the ENS. In fact, both enteric and sympathetic neurons express *Ret*, at least transiently [127, 135]. When *Ret* is knocked out in transgenic mice, the ENS totally fails to develop in the entire bowel, with the exception of the rostral foregut [62, 128]. Since Ret is a functional receptor for GDNF, the fact that a similar lesion occurs in the bowel of knockout mice lacking GDNF [136–138] is not surprising. Neither is the observation surprising that, in contrast to the trophic effects that GDNF exerts on autonomic neuroblasts from control mice, GDNF fails to exert trophic effects on analogous cells from *Ret−/−* animals [131]. Activation of the Ret receptor by GDNF is thus a critical event in the formation of the ENS. Actually, GDNF does not bind directly to the Ret receptor itself. Instead, GDNF binds to a glycosylphosphatidylinositol-linked cell surface protein called GFRα-1, which then complexes with Ret to trigger the autophosphorylation and other actions of Ret [129, 139]. Other growth factors, which are members of the GDNF family of ligands, can also associate with their preferred GFRα proteins to activate Ret [140, 141]. These growth factors include neurturin (GFRα-2), artemin (GFRα-3), and persephin (GFRα-3). Of these, only the combinations of GDNF/GFRα-1 and neurturin/GFRα-2 appear to be important in ENS development [142–144]. Because of its role in GDNF signaling through Ret, GFRα-1 is as essential for ENS (and kidney) development as Ret and GDNF [145].

Despite the fact that most of the bowel is aganglionic in *Ret−/−* mice [128], there are neurons in the portions of the gut that develop from the rostral foregut of these animals [62]. Although the superior cervical ganglion is missing in *Ret−/−* mice, most other sympathetic ganglia do develop. The crest-derived cells that colonize the rostral foregut and the superior cervical ganglion have been traced by injecting a fluorescent dye (DiI) that intercalates into the lipid of the plasma membrane. The DiI-labeled cells that colonize the presumptive esophagus and rostral stomach originate from the same pool of truncal crest cells that gives rise to the sympathetic chain ganglia below the superior cervical ganglion. In contrast, the post-otic vagal crest cells that colonize the entire bowel distal to the rostral foregut also contribute the crest-derived cells that form the superior cervical ganglion. There thus appears to be not one but two common sympathoadrenal-enteric lineages. One of these is *Ret*- and GDNF-dependent, while the other is *Ret*- and GDNF-independent. The bulk of the ENS is constructed of cells in the *Ret*/GDNF-dependent sympathoadrenal-enteric lineage, which evidently also gives rise to the superior cervical ganglion. The *Ret*/GDNF-independent lineage forms the ENS of the rostral foregut and the entire sympathetic chain, except for the superior cervical ganglion. The *Ascl1*-dependent and *Ret*-dependent lineages seem superficially to be opposite sides of a single coin [62]. For example, the ENS of the esophagus, which is totally *Ascl-1*-dependent, happens to be the region of the gut that is *Ret*-independent. In contrast, the ENS of the bowel below the proximal stomach is totally *Ret*-dependent; yet it contains neurons in *Ascl-1* knockout mice. Still, as noted above, there is no region of the ENS that is completely *Ascl-1*-independent. Although there are neurons in the intestines of *Ascl-1* knockout mice, TC cells and all the neurons derived from TC cells are missing. Still to be explained as well is why the presumably *Ret*-independent crest-derived cells of the rostral foregut do not migrate distally in the bowel of *Ret*–/– mice (or mice lacking GDNF). Possibly, the evident inability of the *Ret*-independent cells of the rostral foregut to expand their territory in *Ret*–/– mice is due to an inhibition of their migration. Consistent with this possibility, GDNF signaling has been shown to attract and guide RET-expressing enteric crest-derived cells as they migrate proximo-distally down the developing bowel [146]. GDNF is expressed at high levels early in the mesenchyme of the primordial stomach. As development proceeds, the locus of highest GDNF development moves anally ahead of the front of migrating crest-derived cells until the caecum is reached. Distal progression of GDNF then ceases and the caecum becomes a stable site of high mesenchymal GDNF expression. These observations are consistent with the idea that GDNF acts as a guidance molecule for RET/GFRα-1-expressing cells and is at least partly responsible for the descent of emigres from the vagal crest. A difficulty with this concept is that the accumulation of GDNF in the caecum would trap the migrating crest-derived cells in this segment of the gut. An additional factor has to be postulated that enables enteric crest-derived cells to free themselves from the attraction to GDNF and migrate out of the caecum. Endothelin 3 (EDN3) signaling via the endothelin-B receptor (EDNRB) has been postulated to play this role [147, 148]. Alternatively, all enteric neurons may be GDNF/Ret-dependent but able to survive in the rostral foregut, despite the absence of GDNF or Ret, because a compensatory factor (currently unknown) is expressed only in this region of the bowel.

During development of the ENS, GDNF plays an essential role in survival, proliferation, migration, and neuronal differentiation. Recently, McKeown et al [149] showed that GDNF enhances the ability of enteric neural progenitors to grow as enteric neurospheres and to migrate and generate an ENS. Exposure to GDNF, furthermore, resulted in a 14-fold increases in neurosphere volume and a 12-fold increase in cell number. The GDNF/RET interaction thus shows promise for the future as approaches are sought to replace an ENS when that becomes a clinical necessity.

3.7 The Development of the ENS Is Influenced by a Neurotrophin

For a long time, neurotrophins were thought to play little or no role in the development of the ENS. Unlike developing sensory and sympathetic ganglia, explanted enteric neurons can be cultured without nerve growth factor (NGF) or even in the presence of neutralizing antibodies to NGF [150, 151]. Neuritic outgrowth from organotypic cultures of gut, moreover, is not stimulated by NGF. Autoantibodies to NGF produce severe sensory and sympathetic defects in the progeny of immunized animals [152, 153]; nevertheless, the same autoantibodies to NGF do not induce ENS lesions. These observations, however, suggest only that the development of the ENS is independent of NGF, not that the ENS does not require the action of any neurotrophin. NGF was the first neurotrophin to be discovered and the studies outlined above were carried out before the existence of other neurotrophins became known. NGF, together with brain-derived neurotrophic factor (BDNF), neurotrophin- 3 (NT-3), NT-4/5 [115, 154, 155], and NT-6 [156] are members of a family of small, very basic proteins. Each of these neurotrophins is able to interact independently with a common receptor, p75NTR, and with a specific Trk receptor tyrosine kinase, TrkA for NGF, TrkB for BDNF and NT-4/5, and TrkC for NT-3. At higher concentrations, the neurotrophins become somewhat promiscuous and activate Trks other than their primary receptor. NT-3, for example, activates TrkA and TrkB, but it binds to those receptors with an affinity that is lower than its affinity for its natural ligand, TrkC, or that of NGF or BDNF for TrkA or TrkB, respectively.

The common neurotrophin receptor, p75NTR, regulates many cellular functions [157]. These include an enhancement of the affinity of Trks for their neurotrophins, increasing the rate at which NGF binds to TrkA, and improving the specificity of Trk receptors by decreasing their receptivity to activation by the wrong neurotrophin. p75NTR also affects apoptosis, axonal growth and degeneration, cell proliferation, myelination, and synaptic plasticity [157]. The kaleidoscopic multiplicity of cellular functions that p75NTR governs stems from the equivalent multiplicity of the ligands and co-receptors that associate with p75NTR and modulate its signaling. Survival is promoted through the interactions of p75NTR with Trk receptors; inhibition of axonal regeneration through interactions with the Nogo (Nogo-R) and Lingo-1 receptors, apoptosis is promoted through interactions of p75NTR with sortilin. Signals downstream of the interactions of p75NTR and its various partners are additionally modulated by regulated intramembrane proteolysis of p75NTR and by interactions of the receptors with a wide variety of cytosolic partners.

The first observation to suggest that one or more neurotrophins probably are important in the formation of the ENS was the discovery that the common neurotrophin receptor, p75NTR, is expressed by the crest-derived cells that colonize the fetal mouse and rat gut [71, 72]. The cells that express p75NTR give rise to neurons and glia in vitro [73]. Antibodies to p75NTR specifically immunoselect crest-derived cells from the fetal bowel [158, 159]; moreover, almost no cells able to give rise to neurons or glia remain in dissociated cell populations after p75NTR-expressing cells have been removed by immunoselection. These observations suggest (but do not prove) that all, and not just some, of the crest-derived cells that colonize the gut express p75NTR. No marker has yet been found that reveals a greater number of enteric crest-derived neural precursors than p75NTR. Although p75NTR may not be required for stimulation of cells by a neurotrophin, which can activate a specific Trk, p75NTR is commonly expressed by cells that are neurotrophin-responsive. The fact that enteric neuronal precursors express p75NTR, however, is not the only reason to believe that a neurotrophin plays an important role in the development of enteric neurons and/or glia. The concept that at least one lineage of enteric neurons arises from a common sympathoadrenal-enteric progenitor [57, 90, 160] suggests that at least the enteric neurons of this lineage should share the neurotrophin dependence of their sympathoadrenal equivalents. Sympathetic neural precursors are not at first NGF-dependent [161–164]. Instead, they are supported by NT-3 before they respond to, and become dependent on, NGF [161, 162]. This change in neurotrophin responsivity and dependence is matched in sympathetic neural precursors by a change from TrkC to TrkA expression [162, 163, 165]. This switch in receptor expression may occur spontaneously [165], or it may require the exposure of cells to NT-3 [161]. NT-3 thus promotes the development of sympathoadrenal precursors [161, 163]; moreover, both the knockout of NT-3 in transgenic mice [166, 167] and the administration of neutralizing antibodies to NT-3 impair the normal development of sympathetic neurons [168]. Excessive apoptosis of sympathoadrenal neuroblasts occurs when NT-3 is absent during development [169]. If the enteric neurons that arise from a common sympathoadrenal-enteric progenitor were to diverge from the common lineage before TrkA and NGF dependence are acquired, then the evident NGF independence of virtually all enteric neurons could be explained. In this model, the acquisition of NGF dependence would be considered, for sympathetic neurons the time when their progenitors diverge from the common lineage. Acquisition of NGF dependence would also be an event that does not occur in the enteric microenvironment, where the successors of TC cells lose their catecholaminergic properties and acquire other, gut-specific, phenotypes. Since NT-3 plays such an important role in the early development of sympathoadrenal cells, NT-3 might be expected to play a similar role in the development of those enteric neurons that are derived from the common sympathoadrenal-enteric lineage. NT-3 would be predicted to affect the enteric neuronal progenitors during the predivergent phase, when they share properties with sympathetic neural precursors. Clearly, the logic of this argument suggests that NT-3 would support the development of the subset of enteric neurons that is derived from the *Ascl-1*-dependent TC cells (the common sympathoadrenal-enteric progenitor). What the argument does not suggest is that NT-3 or any other neurotrophin is likely to exert a global effect similar to that of GDNF. GDNF stimulation of the Ret receptor appears to be critical at a very early stage of development, so that the loss of precursor cells that are GDNF/Ret-dependent results in the total failure of both neurons and glia to arise in the affected region of the bowel. The idea that NT-3 is the critical neurotrophin in enteric neuronal development is supported by the observations that TrkC is expressed by enteric neurons, where both full-length and truncated forms of the receptor can be detected in newborn mice [170] and fetal rats [159, 171]. Transcripts encoding TrkC have been shown by in situ hybridization to be located in the developing and mature ENS [171, 172]. mRNA encoding the full-length TrkC (containing a kinase domain) is enriched in purified populations of crest-derived neural and glial precursor cells immunoselected from the fetal rat bowel [159]. NT-3 binding to both full-length and truncated forms of TrkC has been detected in the E13.5 chick gut [173], although affinity labeling has not revealed the presence of significant amounts of NT-3 binding to TrkC in the bowel of newborn mice [173]. NT-3, as well as TrkC, is expressed in the developing gut [174]. The expression of *lacZ* driven by the NT-3 promoter in transgenic mice has enabled cells that express NT-3 to be located and identified in the fetal bowel [174]. The cells that express NT-3 are located in the outer gut mesenchyme of fetal mice. The outer gut mesenchyme is the layer of the bowel within which myenteric ganglia arise, suggesting that NT-3 is secreted in situ, where it can reach and affect TrkC expressed by developing enteric neuronal precursors and/or neurons. NT-3 expression has not been detected in the submucosa. The development of submucosal neurons follows that of myenteric neurons [175, 176] and all submucosal neurons are born late [177]. The neurons of the submucosal plexus, therefore, probably are not derived from the *Ascl-1*-dependent TC cell lineage, which gives rise only to neurons, such as serotonergic cells (of which there are none in the submucosal plexus) that are born early [74]. These considerations are consistent with the idea that a subset of enteric neurons, most likely the *Ascl-1*-dependent TC cell lineage, are affected by NT-3.

3.8 NT-3 and Bone Morphogenetic Proteins Promote the Development of Enteric Neurons

A major breakthrough, which has enabled the effects of growth factors on the development of enteric neurons or glia to be studied in vitro, has been the development of a means of isolating crest-derived cells from within the wall of the fetal bowel. If crest-derived cells are not so isolated, then the direct actions of growth factors on crest-derived neural and/or glial precursors cannot be distinguished from indirect effects of these molecules on other cells of the enteric mesenchyme. The isolation of enteric crest-derived cells takes advantage of the phenomenon that these cells express cell-surface differentiation antigens or markers that are not expressed by non-neuronal cells of the gut wall. Antibodies to these cell surface antigens are utilized for immunoselection of the crest-derived cells. The first differentiation antigen used for the immunoselection of crest-derived cells from the fetal gut of chicks and rats was a protein recognized by HNK-1 monoclonal antibodies [158, 159]. Since then, p75NTR [140] and Ret [89] have each been employed with good effect. In general, the fetal gut is dissociated and the separated cells are incubated with primary antibodies, which selectively decorate the surfaces of the crest-derived cells. The antibody-labeled cells can then be immunoselected with secondary antibodies coupled to magnetic beads, and eventually isolated with a magnet [158, 159]. Alternatively, the primary antibody-labeled cells can be identified with fluorescent secondary antibodies and isolated with a cell sorter [89] or by manual selection [88, 178–180]. The non-immunoselected cells proliferate much more than do the immunoselected crest-derived cells. The crest-derived precursors that colonize the gut are still dividing when they arrive in the bowel [71, 110, 177, 181]; however, crest-derived cells withdraw from the cell cycle when they give rise to neurons. In contrast, the non-neuronal cells of the residual population do not give rise to cells that become postmitotic and thus continue to divide in vitro. The ability of isolated populations of crest-derived cells, immunoselected from the fetal rat gut, to differentiate into neurons and glia is promoted by NT-3 [159, 182]. In contrast to the immunoselected cells, NT-3 has no effect on crest-depleted populations of cells that remain after the crest-derived cells have been removed by immunoselection. In these experiments, it is necessary to identify cells as neurons or glia by demonstrating chemical markers, because the morphological appearance of the cells in culture can be misleading. Neurons can be identified by the expression of the immunoreactivity of specific marker proteins, such as HuC/D [183–186]. Glia can be identified by the expression of the immunoreactivity of markers such as glial fibrillary acidic protein (GFAP), S100, and proteolipid protein 1 (PLP1), which, in contrast to GFAP, is expressed by all enteric glial cells [24, 25]. The ability of NT-3 to promote neuronal and glial development is concentration-dependent and is maximal at 40 ng/ml. In addition to promoting the development of enteric neurons and glia, NT-3 enhances neurite outgrowth, but it is not mitogenic. Similarly, NT-3 does not induce dorsal root ganglion cell precursors to proliferate; on the contrary, when administered early in ontogeny, NT-3 causes sensory neurons to differentiate prematurely, thereby reducing their ultimate numbers [187]. NT-3 thus exerts an effect on the postmigratory crest-derived cells that colonize the bowel and dorsal root ganglia that is different from its action on premigratory crest cells, which are stimulated to proliferate by NT-3 [188, 189]. The action of NT-3 on immunoselected cells, in common with the effects of most growth factors, is associated with the transient induction of the *c-fos* protooncogene in responding cells [159]. Other neurotrophins, such as NGF, BDNF, and NT4/5 affect neither the in vitro development of neurons and glia in populations of immunoselected cells, nor the in vitro proliferation or differentiation of the non-immunoselected cells. NT-3 thus specifically promotes the in vitro differentiation of crest-derived cells as enteric neurons and glia, and may be the only neurotrophin that can do so. Although a physiological role for NT-3 in the normal development of the ENS has not yet been identified, NT-3 has been shown to be able to affect the development of enteric ganglia in vivo. The DBH promoter has been used to direct the overexpression of NT-3 in the developing ENS. When this is done, the myenteric plexus of the small and large intestines of the DBH/NT-3 transgenic animals becomes hyperplastic. There are significant increases in the number of neurons/ganglion, the number of neurons per unit length of gut, the packing density of neurons within ganglia, the proportion area of ganglia, and the size (maximal diameter and volume) of individual neurons. In contrast, none of these parameters are changed in the submucosal plexus and there is no change in the numbers of CGRP-containing neurons (the majority of which are submucosal). CGRP-containing neurons are the latest-born of enteric neurons and are derived from cells in the *Ascl-1*-independent lineage [74, 177]. In fact, the entire set of submucosal neurons tends to be born late. These findings suggest that the late developing *Ascl-1*-independent lineage of enteric neurons is probably not affected by the DBH/NT-3 transgene. Both the myenteric hyperplasia and the increase in neuronal size induced by the overexpression of NT-3 in transgenic mice are thus probably due to a response of the *Ascl-1*-dependent precursor lineage.

An ENS is present in mice that lack NT-3 or TrkC despite the ability of NT-3 to promote enteric neuronal development in vitro [190]. The mere presence of an ENS and the survival of an animal do not, however, demonstrate that the ENS is either normal or complete. Further analysis of mice lacking NT-3 or TrkC demonstrated abnormalities of subsets of enteric neurons. After isolated enteric neurons are exposed to NT-3, the TrkC-expressing subset becomes NT-3 dependent and undergoes apoptosis upon NT-3 withdrawal. Function blocking antibodies to NT-3 inhibit neuronal development in mixed cultures of crest- and non-neural crest-derived cells but do not do so in cultures containing only crest-derived cells isolated from the fetal bowel; therefore, the endogenous source of NT-3 for the support of enteric neuronal development is probably the non-crest-derived mesenchymal cells of the gut wall. Retrograde transport of (125)I-NT-3 reveals the locations and projections of NT-3-responsive neurons in the adult bowel. The submucosal plexus contains NT-3-responsive neurons that project to the mucosa, while the myenteric plexus contains NT-3-responsive interneurons and neurons that innervate distant ganglia, the tertiary plexus and smooth muscle. The numbers of neurons in both plexuses in mice lacking NT-3 or TrkC are less than those of wild-type animals. The neuropoietic cytokine (CNTF) enhances the effect of NT-3 in vitro and can prevent apoptosis of neurons upon NT-3 withdrawal. NT-3 is thus required for the development of a normal ENS although its affects are not as global as those of GDNF.

Another set of regulatory molecules that are important in ENS development is the set of bone morphogenetic proteins (BMPs) [191]. These molecules play a major role early in the morphogenesis of the primordial bowel and are critical in the regulation of mucosal stem cells [192]. Expression of BMP-2 and BMP-4, BMPR-IA (BMP receptor subunit), BMPR-IB, and BMPR-II, and the BMP antagonists, noggin, gremlin, chordin, and follistatin are all expressed in the fetal gut when neurons can first be detected. When applied to crest-derived cells immunopurified from the fetal mouse intestine at E12, moreover, BMP-2 and BMP-4 induce translocation of phosphorylated Smad-1 from cytosol to nucleus, suggesting that these cells are responsive to BMP signaling. Low concentrations of the same BMPs promote neurogenesis from isolated enteric crest-derived cells in vitro, while high concentrations impede neurogenesis because they drive many cells to apoptosis. The BMPs also cause the precocious expression of TrkC in neurons as well as their dependence on TrkC for survival. BMPs synergize with GDNF in enhancing neuronal development; however, the promotion of neuronal development depletes the pool of proliferating precursor cells. Interestingly, when the actions of BMPs 2 and 4 are inhibited by overexpressing noggin in the developing ENS of transgenic mice under the control of the neuron-specific enolase promoter, neuronal numbers in both enteric plexuses are increased throughout the postnatal gut. In contrast to the overall increase in total numbers of neurons, the specific set of neurons that express TrkC are decreased. BMP-2 and/or BMP-4 thus limit the size of the ENS but enhance the development of specific subsets of enteric neurons, such as those that express TrkC. The BMPs thus appear to be differentiating factors that enhance phenotypic expression at the expense of precursor proliferation. These observations of BMP signaling during murine ENS development have been confirmed and extended to the ENS of the avian hindgut [193]. Again, BMP-2, BMP-4, and BMPR-II are strongly expressed in the ENS during hindgut development. The phosphorylated Smad1/5/8 proteins are present in the enteric ganglia, suggesting ongoing BMP signaling. Inhibition of BMP within the developing gut inhibits the normal migration of crest-derived precursor cells and also causes hypoganglionosis and failure of clustering of neurons into ganglionic aggregates.

Evidence that BMPs affect not only neurogenesis and gliogenesis but also migration of crest-derived precursors has come from studies of the neural cell adhesion molecule (Ncam1) [194]. BMP signaling has been found to restrict murine ENS precursors to the outer bowel wall during migration; moreover, inhibition of BMP signaling accelerates colonization of the murine colon but diminishes the formation of ganglionic aggregates and neurite fasciculation. The migration of crest-derived cells through the bowel and the fasciculation of neurites may be related to a BMP-enhanced addition of polysialic acid to Ncam1. Enzymatic removal of polysialic acid from Ncam1 blocks the effects of BMPs on migration of enteric crest-derived cells and the fasciculation of neurites. Additional insight supports a role for BMP regulation of sialyltransferases during ENS development [195]. Transcripts encoding the sialyltransferases, ST8Sia IV (PST) and ST8Sia II (STX), which polysialylate Ncam, have been detected in fetal rat gut by E12 and are downregulated postnatally. Numbers of neurons that express Ncam1with polysialic acid, but not those that express just Ncam, are similarly developmentally regulated. Circular smooth muscle transiently (E16-20) expresses Ncam with polysialic acid at the time when it is traversed by migrating crest-derived cells migrating from the myenteric to the submucosal plexus, which they do under the guidance of netrins [100]. Neurons developing in vitro from crest-derived cells immunoselected at E12 express both Ncam and Ncam polysialic acid [195]. BMP-4 promotes the addition of polysialic acid to neuronal Ncam and the clustering of neurons into ganglionic aggregates. N-butanoylmannosamine, which antagonizes addition of polysialic acid to Ncam, but not N-propanoylmannosamine, which does not, blocks BMP-4-induced formation of ganglionic aggregates. BMP signaling is thus critical in the addition of polysialic acid to Ncam. This process evidently allows crest-derived precursors to migrate and form ganglionic aggregates during ENS development.

Although the migration, differentiation, and survival of enteric neurons during development are reliant on a variety of trophic factors, relatively little is known about the mechanisms that regulate the maturation of enteric neurons in postnatal life. Still, it is now clear that enteric neurons continue to arise in the adult gut [196–198]. One molecule that the maturation of enteric neurons and glia require is a transcriptional cofactor, homeodomain interacting protein kinase 2 (HIPK2) [199]. Deletion of HIPK2 causes distention of the colon and slowing of GI transit. Curiously, loss of HIPK2 does not affect enteric neurons in prenatal life; however, in Hipk2-/- mice, there is a progressive postnatal loss of enteric neurons. Enteric dopaminergic neurons are lost preferentially. The action of HIPK2 in postnatal ENS development is intertwined with the response of enteric neuronal BMPs. The proportion of enteric neurons in Hipk2-/- mutants that have a high level of phosphorylated Smad1/5/8 is greater than that in wild-type animals. Smad protein 1/5/8 are pivotal in BMP signaling. Gliogenesis is also increased in the ENS of Hipk2-/- mutants, suggesting that a diminution of neurogenesis in the adult ENS in Hipk2-/- mutants is compensated by an increase in gliogenesis. Autophagy is increased in enteric neurons in Hipk2-/- mutants and synaptic maturation is impaired. HIPK2 is thus an important transcriptional cofactor in the regulation of BMP signaling during enteric neuronal and glial maintenance. The development of the ENS thus does not cease at birth.

3.9 The Development of the ENS Is Influenced by Neuropoietic Cytokines

Ciliary neurotrophic factor (CNTF) was first identified as a factor in the eye that promotes the survival of chick ciliary ganglion neurons [200]. CNTF has since been purified, cloned, and found to affect many different neurons, both developing and mature [201]. CNTF does not resemble any of the neurotrophins and is a member of the cytokine family, which includes distantly related molecules, such as leukemia inhibitory factor (LIF), interleukin-6 (IL-6), interleukin-11 (IL-11), oncostatin M (OSM), cardiotrophin-1, neuropoietin (formerly known as cardiotrophin 2), and cardiotrophin-like factor (CLCF1) [201–204]. CNTF primarily acts on neurons and skeletal muscle [205], while the actions of the other cytokines are exerted on many other types of cell. The active CNTF receptor (CNTFR) is an assembly of three molecular components, only one of which, CNTFRα, actually binds CNTF [206]. There are two β receptor subunits, gp130 and LIFRβ. These are signal-transducing molecules and also serve as components of receptors for cytokine relatives of CNTF, such as LIF and IL-6 [203, 205, 207–209]. The three molecular components are not initially associated with one another on cell surfaces but are recruited to form a complex when stimulated by CNTF. CNTF binds first to CNTFRα and the β components then join to form the tripartite complex [209]. The signal transduction process thus begins with formation of the CNTFRα/LIFRβ/gp130 complex, involves the dimerization of LIFRβ with gp130, and proceeds by activating Jak tyrosine kinases, which are constitutively associated with the cytosolic tails of each of the β components [210, 211]. CNTF neither binds to, nor activates the β components in the absence of CNTFRα. CNTFRα, moreover, is restricted to the nervous system and skeletal muscle, which thus explains the relative neural specificity of the actions of CNTF [205]. Other cytokines have different specificity determinants, which are expressed extraneuronally. Levels of CNTF in embryonic and fetal animals are very low [201], although expression of mRNA encoding CNTF can be detected in the developing bowel by using reverse transcriptase and the polymerase chain reaction. In contrast to CNTF, CNTFRα is expressed by many cells of the developing nervous system, including the ENS [212]. The natural or targeted knockout of genes encoding CNTF does not cause notable developmental defects in mice [213] or humans (about 2.5% of the Japanese population) [214]. CNTF, furthermore, unlike the majority of secreted proteins, lacks a signal sequence and thus is probably cytosolic. In the absence of cell death, such a protein requires a chaperone to be secreted [204]. CNTF has thus been proposed to be an emergency factor, which is released only in response to injury; moreover, mice that lack CNTF appear normal at birth but lose motor neurons excessively as they age, further supporting the idea that CNTF is helpful in protecting neurons from injury [205].

In situ, all myenteric ganglia of the fetal stomach and intestine express the immunoreactivity of CNTFRα by E16-E18 [215]. In vitro, CNTF and LIF cause nuclear translocation of signal transducer and activator of transcription 3 (STAT3), a concentration-dependent increase in neurons and glia, and a decrease in expression of the precursor marker, nestin. CNTF and LIF were additive with NT-3 in the ability to enhance neuronal but not glial development. Specifically, the development of NOS-expressing neurons (a marker of inhibitory motor neurons) was promoted by CNTF and NT-3. These observations suggest that a ligand for the tripartite CNTF receptor complex plays a role in ENS development; however, the identity of that ligand is not yet clear.

In contrast to the relatively normal development of CNTF knockout mice, there are profound motor and other defects at birth in animals with targeted deletions of CNTFRα [202]. Mice lacking CNTFRα fail to feed and die with a massive dilation of the bowel during the perinatal period. Neurons immunoreactive for substance P (SP) and NOS are markedly reduced in the enteric plexuses of these animals. Almost no SP- or NOS-immunoreactive axons are found in the circular muscle of CNTFRα knockout mice. Motor neurons that excite smooth muscle contain SP [216] and motor neurons that relax smooth muscle contain NOS [217–221]. An identical defect is seen in the gut of mice in which the expression of *LIFRβ* has been knocked out. These observations suggest that the tripartite CNTFR, and particularly its α component, plays a vital role in the development of enteric motor neurons. Although enteric ganglia are present in mice that lack CNTFRα or LIFRβ, the ENS cannot function in the absence of motor neurons. Since a similar effect is not seen in mice lacking CNTF, there may be another endogenous ligand in the fetal gut that can bind to CNTFRα. This yet-to-be-identified ligand is essential for the development of enteric motor neurons. Many relatives of CNTF, LIF, OSM, IL-6, IL-11, and cardiotrophin-1, do not require CNTFRα and thus are unlikely to be the unknown CNTFRα ligand [202]. In contrast, neuropoietin (formerly known as cardiotrophin

2) and cardiotrophin-like factor (CLCF1) bind to CNTFRα and activate the tripartite CNTF receptor [204]. A role for these agents in ENS development may thus be important and should be investigated. Mice that lack CLCF1 die perinatally due to a suckling defect. The state of the ENS in these animals has not yet been described but may well be deficient.

3.10 An Aganglionosis Similar to That in Hirschsprung Disease Occurs in *ls/ls* and *sl/sl* Mice

The terminal colon of lethal spotted (*ls/ls*) and piebald lethal mutant mice (*sl/sl*) becomes aganglionic [222]. These murine aganglionoses, inherited as autosomal recessives, provide the best-known spontaneous animal models of Hirschsprung disease [223]. Related models in other species have now been discovered. These include megacolon inherited as a recessive trait in the spotting lethal rat (*sl/sl*) [10, 224–228], white patterned foals [229], and the homozygous spotted rabbit (en/en) [230]. What all of these models have in common, whether they are inherited as a recessive or a dominant trait, is that the terminal region of the gut is aganglionic, megacolon develops, and the animals exhibit a spotted coat. The megacolon can be attributed to a loss of the reflexes normally mediated by the ENS. The presence of nerve fibers thus does not compensate for the aganglionosis which contain the neural circuitry responsible for enteric reflexes. The spotted coat color reflects an abnormality of melanocytes, which like enteric neurons are derivatives of the neural crest. The defects in the animal models, however, like that which occurs in patients with Hirschsprung disease, do not extend to all derivatives of the neural crest, or even to all crest-derived neurons. The constant association of enteric neuronal and melanocytic deficiencies thus suggests that there is a common factor or requirement for normal differentiation that the ENS of the terminal gut shares with melanocytes; this common factor is the signaling of endothelin 3 and its receptor endothelin B.

3.11 Genetic Abnormalities in Genes Encoding Endothelin-3 and Its Receptor, Endothelin-B, Are Associated with Spotted Coats and Aganglionosis

The genes that are abnormal in lethal spotted (*ls/ls*) and piebald lethal (*sl/sl*) mice, as well as the spotting lethal rat, have recently been identified. The loci that are involved in these models are also abnormal in a subset of patients with Hirschsprung disease. Aganglionosis in *ls/ls* mice is associated with a mutation in the gene encoding the peptide hormone, endothelin-3 (EDN3) [231], while the somewhat more severe aganglionosis that occurs in *sl/sl* mice [232], spotting lethal rats [225, 227, 228], white patterned foals [233], and some patients with Hirschsprung disease [234] is linked to abnormalities of genes encoding the endothelin-B receptor (EDNRB). This is the receptor normally activated by EDN3. The discovery that EDN3 and EDNRB are important in the development of the ENS (at least in the colon) was made as a result of analyses of the effects of knockouts of the genes that encode these molecules in mice. Endothelins 1–3 represent a family of peptides, each with a chain length of 21 amino acids that activate one or both of two serpentine (G-protein coupled) receptors, endothelin-A (EDNRA) and/or EDNRB [235, 236]. Each of the endothelins has an equivalent potency for stimulating EDNRB, but that for activating EDNRA is EDN1 > EDN2 >> EDN3 [237]. EDN1 was discovered as a product of vascular endothelial cells that is a strong vasoconstrictor [238]. Since their initial discovery, however, the endothelins and the EDNRs have been found to be widely distributed [235]. The endothelins are initially synthesized with a signal sequence (a preproendothelin) that is responsible for translocation of the proteins across the membranes of the rough endoplasmic reticulum into the cisternal space. This translocation enables the proteins to be packaged for secretion. The signal sequence is removed cotranslationally to yield an inactive precursor, called a big endothelin, which is secreted. Big endothelins, in turn, are again cleaved by a specific membrane-bound metalloprotease, the endothelin-converting enzyme-1 (ECE-1), to produce the smaller active peptides [239]. Craniofacial defects arise in transgenic knockout mice that fail to produce EDN1 due to the abnormal development of first branchial arch derivatives [240]. Missense mutations in *ednrb* occur in *sl/sl* mice [232]. Similar mutations can be found in *EDNRB*, which is the analogous human locus, in patients with Hirschsprung disease [234]. When *ednrb* is knocked out by homologous recombination, an aganglionosis of the colon develops that is identical to that seen in *sl/sl* mice [232]. More recently, lethal spotting in rats has also been demonstrated to arise as a result of an interstitial deletion in an exon of the *ednrb* gene that prevents expression of the rat EDNRB [225, 227]. The *edn3* gene is mutated in *ls/ls* mice ($EDN3^{ls/ls}$) so that an arginine is replaced with a tryptophan residue in the C-terminus of big EDN3 [231]. This defect prevents the conversion of big EDN3 to the active EDN3 by ECE-1. In an analogous fashion, the knockout of *edn3* also causes the terminal colon to become aganglionic. It is thus clear that the receptor, EDNRB; the ligand, EDN3; and the converting enzyme, ECE-1, play critical roles in the development of the ENS. The nature of these roles, however, remains to be fully explained. The genetic loss of EDN3 stimulation could, in theory, lead to aganglionosis by affecting the crest-derived precursors of enteric neurons themselves. Alternatively, the effect of EDN3 could be mediated indirectly, through an action on another cell type that interacts with crest-derived cells in a manner that is essential for neuronal and/or glial development. Why the absence of EDN3 interferes with the development of neurons only in the colon is also an issue that must be resolved. The inability of EDN1 or EDN2 to compensate for the loss of active EDN3 in $EDN3^{ls/ls}$ or *edn3* knockout mice [231] is also hard to understand, in view of the fact that all endothelins are equally good as ligands for the EDNRB [237]. The effects of EDN3, therefore, must be quite local and the circulating concentrations of EDN1 and EDN2 must be too low to be effective at those EDNRBs that are critical for development of the ENS of the terminal bowel.

3.12 An Action of EDN3 on Crest-Derived Precursors Does Not, by Itself, Account for the Pathogenesis of Aganglionosis

Several hypotheses have been advanced to explain the critical role played by EDN3 on the development of enteric neurons. One idea is that EDN3 is an autocrine growth factor [231]. This proposal considers (1) that EDN3 is essential for the development of migrating crest-derived cells as enteric neurons or melanocytes, and (2) that the crest-derived cells themselves are both the source and target of EDN3. The nice feature of this hypothesis is that it explains why the coats of all of the animal models of Hirschsprung disease are spotted or white. The lack of EDN3 deprives both the precursors of melanocytes and enteric neurons of a necessary growth factor. The hypothesis postulates that the migrating crest-derived cells that colonize the bowel synthesize big EDN3, convert it to active EDN3, and express EDNRBs. A problem for this autocrine hypothesis is that it fails to explain why the development of enteric neurons in mice lacking EDN3 [231] and in both piebald mice [232, 241] and spotting lethal rats [225, 227, 228] that lack EDNRBs only becomes abnormal in the colon. If no factors other than the crest-derived cells themselves were to be involved, then there is no obvious reason why enteric neuronal development should be independent of EDN3 in the esophagus, stomach, and small intestine but EDN3-dependent in the terminal colon. An idea that has been advanced to account for this problem is to assume that the ability of the vagal population of crest-derived cells to migrate as far as the terminal colon requires that the starting population be large and proliferating [109, 242]. This hypothesis postulates that EDN3 is a mitogen that is required to provoke vagal crest cells to multiply sufficiently to generate a population that is large enough to colonize the entire bowel. EDN3, in fact, has been demonstrated to be a mitogen for cells cultured from the premigratory neural crest [243]. Addition of EDN3 causes these cells to proliferate massively; however, following their multiplication, the cultured crest cells go on to develop primarily as melanocytes. The neural crest cells, therefore, do not respond to EDN3 exactly as predicted by the hypothesis that EDN3 is required to generate adequate numbers of neural precursors to colonize the entire gut. EDN3 promotes the formation of melanocytes, not neurons, suggesting that, at least in culture, the precursors that proliferate in response to EDN3 are not neurogenic but melanogenic. The data are even consistent with the possibility that EDN3 shifts the originally pluripotent neural crest population toward the melanocytic lineage. Unless EDN3, therefore, were to exert a different effect in vivo, this outcome would not enhance the formation of neurons in the colon. The proliferative action of EDN3 on premigratory crest cells in vitro thus is consistent with the idea that its mitogenic properties are needed to enlarge the number of melanogenic precursors enough to colonize the skin, but the data do not support the concept that the mitogenic properties of EDN3 are needed for the formation of the ENS. To apply the hypothesis to the ENS, it is necessary to assume that the effects of EDN3 on crest-derived cells that have colonized the gut are different from those which EDN3 exerts on cells isolated from the neural crest itself. There are no longer any cells with a melanogenic potential in the crest-derived cell population that colonizes the bowel; moreover, the cohort of crest-derived cells that colonizes the gut is still proliferating [71, 72, 181].

To identify enteric cells that express EDN3 and EDNRB, the fetal mouse gut was dissociated at E11-13, and positive and negative immunoselection with antibodies to p75NTR were used to isolate neural crest- and non-crest-derived cells [111] Transcripts encoding EDNRB were detected in both crest-and non-crest-derived cells; however, transcripts encoding preproendothelin-3 were exclusively found in the non-crest-derived population. These data suggest that both crest- and non-crest-derived cells express EDNRB, but that EDN3 is produced by non-neuronal cells of the gut wall and is thus a factor of the enteric microenvironment. Neurons and glia develop in cultures of crest-derived cells isolated from the bowel in the absence of EDN3 and even in the presence of the EDN3 antagonist, BQ 788 [111]. EDN3 is thus not an autocrine factor that is required for the development of enteric neurons. In fact, the addition of EDN3 or the EDNRB agonist, IRL 1620, actually inhibits neuronal development, an effect that BQ 788 antagonizes. The ability of EDN signaling to inhibit enteric neurogenesis has been confirmed [112, 147, 244]. Neurons do not develop in explants of the terminal bowel of E12 $EDN3^{ls/ls}$ mice, but addition of extrinsic EDN3 makes them do so if a source of crest-derived cells is present in the bowel proximal to the aganglionic region. These observations are compatible with the suggestion that EDN3/ECNRB signaling prevents premature differentiation of crest-derived precursors [111, 147, 244]. The underlying assumption is that precursors migrate while post-mitotic neurons do not. The inhibitory effect of EDN3/ECNRB signaling thus enables the precursor population to persist long enough to finish colonizing the bowel. In fact, when EDNRB is selectively deleted only in crest-derived cells, the bowel is still aganglionic; thus, although both crest- and non-crest-derived cells express EDNRB, the expression by the crest-derived cells is necessary for the terminal bowel to become ganglionated [245].

EDN3/EDNRB signaling plays additional roles in the developing gut. EDN3 opposes the attraction of Ret-expressing crest-derived cells to sources of GDNF [147]. This allows crest-derived cells to avoid becoming trapped in the cecum, where GDNF expression peaks. EDN3 also opposes the accumulation of semaphorin 3A in the colon [246]. When EDN3 is deleted, semaphorin 3A accumulates in the presumptive aganglionic bowel. Given the ability of semaphorin 3A to repel migrating crest-derived cells, it is likely that the excess of semaphorin 3A in the terminal gut of mice lacking EDNRB contributes to the development of the aganglionosis. Such an effect is compatible with the in vitro observation that the presumptive aganglionic bowel of $EDN3^{ls/ls}$ mice can be colonized in vitro if extrinsic EDN3 is provided [111]. Presumably, the EDN can rescue the gut by suppressing the overabundance of semaphorin 3A.

3.13 The Pathogenesis of Aganglionosis Is Not Explained by an Abnormality Limited to Crest-Derived Neural Precursors

The enteric microenvironment may become inhospitable for colonization by crest-derived cells if EDN3 is deficient or if the EDNRB is lacking [68, 70, 241, 247]. Such an effect could be the result of an action of EDN3 on EDNRBs expressed by non-neuronal cells of the bowel wall. Alternatively, the crest-derived cells themselves may respond to EDN3 by secreting a factor that stimulates their non-neuronal neighbors to make the enteric microenvironment tractable for invasion by crest-derived emigres. As noted above, the advancing front of crest-derived cells in the developing gut cannot be recognized by the expression of neural or glial markers, but can be detected indirectly by explanting and culturing the bowel [51, 248, 249]. Neurons develop in cultures of the normal murine terminal colon explanted after stage 33, but not before [250]. In contrast, neurons never arise in the terminal 2 mm of an EDN3-deficient (*EDN3$^{ls/ls}$*) gut, no matter what the stage of the fetus at the time of explantation [248, 249]. These observations establish that the final segment of the *EDN3$^{ls/ls}$* bowel is the presumptive aganglionic region and they suggest that viable crest-derived cells do not enter this zone. In co-culture experiments, crest-derived cells from a variety of sources, including the ganglionated proximal gut of *EDN3$^{ls/ls}$* mice, have been shown to enter explants of the terminal bowel from control mice and give rise to neurons; however, no source of crest-derived cells migrates into an *EDN3$^{ls/ls}$* terminal colon [250]. In contrast to the normal colon, moreover, the *EDN3$^{ls/ls}$* colon also fails to promote the acquisition of gut-appropriate phenotypes when it is co-cultured with sources of crest cells [53]. These observations suggest that there may be non-neuronal EDNRB-expressing targets of EDN3 in the colon. The EDNRB that non-neuronal cells express as well as that expressed by crest-derived cells may contribute to making it possible for crest-derived cells to complete their colonization of the bowel. The possibility that EDN3 acts on non-neuronal cells of the gut wall has received strong experimental support. Aganglionosis does not occur in *EDN3$^{ls/ls}$* × C3H aggregation chimeric mice, as long as >5% of enteric cells are of C3H origin; moreover, *EDN3$^{ls/ls}$* neurons, identified with an endogenous marker (β-glucuronidase activity), are found even in the most distal enteric ganglia [247]. Similarly, ganglia containing mutant neurons (marked by the expression of a transgene, *lacZ* driven by the DBH promoter) develop in the terminal colon of aggregation chimeras constructed between wild-type and either *EDN3$^{ls/ls}$* [69, 70] or *sl/sl* embryos [241]. It has been postulated that intercellular signals "downstream" from the EDNRB mediate colonization of the terminal gut by crest-derived cells [241]. An alternative hypothesis is that there is an additional, non-neuronal cell in the wall of the colon that expresses the EDNRB and must be stimulated by EDN3 in order to open the colon to colonization by crest-derived neuronal precursors. This latter idea is supported by the observation that the migration of vagal crest-derived cells, visualized by their expression of the *DBH/lacZ* transgene, is entirely normal in *EDN3$^{ls/ls}$* mice until the cells reach the colon; however, the migration of vagal crest-derived cells becomes abnormal within the colon, which is not fully colonized [68, 70]. These observations imply that the ability of crest-derived cells to migrate within the colon is influenced by the enteric microenvironment, which is abnormal in EDN3-deficient *EDN3$^{ls/ls}$* mice. This suggestion has been confirmed by back-transplantation experiments [247]. When segments of wild-type or *EDN3$^{ls/ls}$* colon are placed in a neural crest migration pathway of a quail embryo, the avian crest-derived cells enter wild-type, but not *EDN3$^{ls/ls}$* grafts. There is no reason to suppose that the quail crest-derived cells in these experiments fail to express either EDN3 or the EDNRB. Their inability to enter the *EDN3$^{ls/ls}$* colon, therefore, cannot be explained by an autocrine hypothesis; furthermore, the back-transplantation experiment demonstrates that the absence of active EDN3 in the aganglionic *EDN3$^{ls/ls}$* colon has produced an environment that crest-derived cells will not enter even if they are themselves normal. In sum, the accumulated evidence suggests that crest-derived cells are capable of colonizing the gut and forming enteric neurons whether or not they produce EDN3 but that the enteric microenvironment becomes abnormal in the absence of EDN3/EDNRB stimulation, so that the colon becomes resistant to colonization by crest-derived cells. In fact, extracellular matrix abnormalities have been described, both in the colon of $EDN3^{ls/ls}$ mice and in human patients with Hirschsprung disease.

3.14 The Extracellular Matrix Is Abnormal in the Presumptive Aganglionic Bowel of *EDN3*$^{ls/ls}$ Mice

A variety of defects involving components of the extracellular matrix have been found in mice with deficient EDNRB signaling [113, 251–254] and in human patients with Hirschsprung disease [255, 256]. A common feature that unites these abnormalities is that they all involve an over-abundance and/or maldistribution of constituents of basal laminae. Molecules that have been noted to be over-abundant include laminin, collagen type IV, nidogen non-sulfated glycosaminoglycans, and proteoglycans. In the developing colon of fetal $EDN3^{ls/ls}$ mice, the abnormal molecules are diffusely distributed throughout the mesenchyme of the colon and the surrounding pelvis and are not, for the most part, aggregated in formed basal laminae [251–253]. The mucosal basal lamina of the terminal and distal colon, however, is also thickened relative to that of a wild-type fetus of the same age. The location of the accumulated molecules of the extracellular matrix is in the paths both of vagal crest-derived cells migrating down the bowel [257] and of sacral crest-derived cells approaching the gut [258]. Double-label electron microscopic immunocytochemistry, moreover, has revealed that crest-derived cells, identified by their expression of HNK-1 immunoreactivity, migrate through the enteric mesenchyme of the developing bowel in contact with what appears to be diffuse tufts of electron-opaque material that is laminin-immunoreactive [259].

The over-abundance of laminin and type IV collagen can be detected in the colon of $EDN3^{ls/ls}$ mice at an earlier age [251] than that when crest-derived cells colonize the terminal colon in wild-type mice [250]. This timing and the fact that the extracellular matrix molecules accumulate in the path of incoming crest-derived cells are consistent with the possibility that the abnormal extracellular matrix in $EDN3^{ls/ls}$ mice (and by analogy, in patients with Hirschsprung disease) contributes to the pathogenesis of aganglionosis. This suggestion, however, presumes that the accumulation of laminin and other constituents of the extracellular matrix is a primary event rather than a secondary response to the absence of neurons and/or their precursors.

Studies with $EDN3^{ls/ls}$ mice have indicated that, at least in that model, the accumulation of molecules of the extracellular matrix in the fetal bowel is probably due to an increase in their biosynthesis [253]. Transcripts encoding the $\beta1$ and $\gamma1$ subunits of laminin, as well as the $\alpha1$ and $\alpha2$ chains of collagens type IV, were found to be overly abundant in the colons of $EDN3^{ls/ls}$ mice. Transcripts encoding laminin $\alpha1$ were also found to be increased; however, the abundance of transcripts encoding the $\alpha1$ chain was so much less than that of the $\beta1$ and $\gamma1$ subunits that the $\alpha1$ protein had to be evaluated quantitatively with reverse transcription and the competitive polymerase chain reaction (RT-cPCR). The abundance of mRNA encoding laminin $\alpha1$ was developmentally regulated and declined as a function of age after E11; nevertheless, at all ages, the abundance of mRNA encoding laminin $\alpha1$ was higher in the $EDN3^{ls/ls}$ colon than in an age-matched wild-type colon or in the small intestine of the same $EDN3^{ls/ls}$ animals. The location of the cells responsible for the bulk of the biosynthesis of laminin α 1 and $\beta1$ and the $\alpha2$ chain of collagen type IV was found by in situ hybridization (with 35S-labeled antisense riboprobes) to change as a function of developmental age. In the fetal colon, transcripts encoding these molecules are first concentrated in the endodermal epithelium; however, by day E15, the transcripts are more abundant in mesenchymal cells of the outer gut wall than in the epithelium. More mRNA was found in the colonic mesenchyme of the *EDN3*$^{ls/ls}$ colon than in the wild-type colon at an equivalent age.

To determine whether the increase in transcripts encoding subunits of laminin is a primary or secondary event, the expression of laminin-111 in E15 and newborn *Ret* knockout mice were compared with that in age-matched *EDN3*$^{ls/ls}$ and wild-type animals. The assumption behind this comparison was that the aganglionosis that occurs in both *EDN3*$^{ls/ls}$ and *Ret* knockout mice does so for different genetic reasons. In *Ret* knockout mice, the entire bowel distal to the rostral foregut becomes aganglionic because early crest-derived precursors lack functional Ret receptors and thus cannot respond to GDNF [128–131, 136]. In the *EDN3*$^{ls/ls}$ mice, the animals lack EDN3 and the aganglionic region is restricted to the colon [231]. If the increase in transcripts of laminin and the associated accumulation of laminin and other molecules of the extracellular matrix in the colon of *EDN3*$^{ls/ls}$ mice were to be a secondary response to the absence of neural precursors, then one would expect to see the same increase in the aganglionic bowel of *Ret* knockout mice. In contrast, the increase in mRNA encoding laminin subunits should not occur in the aganglionic bowel of *Ret* knockout mice if the change is *EDN3*$^{ls/ls}$ -specific and related to an effect of the absence of EDN3 on the colonic mesenchyme. No difference from controls either at E15 or in newborn mice was detected by RT-cPCR in the abundance of mRNA encoding laminin $\alpha 1$ in the *Ret* knockout colon [253]; furthermore, the overabundance of immunocytochemically visualizable laminin characteristic of the *EDN3*$^{ls/ls}$ colon was not seen in *Ret* knockout mice.

The results of these experiments suggest that the increase in abundance of transcripts encoding components of the extracellular matrix occurs in *EDN3*$^{ls/ls}$ mice as a primary effect of the genetic defect in EDN3, and is not a consequence of the aganglionosis. The observations also suggest that at least one isoform of laminin that is present in excess in the *EDN3*$^{ls/ls}$ mouse is laminin-111 ($\alpha 1$-$\beta 1$-$\gamma 1$). It should be noted that the accumulation of laminin-111 and other molecules of the extracellular matrix is not limited to the colon, although it occurs there. The excess of these molecules is also found in the pelvic mesenchyme that surrounds the terminal bowel. As a result, the abnormal extracellular matrix is located in the paths both of the vagal crest-derived cells that descend within the gut and of the sacral crest-derived cells that approach the bowel within the pelvis. The location, as well as the *EDN3*$^{ls/ls}$ specificity of the abnormal matrix, therefore, are compatible with the possibility that it contributes to the pathogenesis of aganglionosis. Suggestive evidence has been found showing that the effect of laminin-111, which normally enhances migration of crest-derived cells, changes to inhibition in the terminal bowel of EDNRB-deficient mice [113, 254]. Whether the extracellular matrix defects are actually contributory to the condition, however, remains to be confirmed.

Although molecules of the extracellular matrix have been demonstrated to inhibit the migration of crest cells in a number of locations, including the dorsolateral path between the ectoderm and the somites [260, 261], the posterior sclerotome [262, 263], and the perinotochordal mesenchyme [264], in none of these regions have the inhibitory effects been linked to accumulations of components of basal laminae [260, 263, 265]. In fact, the extracellular matrix in these regions behaves rather differently from that of either the aganglionic *EDN3*$^{ls/ls}$ [175] or Hirschsprung bowel [7, 266]. The aganglionic bowel in each of these conditions is heavily innervated both by axons of neurons from the more rostral hypoganglionic gut and from extrinsic ganglia [175]. The defect in the colon of *EDN3*$^{ls/ls}$ mice and patients with Hirschsprung disease thus impedes its colonization by crest-derived cells, but it does not antagonize the ingrowth of axons.

In contrast, the other regions that normally exclude crest-derived cells also inhibit the outgrowth of axons [265]. It seems paradoxical that laminin-111 should be one of the molecules that is overly abundant in a zone where crest-derived cells fail to migrate. Laminin is a favorable substrate for the adherence of crest-derived cells [98, 267]; moreover, laminin-111 also stimulates the migration of cells away from the neural crest itself [99, 268]. Antibodies to integrins that block attachment of crest-derived cells to laminin [269, 270], as well as antibodies that bind to a laminin-proteoglycan complex [271] inhibit cranial crest cell migration in vivo. The abundance of laminin in the aganglionic *EDN3*$^{ls/ls}$ colon, therefore, might be expected to promote rather than inhibit the colonization of this region of the bowel by cells from the neural crest. On the other hand, the abundance of laminin-111 in the aganglionic colon of *EDN3*$^{ls/ls}$ mice and human patients with Hirschsprung disease could explain why this region of the gut is so well innervated by extrinsic axons; laminin promotes neurite extension and axonal growth [272–277].

3.15 Laminin-111 Promotes the Development of Neurons from Enteric Cells of Neural Crest Origin

Molecules of the extracellular matrix have been demonstrated to be biologically active and able to alter the fate of stem cells from the neural crest in vitro [278]. Extracellular matrix molecules, therefore, can provide more than just an adhesive substrate for crest-derived cells; they are also able to provide signaling information and are, at least potentially, capable of influencing the differentiation of crest-derived cells. Specifically, with respect to crest-derived cells that colonize the bowel, a substrate that includes laminin-111 has been found to increase the in vitro development of neurons relative to that which occurs on substrates of tissue culture plastic or type I collagen [158]. Neurons in these studies were defined as cells that express markers (such as peripherin, neurofilament proteins, neuron-specific enolase, or PGP9.5) that were visualized by immunocytochemistry. The ability of laminin-111 to promote the development of enteric neurons was initially observed in cultures of crest-derived cells immunoselected from the developing avian or rat gut with HNK-1 monoclonal antibodies. An even more pronounced effect of laminin-111 is seen in cultures of cells immunoselected from the mouse gut with antibodies to a cell-surface laminin-binding protein, known as LBP110 [273, 279, 280].

3.16 The Effect of Laminin-111 on Enteric Neuronal Development Depends on the Binding of Its α1 Chain to LBP110

LBP110 is not an integrin, but is similar to β-amyloid precursor protein [281]. Given the relationship of LBP110 to β-amyloid precursor protein, it is interesting that a recent whole genome mapping study has implicated β-amyloid precursor protein in susceptibility to Hirschsprung disease [282]. Specifically, alterations in β-secretase (BACE1) signaling via β -amyloid precursor protein and BACE2 have been proposed as contributors to the pathogenesis of Hirschsprung disease.

The domain of laminin that binds to LBP110 contains an isoleucine-lysine-valine-alanine-valine (IKVAV) sequence and is located on the laminin α1 chain, near its globular C-terminal end [283–285]. The IKVAV peptide also binds to integrins [286] and nucleolin [287]. Expression of LBP110 by PC12 cells is downregulated by transfection of the cells with an antisense amyloid precursor protein cDNA [281, 283]. The ability of NGF to induce neurite extension on a laminin-111 substrate is reduced in such antisense-treated PC12 cells. Kleinman and colleagues have concluded that LBP110 is a laminin-111 receptor that mediates the effects of laminin-111 on neurite outgrowth and also is responsible for controlling a variety of behaviors in non-neuronal cells [281, 283, 288–293]. The only cells in the bowel that express LBP110 are those of neural crest origin; therefore, LBP110 immunoreactivity co-localizes in the gut with crest markers [259] and cells immunoselected from the fetal mouse gut with antibodies to LBP110 preferentially differentiate as neurons or glia [158]. The ability of laminin-111 to promote the development of crest-derived cells as neurons or glia is specifically blocked by a synthetic peptide that contains the IKVAV sequence (IKVAV peptide). A variety of control peptides exert no effect on neuronal differentiation, including a nonsense peptide, a peptide with the same amino acids in a different sequence, or a peptide with a sequence found elsewhere in the laminin-1 molecule. The

IKVAV peptide, moreover, does not affect the development of neurons and glia when similar populations of anti-LBP110-immunoselected crest-derived cells are cultured on poly-d-lysine or fibronectin. The IKVAV peptide, therefore, does not exert a generally inhibitory action on the development of enteric neurons, but only blocks the increment in neuronal development that is a response to laminin-111. Since the addition of an IKVAV peptide does not reduce the total number of cells in culture, the IKVAV peptide appears not to antagonize the adhesion of cells to laminin-111. Adhesion is probably integrin-dependent [269, 270] and independent of LBP110 [283].

Further evidence that the IKVAV peptide does not interfere selectively with the attachment of a small neurogenic subset of crest-derived cells (which could be too small to affect the total number of cells counted in the cultures) has come from the observation that laminin-111 is just as effective when added in soluble form to already adherent cells as it is when it is used as the substrate upon which cells are plated. Soluble laminin is also equally efficacious when applied to cells immunoselected from the fetal mouse gut with antibodies to p75NTR as when it is applied to cells immunoselected with antibodies to LBP110. The effectiveness of soluble laminin-111 does not necessarily indicate that laminin-111, in a soluble form, is able to activate the receptors responsible for its effect on enteric neuronal development. Even when added as a soluble molecule, laminin-111 might bind to the substrate and then, after becoming bound, activate the receptors on cell surfaces that mediate its effects; nevertheless, the observation that laminin-111 retains its efficacy many hours after cells have adhered to poly-d-lysine, indicates that the ability of laminin-111 to increase the numbers of neurons developing in vitro is not due to the selective adherence of neurogenic crest-derived cells to laminin-111 at the time of plating.

As is true of the responses of cells to the addition of a growth factor, the response of immunoselected crest-derived cells to laminin-111 is associated with a rapid, but transient induction of the expression of the *c-fos* protooncogene. The effect of laminin-111 on *c-fos* expression is evident within one hour of adding laminin-111 and is no longer detectable by 24 hours. The *c-fos* response to laminin-1, like the promotion by laminin-111 of neuronal development, is abolished by the IKVAV peptide, but not by control peptides. The specific antagonism by the IKVAV peptide of both the laminin-111-induced development of neurons and the expression of *c-fos* suggests that both of these responses are mediated by LBP110, which is the cellular binding site for the IKVAV domain of laminin-1. Since the IKVAV peptide is an antagonist, and not an agonist, the observations also imply that activation of the putative receptor function of LBP110 requires more than simply its binding to the IKVAV domain of laminin α1. It is likely that the binding of the IKVAV domain to laminin-111 is necessary but not sufficient to stimulate the LBP110 receptor. Other sequences of laminin-111 and/or the whole laminin-111 molecule must be required for agonist activity. Although the IKVAV peptide does not stimulate LBP110, however, its presence in excess in the medium indicates that it probably occupies IKVAV binding sites on LBP110 and competitively antagonizes the binding of laminin-111.

These ideas have recently been supported by additional experiments that have shown that an antipeptide neutralizing antibody directed against the IKVAV domain of the α1 chain of laminin-111 mimics the effect of the IKVAV peptide and blocks the promotion of the development of enteric neurons in vitro by laminin-111 [294]. In contrast, precipitating antibodies to the β1 chain of laminin-111, applied in the same manner, fail to interfere with the in vitro differentiation of enteric neurons. Neither the antibodies to the α1 chain, nor those to the β1 chain, cause cells to detach from a laminin-111-containing substrate. Laminin-111 promotes the extension of neurites, as well as the development of neurons. This action is also specifically antagonized by an IKVAV peptide and by antibodies to the IKVAV domain of laminin α1.

3.17 The Effects of Laminin-111 on Crest-Derived Cells Immunoselected from the Fetal Bowel Are Different from Those of Laminin-111 on Cells Isolated from the Crest Itself

In contrast to its action on crest-derived cells immunoselected from the fetal gut, laminin-111 does not induce neural crest stem cells to differentiate as neurons [278, 295]. The ability of crest-derived neuronal precursors to respond to laminin-111 must thus be a characteristic the cells acquire, either while migrating to the bowel, or after they enter it. The difference in responsivity to laminin-111 between neural crest stem cells and their crest-derived successors, could be accounted for by the timing of LBP110 expression. Although premigratory and early-migrating crest cells express integrins, and thus are able to bind to laminin [98, 267, 268, 270, 271], which is abundant in the embryonic mesenchyme and basal laminae [258, 259, 296, 297], premigratory and early-migrating crest cells do not express LBP110 [259]. LBP110 is expressed only in target organs; moreover, the crest-derived emigres that colonize the bowel express LBP110 for the first time within the gut itself. If the induction of neuronal development by laminin-111 depends on the interaction of LBP110 with the IKVAV domain of the α1 chain of laminin-111, as suggested by the in vitro studies outlined above, then enteric neuronal precursors could adhere to laminin-111 while migrating to the bowel without being induced to prematurely differentiate into neurons. The premature differentiation of crest-derived cells into neurons prior to their arrival in the gut would prevent them from colonizing the bowel. Neurons are not notably migratory; thus, for ganglia to develop within a given region of the bowel, that region must first be colonized by crest-derived neural precursors. Crest-derived cells, within the gut, acquire LBP110 asynchronously. Some of the vagal crest-derived emigres express LBP110 as soon they enter the proximal bowel. Others, however, acquire LBP110 later and by the time they express LBP110, they have moved distally [259]. This asynchronous delay in the timing of LBP110 expression may enable the late-responding crest-derived cells to make their way distally into the caudal bowel before they differentiate and cease migrating.

3.18 Premature Neuronal Differentiation May Result When Inadequately Resistant Progenitors Encounter an Excessively Permissive Extracellular Matrix

The expression of LBP110 and the evidently related ability of laminin-111 to promote enteric neuronal development from crest-derived precursors may explain the seemingly paradoxical association of an excess of laminin-111 with aganglionosis in the terminal colon of EDN3-deficient *EDN3*$^{ls/ls}$ mice and human patients with Hirschsprung disease. As has been noted previously, it is possible that the deficiency of EDN3 removes an inhibitory influence on neuronal differentiation [111, 113, 254]. By simultaneously leading to an excess laminin-111 in the colonic mesenchyme, the lack of EDN3 also causes crest-derived cells to become exposed to an overabundance of laminin-111, a signal that promotes neuronal development. On the one hand, a brake (EDN3) to neuronal differentiation is absent, while on the other hand, a drive to differentiate (laminin-111) is enhanced. The consequence of the combined effect may be the premature differentiation of crest-derived emigres as neurons. Premature differentiation in turn causes the cells to cease migrating before colonization of the gut is complete. The genetic deficiency of EDN3 may thus exert both direct and indirect effects, which combine synergistically to prevent the formation of ganglia in the terminal bowel. Effects of EDN3 deficiency include allowing crest-derived cells to become trapped by their attraction to GDNF in the caecum, allowing accumulation of semaphorin A, enhancing synthesis of laminin-111, allowing exhaustion of the supply of proliferating precursor cells to occur, enabling premature neuronal differentiation. These ideas predict that vagal crest-derived cells of $EDN3^{ls/ls}$ mice (or the subset of patients with Hirschsprung disease with defects in EDN3 or the EDNRB) would encounter an abnormally strong inducement to differentiate (the over-abundance of laminin-111) when they enter the proximal colon. Consistent with this prediction is the observation that the progression of crest-derived cells, visualized in $EDN3^{ls/ls}$ mice by their expression of the *DBH-lacZ* transgene, is comparable to that in wild-type animals until the cells cross the ileocecal threshold, but becomes abnormal immediately thereafter [70].

Since laminin-111 is present in excess in the pelvic mesenchyme that surrounds the bowel, the hypothesis also predicts that sacral crest-derived precursors will not even enter the gut [251]. This prediction too has been confirmed, in that unique ectopic ganglia are present outside the terminal bowel in $EDN3^{ls/ls}$ mice [175, 248]. It is likely that these extra-enteric ganglia are formed by migrating sacral crest-derived cells that prematurely differentiate and stop before entering the gut. In the hypoganglionic region of the $EDN3^{ls/ls}$ colon, the aberrant ganglia actually pierce the longitudinal muscle and fuse with ganglia of the myenteric plexus. This peculiar configuration of ganglia, partly in and partly out of the gut, provides strong support for the idea that sacral crest-derived cells cease migrating short of their destination in the $EDN3^{ls/ls}$ bowel. This concept, that the aganglionosis of EDN3 deficiency (or absence of EDNRB) has a dual origin in an abnormal extracellular matrix driving an inadequately resistant crest-derived progenitor, would account for the observations that the failure of neurogenesis in the terminal bowel in these conditions is not neural crest-autonomous.

3.19 Both Crest-Derived and Non-neuronal Cells of the Colon Probably Respond to EDN3

There is evidence that EDN3 affects both crest-derived and non-crest-derived cells in the colon. Clearly, the excess of laminin-111, which occurs independently of crest-derived cells in the $EDN3^{ls/ls}$ bowel, is most easily explained by the postulate that EDN3 normally acts on one or more of the cells of the fetal enteric mesenchyme to downregulate their secretion of laminin-111. This postulate assumes that the EDNRB must be expressed, not only by crest-derived cells, but also by other cells of the fetal mesenchyme. Smooth muscle precursors and cells that form interstitial cells of Cajal (ICCs) are each candidates. In the mature gut, EDNRBs have been demonstrated to be expressed by the smooth muscle cells of the muscularis externa of both the large intestine [298] and small intestine [299]; moreover, intestinal smooth muscle responds directly to EDN3. When, during development, smooth muscle cells acquire EDNRBs is unknown. Transcripts encoding EDN3 and those encoding EDNRB are each found in the totally aganglionic bowel of *Ret* knockout, confirming (albeit indirectly) that enteric neuronal and glial precursors are not the only cells in the bowel wall that synthesize these molecules.

Direct evidence that non-neuronal cells contain mRNA encoding the EDNRB has been provided by in situ hybridization carried out in mice in which the crest-derived cells are marked by their expression of the *DBHlacZ* transgene (Kapur R and Yanagisawa M, reported at the 1996 Meeting of the American Motility Society). Both the *lacZ*-expressing crest-derived cells in primordial myenteric ganglia and non-*lacZ*-expressing cells that surround the ganglia were found to express the EDNRB. The location of the *lacZ*-negative cells that contain mRNA encoding the EDNRB is compatible with the idea that these cells are ICCs. That possibility must still be confirmed; however, ICCs have been found to be abnormal in patients with Hirschsprung disease [300, 301].

3.20 Interstitial Cells of Cajal Are Present, but Abnormal, in the Aganglionic Bowel of Hirschsprung Disease

The nature of the ICC has long been the subject of debate [302, 303]. An old idea that ICCs might be fibroblasts [304] has now been discarded [304]. A more recent suggestion is that

ICCs are modified or primitive smooth muscle cells [305, 306]. Whether or not they are related to smooth muscle, ICCs can be identified as a distinct cell type by their expression of, and dependence on, the *ckit* protooncogene [307–309]. *c-kit* encodes a receptor tyrosine kinase (Kit) and is allelic with *White Spotting* (*W*) [310]. Kit ligand (KL; also known as *Steel* factor or stem cell factor) is allelic with *Steel* (*Sl*). Activation of Kit by KL is probably critical for the development and/or maintenance of ICCs, because *W* [307, 311] and *Sl* [308] mutations interfere with the appearance of ICCs, the injection of neutralizing antibodies to Kit causes ICCs to disappear [309, 312], and the development of Kit-expressing ICCs in vitro is dependent on KL in the culture medium [260]. ICCs appear to be the pacemakers for myogenic intestinal slow waves because these waves are impaired when the network of ICCs is lost or fails to develop [307–309, 311, 312]. Once the ICC network is disrupted and slow waves are lost, intestinal motility becomes abnormal and the bowel dilates in a manner that is not dissimilar to that seen in aganglionosis.

During fetal development and, in some regions (the longitudinal muscle) extending into postnatal life, ICCs express markers in common with smooth muscle cells [302]. These markers include the intermediate filament protein, desmin, and smooth muscle isoforms of actin and myosin. ICCs never express Ret, which can serve as a marker for crest-derived cells in the wall of the gut [127, 128, 135]. These observations suggest that ICCs are not crest-derived cells, but that instead, they share a common precursor with smooth muscle. A similar conclusion has been reached from studies of stably marked crest-derived cells in avian interspecies chimeras [313]. Interestingly, Kit-immunoreactive ICCs assume a variety of shapes in different locations in the intestinal wall and may be divided by the timing of their divergence from the common smooth muscle/ICC precursor into subtypes of ICC [302]. It has been proposed that those ICCs that surround myenteric ganglia and those that are found within the deep muscle plexus, circular, and longitudinal muscle layers constitute functionally distinct cell classes [314].

Since ICCs are not crest-derived cells, it follows that their abnormality in the affected region of the bowel of patients with Hirschsprung disease [300, 301, 314, 315] demonstrates that the genetic lesion in these patients affects more cells than just neurons and their precursors. ICCs, however, are reduced in number and disrupted in pattern, but they are not totally absent from the aganglionic region of the colon in Hirschsprung disease. ICCs are also found in the terminal colon of *ls/ls* mice and in the aganglionic bowel of *Ret* knockout mice, although again, their numbers are reduced in comparison to those of wild-type mice, and the distribution pattern of ICCs is abnormal. These observations indicate that ICCs can develop in the absence of EDN3 and even in the absence of neurons. Conceivably, the abnormal numbers and distribution of ICCs in the aganglionic bowel of patients with Hirschsprung disease and *ls/ls* mice are secondary effects, resulting from the aganglionosis. Supporting this possibility, in situ hybridization has indicated that enteric neurons do contain transcripts encoding KL [302]. Enteric neurons thus are likely to be a source of KL; moreover, the physiologically active form of KL is not the secreted protein, but a membrane-bound ligand [316, 317]. To be stimulated by neuronal KL, therefore, neurons probably must come into contact with target cells so that the Kit receptors of the targets can be activated by the KL bound to neuronal surfaces. The requirement that cell-to-cell contact must occur for the KL/Kit interaction to take place could explain the close spatial relationship of a subset of ICCs to myenteric ganglia. It could also explain the paucity of ICC of the myenteric type in the aganglionic region of the Hirschsprung bowel [314, 315].

The aganglionosis of Hirschsprung disease and that of $EDN3^{ls/ls}$ mice, therefore, might each be expected to be associated with ICC abnormalities; the KL-dependent ICCs would be deprived of neuronal KL in the aganglionic bowel in these conditions. Neurons, however, are probably not the only source of KL in the bowel. First, if they were, then ICCs would be expected to be totally absent from the aganglionic zone of the Hirschsprung and $EDN3^{ls/ls}$ colon, but they are not. Second, ICCs develop in the *Ret* knockout gut, which contains no neurons at all; moreover, mRNA encoding KL (as well as that encoding Kit) can be detected in this tissue. It is possible that ICCs do not require EDN3 for their development, but they might still express the EDNRB and be EDN3-responsive. The abnormalities noted in the numbers and distribution of ICCs in the aganglionic regions of the Hirschsprung and *EDN3*$^{ls/ls}$ colons are consistent with this idea. Certainly, the location of the non-neuronal cells of the colon of *DBH-lacZ* mice found by in situ hybridization to contain mRNA encoding the EDNRB conforms to the known location of Kit-immunoreactive ICCs in the bowel. One might speculate that EDN3 speeds the development of ICCs or smooth muscle. In its absence, the respective precursors might remain secretory for a longer period of time than normal and secrete more laminin-111. As the cells mature as smooth muscle and/or ICCs, laminin-111 secretion diminishes. This hypothesis is consistent with the observed developmental regulation of laminin-111 and the slower than normal rate of decline found in its expression in the *EDN3*$^{ls/ls}$ colon [253].

3.21 Serotonin (5-HT) and Cross-talk Between Progenitors in the Developing ENS

Crest-derived precursors of enteric neurons interact, not only with the microenvironment they encounter as they migrate to and within the bowel, but they also interact with one another. Serotonergic neurons, which are among the first neurons to arise during ontogeny [104], synapse on dividing precursors in the developing guinea pig ENS [318]; moreover, in mice that lack tryptophan hydroxylase 2, which is essential for neuronal biosynthesis of 5-HT, the ENS is profoundly hypoplastic [319]. The same defect, a hypoplastic ENS, also occurs in mice with a gain-of-function mutation (G56A) in the serotonin transporter (SERT; *Slc6a4*). SERT takes up 5-HT, which has the effect of removing it from its receptors. The overly active G56A isoform of SERT removes 5-HT so fast that it does not have the opportunity to activate its receptors adequately [320]. In contrast, a hyperplastic ENS develops in mice that lack SERT or which have been treated during gestation with a selective serotonin-reuptake inhibitor (SSRI) [320]. ENS hyper- and hypoplasia each cause gastrointestinal motility to be abnormal.

Many subtypes of 5-HT receptor are expressed in the bowel during ontogeny and in adult life. Of these, the 5-HT$_4$ receptor has been most extensively studied with respect to mediation of the developmental effects of 5-HT. Both 5-HT and 5-HT$_4$ receptor agonists, such as tegaserod and prucalopride, enhance enteric neurogenesis when they are applied to isolated enteric crest-derived cells in vitro; moreover, the neurogenic effects of each are blocked by 5-HT$_4$ receptor antagonists [196, 319]. Similarly, 5-HT and 5-HT$_4$ agonists promote enteric neurogenesis, even in adult bowel *in vivo*, and again, 5-HT$_4$-promoted neurogenesis is 5-blocked by HT$_4$ antagonists [196, 321, 322]. These observations imply that 5-HT from enteric serotonergic neurons is necessary for adequate neurogenesis in the developing and mature ENS. Importantly a 5-HT$_4$ receptor agonist, such as prucalopride, rescues ENS development and prevents abnormal gastrointestinal motility in mice that carry the overly active G56A isoform of SERT [320]. Early-born enteric serotonergic neurons may thus unwittingly be affected by drugs used during pregnancy. Depression is commonly treated with tricyclic antidepressants or SSRIs and drugs of abuse (cocaine, for example) may be taken by pregnant or lactating women. These compounds all alter the function of serotonergic neurons and thus, by changing the development of the ENS, the drugs may lead to unanticipated and long-lasting effects on the ENS of offspring [320, 323].

SERT is transiently expressed during CNS development in glutamatergic neurons [324–327]. Although these neurons do not synthesize 5-HT, their ability to take it up enables them to utilize 5-HT, which they do to help pattern the innervation of the sensory cortex. It is likely that SERT expression in the developing ENS is also not limited to serotonergic neurons. The role of SERT-mediated 5-HT uptake in ENS development appears to be important but has not yet been fully explored. SERT is expressed in the gut, not only in the ENS, but also in the enterocytes of the fetal and adult gastrointestinal mucosa; moreover, SERT is functional in the early fetal endoderm and ENS even before 5-HT itself can be detected [328]. Epithelial SERT probably helps to compartmentalize the bowel wall and prevent the ENS from becoming swamped by the very large amount of 5-HT that mucosal enterochromaffin cells constitutively secrete. If it were to reach the ENS, mucosal 5-HT would make it impossible for the much smaller quantity of enteric neuronal 5-HT to function properly [329]. 5-HT is a multifunctional molecule. It is not only a neurotransmitter, a paracrine factor, and a hormone [329], but also a growth factor that is critical for ENS ontogeny and its clinical effects, though currently unknown, may be highly significant.

3.22 Deficiency of Platelet-Derived Growth Factor Receptor-α-Expressing Cells in Hirschsprung Disease Colon

Gastrointestinal smooth muscle contraction is controlled by coordinated interaction of three main cell types: enteric nerve cells, intestinal cells of Cajal (ICCs), and smooth muscle cells (SMCs). In recent years, a fourth cell type has been described as forming part of this complex network, namely platelet-derived growth factor receptor alpha-positive cells (PDGFRα$^+$-cells). These PDGFRα$^+$-cells were, for many years, known as "fibroblast-like cells" or "ICC-like" cells, as they resembled ICCs morphologically, but were c-kit negative [330]. More recently, enhanced green fluorescent protein (eGFP) labeling of these cells, as well as commercial availability of antibodies directed against PDGFRα, has enabled specific and reliable identification of this cell type [331]. PDGFRα$^+$-cells form discrete networks in the region of the myenteric plexus and within the circular and longitudinal muscle layers [332]. PDGFRα$^+$-cells express the small-conductance Ca^{2+}-activated K^+ channel (SK3), which is an important mediator of purinergic neurotransmission in gastrointestinal smooth muscle [332, 333].

Many studies have investigated the expression of PDGFRα$^+$-cells in the gastrointestinal tract of various animals in recent years. Iino et al. [330] who were the first authors to examine PDGFRα$^+$-cells found that they form a cellular network with their ramified processes and encompass myenteric ganglia. Kurahashi et al. [334] were the first group to confirm a functional role for PDGFRα$^+$-cells in gastrointestinal smooth muscle using transgenic mice with constitutive expression of enhanced green fluorescent protein (eGFP) in PDGFRα$^+$-cells. The eGFP label allowed the authors to isolate and study the function of PDGFRα$^+$-cells. They found that PDGFRα$^+$-cells expressed appropriate receptors and effectors to receive and transduce purinergic neural signals [334]. O'Donnell et al. [335] have verified that the mucosal PDGFRα$^+$-cells in the human colon, like that of the mouse, also express TLR4, TLR5 and P2RY1, suggesting a role for these cells in the immune response and in purinergic neurotransmission. The results of their study have revealed that there are many fewer PDGFRα$^+$-cells in both ganglionic and aganglionic regions of the bowel in patients with Hirschsprung disease than in control colon [335]. The same authors have also shown that the expression of both ICCs and small conductance Ca^{2+}-activated K^+ (SK3) channels is much less than normal in Hirschsprung disease colon [315, 336]. The reduced expression of PDGFRα$^+$-cells is consistent with the existence of a deficiency in inhibitory neurotransmission in Hirschsprung disease bowel and may contribute to the state of tonic contraction of aganglionic segments of gut [335].

3.23 Hirschsprung Disease Is Associated with Many Different Genetic Abnormalities: Conclusion from Animal Models

Congenital neuromuscular disorders of the gut are commonly encountered during the neonatal period. These conditions include, in addition to

Hirschsprung disease (long- and short-segment varieties), the allied disorders, hypoganglionosis, neuronal intestinal dysplasia (hyperganglionosis), ganglion cell immaturity, and dysganglionoses. There are also additional defects such as hypertrophic pyloric stenosis, volvulus, and intussusception that may also involve abnormalities of the development of the ENS. HSCR is quite common and occurs in up to 1 in 5000 live births [337]. The major susceptibility gene is the *RET* protooncogene [47, 337–345]. Hirschsprung disease has been shown to be associated with loss-of-function mutations in the coding sequence of *RET* mutations [337–339] or with non-coding regions that reduce expression of RET protein [47, 342–345]. Both long- and short-segment Hirschsprung disease can occur in patients with identical *RET* abnormalities and patients may also exhibit other problems, including multiple endocrine neoplasia type A (more commonly associated with gain-of-function mutations in *RET*), maternal deafness, talipes, and malrotation of the gut. Identical mutations in *RET* may thus give rise to distinctly different phenotypes in affected individuals. Unfortunately, there is no obvious relationship between the *RET* genotype and the Hirschsprung phenotype; moreover, the frequency of coding mutations of *RET* in Hirschsprung disease is sufficiently low that other genetic and/ or environmental conditions must be invoked to explain susceptibility to Hirschsprung disease in the majority of patients. Another genetic defect that has been associated with Hirschsprung disease involves mutations in *EDNRB,* which accounts for many fewer instances of the disorder than *RET* (<5% of isolated cases) [234, 346]. Again, many patients with Hirschsprung disease do not exhibit mutations of *EDNRB* or *RET* and there are individuals who carry these mutations (and also those of *RET*) who do not express the Hirschsprung disease phenotype [234]. As might be expected, not only are some cases of Hirschsprung disease linked to mutations in *EDNRB*, but mutations of genes encoding the ligand, EDN3, are also associated with Hirschsprung disease, albeit rarely [346]. In the case of the *EDN3* mutations, the phenotype is reminiscent of that which is seen in $EDN3^{ls/ls}$ mice. Hirschsprung disease occurs together with pigmentary abnormalities and is combined with a Waardenburg type 4 or 2 phenotype (Shah-Waardenburg syndrome) [346–348]. Hirschsprung disease is thus a multigene abnormality and a wide variety of mutations (many of which are still to be identified) predispose toward it [47, 234, 282, 337, 342–345]. The environmental background within which these mutations operate also influences the phenotypic outcome. A major whole-genome sequencing study has recently expanded the known genes that increase the risk for Hirschsprung disease [282]. This study identified 4 susceptibility loci, including one in the phospholipase D1 gene. The patients in the new whole genome analysis had a significant excess of rare protein-altering variants in genes that were already known to be associated with Hirschsprung disease, but an excess was also found in the gene encoding BACE2. Many common and distinct pathways were identified that enhanced risk of Hirschsprung disease when they were associated with variants in RET. The study linked BACE-1, β-amyloid precursor protein and BACE-2 to Hirschsprung disease.

3.24 Conclusion

The ENS is a complex and independent nervous system that is formed by precursors that migrate to the bowel from vagal, truncal, and sacral regions of the neural crest. Very recently, a claim has been made that endodermal pancreatic duodenal homeobox-1-expressing cells also contribute to the murine ENS [349]. The crest-derived enteric neuronal progenitors are initially multipotent; however, their developmental potential decreases as a function of time and place during ontogeny [350]. The crest-derived emigres that arrive in the bowel have lost the potential to give rise to some derivatives, such as ectomesenchyme and melanocytes, but the emigres retain a high degree of multipotency and their ultimate fate is influenced by the enteric microenvironment. The effects of the microenvironment are played out on cells that vary in their receptivity according to the lineages and sublineages into which they have been sorted. One set of neurons is born early, is transiently catecholaminergic, is dependent on expression of the *Ascl-1* gene, and gives rise to serotonergic neurons. The other, from which CGRP-containing neurons are derived, is born late, is never catecholaminergic, and is *Ascl-1*-independent. A variety of signals have been identified that influence the differentiation and/or survival of enteric neurons. An early-acting factor is GDNF, which activates the Ret receptor. Other factors, such as EDN3, the neurotrophin, NT-3, neuropoietic cytokines, and laminin-111 act later.

Natural or targeted mutations in genes that encode factors required by crest-derived precursors early in development affect cells that are still relatively multipotent; therefore, the resulting defects tend to be large, such as those associated with the deletion of GDNF or Ret. Later-acting factors give rise to many fewer global abnormalities, although even a small loss of a critical neuron may be lethal. Knockout of CNTFRα, which results in an apparent loss of motor fibers to smooth muscle, is an example. A still more localized abnormality occurs in mice lacking EDN3 or EDNRB. The terminal colon of these animals becomes aganglionic. This defect may result from an effect of the mutation both on the crest-derived precursors of enteric neurons and on the non-neuronal cells of the bowel wall that produce the matrix through which crest-derived cells must migrate to colonize the gut. There is an excess of laminin-111 in the colon of EDNRB signaling-deficient animals and humans that may combine with the loss of the effect of EDN3 on crest-derived cells to cause premature differentiation of precursors as neurons. Since neurons do not migrate, the consequence of premature differentiation is an early cessation of migration leading to a distal aganglionosis. Many mutations have been associated with Hirschsprung disease, although the most important contributing gene is *RET* [282].

Hirschsprung disease is a multigene abnormality that cannot be completely accounted for by known mutations or easily identified by genetic testing [282, 342, 343]. Each of the many factors that are critical for the formation of the normal ENS [114] are potential targets of mutations that might cause Hirschsprung disease or other birth defects in humans. Future research should begin to reveal genes that, when abnormal, cause not just an aganglionosis, but hypoganglionosis, neuronal intestinal dysplasia, and intestinal dysganglionoses, as well as additional contributors to Hirschsprung disease. Hopefully, progress made in understanding the pathogenesis of Hirschsprung disease and allied disorders will provide better means of treating these conditions and, better yet, preventing them.

During the last decade, there has been much progress in the understanding of ENS development including how neural crest-derived progenitors migrate and colonize the bowel, the formation of ganglionated plexuses, and the molecular mechanisms of enteric neural and glial diversification [12, 47, 114, 282, 351]. Recent advances have highlighted the potential of enteric neural stem cell transplantation as a possible treatment option for enteric neuropathies including Hirschsprung disease [352]. Much research has already resulted in the development of robust and reproducible methodologies to facilitate the harvesting and propagation of neural stem cells, their potential and safety in murine models. Recent studies have transplanted human enteric neural progenitors into the mouse colon and shown engraftment [352, 353]. The identification and isolation of neuronal progenitor cells from the human postnatal intestine raise the possibility of transplanting these cells to replace missing neurons in patients with Hirschsprung disease.

References

1. Teitelbaum DH. Hirschsprung's disease in children. Curr Opin Pediatr. 1995;7(3):316–22.
2. Larsson LT. Hirschsprung's disease – immunohistochemical findings. Histol Histopathol. 1994;9(3):615–29.
3. Furness JB. The enteric nervous system. Malden: Blackwell Publishing; 2006. p. 1–274.
4. Wood JD. Excitation of intestinal muscle by atropine, tetrodotoxin, and xylocaine. Am J Physiol. 1972;222(1):118–25.
5. Sullivan PB. Hirschprung's disease. Arch Dis Child. 1996;74(1):5–7.
6. Skinner MA. Hirschsprung's disease. Curr Probl Surg. 1996;33(5):389–460.

7. Holschneider AM, Meier-Ruge W, Ure BM. Hirschsprung's disease and allied disorders – a review. Eur J Pediatr Surg. 1994;4(5):260–6.
8. Qualman SJ, Murray R. Aganglionosis and related disorders. Hum Pathol. 1994;25(11):1141–9.
9. Rogawski MA, Goodrich JT, Gershon MD, Touloukian RJ. Hirschsprung's disease: absence of serotonergic neurons in the aganglionic colon. J Pediatr Surg. 1978;13(6D):608–15.
10. Teramoto M, Domoto T, Tanigawa K, Yasui Y, Tamura K. Distribution of nitric oxide synthase-containing nerves in the aganglionic intestine of mutant rats: a histochemical study. J Gastroenterol. 1996;31(2):214–23.
11. Tomita R, Munakata K, Kurosu Y, Tanjoh K. A role of nitric oxide in Hirschsprung's disease. J Pediatr Surg. 1995;30(3):437–40.
12. Nagy N, Goldstein AM. Enteric nervous system development: a crest cell's journey from neural tube to colon. Semin Cell Dev Biol. 2017;66:94–106.
13. Gershon MD. The second brain. Harper Collins: New York; 1998. 312 p.
14. Bayliss WM, Starling EH. The movements and innervation of the small intestine. J Physiol (Lond). 1899;24:99–143.
15. Bayliss WM, Starling EH. The movements and innervation of the small intestine. J Physiol (Lond). 1900;26:125–38.
16. Trendelenburg P. Physiologische und pharmakologische Versuche über die Dünndarm Peristaltick. Naunyn-Schmiedebergs Arch Exp Pathol Pharmakol. 1917;81:55–129.
17. Langley JN. The autonomic nervous system, part 1. Cambridge: W. Heffer; 1921.
18. Bayliss WM, Starling EH. The movements and innervation of the small intestine. J Physiol. 1899;24(2):99–143.
19. Bayliss WM, Starling EH. The movements and the innervation of the large intestine. J Physiol. 1900;26(1-2):107–18.
20. Trendelenburg P. Physiological and pharmacological investigations of small intestinal peristalsis. Translation of the article "Physiologische und pharmakologische Versuche uber die Dunndarmperistaltik", Arch Exp Pathol Pharmakol 81:55–129, 1917. Naunyn Schmiedebergs Arch Pharmacol. 2006;373(2):101–33.
21. Gabella G. Glial cells in the myenteric plexus. Z Naturforsch B. 1971;26(3):244–5.
22. Gabella G. Ultrastructure of the nerve plexuses of the mammalian intestine: the enteric glial cells. Neuroscience. 1981;6(3):425–36.
23. Gershon MD, Rothman TP. Enteric glia. Glia. 1991;4(2):195–204.
24. Rao M, Nelms BD, Dong L, Salinas-Rios V, Rutlin M, Gershon MD, et al. Enteric glia express proteolipid protein 1 and are a transcriptionally unique population of glia in the mammalian nervous system. Glia. 2015;11:2042–57.
25. Rao M, Rastelli D, Dong L, Chiu S, Setlik W, Gershon MD, et al. Enteric glia regulate gastrointestinal motility but are not required for maintenance of the epithelium in mice. Gastroenterology. 2017;153(4):1068–81.67.
26. Cooke HJ. Role of the "little brain" in the gut in water and electrolyte homeostasis. FASEB J. 1989;3(2):127–38.
27. Furness JB, Stebbing MJ. The first brain: Species comparisons and evolutionary implications for the enteric and central nervous systems. Neurogastroenterol Motil. 2018;30(2) https://doi.org/10.1111/nmo.13234.
28. Crowcroft PJ, Holman ME, Szurszewski JH. Excitatory input from the distal colon to the inferior mesenteric ganglion in the guinea-pig. J Physiol. 1971;219(2):443–61.
29. Kreulen DL, Szurszewski JH. Reflex pathways in the abdominal prevertebral ganglia: evidence for a colocolonic inhibitory reflex. J Physiol. 1979;295:21–32.
30. Szurszewski JH. Physiology of mammalian prevertebral ganglia. Annu Rev Physiol. 1981;43:53–68.
31. Mawe GM, Gershon MD. Structure, afferent innervation, and transmitter content of ganglia of the guinea pig gallbladder: relationship to the enteric nervous system. J Comp Neurol. 1989;283(3):374–90.
32. Kirchgessner AL, Gershon MD. Innervation of the pancreas by neurons in the gut. J Neurosci. 1990;10(5):1626–42.
33. Kirchgessner AL, Gershon MD. Presynaptic inhibition by serotonin of nerve-mediated secretion of pancreatic amylase. Am J Physiol. 1995;268(2 Pt 1):G339–45.
34. Gershon MD. Developmental determinants of the independence and complexity of the enteric nervous system. Trends Neurosci. 2010;33(10):446–56.
35. Scheuermann DW, Stach W. Fluorescence microscopic study of the architecture and structure of an adrenergic network in the plexus myentericus (Auerbach), plexus submucosus externus (Schabadasch) and plexus submucosus internus (Meissner) of the porcine small intestine. Acta Anat (Basel). 1984;119(1):49–59.
36. Timmermans JP, Scheuermann DW, Stach W, Adriaensen D, De Groodt-Lasseel MH. Distinct distribution of CGRP-, enkephalin-, galanin-, neuromedin U-, neuropeptide Y-, somatostatin-, substance P-, VIP- and serotonin-containing neurons in the two submucosal ganglionic neural networks of the porcine small intestine. Cell Tissue Res. 1990;260(2):367–79.
37. Bulbring E, Lin RC, Schofield G. An investigation of the peristaltic reflex in relation to anatomical observations. Q J Exp Physiol Cogn Med Sci. 1958;43(1):26–37.
38. Kirchgessner AL, Tamir H, Gershon MD. Identification and stimulation by serotonin of intrinsic sensory neurons of the submucosal plexus of the guinea pig gut: activity-induced expression of Fos immunoreactivity. J Neurosci. 1992;12(1):235–48.
39. Bornstein JC, Furness JB. Correlated electrophysiological and histochemical studies of submucous neurons and their contribution to understanding enteric neural circuits. J Auton Nerv Syst. 1988;25(1):1–13.

40. Frieling T, Cooke HJ, Wood JD. Electrophysiological properties of neurons in submucosal ganglia of guinea pig distal colon. Am J Physiol. 1991;260(6 Pt 1):G835–41.
41. Jiang MM, Kirchgessner A, Gershon MD, Surprenant A. Cholera toxin-sensitive neurons in guinea pig submucosal plexus. Am J Physiol. 1993;264(1 Pt 1):G86–94.
42. Hendriks R, Bornstein JC, Furness JB. An electrophysiological study of the projections of putative sensory neurons within the myenteric plexus of the guinea pig ileum. Neurosci Lett. 1990;110:286–90.
43. Kunze WA, Bornstein JC, Furness JB. Identification of sensory nerve cells in a peripheral organ (the intestine) of a mammal. Neuroscience. 1995;66:1–4.
44. Wattchow DA, Brookes SJ, Costa M. The morphology and projections of retrogradely labeled myenteric neurons in the human intestine. Gastroenterology. 1995;109(3):866–75.
45. Rao M, Gershon MD. The bowel and beyond: the enteric nervous system in neurological disorders. Nat Rev Gastroenterol Hepatol. 2016;13(9):517–28.
46. Kuntz A. The autonomic nervous system. Philadelphia: Lea and Febiger; 1953.
47. Bondurand N, Southard-Smith EM. Mouse models of Hirschsprung disease and other developmental disorders of the enteric nervous system: old and new players. Dev Biol. 2016;417(2):139–57.
48. Yntema CL, Hammond WS. The origin of intrinsic ganglia of trunk viscera from vagal neural crest in the chick embryo. J Comp Neurol. 1954;101(2):515–41.
49. Le Douarin NM, Teillet MA. The migration of neural crest cells to the wall of the digestive tract in avian embryo. J Embryol Exp Morphol. 1973;30(1):31–48.
50. Allan IJ, Newgreen DF. The origin and differentiation of enteric neurons of the intestine of the fowl embryo. Am J Anat. 1980;157(2):137–54.
51. Rothman TP, Gershon MD. Phenotypic expression in the developing murine enteric nervous system. J Neurosci. 1982;2(3):381–93.
52. Gershon MD, Chalazonitis A, Rothman TP. From neural crest to bowel: development of the enteric nervous system. J Neurobiol. 1993;24(2):199–214.
53. Coulter HD, Gershon MD, Rothman TP. Neural and glial phenotypic expression by neural crest cells in culture: effects of control and presumptive aganglionic bowel from ls/ls mice. J Neurobiol. 1988;19(6):507–31.
54. Mackey HM, Payette RF, Gershon MD. Tissue effects on the expression of serotonin, tyrosine hydroxylase and GABA in cultures of neurogenic cells from the neuraxis and branchial arches. Development. 1988;104(2):205–17.
55. Serbedzija GN, Burgan S, Fraser SE, Bronner-Fraser M. Vital dye labelling demonstrates a sacral neural crest contribution to the enteric nervous system of chick and mouse embryos. Development. 1991;111(4):857–66.
56. Pomeranz HD, Rothman TP, Gershon MD. Colonization of the post-umbilical bowel by cells derived from the sacral neural crest: direct tracing of cell migration using an intercalating probe and a replication-deficient retrovirus. Development. 1991;111(3):647–55.
57. Espinosa-Medina I, Jevans B, Boismoreau F, Chettouh Z, Enomoto H, Muller T, et al. Dual origin of enteric neurons in vagal Schwann cell precursors and the sympathetic neural crest. Proc Natl Acad Sci U S A. 2017;114(45):11980–5.
58. Uesaka T, Young HM, Pachnis V, Enomoto H. Development of the intrinsic and extrinsic innervation of the gut. Dev Biol. 2016;417(2):158–67.
59. Uesaka T, Nagashimada M, Enomoto H. Neuronal differentiation in Schwann cell lineage underlies postnatal neurogenesis in the enteric nervous system. J Neurosci. 2015;35(27):9879–88.
60. Tam PK, Lister J. Development profile of neuron-specific enolase in human gut and its implications in Hirschsprung's disease. Gastroenterology. 1986;90(6):1901–6.
61. Toyohara T, Nada O, Nagasaki A, Goto S, Ikeda K. An immunohistochemical study of serotoninergic nerves in the colon and rectum of children with Hirschsprung's disease. Acta Neuropathol. 1985;68(4):306–10.
62. Durbec PL, Larsson-Blomberg LB, Schuchardt A, Costantini F, Pachnis V. Common origin and developmental dependence on c-ret of subsets of enteric and sympathetic neuroblasts. Development. 1996;122(1):349–58.
63. Epstein ML, Mikawa T, Brown AM, McFarlin DR. Mapping the origin of the avian enteric nervous system with a retroviral marker. Dev Dyn. 1994;201(3):236–44.
64. Kuo BR, Erickson CA. Regional differences in neural crest morphogenesis. Cell Adh Migr. 2010;4(4):567–85.
65. Barlow AJ, Wallace AS, Thapar N, Burns AJ. Critical numbers of neural crest cells are required in the pathways from the neural tube to the foregut to ensure complete enteric nervous system formation. Development. 2008;135(9):1681–91.
66. Rothman TP, Le Douarin NM, Fontaine-Perus JC, Gershon MD. Developmental potential of neural crest-derived cells migrating from segments of developing quail bowel back-grafted into younger chick host embryos. Development. 1990;109(2):411–23.
67. Rothman TP, Le Douarin NM, Fontaine-Perus JC, Gershon MD. Colonization of the bowel by neural crest-derived cells re-migrating from foregut backtransplanted to vagal or sacral regions of host embryos. Dev Dyn. 1993;196(3):217–33.
68. Kapur RP, Yost C, Palmiter RD. A transgenic model for studying development of the enteric nervous system in normal and aganglionic mice. Development. 1992;116(1):167–75.
69. Kapur RP, Yost C, Palmiter RD. Aggregation chimeras demonstrate that the primary defect responsible for aganglionic megacolon in lethal spotted

mice is not neuroblast autonomous. Development. 1993;117(3):993–9.
70. Coventry S, Yost C, Palmiter RD, Kapur RP. Migration of ganglion cell precursors in the ileoceca of normal and lethal spotted embryos, a murine model for Hirschsprung disease. Lab Invest. 1994;71(1):82–93.
71. Baetge G, Gershon MD. Transient catecholaminergic (TC) cells in the vagus nerves and bowel of fetal mice: relationship to the development of enteric neurons. Dev Biol. 1989;132(1):189–211.
72. Baetge G, Pintar JE, Gershon MD. Transiently catecholaminergic (TC) cells in the bowel of the fetal rat: precursors of noncatecholaminergic enteric neurons. Dev Biol. 1990;141(2):353–80.
73. Baetge G, Schneider KA, Gershon MD. Development and persistence of catecholaminergic neurons in cultured explants of fetal murine vagus nerves and bowel. Development. 1990;110(3):689–701.
74. Blaugrund E, Pham TD, Tennyson VM, Lo L, Sommer L, Anderson DJ, et al. Distinct subpopulations of enteric neuronal progenitors defined by time of development, sympathoadrenal lineage markers and Mash-1-dependence. Development. 1996;122(1):309–20.
75. Kuo BR, Erickson CA. Vagal neural crest cell migratory behavior: a transition between the cranial and trunk crest. Dev Dyn. 2011;240(9):2084–100.
76. Birchmeier C. ErbB receptors and the development of the nervous system. Exp Cell Res. 2009;315(4):611–8.
77. Chalazonitis A, D'Autreaux F, Pham TD, Kessler JA, Gershon MD. Bone morphogenetic proteins regulate enteric gliogenesis by modulating ErbB3 signaling. Dev Biol. 2011;350(1):64–79.
78. Rothman TP, Sherman D, Cochard P, Gershon MD. Development of the monoaminergic innervation of the avian gut: transient and permanent expression of phenotypic markers. Dev Biol. 1986;116(2):357–80.
79. Fontaine-Perus J, Chanconie M, Le Douarin NM. Developmental potentialities in the nonneuronal population of quail sensory ganglia. Dev Biol. 1988;128(2):359–75.
80. Duff RS, Langtimm CJ, Richardson MK, Sieber-Blum M. In vitro clonal analysis of progenitor cell patterns in dorsal root and sympathetic ganglia of the quail embryo. Dev Biol. 1991;147(2):451–9.
81. Ito K, Morita T, Sieber-Blum M. In vitro clonal analysis of mouse neural crest development. Dev Biol. 1993;157(2):517–25.
82. Sieber-Blum M, Cohen AM. Clonal analysis of quail neural crest cells: they are pluripotent and differentiate in vitro in the absence of noncrest cells. Dev Biol. 1980;80(1):96–106.
83. Baroffio A, Dupin E, Le Douarin NM. Clone-forming ability and differentiation potential of migratory neural crest cells. Proc Natl Acad Sci U S A. 1988;85(14):5325–9.
84. Sextier-Sainte-Claire Deville F, Ziller C, Le Douarin N. Developmental potentialities of cells derived from the truncal neural crest in clonal cultures. Brain Res Dev Brain Res. 1992;66(1):1–10.
85. Bronner-Fraser M, Fraser S. Developmental potential of avian trunk neural crest cells in situ. Neuron. 1989;3(6):755–66.
86. Bronner-Fraser M, Fraser SE. Cell lineage analysis reveals multipotency of some avian neural crest cells. Nature. 1988;335(6186):161–4.
87. Fraser SE, Bronner-Fraser M. Migrating neural crest cells in the trunk of the avian embryo are multipotent. Development. 1991;112(4):913–20.
88. Sextier-Sainte-Claire Deville F, Ziller C, Le Douarin NM. Developmental potentials of enteric neural crest-derived cells in clonal and mass cultures. Dev Biol. 1994;163(1):141–51.
89. Lo L, Anderson DJ. Postmigratory neural crest cells expressing c-RET display restricted developmental and proliferative capacities. Neuron. 1995;15(3):527–39.
90. Espinosa-Medina I, Saha O, Boismoreau F, Chettouh Z, Rossi F, Richardson WD, et al. The sacral autonomic outflow is sympathetic. Science. 2016;354(6314):893–7.
91. Kennedy TE, Serafini T, de la Torre JR, Tessier-Lavigne M. Netrins are diffusible chemotropic factors for commissural axons in the embryonic spinal cord. Cell. 1994;78(3):425–35.
92. Serafini T, Kennedy TE, Galko MJ, Mirzayan C, Jessell TM, Tessier-Lavigne M. The netrins define a family of axon outgrowth-promoting proteins homologous to C. elegans UNC-6. Cell. 1994;78(3):409–24.
93. Colamarino SA, Tessier-Lavigne M. The axonal chemoattractant netrin-1 is also a chemorepellent for trochlear motor axons. Cell. 1995;81(4):621–9.
94. Luo Y, Raible D, Raper JA. Collapsin: a protein in brain that induces the collapse and paralysis of neuronal growth cones. Cell. 1993;75(2):217–27.
95. Messersmith EK, Leonardo ED, Shatz CJ, Tessier-Lavigne M, Goodman CS, Kolodkin AL. Semaphorin III can function as a selective chemorepellent to pattern sensory projections in the spinal cord. Neuron. 1995;14(5):949–59.
96. Kolodkin AL. Semaphorins: mediators of repulsive growth cone guidance. Trends Cell Biol. 1996;6(1):15–22.
97. Guthrie S. Axon guidance: starting and stopping with Slit. Curr Biol. 1999;9:R432–R5.
98. Lallier T, Deutzmann R, Perris R, Bronner-Fraser M. Neural crest cell interactions with laminin: structural requirements and localization of the binding site for alpha 1 beta 1 integrin. Dev Biol. 1994;162(2):451–64.
99. Perris R, Paulsson M, Bronner-Fraser M. Molecular mechanisms of avian neural crest cell migration on fibronectin and laminin. Dev Biol. 1989;136(1):222–38.
100. Jiang Y, Liu M, Gershon MD. Netrins and DCC in the guidance of migrating neural crest-derived cells in the developing bowel and pancreas. Dev Biol. 2003;258(2):364–84.
101. Ratcliffe EM, D'Autreaux F, Gershon MD. Laminin terminates the Netrin/DCC mediated attrac-

tion of vagal sensory axons. Dev Neurobiol. 2008;68(7):960–71.
102. Ratcliffe EM, Fan L, Mohammed TJ, Anderson M, Chalazonitis A, Gershon MD. Enteric neurons synthesize netrins and are essential for the development of the vagal sensory innervation of the fetal gut. Dev Neurobiol. 2011;71(5):362–73.
103. Lasrado R, Boesmans W, Kleinjung J, Pin C, Bell D, Bhaw L, et al. Lineage-dependent spatial and functional organization of the mammalian enteric nervous system. Science. 2017;356(6339):722–6.
104. Pham TD, Gershon MD, Rothman TP. Time of origin of neurons in the murine enteric nervous system. J Comp Neurol. 1991;314:789–98.
105. Kabouridis PS, Lasrado R, McCallum S, Chng SH, Snippert HJ, Clevers H, et al. Microbiota controls the homeostasis of glial cells in the gut lamina propria. Neuron. 2015;85(2):289–95.
106. Obata Y, Pachnis V. The effect of microbiota and the immune system on the development and organization of the enteric nervous system. Gastroenterology. 2016;151(5):836–44.
107. Zuhdi N, Ortega B, Giovannone D, Ra H, Reyes M, Asencion V, et al. Slit molecules prevent entrance of trunk neural crest cells in developing gut. Int J Dev Neurosci. 2015;41:8–16.
108. De Bellard ME, Rao Y, Bronner-Fraser M. Dual function of Slit2 in repulsion and enhanced migration of trunk, but not vagal, neural crest cells. J Cell Biol. 2003;162(2):269–79.
109. Simpson MJ, Zhang DC, Mariani M, Landman KA, Newgreen DF. Cell proliferation drives neural crest cell invasion of the intestine. Dev Biol. 2007;302(2):553–68.
110. Young HM, Bergner AJ, Anderson RB, Enomoto H, Milbrandt J, Newgreen DF, et al. Dynamics of neural crest-derived cell migration in the embryonic mouse gut. Dev Biol. 2004;270(2):455–73.
111. Wu JJ, Chen J-X, Rothman TP, Gershon MD. Inhibition of *in vitro* enteric neuronal development by endothelin-3: mediation by endothelin B receptors. Development. 1999;126(6):1161–73.
112. Hearn CJ, Murphy M, Newgreen D. GDNF and ET-3 differentially modulate the numbers of avian enteric neural crest cells and enteric neurons *in vitro*. Dev Biol. 1998;197:93–105.
113. Fujiwara N, Nakazawa-Tanaka N, Miyahara K, Arikawa-Hirasawa E, Akazawa C, Yamataka A. Altered expression of laminin alpha1 in aganglionic colon of endothelin receptor-B null mouse model of Hirschsprung's disease. Pediatr Surg Int. 2018;34(2):137–41.
114. Memic F, Knoflach V, Morarach K, Sadler R, Laranjeira C, Hjerling-Leffler J, et al. Transcription and signaling regulators in developing neuronal subtypes of mouse and human enteric nervous system. Gastroenterology. 2018;154(3):624–36.
115. Pattyn A, Morin X, Cremer H, Goridis C, Brunet J-F. The homeobox gene *Phox2b* is essential for the development of autonomic neural crest derivatives. Nature. 1999;399:366–70.
116. Nagashimada M, Ohta H, Li C, Nakao K, Uesaka T, Brunet JF, et al. Autonomic neurocristopathy-associated mutations in PHOX2B dysregulate Sox10 expression. J Clin Invest. 2012;122(9):3145–58.
117. Amiel J, Laudier B, Attie-Bitach T, Trang H, de Pontual L, Gener B, et al. Polyalanine expansion and frameshift mutations of the paired-like homeobox gene PHOX2B in congenital central hypoventilation syndrome. Nat Genet. 2003;33(4):459–61.
118. Weese-Mayer DE, Berry-Kravis EM, Zhou L, Maher BS, Silvestri JM, Curran ME, et al. Idiopathic congenital central hypoventilation syndrome: analysis of genes pertinent to early autonomic nervous system embryologic development and identification of mutations in PHOX2b. Am J Med Genet A. 2003;123A(3):267–78.
119. Lane PW, Liu HM. Association of megacolon with a new dominant spotting gene (Dom) in the mouse. J Hered. 1984;75(6):435–9.
120. Herbarth B, Pingault V, Bondurand N, Kuhlbrodt K, Hermans-Borgmeyer I, Puliti A, et al. Mutation of the Sry-related Sox10 gene in Dominant megacolon, a mouse model for human Hirschsprung disease. Proc Natl Acad Sci U S A. 1998;95(9):5161–5.
121. Southard-Smith EM, Kos L, Pavan WJ. Sox10 mutation disrupts neural crest development in Dom Hirschsprung mouse model. Nat Genet. 1998;18(1):60–4.
122. Britsch S, Goerich DE, Riethmacher D, Peirano RI, Rossner M, Nave KA, et al. The transcription factor Sox10 is a key regulator of peripheral glial development. Genes Dev. 2001;15(1):66–78.
123. Pingault V, Bondurand N, Kuhlbrodt K, Goerich DE, Prehu MO, Puliti A, et al. SOX10 mutations in patients with Waardenburg-Hirschsprung disease. Nat Genet. 1998;18(2):171–3.
124. Paratore C, Goerich DE, Suter U, Wegner M, Sommer L. Survival and glial fate acquisition of neural crest cells are regulated by an interplay between the transcription factor Sox10 and extrinsic combinatorial signaling. Development. 2001;128(20):3949–61.
125. Kim J, Lo L, Dormand E, Anderson DJ. SOX10 maintains multipotency and inhibits neuronal differentiation of neural crest stem cells. Neuron. 2003;38(1):17–31.
126. Musser MA, Correa H, Southard-Smith EM. Enteric neuron imbalance and proximal dysmotility in ganglionated intestine of the Sox10(Dom/+) Hirschsprung mouse model. Cell Mol Gastroenterol Hepatol. 2015;(1, 1):87–101.
127. Pachnis V, Mankoo B, Costantini F. Expression of the c-ret proto-oncogene during mouse embryogenesis. Development. 1993;119(4):1005–17.
128. Schuchardt A, D'Agati V, Larsson-Blomberg L, Costantini F, Pachnis V. Defects in the kidney and

enteric nervous system of mice lacking the tyrosine kinase receptor Ret. Nature. 1994;367(6461):380–3.
129. Jing S, Wen D, Yu Y, Holst PL, Luo Y, Fang M, et al. GDNF-induced activation of the ret protein tyrosine kinase is mediated by GDNFR-alpha, a novel receptor for GDNF. Cell. 1996;85(7):1113–24.
130. Trupp M, Arenas E, Fainzilber M, Nilsson AS, Sieber BA, Grigoriou M, et al. Functional receptor for GDNF encoded by the c-ret proto-oncogene. Nature. 1996;381(6585):785–9.
131. Durbec P, Marcos-Gutierrez CV, Kilkenny C, Grigoriou M, Wartiowaara K, Suvanto P, et al. GDNF signalling through the Ret receptor tyrosine kinase. Nature. 1996;381(6585):789–93.
132. Lin LF, Doherty DH, Lile JD, Bektesh S, Collins F. GDNF: a glial cell line-derived neurotrophic factor for midbrain dopaminergic neurons. Science. 1993;260(5111):1130–2.
133. Trupp M, Ryden M, Jornvall H, Funakoshi H, Timmusk T, Arenas E, et al. Peripheral expression and biological activities of GDNF, a new neurotrophic factor for avian and mammalian peripheral neurons. J Cell Biol. 1995;130(1):137–48.
134. Choi-Lundberg DL, Bohn MC. Ontogeny and distribution of glial cell line-derived neurotrophic factor (GDNF) mRNA in rat. Brain Res Dev Brain Res. 1995;85(1):80–8.
135. Tsuzuki T, Takahashi M, Asai N, Iwashita T, Matsuyama M, Asai J. Spatial and temporal expression of the ret proto-oncogene product in embryonic, infant and adult rat tissues. Oncogene. 1995;10(1):191–8.
136. Sanchez MP, Silos-Santiago I, Frisen J, He B, Lira SA, Barbacid M. Renal agenesis and the absence of enteric neurons in mice lacking GDNF. Nature. 1996;382(6586):70–3.
137. Moore MW, Klein RD, Farinas I, Sauer H, Armanini M, Phillips H, et al. Renal and neuronal abnormalities in mice lacking GDNF. Nature. 1996;382(6586):76–9.
138. Pichel JG, Shen L, Sheng HZ, Granholm AC, Drago J, Grinberg A, et al. Defects in enteric innervation and kidney development in mice lacking GDNF. Nature. 1996;382(6586):73–6.
139. Treanor JJ, Goodman L, de Sauvage F, Stone DM, Poulsen KT, Beck CD, et al. Characterization of a multicomponent receptor for GDNF. Nature. 1996;382(6586):80–3.
140. Airaksinen MS, Saarma M. The GDNF family: signalling, biological functions and therapeutic value. Nat Rev Neurosci. 2002;3(5):383–94.
141. Bespalov MM, Saarma M. GDNF family receptor complexes are emerging drug targets. Trends Pharmacol Sci. 2007;28(2):68–74.
142. Heuckeroth RO, Enomoto H, Grider JR, Golden JP, Hanke JA, Jackman A, et al. Gene targeting reveals a critical role for neurturin in the development and maintenance of enteric, sensory, and parasympathetic neurons. Neuron. 1999;22:253–63.
143. Heuckeroth RO, Lampe PA, Johnson EM, Milbrandt J. Neurturin and GDNF promote proliferation and survival of enteric neuron and glial progenitors in vitro. Dev Biol. 1998;200(1):116–29.
144. Yan H, Bergner AJ, Enomoto H, Milbrandt J, Newgreen DF, Young HM. Neural cells in the esophagus respond to glial cell line-derived neurotrophic factor and neurturin, and are RET-dependent. Dev Biol. 2004;272(1):118–33.
145. Cacalano G, Fariñas I, Wang LC, Hagler K, Forgie A, Moore M, et al. GFRa-1 is an essential receptor component for GDNF in the developing nervous system and kidney. Neuron. 1998;21:53–62.
146. Barlow A, de Graaff E, Pachnis V. Enteric nervous system progenitors are coordinately controlled by the G protein-coupled receptor EDNRB and the receptor tyrosine kinase RET. Neuron. 2003;40(5):905–16.
147. Nagy N, Goldstein AM. Endothelin-3 regulates neural crest cell proliferation and differentiation in the hindgut enteric nervous system. Dev Biol. 2006;293(1):203–17.
148. Lee HO, Levorse JM, Shin MK. The endothelin receptor-B is required for the migration of neural crest-derived melanocyte and enteric neuron precursors. Dev Biol. 2003;259(1):162–75.
149. McKeown SJ, Mohsenipour M, Bergner AJ, Young HM, Stamp LA. Exposure to GDNF enhances the ability of enteric neural progenitors to generate an enteric nervous system. Stem Cell Reports. 2017;8(2):476–88.
150. Dreyfus CF, Bornstein MB. Synthesis of serotonin by neurons of the myenteric plexus in situ and in organotypic tissue culture. Brain Res. 1977;128(1):125–39.
151. Dreyfus CF, Sherman DL, Gershon MD. Uptake of serotonin by intrinsic neurons of the myenteric plexus grown in organotypic tissue culture. Brain Res. 1977;128(1):109–23.
152. Johnson EM Jr, Osborne PA, Rydel RE, Schmidt RE, Pearson J. Characterization of the effects of autoimmune nerve growth factor deprivation in the developing guinea-pig. Neuroscience. 1983;8(3):631–42.
153. Pearson J, Johnson EM, Brandeis L. Effects of antibodies to nerve growth factor on intrauterine development of derivatives of cranial neural crest and placode in the guinea pig. Dev Biol. 1983;96(1):32–6.
154. Chao MV, Hempstead BL. p75 and Trk: a two-receptor system. Trends Neurosci. 1995;18(7): 321–6.
155. Lindsay RM, Wiegand SJ, Altar CA, DiStefano PS. Neurotrophic factors: from molecule to man. Trends Neurosci. 1994;17(5):182–90.
156. Gotz R, Koster R, Winkler C, Raulf F, Lottspeich F, Schartl M, et al. Neurotrophin-6 is a new member of the nerve growth factor family. Nature. 1994;372(6503):266–9.
157. Kraemer BR, Yoon SO, Carter BD. The biological functions and signaling mechanisms of the

p75 neurotrophin receptor. Handb Exp Pharmacol. 2014;220:121–64.
158. Pomeranz HD, Rothman TP, Chalazonitis A, Tennyson VM, Gershon MD. Neural crest-derived cells isolated from the gut by immunoselection develop neuronal and glial phenotypes when cultured on laminin. Dev Biol. 1993;156(2):341–61.
159. Chalazonitis A, Rothman TP, Chen J, Lamballe F, Barbacid M, Gershon MD. Neurotrophin-3 induces neural crest-derived cells from fetal rat gut to develop in vitro as neurons or glia. J Neurosci. 1994;14(11 Pt 1):6571–84.
160. Carnahan JF, Anderson DJ, Patterson PH. Evidence that enteric neurons may derive from the sympathoadrenal lineage. Dev Biol. 1991;148:552–61.
161. Verdi JM, Anderson DJ. Neurotrophins regulate sequential changes in neurotrophin receptor expression by sympathetic neuroblasts. Neuron. 1994;13(6):1359–72.
162. Birren SJ, Lo L, Anderson DJ. Sympathetic neuroblasts undergo a developmental switch in trophic dependence. Development. 1993;119(3):597–610.
163. DiCicco-Bloom E, Friedman WJ, Black IB. NT-3 stimulates sympathetic neuroblast proliferation by promoting precursor survival. Neuron. 1993;11(6):1101–11.
164. Black IB. Regulation of autonomic development. Annu Rev Neurosci. 1978;1:183–214.
165. Wyatt S, Davies AM. Regulation of nerve growth factor receptor gene expression in sympathetic neurons during development. J Cell Biol. 1995;130(6):1435–46.
166. Ernfors P, Lee KF, Kucera J, Jaenisch R. Lack of neurotrophin-3 leads to deficiencies in the peripheral nervous system and loss of limb proprioceptive afferents. Cell. 1994;77(4):503–12.
167. Farinas I, Jones KR, Backus C, Wang XY, Reichardt LF. Severe sensory and sympathetic deficits in mice lacking neurotrophin-3. Nature. 1994;369(6482):658–61.
168. Zhou XF, Rush R. Sympathetic neurons in neonatal rats require endogenous neurotrophin-3 for survival. J Neurosci. 1995;15(10):6521–30.
169. ElShamy WM, Linnarsson S, Lee KF, Jaenisch R, Ernfors P. Prenatal and postnatal requirements of NT-3 for sympathetic neuroblast survival and innervation of specific targets. Development. 1996;122(2):491–500.
170. Tsoulfas P, Soppet D, Escandon E, Tessarollo L, Mendoza-Ramirez JL, Rosenthal A, et al. The rat trkC locus encodes multiple neurogenic receptors that exhibit differential response to neurotrophin-3 in PC12 cells. Neuron. 1993;10(5):975–90.
171. Lamballe F, Smeyne RJ, Barbacid M. Developmental expression of trkC, the neurotrophin-3 receptor, in the mammalian nervous system. J Neurosci. 1994;14(1):14–28.
172. Tessarollo L, Tsoulfas P, Martin-Zanca D, Gilbert DJ, Jenkins NA, Copeland NG, et al. trkC, a receptor for neurotrophin-3, is widely expressed in the developing nervous system and in non-neuronal tissues. Development. 1993;118(2):463–75.
173. Escandon E, Soppet D, Rosenthal A, Mendoza-Ramirez JL, Szonyi E, Burton LE, et al. Regulation of neurotrophin receptor expression during embryonic and postnatal development. J Neurosci. 1994;14(4):2054–68.
174. Tojo H, Kaisho Y, Nakata M, Matsuoka K, Kitagawa M, Abe T, et al. Targeted disruption of the neurotrophin-3 gene with lacZ induces loss of trkC-positive neurons in sensory ganglia but not in spinal cords. Brain Res. 1995;669(2): 163–75.
175. Payette RF, Tennyson VM, Pham TD, Mawe GM, Pomeranz HD, Rothman TP, et al. Origin and morphology of nerve fibers in the aganglionic colon of the lethal spotted (ls/ls) mutant mouse. J Comp Neurol. 1987;257(2):237–52.
176. Payette RF, Bennett GS, Gershon MD. Neurofilament expression in vagal neural crest-derived precursors of enteric neurons. Dev Biol. 1984;105(2): 273–87.
177. Pham TD, Gershon MD, Rothman TP. Time of origin of neurons in the murine enteric nervous system: sequence in relation to phenotype. J Comp Neurol. 1991;314(4):789–98.
178. Kruger GM, Mosher JT, Bixby S, Joseph N, Iwashita T, Morrison SJ. Neural crest stem cells persist in the adult gut but undergo changes in self-renewal, neuronal subtype potential, and factor responsiveness. Neuron. 2002;35(4):657–69.
179. Joseph NM, He S, Quintana E, Kim YG, Nunez G, Morrison SJ. Enteric glia are multipotent in culture but primarily form glia in the adult rodent gut. J Clin Invest. 2011;121(9):3398–411.
180. Bixby S, Kruger GM, Mosher JT, Joseph NM, Morrison SJ. Cell-intrinsic differences between stem cells from different regions of the peripheral nervous system regulate the generation of neural diversity. Neuron. 2002;35(4):643–56.
181. Teitelman G, Gershon MD, Rothman TP, Joh TH, Reis DJ. Proliferation and distribution of cells that transiently express a catecholaminergic phenotype during development in mice and rats. Dev Biol. 1981;86(2):348–55.
182. Chalazonitis A. Neurotrophin-3 as an essential signal for the developing nervous system. Mol Neurobiol. 1996;12(1):39–53.
183. Chu G, Wilson PC, Carter CD, Lennon VA, Roberts-Thomson IC. Intestinal pseudo-obstruction, type 1 anti-neuronal nuclear antibodies and small-cell carcinoma of the lung. J Gastroenterol Hepatol. 1993;8(6):604–6.
184. Fairman CL, Clagett-Dame M, Lennon VA, Epstein ML. Appearance of neurons in the developing chick gut. Dev Dyn. 1995;204(2):192–201.
185. King PH, Redden D, Palmgren JS, Nabors LB, Lennon VA. Hu antigen specificities of ANNA-I

autoantibodies in paraneoplastic neurological disease. J Autoimmun. 1999;13(4):435–43.
186. Lennon VA. The case for a descriptive generic nomenclature: clarification of immunostaining criteria for PCA-1, ANNA-1, and ANNA-2 autoantibodies. Neurology. 1994;44(12):2412–5.
187. Ockel M, Lewin GR, Barde YA. In vivo effects of neurotrophin-3 during sensory neurogenesis. Development. 1996;122(1):301–7.
188. Kalcheim C, Carmeli C, Rosenthal A. Neurotrophin 3 is a mitogen for cultured neural crest cells. Proc Natl Acad Sci U S A. 1992;89(5):1661–5.
189. Pinco O, Carmeli C, Rosenthal A, Kalcheim C. Neurotrophin-3 affects proliferation and differentiation of distinct neural crest cells and is present in the early neural tube of avian embryos. J Neurobiol. 1993;24(12):1626–41.
190. Chalazonitis A, Pham TD, Rothman TP, DiStefano PS, Bothwell M, Blair-Flynn J, et al. Neurotrophin-3 is required for the survival-differentiation of subsets of developing enteric neurons. J Neurosci. 2001;21(15):5620–36.
191. Chalazonitis A, D'Autreaux F, Guha U, Pham TD, Faure C, Chen JJ, et al. Bone morphogenetic protein-2 and -4 limit the number of enteric neurons but promote development of a TrkC-expressing neurotrophin-3-dependent subset. J Neurosci. 2004;24(17):4266–82.
192. Thompson CA, DeLaForest A, Battle MA. Patterning the gastrointestinal epithelium to confer regional-specific functions. Dev Biol. 2018;435(2):97–108.
193. Goldstein AM, Brewer KC, Doyle AM, Nagy N, Roberts DJ. BMP signaling is necessary for neural crest cell migration and ganglion formation in the enteric nervous system. Mech Dev. 2005;122(6):821–33.
194. Fu M, Vohra BP, Wind D, Heuckeroth RO. BMP signaling regulates murine enteric nervous system precursor migration, neurite fasciculation, and patterning via altered Ncam1 polysialic acid addition. Dev Biol. 2006;299(1):137–50.
195. Faure C, Chalazonitis A, Rheaume C, Bouchard G, Sampathkumar SG, Yarema KJ, et al. Gangliogenesis in the enteric nervous system: roles of the polysialylation of the neural cell adhesion molecule and its regulation by bone morphogenetic protein-4. Dev Dyn. 2007;236(1):44–59.
196. Liu MT, Kuan YH, Wang J, Hen R, Gershon MD. 5-HT4 receptor-mediated neuroprotection and neurogenesis in the enteric nervous system of adult mice. J Neurosci. 2009;29(31):9683–99.
197. Laranjeira C, Sandgren K, Kessaris N, Richardson W, Potocnik A, Vanden Berghe P, et al. Glial cells in the mouse enteric nervous system can undergo neurogenesis in response to injury. J Clin Invest. 2011;121(9):3412–24.
198. Kulkarni S, Micci MA, Leser J, Shin C, Tang SC, Fu YY, et al. Adult enteric nervous system in health is maintained by a dynamic balance between neuronal apoptosis and neurogenesis. Proc Natl Acad Sci U S A. 2017;114(18):E3709–E18.
199. Chalazonitis A, Tang AA, Shang Y, Pham TD, Hsieh I, Setlik W, et al. Homeodomain interacting protein kinase 2 regulates postnatal development of enteric dopaminergic neurons and glia via BMP signaling. J Neurosci. 2011;31(39):13746–57.
200. Adler R, Landa KB, Manthorpe M, Varon S. Cholinergic neuronotrophic factors: intraocular distribution of trophic activity for ciliary neurons. Science. 1979;204(4400):1434–6.
201. Sendtner M, Carroll P, Holtmann B, Hughes RA, Thoenen H. Ciliary neurotrophic factor. J Neurobiol. 1994;25(11):1436–53.
202. DeChiara TM, Vejsada R, Poueymirou WT, Acheson A, Suri C, Conover JC, et al. Mice lacking the CNTF receptor, unlike mice lacking CNTF, exhibit profound motor neuron deficits at birth. Cell. 1995;83(2):313–22.
203. Pennica D, Shaw KJ, Swanson TA, Moore MW, Shelton DL, Zioncheck KA, et al. Cardiotrophin-1. Biological activities and binding to the leukemia inhibitory factor receptor/gp130 signaling complex. J Biol Chem. 1995;270(18):10915–22.
204. Sims NA. Cardiotrophin-like cytokine factor 1 (CLCF1) and neuropoietin (NP) signalling and their roles in development, adulthood, cancer and degenerative disorders. Cytokine Growth Factor Rev. 2015;26(5):517–22.
205. Sleeman MW, Anderson KD, Lambert PD, Yancopoulos GD, Wiegand SJ. The ciliary neurotrophic factor and its receptor, CNTFR alpha. Pharm Acta Helv. 2000;74(2–3):265–72.
206. Davis S, Aldrich TH, Valenzuela DM, Wong VV, Furth ME, Squinto SP, et al. The receptor for ciliary neurotrophic factor. Science. 1991;253(5015):59–63.
207. Gearing DP, Thut CJ, VandeBos T, Gimpel SD, Delaney PB, King J, et al. Leukemia inhibitory factor receptor is structurally related to the IL-6 signal transducer, gp130. EMBO J. 1991;10(10):2839–48.
208. Gearing DP, Comeau MR, Friend DJ, Gimpel SD, Thut CJ, McGourty J, et al. The IL-6 signal transducer, gp130: an oncostatin M receptor and affinity converter for the LIF receptor. Science. 1992;255(5050):1434–7.
209. Davis S, Aldrich TH, Stahl N, Pan L, Taga T, Kishimoto T, et al. LIFR beta and gp130 as heterodimerizing signal transducers of the tripartite CNTF receptor. Science. 1993;260(5115):1805–8.
210. Kishimoto T, Taga T, Akira S. Cytokine signal transduction. Cell. 1994;76(2):253–62.
211. Stahl N, Boulton TG, Farruggella T, Ip NY, Davis S, Witthuhn BA, et al. Association and activation of Jak-Tyk kinases by CNTF-LIF-OSM-IL-6 beta receptor components. Science. 1994;263(5143):92–5.
212. Ip NY, McClain J, Barrezueta NX, Aldrich TH, Pan L, Li Y, et al. The alpha component of the CNTF receptor is required for signaling and defines poten-

tial CNTF targets in the adult and during development. Neuron. 1993;10(1):89–102.
213. Masu Y, Wolf E, Holtmann B, Sendtner M, Brem G, Thoenen H. Disruption of the CNTF gene results in motor neuron degeneration. Nature. 1993;365(6441):27–32.
214. Takahashi R, Yokoji H, Misawa H, Hayashi M, Hu J, Deguchi T. A null mutation in the human CNTF gene is not causally related to neurological diseases. Nat Genet. 1994;7(1):79–84.
215. Chalazonitis A, Rothman TP, Chen J, Vinson EN, MacLennan AJ, Gershon MD. Promotion of the development of enteric neurons and glia by neuropoietic cytokines: interactions with neurotrophin-3. Dev Biol. 1998;198(2):343–65.
216. Brookes SJ, Steele PA, Costa M. Identification and immunohistochemistry of cholinergic and non-cholinergic circular muscle motor neurons in the guinea-pig small intestine. Neuroscience. 1991;42(3):863–78.
217. Bult H, Boeckxstaens GE, Pelckmans PA, Jordaens FH, Van Maercke YM, Herman AG. Nitric oxide as an inhibitory non-adrenergic non-cholinergic neurotransmitter. Nature. 1990;345(6273):346–7.
218. Costa M, Furness JB, Pompolo S, Brookes SJ, Bornstein JC, Bredt DS, et al. Projections and chemical coding of neurons with immunoreactivity for nitric oxide synthase in the guinea-pig small intestine. Neurosci Lett. 1992;148(1–2):121–5.
219. Konturek SJ, Bilski J, Konturek PK, Cieszkowski M, Pawlik W. Role of endogenous nitric oxide in the control of canine pancreatic secretion and blood flow. Gastroenterology. 1993;104(3): 896–902.
220. Stark ME, Bauer AJ, Szurszewski JH. Effect of nitric oxide on circular muscle of the canine small intestine. J Physiol. 1991;444:743–61.
221. Young HM, McConalogue K, Furness JB, De Vente J. Nitric oxide targets in the guinea-pig intestine identified by induction of cyclic GMP immunoreactivity. Neuroscience. 1993;55(2):583–96.
222. Lane PW. Association of megacolon with two recessive spotting genes in the mouse. J Hered. 1966;57(1):29–31.
223. Bolande RP. Hirschsprung's disease, aganglionic or hypoganglionic megacolon. Animal model: aganglionic megacolon in piebald and spotted mutant mouse strains. Am J Pathol. 1975;79(1):189–92.
224. Watanabe Y, Ito T, Harada T, Kobayashi S, Ozaki T, Nimura Y. Spatial distribution and pattern of extrinsic nerve strands in the aganglionic segment of congenital aganglionosis: stereoscopic analysis in spotting lethal rats. J Pediatr Surg. 1995;30(10): 1471–6.
225. Karaki H, Mitsui-Saito M, Takimoto M, Oda K, Okada T, Ozaki T, et al. Lack of endothelin ETB receptor binding and function in the rat with a mutant ETB receptor gene. Biochem Biophys Res Commun. 1996;222(1):139–43.
226. Watanabe Y, Ito T, Harada T, Takahashi M, Kobayashi S, Ozaki T, et al. Expression of ret protooncogene products in the hypoganglionic segment of the small intestine of congenital aganglionosis rats. J Pediatr Surg. 1995;30(5):641–5.
227. Ceccherini I, Zhang AL, Matera I, Yang G, Devoto M, Romeo G, et al. Interstitial deletion of the endothelin-B receptor gene in the spotting lethal (sl) rat. Hum Mol Genet. 1995;4(11):2089–96.
228. Gariepy CE, Cass DT, Yanagisawa M. Null mutation of endothelin receptor type B gene in spotting lethal rats causes aganglionic megacolon and white coat color. Proc Natl Acad Sci U S A. 1996;93(2):867–72.
229. Murray MJ, Parker GA, White NA. Megacolon with myenteric hypoganglionosis in a foal. J Am Vet Med Assoc. 1988;192(7):917–9.
230. Bodeker D, Turck O, Loven E, Wieberneit D, Wegner W. Pathophysiological and functional aspects of the megacolon-syndrome of homozygous spotted rabbits. Zentralbl Veterinarmed A. 1995;42:549–59.
231. Baynash AG, Hosoda K, Giaid A, Richardson JA, Emoto N, Hammer RE, et al. Interaction of endothelin-3 with endothelin-B receptor is essential for development of epidermal melanocytes and enteric neurons. Cell. 1994;79(7):1277–85.
232. Hosoda K, Hammer RE, Richardson JA, Baynash AG, Cheung JC, Giaid A, et al. Targeted and natural (piebald-lethal) mutations of endothelin-B receptor gene produce megacolon associated with spotted coat color in mice. Cell. 1994;79(7):1267–76.
233. Santschi EM, Vrotsos PD, Purdy AK, Mickelson JR. Incidence of the endothelin receptor B mutation that causes lethal white foal syndrome in white-patterned horses. Am J Vet Res. 2001;62(1):97–103.
234. Puffenberger EG, Hosoda K, Washington SS, Nakao K, deWit D, Yanagisawa M, et al. A missense mutation of the endothelin-B receptor gene in multigenic Hirschsprung's disease. Cell. 1994;79(7):1257–66.
235. Rubanyi GM, Polokoff MA. Endothelins: molecular biology, biochemistry, pharmacology, physiology, and pathophysiology. Pharmacol Rev. 1994;46(3):325–415.
236. Sakamoto A, Yanagisawa M, Sawamura T, Enoki T, Ohtani T, Sakurai T, et al. Distinct subdomains of human endothelin receptors determine their selectivity to endothelinA-selective antagonist and endothelinB-selective agonists. J Biol Chem. 1993;268(12):8547–53.
237. Yanagisawa M. The endothelin system. A new target for therapeutic intervention. Circulation. 1994;89(3):1320–2.
238. Yanagisawa M, Kurihara H, Kimura S, Tomobe Y, Kobayashi M, Mitsui Y, et al. A novel potent vasoconstrictor peptide produced by vascular endothelial cells. Nature. 1988;332(6163):411–5.
239. Xu D, Emoto N, Giaid A, Slaughter C, Kaw S, deWit D, et al. ECE-1: a membrane-bound metalloprotease that catalyzes the proteolytic activation of big endothelin-1. Cell. 1994;78(3):473–85.

240. Kurihara Y, Kurihara H, Suzuki H, Kodama T, Maemura K, Nagai R, et al. Elevated blood pressure and craniofacial abnormalities in mice deficient in endothelin-1. Nature. 1994;368(6473):703–10.
241. Kapur RP, Sweetser DA, Doggett B, Siebert JR, Palmiter RD. Intercellular signals downstream of endothelin receptor-B mediate colonization of the large intestine by enteric neuroblasts. Development. 1995;121(11):3787–95.
242. Simkin JE, Zhang D, Rollo BN, Newgreen DF. Retinoic acid upregulates ret and induces chain migration and population expansion in vagal neural crest cells to colonise the embryonic gut. PLoS One. 2013;8(5):e64077.
243. Lahav R, Ziller C, Dupin E, Le Douarin NM. Endothelin 3 promotes neural crest cell proliferation and mediates a vast increase in melanocyte number in culture. Proc Natl Acad Sci U S A. 1996;93(9):3892–7.
244. Bondurand N, Natarajan D, Barlow A, Thapar N, Pachnis V. Maintenance of mammalian enteric nervous system progenitors by SOX10 and endothelin 3 signalling. Development. 2006;133(10):2075–86.
245. Druckenbrod NR, Powers PA, Bartley CR, Walker JW, Epstein ML. Targeting of endothelin receptor-B to the neural crest. Genesis. 2008;46(8):396–400.
246. Fujiwara N, Miyahara K, Nakazawa-Tanaka N, Akazawa C, Yamataka A. Increased expression of Semaphorin 3A in the endothelin receptor-B null mouse model of Hirschsprung disease. J Pediatr Surg. 2018;53(2):326–9.
247. Rothman TP, Goldowitz D, Gershon MD. Inhibition of migration of neural crest-derived cells by the abnormal mesenchyme of the presumptive aganglionic bowel of ls/ls mice: analysis with aggregation and interspecies chimeras. Dev Biol. 1993;159(2):559–73.
248. Rothman TP, Gershon MD. Regionally defective colonization of the terminal bowel by the precursors of enteric neurons in lethal spotted mutant mice. Neuroscience. 1984;12(4):1293–311.
249. Rothman TP, Tennyson VM, Gershon MD. Colonization of the bowel by the precursors of enteric glia: studies of normal and congenitally aganglionic mutant mice. J Comp Neurol. 1986;252(4):493–506.
250. Jacobs-Cohen RJ, Payette RF, Gershon MD, Rothman TP. Inability of neural crest cells to colonize the presumptive aganglionic bowel of ls/ls mutant mice: requirement for a permissive microenvironment. J Comp Neurol. 1987;255(3):425–38.
251. Payette RF, Tennyson VM, Pomeranz HD, Pham TD, Rothman TP, Gershon MD. Accumulation of components of basal laminae: association with the failure of neural crest cells to colonize the presumptive aganglionic bowel of ls/ls mutant mice. Dev Biol. 1988;125(2):341–60.
252. Tennyson VM, Payette RF, Rothman TP, Gershon MD. Distribution of hyaluronic acid and chondroitin sulfate proteoglycans in the presumptive aganglionic terminal bowel of ls/ls fetal mice: an ultrastructural analysis. J Comp Neurol. 1990;291(3):345–62.
253. Rothman TP, Chen J, Howard MJ, Costantini F, Schuchardt A, Pachnis V, et al. Increased expression of laminin-1 and collagen (IV) subunits in the aganglionic bowel of ls/ls, but not c-ret -/- mice. Dev Biol. 1996;178(2):498–513.
254. Nakazawa-Tanaka N, Fujiwara N, Miyahara K, Nakada S, Arikawa-Hirasawa E, Akazawa C, et al. The effect of laminin-1 on enteric neural crest-derived cell migration in the Hirschsprung's disease mouse model. Pediatr Surg Int. 2018;34(2):143–7.
255. Parikh DH, Tam PK, Van Velzen D, Edgar D. Abnormalities in the distribution of laminin and collagen type IV in Hirschsprung's disease. Gastroenterology. 1992;102(4 Pt 1):1236–41.
256. Parikh DH, Leibl M, Tam PK, Edgar D. Abnormal expression and distribution of nidogen in Hirschsprung's disease. J Pediatr Surg. 1995;30(12):1687–93.
257. Tucker GC, Ciment G, Thiery JP. Pathways of avian neural crest cell migration in the developing gut. Dev Biol. 1986;116(2):439–50.
258. Pomeranz HD, Gershon MD. Colonization of the avian hindgut by cells derived from the sacral neural crest. Dev Biol. 1990;137(2):378–94.
259. Pomeranz HD, Sherman DL, Smalheiser NR, Tennyson VM, Gershon MD. Expression of a neurally related laminin binding protein by neural crest-derived cells that colonize the gut: relationship to the formation of enteric ganglia. J Comp Neurol. 1991;313(4):625–42.
260. Oakley RA, Lasky CJ, Erickson CA, Tosney KW. Glycoconjugates mark a transient barrier to neural crest migration in the chicken embryo. Development. 1994;120(1):103–14.
261. Erickson CA, Duong TD, Tosney KW. Descriptive and experimental analysis of the dispersion of neural crest cells along the dorsolateral path and their entry into ectoderm in the chick embryo. Dev Biol. 1992;151(1):251–72.
262. Rickmann M, Fawcett JW, Keynes RJ. The migration of neural crest cells and the growth of motor axons through the rostral half of the chick somite. J Embryol Exp Morphol. 1985;90:437–55.
263. Norris WE, Stern CD, Keynes RJ. Molecular differences between the rostral and caudal halves of the sclerotome in the chick embryo. Development. 1989;105(3):541–8.
264. Pettway Z, Guillory G, Bronner-Fraser M. Absence of neural crest cells from the region surrounding implanted notochords in situ. Dev Biol. 1990;142(2):335–45.
265. Oakley RA, Tosney KW. Peanut agglutinin and chondroitin-6-sulfate are molecular markers for tissues that act as barriers to axon advance in the avian embryo. Dev Biol. 1991;147(1):187–206.
266. Miura H, Ohi R, Tseng SW, Takahashi T. The structure of the transitional and aganglionic zones of Auerbach's plexus in patients with

Hirschsprung's disease: a computer-assisted three-dimensional reconstruction study. J Pediatr Surg. 1996;31(3):420–6.
267. Lallier T, Bronner-Fraser M. Avian neural crest cell attachment to laminin: involvement of divalent cation dependent and independent integrins. Development. 1991;113(4):1069–84.
268. Bilozur ME, Hay ED. Neural crest migration in 3D extracellular matrix utilizes laminin, fibronectin, or collagen. Dev Biol. 1988;125(1):19–33.
269. Bronner-Fraser M. Alterations in neural crest migration by a monoclonal antibody that affects cell adhesion. J Cell Biol. 1985;101(2):610–7.
270. Bronner-Fraser M. An antibody to a receptor for fibronectin and laminin perturbs cranial neural crest development in vivo. Dev Biol. 1986;117(2):528–36.
271. Bronner-Fraser M, Lallier T. A monoclonal antibody against a laminin-heparan sulfate proteoglycan complex perturbs cranial neural crest migration in vivo. J Cell Biol. 1988;106(4):1321–9.
272. Engvall E, Davis GE, Dickerson K, Ruoslahti E, Varon S, Manthorpe M. Mapping of domains in human laminin using monoclonal antibodies: localization of the neurite-promoting site. J Cell Biol. 1986;103(6 Pt 1):2457–65.
273. Kleinman HK, Ogle RC, Cannon FB, Little CD, Sweeney TM, Luckenbill-Edds L. Laminin receptors for neurite formation. Proc Natl Acad Sci U S A. 1988;85(4):1282–6.
274. Lander AD, Fujii DK, Reichardt LF. Laminin is associated with the "neurite outgrowth-promoting factors" found in conditioned media. Proc Natl Acad Sci U S A. 1985;82(7):2183–7.
275. Liesi P, Narvanen A, Soos J, Sariola H, Snounou G. Identification of a neurite outgrowth-promoting domain of laminin using synthetic peptides. FEBS Lett. 1989;244(1):141–8.
276. Manthorpe M, Engvall E, Ruoslahti E, Longo FM, Davis GE, Varon S. Laminin promotes neuritic regeneration from cultured peripheral and central neurons. J Cell Biol. 1983;97(6):1882–90.
277. Calof AL, Reichardt LF. Response of purified chick motoneurons to myotube conditioned medium: laminin is essential for the substratum-binding, neurite outgrowth-promoting activity. Neurosci Lett. 1985;59(2):183–9.
278. Stemple DL, Anderson DJ. Isolation of a stem cell for neurons and glia from the mammalian neural crest. Cell. 1992;71(6):973–85.
279. Douville PJ, Harvey WJ, Carbonetto S. Isolation and partial characterization of high affinity laminin receptors in neural cells. J Biol Chem. 1988;263(29):14964–9.
280. Kleinman HK, Weeks BS. Laminin: structure, functions and receptors. Curr Opin Cell Biol. 1989;1(5):964–7.
281. Kibbey MC, Jucker M, Weeks BS, Neve RL, Van Nostrand WE, Kleinman HK. beta-Amyloid precursor protein binds to the neurite-promoting IKVAV site of laminin. Proc Natl Acad Sci U S A. 1993;90(21):10150–3.
282. Tang CS, Li P, Lai FP, Fu AX, Lau ST, So MT, et al. Identification of genes associated with Hirschsprung disease, based on whole-genome sequence analysis, and potential effects on enteric nervous system development. Gastroenterology. 2018;155(6):1908–22 e5.
283. Kleinman HK, Weeks BS, Cannon FB, Sweeney TM, Sephel GC, Clement B, et al. Identification of a 110-kDa nonintegrin cell surface laminin-binding protein which recognizes an A chain neurite-promoting peptide. Arch Biochem Biophys. 1991;290(2):320–5.
284. Sephel GC, Tashiro K, Sasaki M, Kandel S, Yamada Y, Kleinman HK. A laminin-pepsin fragment with cell attachment and neurite outgrowth activity at distinct sites. Dev Biol. 1989;135(1):172–81.
285. Sephel GC, Tashiro KI, Sasaki M, Greatorex D, Martin GR, Yamada Y, et al. Laminin A chain synthetic peptide which supports neurite outgrowth. Biochem Biophys Res Commun. 1989;162(2):821–9.
286. Freitas VM, Vilas-Boas VF, Pimenta DC, Loureiro V, Juliano MA, Carvalho MR, et al. SIKVAV, a laminin alpha1-derived peptide, interacts with integrins and increases protease activity of a human salivary gland adenoid cystic carcinoma cell line through the ERK 1/2 signaling pathway. Am J Pathol. 2007;171(1):124–38.
287. Kibbey MC, Johnson B, Petryshyn R, Jucker M, Kleinman HK. A 110-kD nuclear shuttling protein, nucleolin, binds to the neurite-promoting IKVAV site of laminin-1. J Neurosci Res. 1995;42(3):314–22.
288. Bresalier RS, Schwartz B, Kim YS, Duh QY, Kleinman HK, Sullam PM. The laminin alpha 1 chain Ile-Lys-Val-Ala-Val (IKVAV)-containing peptide promotes liver colonization by human colon cancer cells. Cancer Res. 1995;55(11):2476–80.
289. Corcoran ML, Kibbey MC, Kleinman HK, Wahl LM. Laminin SIKVAV peptide induction of monocyte/macrophage prostaglandin E2 and matrix metalloproteinases. J Biol Chem. 1995;270(18):10365–8.
290. Haralabopoulos GC, Grant DS, Kleinman HK, Lelkes PI, Papaioannou SP, Maragoudakis ME. Inhibitors of basement membrane collagen synthesis prevent endothelial cell alignment in matrigel in vitro and angiogenesis in vivo. Lab Invest. 1994;71(4):575–82.
291. Kibbey MC, Corcoran ML, Wahl LM, Kleinman HK. Laminin SIKVAV peptide-induced angiogenesis in vivo is potentiated by neutrophils. J Cell Physiol. 1994;160(1):185–93.
292. Nomizu M, Weeks BS, Weston CA, Kim WH, Kleinman HK, Yamada Y. Structure-activity study of a laminin alpha 1 chain active peptide segment Ile-Lys-Val-Ala-Val (IKVAV). FEBS Lett. 1995;365(2-3):227–31.
293. Weeks BS, Holloway E, Klotman PE, Akiyama SK, Schnaper HW, Kleinman HK. 12-O-tetradecanoylphorbol 13-acetate stimulates human T-lymphocyte adherence to the fibronectin RGD domain and the laminin IKVAV domain. Cell Immunol. 1994;153(1):94–104.

294. Chalazonitis A, Tennyson VM, Kibbey MC, Rothman TP, Gershon MD. The a-1 subunit of laminin-1 promotes the development of neurons by interacting with LBP110 expressed by neural crest-derived cells immunoselected from the fetal mouse gut. J Neurobiol. 1997;33:118–38.
295. Stemple DL, Anderson DJ. Lineage diversification of the neural crest: in vitro investigations. Dev Biol. 1993;159(1):12–23.
296. Erickson CA, Loring JF, Lester SM. Migratory pathways of HNK-1-immunoreactive neural crest cells in the rat embryo. Dev Biol. 1989;134(1):112–8.
297. Martins-Green M, Erickson CA. Basal lamina is not a barrier to neural crest cell emigration: documentation by TEM and by immunofluorescent and immunogold labelling. Development. 1987;101(3):517–33.
298. Okabe H, Chijiiwa Y, Nakamura K, Yoshinaga M, Akiho H, Harada N, et al. Two endothelin receptors (ETA and ETB) expressed on circular smooth muscle cells of guinea pig cecum. Gastroenterology. 1995;108(1):51–7.
299. Yoshinaga M, Chijiiwa Y, Misawa T, Harada N, Nawata H. EndothelinB receptor on guinea pig small intestinal smooth muscle cells. Am J Physiol. 1992;262(2 Pt 1):G308–11.
300. Vanderwinden JM, Rumessen JJ, Liu H, Descamps D, De Laet MH, Vanderhaeghen JJ. Interstitial cells of Cajal in human colon and in Hirschsprung's disease. Gastroenterology. 1996;111(4):901–10.
301. Yamataka A, Kato Y, Tibboel D, Murata Y, Sueyoshi N, Fujimoto T, et al. A lack of intestinal pacemaker (c-kit) in aganglionic bowel of patients with Hirschsprung's disease. J Pediatr Surg. 1995;30(3):441–4.
302. Torihashi S, Ward SM, Sanders KM. Development of c-Kit-positive cells and the onset of electrical rhythmicity in murine small intestine. Gastroenterology. 1997;112(1):144–55.
303. Kobayashi S, Furness JB, Smith TK, Pompolo S. Histological identification of the interstitial cells of Cajal in the guinea-pig small intestine. Arch Histol Cytol. 1989;52(3):267–86.
304. Cook RD, Burnstock G. The ultrastructure of Auerbach's plexus in the guinea-pig. II. Non-neuronal elements. J Neurocytol. 1976;5(2):195–206.
305. Faussone-Pellegrini MS. Cytodifferentiation of the interstitial cells of Cajal related to the myenteric plexus of mouse intestinal muscle coat. An E.M. study from foetal to adult life. Anat Embryol. 1985;171(2):163–9.
306. Torihashi S, Kobayashi S, Gerthoffer WT, Sanders KM. Interstitial cells in deep muscular plexus of canine small intestine may be specialized smooth muscle cells. Am J Physiol. 1993;265(4 Pt 1):G638–45.
307. Ward SM, Burns AJ, Torihashi S, Sanders KM. Mutation of the proto-oncogene c-kit blocks development of interstitial cells and electrical rhythmicity in murine intestine. J Physiol. 1994;480(Pt 1):91–7.
308. Ward SM, Burns AJ, Torihashi S, Harney SC, Sanders KM. Impaired development of interstitial cells and intestinal electrical rhythmicity in steel mutants. Am J Physiol. 1995;269(6 Pt 1): C1577–85.
309. Torihashi S, Ward SM, Nishikawa S, Nishi K, Kobayashi S, Sanders KM. c-kit-dependent development of interstitial cells and electrical activity in the murine gastrointestinal tract. Cell Tissue Res. 1995;280(1):97–111.
310. Besmer P. The kit ligand encoded at the murine Steel locus: a pleiotropic growth and differentiation factor. Curr Opin Cell Biol. 1991;3(6):939–46.
311. Huizinga JD, Thuneberg L, Kluppel M, Malysz J, Mikkelsen HB, Bernstein A. W/kit gene required for interstitial cells of Cajal and for intestinal pacemaker activity. Nature. 1995;373(6512):347–9.
312. Maeda H, Yamagata A, Nishikawa S, Yoshinaga K, Kobayashi S, Nishi K, et al. Requirement of c-kit for development of intestinal pacemaker system. Development. 1992;116(2):369–75.
313. Lecoin L, Gabella G, Le Douarin N. Origin of the c-kit-positive interstitial cells in the avian bowel. Development. 1996;122(3):725–33.
314. Gfroerer S, Rolle U. Interstitial cells of Cajal in the normal human gut and in Hirschsprung disease. Pediatr Surg Int. 2013;29(9):889–97.
315. Rolle U, Piotrowska AP, Nemeth L, Puri P. Altered distribution of interstitial cells of Cajal in Hirschsprung disease. Arch Pathol Lab Med. 2002;126(8):928–33.
316. Miyazawa K, Williams DA, Gotoh A, Nishimaki J, Broxmeyer HE, Toyama K. Membrane-bound Steel factor induces more persistent tyrosine kinase activation and longer life span of c-kit gene-encoded protein than its soluble form. Blood. 1995;85(3): 641–9.
317. Wehrle-Haller B, Weston JA. Soluble and cell-bound forms of steel factor activity play distinct roles in melanocyte precursor dispersal and survival on the lateral neural crest migration pathway. Development. 1995;121(3):731–42.
318. Gershon MD, Sherman D, Gintzler A. An ultrastructural analysis of the developing enteric nervous system of the guinea pig small intestine. J Neurocytol. 1981;10:271–96.
319. Li Z, Chalazonitis A, Huang YY, Mann JJ, Margolis KG, Yang QM, et al. Essential roles of enteric neuronal serotonin in gastrointestinal motility and the development/survival of enteric dopaminergic neurons. J Neurosci. 2011;31(24):8998–9009.
320. Margolis KG, Li ZS, Stevanovic K, Saurman V, Israelyan N, Anderson GM, et al. Serotonin transporter variant drives preventable gastrointestinal abnormalities in development and function. J Clin Investig. 2016;126(6):2221–35.

321. Belkind-Gerson J, Hotta R, Nagy N, Thomas AR, Graham H, Cheng L, et al. Colitis induces enteric neurogenesis through a 5-HT4-dependent mechanism. Inflamm Bowel Dis. 2015;21(4):870–8.
322. Goto K, Kawahara I, Inada H, Misawa H, Kuniyasu H, Nabekura J, et al. Activation of 5-HT4 receptors facilitates neurogenesis from transplanted neural stem cells in the anastomotic ileum. J Physiol Sci. 2016;66(1):67–76.
323. Li Z, Margolis KG, Israelyan N, Sturgeon S, Blakely RD, Gershon MD. Cholinergic neuronal regulation of enteric neurogenesis, GI motility, and mucosal homeostasis: insights from mice that under-or overexpress the presynaptic choline transporter. Gastroenterology. 2016;150(4):S343.
324. Gaspar P, Cases O, Maroteaux L. The developmental role of serotonin: news from mouse molecular genetics. Nat Rev Neurosci. 2003;4(12):1002–12.
325. D'Amato RJ, Largent BL, Snowman AM, Snyder SH. Selective labeling of serotonin uptake sites in rat brain by [3H]citalopram contrasted to labeling of multiple sites by [3H]imipramine. J Pharmacol Exp Ther. 1987;242(1):364–71.
326. Lebrand C, Cases O, Wehrle R, Blakely RD, Edwards RH, Gaspar P. Transient developmental expression of monoamine transporters in the rodent forebrain. J Comp Neurol. 1998;401(4):506–24.
327. Chen X, Ye R, Gargus JJ, Blakely RD, Dobrenis K, Sze JY. Disruption of transient serotonin accumulation by non-serotonin-producing neurons impairs cortical map development. Cell Rep. 2015;10(3):346–58.
328. Rothman TP, Ross LL, Gershon MD. Separately developing axonal uptake of 5-hydroxytryptamine and norepinephrine in the ileum of the rabbit. Brain Res. 1976;115:437–56.
329. Gershon MD. 5-Hydroxytryptamine (serotonin) in the gastrointestinal tract. Curr Opin Endocrinol Diabetes Obes. 2013;20(1):14–21.
330. Iino S, Horiguchi K, Horiguchi S, Nojyo Y. c-Kit-negative fibroblast-like cells express platelet-derived growth factor receptor alpha in the murine gastrointestinal musculature. Histochem Cell Biol. 2009;131(6):691–702.
331. Kurahashi M, Nakano Y, Peri LE, Townsend JB, Ward SM, Sanders KM. A novel population of subepithelial platelet-derived growth factor receptor alpha-positive cells in the mouse and human colon. Am J Physiol Gastrointest Liver Physiol. 2013;304(9):G823–34.
332. Kurahashi M, Nakano Y, Hennig GW, Ward SM, Sanders KM. Platelet-derived growth factor receptor alpha-positive cells in the tunica muscularis of human colon. J Cell Mol Med. 2012;16(7):1397–404.
333. Coyle D, O'Donnell AM, Puri P. Altered distribution of small-conductance calcium-activated potassium channel SK3 in Hirschsprung's disease. J Pediatr Surg. 2015;50(10):1659–64.
334. Kurahashi M, Zheng H, Dwyer L, Ward SM, Koh SD, Sanders KM. A functional role for the 'fibroblast-like cells' in gastrointestinal smooth muscles. J Physiol. 2011;589(Pt 3):697–710.
335. O'Donnell AM, Coyle D, Puri P. Deficiency of platelet-derived growth factor receptor-alpha-positive cells in Hirschsprung's disease colon. World J Gastroenterol. 2016;22(12):3335–40.
336. Piotrowska AP, Rolle U, Chertin B, De Caluwe D, Bianchi A, Puri P. Alterations in smooth muscle contractile and cytoskeleton proteins and interstitial cells of Cajal in megacystis microcolon intestinal hypoperistalsis syndrome. J Pediatr Surg. 2003;38(5):749–55.
337. Angrist M, Bolk S, Thiel B, Puffenberger EG, Hofstra RM, Buys CH, et al. Mutation analysis of the RET receptor tyrosine kinase in Hirschsprung disease. Hum Mol Genet. 1995;4(5):821–30.
338. Edery P, Lyonnet S, Mulligan LM, Pelet A, Dow E, Abel L, et al. Mutations of the RET proto-oncogene in Hirschsprung's disease. Nature. 1994;367(6461):378–80.
339. Romeo G, Ronchetto P, Luo Y, Barone V, Seri M, Ceccherini I, et al. Point mutations affecting the tyrosine kinase domain of the RET proto-oncogene in Hirschsprung's disease. Nature. 1994;367(6461):377–8.
340. Pasini B, Borrello MG, Greco A, Bongarzone I, Luo Y, Mondellini P, et al. Loss of function effect of RET mutations causing Hirschsprung disease. Nat Genet. 1995;10(1):35–40.
341. Borrello MG, Smith DP, Pasini B, Bongarzone I, Greco A, Lorenzo MJ, et al. RET activation by germline MEN2A and MEN2B mutations. Oncogene. 1995;11(11):2419–27.
342. Heuckeroth RO. Even when you know everything, there is still more to learn about Hirschsprung disease. Gastroenterology. 2018;155(6):1681–4.
343. Heuckeroth RO. Hirschsprung disease – integrating basic science and clinical medicine to improve outcomes. Nat Rev Gastroenterol Hepatol. 2018;15(3):152–67.
344. McKeown SJ, Stamp L, Hao MM, Young HM. Hirschsprung disease: a developmental disorder of the enteric nervous system. Wiley Interdiscip Rev Dev Biol. 2013;2(1):113–29.
345. Amiel J, Sproat-Emison E, Garcia-Barcelo M, Lantieri F, Burzynski G, Borrego S, et al. Hirschsprung disease, associated syndromes and genetics: a review. J Med Genet. 2008;45(1):1–14.
346. Bondurand N, Dufour S, Pingault V. News from the endothelin-3/EDNRB signaling pathway: role during enteric nervous system development and involvement in neural crest-associated disorders. Dev Biol. 2018;444(Suppl 1):S156–69.
347. Hofstra RM, Osinga J, Tan-Sindhunata G, Wu Y, Kamsteeg EJ, Stulp RP, et al. A homozygous mutation in the endothelin-3 gene associated with a

combined Waardenburg type 2 and Hirschsprung phenotype (Shah-Waardenburg syndrome). Nat Genet. 1996;12(4):445–7.
348. Edery P, Attie T, Amiel J, Pelet A, Eng C, Hofstra RM, et al. Mutation of the endothelin-3 gene in the Waardenburg-Hirschsprung disease (Shah-Waardenburg syndrome). Nat Genet. 1996;12(4):442–4.
349. Brokhman I, Xu J, Coles BLK, Razavi R, Engert S, Lickert H, et al. Dual embryonic origin of the mammalian enteric nervous system. Dev Biol. 2018;445(2):256–70.
350. Zhang D, Rollo BN, Nagy N, Stamp L, Newgreen DF. The enteric neural crest progressively loses capacity to form enteric nervous system. Dev Biol. 2019;446(1):34–42.
351. Avetisyan M, Schill EM, Heuckeroth RO. Building a second brain in the bowel. J Clin Invest. 2015;125(3):899–907.
352. McCann CJ, Thapar N. Enteric neural stem cell therapies for enteric neuropathies. Neurogastroenterol Motil. 2018;30(10):e13369.
353. Fattahi F, Steinbeck JA, Kriks S, Tchieu J, Zimmer B, Kishinevsky S, et al. Deriving human ENS lineages for cell therapy and drug discovery in Hirschsprung disease. Nature. 2016;531(7592):105–9.

Normal Colonic Motor Function and Structure

4

Philip K. Frykman, Stephanie Chen, Deven C. Patel, and James Christensen

Contents

P. K. Frykman (✉)
Pacific Coast Pediatric Surgery, Thousand Oaks, CA, USA

Division of Pediatric Surgery, Department of Surgery, Cedars-Sinai Medical Center, Los Angeles, CA, USA
https://www.pacificcoastpediatricsurgery.com

S. Chen · D. C. Patel
Division of Pediatric Surgery, Department of Surgery, Cedars-Sinai Medical Center, Los Angeles, CA, USA

J. Christensen
Department of Internal Medicine, University of Iowa Carver College of Medicine, Iowa City, IA, USA

4.1 Introduction

In all mammals, a segment at the caudal end of the gastrointestinal tract exhibits morphological and functional distinctions that justify its designation as a structure fundamentally different from the other parts of the tract [1]. Its special functions seem to relate to three particular needs of the bodily economy: for the conservation of water, for the maximal utilization of nutrients, and for the voluntary control of defecation.

The need for the conservation of water is suspected to have originated, along with specialization in the kidney, in the adaptation of mammals to terrestrial life. The need to maximize the utilization of nutrients arose with the adaptation of mammals to herbivorous diets where intralumi-

P. Puri (ed.), *Hirschsprung's Disease and Allied Disorders*,
https://doi.org/10.1007/978-3-030-15647-3_4

nal bacteria came to provide for the digestion of substances from plants that resist mammalian digestive enzymes. The voluntary control of defecation may have come about in response to animal predation: both as a means for predators to identify hunting territories and as a possible means for those being hunted to elude tracking. These needs are met by the functions of the large intestine, which derive especially from the unique motility of that organ. Throughout the entire colon, contractions produce very slow antegrade flows that facilitate the mucosal extraction of water from the fecal mass while supporting bacterial proliferation. In the most distal part of the large intestine, there are few spontaneous contractions and fecal flow can be suspended at will to provide for the voluntary control of defecation.

Not surprisingly, these specialized motor functions are distinct from those of the small intestine and other parts of the gastrointestinal tract, and as such, the colon has specialized neural and muscular structures controlling contractions and flow. This chapter describes the specialized morphology and motor functions of the large intestine.

4.2 Morphology

4.2.1 Gross Anatomy

4.2.1.1 Structure of the Large Intestine

The human large intestine, 1.5 m long, forms an arch in the abdomen, beginning in the right iliac region, running cephalad to the caudal surface of the liver, passing across the midline to the left hypochondrium, descending into the left iliac region, and then curving to the midline to pass along the posterior pelvic wall to the anus. This configuration provides a set of terms used for the various parts of the human large intestine (Fig. 4.1). The large intestine comprises five parts: the appendix, cecum, colon, rectum, and

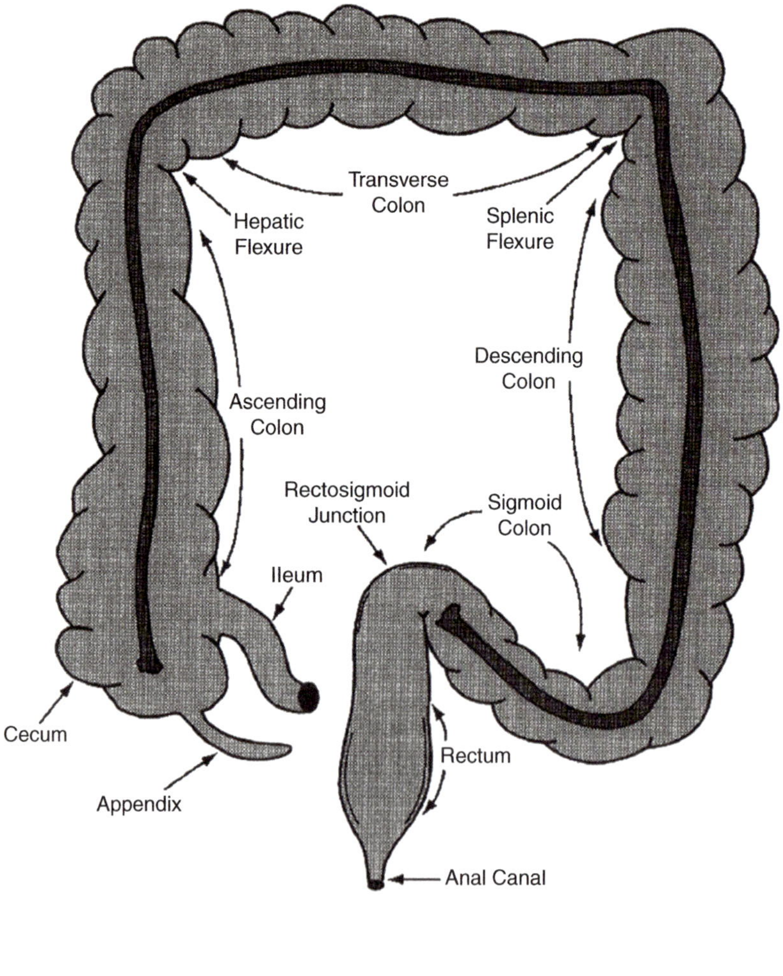

Fig. 4.1 The human large intestine with its parts and landmarks

anal canal. The colon has four parts: the ascending colon on the right side of the abdomen, the transverse colon, the descending colon on the left side of the abdomen, and the sigmoid colon. Key landmarks associated with the colon are the ileocecal junction, the hepatic flexure, the splenic flexure, and the rectosigmoid junction (Fig. 4.1).

The ileocecal junction, also known as the ileocecal valve, separates the terminal ileum from the large intestine. The cecum is the blind pouch of the large intestine that extends upstream from the ileocecal junction. It usually contacts the iliac muscle posteriorly and the abdominal wall anteriorly, but its mobility derives from the breadth of its mesentery allowing for great variation in its exact position within the abdomen. The cecum may extend into the pelvis to contact the rectum, extend across the midline into left iliac fossa, or even extend cephalad to the iliac fossa. The vermiform appendix is a worm-like, blind tube 10–20 cm long and 10 mm in diameter that extends from the apex of the cecum. Its position within the abdomen may vary greatly due to its mesentery.

The ascending colon, extending from the ileocecal junction to the hepatic flexure (the angulation formed by the colon on the caudal surface of the liver), lacks a mesentery. The investing peritoneum tethers the colon to the iliopsoas muscle, quadratus lumborum muscle, aponeurotic origin of the transverse abdominal muscles, and the ventrolateral surface of the right kidney. The transverse colon extends from the colic impression on the caudal surface of the liver to the spleen, crosses the midline in a caudal direction, and extends below the interiliac line. The abundant mesentery in this region, known as the mesocolon, allows for a large degree of mobility of the transverse colon, and thus, its position within the abdomen can vary. The acute angulation formed by the colon just below the spleen, the splenic flexure, demarcates the beginning of the descending colon. The splenic flexure of the colon usually touches both the spleen and the tail of the pancreas. The splenic flexure is relatively fixed as it is held in place by the phrenicocolic ligament, a peritoneal fold attaching both the splenic flexure and the spleen to the diaphragm opposite the tenth and 11th ribs. The *descending colon*, running caudad from the spleen to the pelvis, lacks a mesentery, the investing peritoneum holding it close against the iliopsoas and quadratus lumborum muscles, the left kidney, and the aponeurotic origin of the transverse abdominal muscles. The descending colon curves medially in the left iliac fossa ventral to the iliopsoas muscle to form a loop, the *sigmoid colon*. This loop, beginning at about the level of the upper aperture of the lesser pelvis, is suspended from a mesentery, the sigmoid mesocolon, which also confers a considerable amount of mobility. The sigmoid colon ends in the midline on the ventral surface of the sacrum at the level of the third sacral vertebra where it becomes the rectosigmoid junction.

The relatively straight course of the part of the large intestine that lies between the level of the third sacral vertebra and the pelvic floor dictates its name, the rectum. The segment, about 12 cm long, actually exhibits a slight dorsoventral curvature. It widens a little just above the pelvic floor to form the rectal ampulla. Three fixed semilunar folds, the valves of Houston, indent its lumen. The rectum lies within the peritoneal cavity at its rostral end, lacking a mesentery but invested by peritoneum. This peritoneal covering is reflected about 7.5 cm above the anal canal in men and 5.5 cm above the anal canal in women. Below that point lies the rectum which is bordered dorsally by the coccyx and sacrum and ventrally by the bladder and vagina in women or the bladder, prostate, and seminal vesicles in men.

The anal canal extends from the end of the rectal ampulla (at about the apex of the prostate in men) to the external anal orifice. The rectum joins the anal canal at an obtuse angle pointing anteriorly. That is, the axis of the anal canal points ventrally toward the umbilicus, while the axis of the rectum points dorsally toward the sacroiliac joint. The anal canal is 2.5–4 cm long and lies entirely within the pelvic floor, surrounded by the levator ani muscle and the external anal sphincter. A fibromuscular wedge, the perineal body, separates the anal canal from the urogenital structures ventrally. A similar structure, the postanal plate, separates it from the coccyx dorsally. The mucosa of the anal canal lies in longitudinal folds, the columns of Morgagni, separated

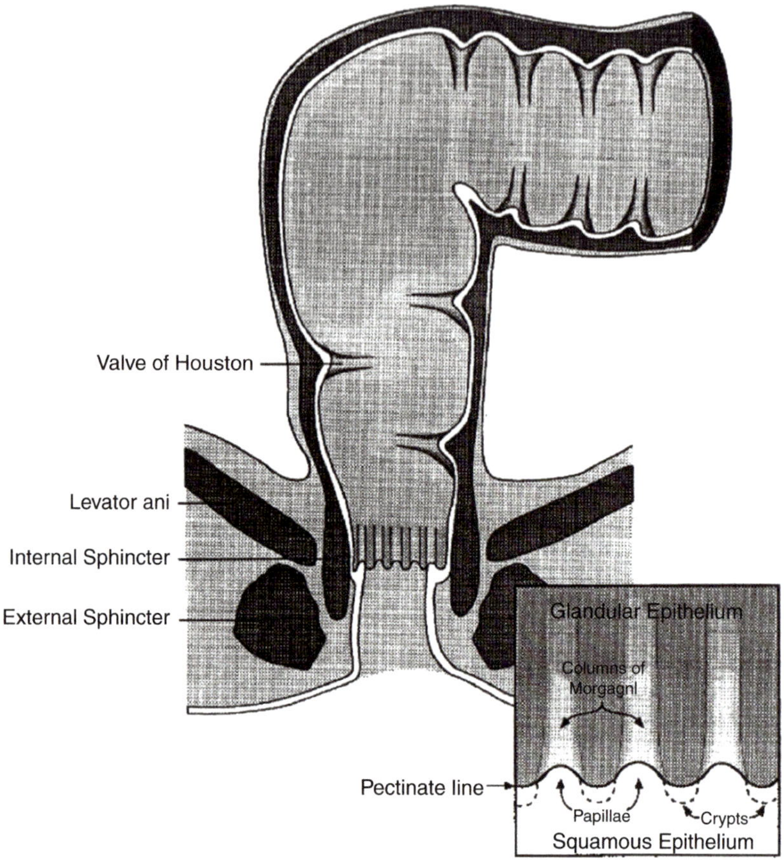

Fig. 4.2 The rectum and anal canal

by valleys, the rectal sinuses (Fig. 4.2). Each column ends at the external anal orifice as a triangular nipple. These nipples, the anal papillae, covered with squamous epithelium, form a row which marks the squamocolumnar epithelial border (pectinate line). Thin epithelial folds, the anal valves, link the adjacent anal papillae and form a row of tiny pockets known as the anal crypts or sinuses between the papillae.

The large intestine grossly has a markedly different appearance from the relatively smooth appearance of the small bowel (Fig. 4.3). This irregular configuration of the large intestine arises from the thickening of the longitudinal musculature of the large intestine into three bundles, the *taeniae coli*, one lying along the mesenteric insertion and the other two approximately equidistant from it. Between the three taeniae, the walls of the colon are elongated and bulge. Thin rings of the circular muscle layer interrupt the bulging walls at intervals to form the lumen into a chain of saccules or pockets, the haustra. This sacculated appearance characterizes the cecum and the colon as far as the rectosigmoid junction. The rectum itself is a more uniform cylinder, with indentations produced by the valves of Houston.

4.2.1.2 The Comparative Anatomy of the Large Intestine

The form of the large intestine varies enormously among mammals, especially in respect to the size of the cecum and to the extent and distribution of sacculation or haustration [2, 3]. The simplest mammalian large intestine, as seen in the mink and similar animals, has no cecum and a smooth, cylindrical colon without redundancies or pockets. Complex large intestines, like that of the horse, for example, possess a voluminous cecum with haustration extending all the way to the rectum. These variations in complexity seem to be related to diet, herbivores having complex colons, carnivores simple ones, and omnivores colons of intermediate complexity. But some omnivores (such as the pig) have very complex

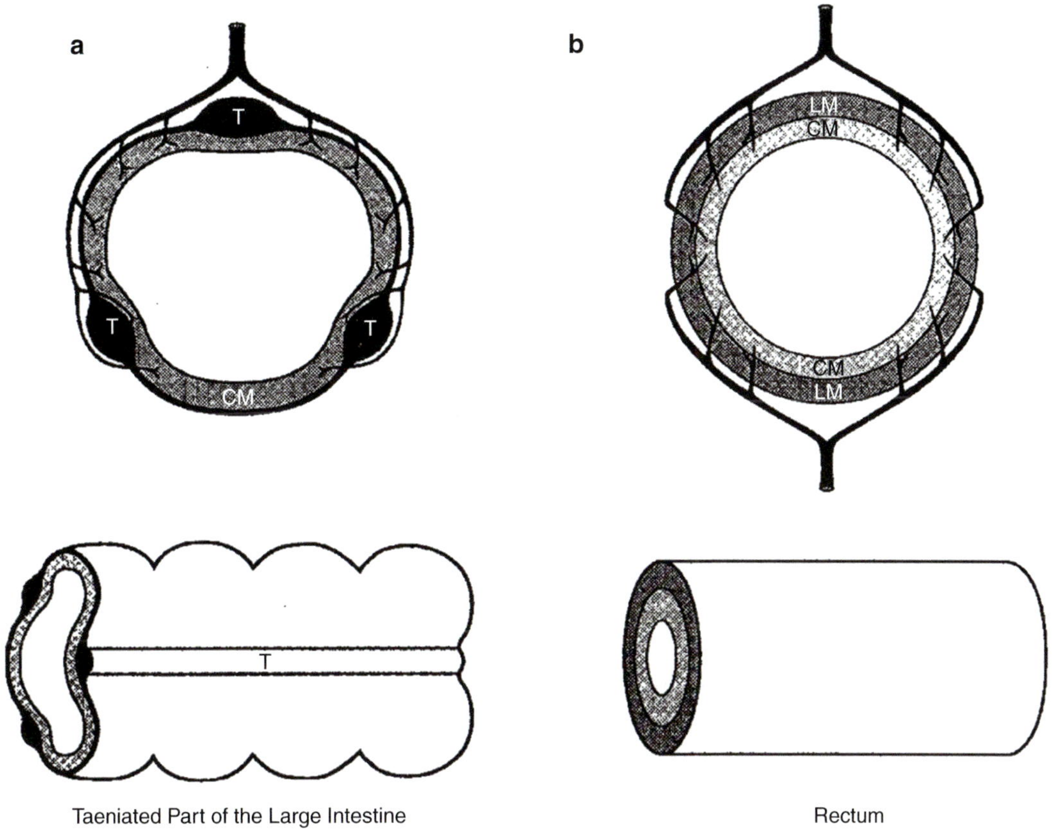

Fig. 4.3 (**a**) The sacculated configuration that characterizes most of the large intestine in humans. (**b**) The cylindrical configuration that characterizes the rectum

colons, while others (such as the rat) have very simple ones. The reason for this may be that the diet changed more easily than did colonic morphology in mammalian evolution. Omnivores with simple colons likely evolved from carnivorous antecedents, while omnivores with complex colons had herbivorous ancestors. In humans, there is wide variation in colorectal anatomy of adults depending on age, gender, and body mass index [4].

4.2.2 Histology

4.2.2.1 The Structure of the Wall of the Large Intestine

The colon is composed of four layers: the *mucosa,* the *submucosa*, the *muscularis propria*, and the *serosa*. The mucosa consists of three layers: the *epithelium*, the *lamina propria*, and the *muscularis mucosae.* The *muscularis propria* also contains three layers: the *circular muscle layer*, the *intermuscular space*, and the *longitudinal muscle layer*.

The epithelium constitutes a single layer composed mainly of *columnar absorptive cells* and *goblet cells.* The columnar absorptive cell of the colon is similar to that found in the small intestine except that its microvilli are rudimentary. Colonic goblet cells also resemble those of the small intestine; however, they are more numerous. The colonic *enteroendocrine cells* of the colon are solitary compared to aggregated as they are in the small intestine. These three cell types develop from undifferentiated cells that line the colonic epithelial crypts.

The lamina propria is the space between the epithelium and the muscularis mucosae and is a loose stroma of collagen fibers, fibroblasts, lymphocytes, plasma cells, macrophages, and eosinophils. The lamina propria also contains large lymphoid aggregates that can protrude into the submucosa.

The muscularis mucosae, a continuous thin sheet of visceral muscle at the base of the lamina propria, constitutes a network of collagen and elastin fibers that supports about four to six layers of smooth muscle cells. Most of these muscle cells lie with their long axes in the longitudinal axis on the serosal side of the layer and in the circular axis on the mucosal side.

The submucosa in the large intestine makes up about half the total wall thickness, a proportion that exceeds that found in other parts of the gut. The loose stroma of collagen and elastin fibers in the submucosa contains fibroblasts, lymphocytes, plasma cells, macrophages, and eosinophils. The submucosa is also rich in arterioles and venules which branch into the adjacent mucosa and muscularis propria. In addition, the submucosa contains an extensive submucosal nerve plexus of nerve fascicles, nerve process bundles, interconnecting ganglia, and nerve cell bodies.

The muscularis propria, the major muscular component of the large intestine, constitutes two distinct layers of smooth muscle with an intervening intermuscular space. The inner circular layer of muscle constitutes bundles of smooth muscle cells oriented so that their long axes follow the circumference of the organ. The circular muscle layer is uniformly thick along most of the organ until it thickens at the anal canal to form the internal anal sphincter. The inner submucosal surface of this muscle layer is covered by a specialized structure known as Stach's plexus, which represents a dense, two-dimensional network of specialized mesenchymal cells called the interstitial cells of Cajal (ICC).

The intermuscular space, about 100 μm thick, contains the myenteric plexus, large ganglia joined together by interganglionic bundles of fascicles of nerve processes. The intermuscular space also contains a scattering of interstitial cells of Cajal as well as a sparse network of blood vessels.

The longitudinal outer muscle layer, a loose stroma of collagen and elastin fibers containing smooth muscle cells, is much thinner than the inner circular muscle layer. As described above, in most of the human colon, this layer is clustered mainly into three major bundles that run closely and parallel to one another, the taeniae coli.

The *serosa,* a continuous sheet of squamous epithelial cells, invests the colon in whole or in part, being separated from the longitudinal muscle layer by a thin connective tissue stroma. This stroma contains blood vessels and a few nerve fibers. It also contains fatty nodules, the *appendices epiploicae*, which can be quite large.

4.2.2.2 Structure of Gut Smooth Muscle

Gastrointestinal visceral (or smooth) muscle closely resembles vascular and other smooth muscle [5]. Each fusiform cell, about 500–700 μm long and 5–15 μm broad, contains a single elongated nucleus near the midpoint of the cell (Fig. 4.4). The nuclear silhouette usually appears smooth and uniform because of the stretch applied to tissue before fixation, but inspection of unstretched tissues reveals wrinkling of the nucleus. Usually two or more nucleoli stand out in the nucleus, lying within a delicate aggregation of nuclear chromatin fairly uniformly dispersed in the nucleoplasm with some condensation just inside the nuclear envelope.

One muscle cell overlaps the next so that the thickest part of one cell lies next to the thin extremities of its neighbors. Thus, the nuclei in the smooth muscle mass appear to be staggered rather than aligned. The muscle cell cytoplasm or sarcoplasm, viewed at light microscopy, seems essentially devoid of structure, hence the adjective, "smooth." The muscle cells lie closely apposed in bundles, delineated and bound together by bands or sheets of connective tissue. Thus, a cross-section shows the muscle as a series of tightly packed palisades of muscle cells separated by connective tissue septa. The muscle bundles join, separate, and join again along their course throughout the muscle. This arrangement ensures the uniform transmission of contractile forces throughout the whole mass in a smooth muscle.

Gut smooth muscle is a relatively dense tissue, the proportion of tissue volume that is extracellular space being about 10–30%. Most of the mass constitutes muscle cells, and for the other constituents, fibroblasts and nerve processes make up a very small proportion. The size and spacing of the muscle cells makes for a high surface-to-volume ratio of the muscle cells. About 1.5 m^2 of muscle cell surface is available for exchange with the extracellular space in each gram of muscle tissue.

The cell membrane in smooth muscle possesses many invaginations, the *caveolae*, each about

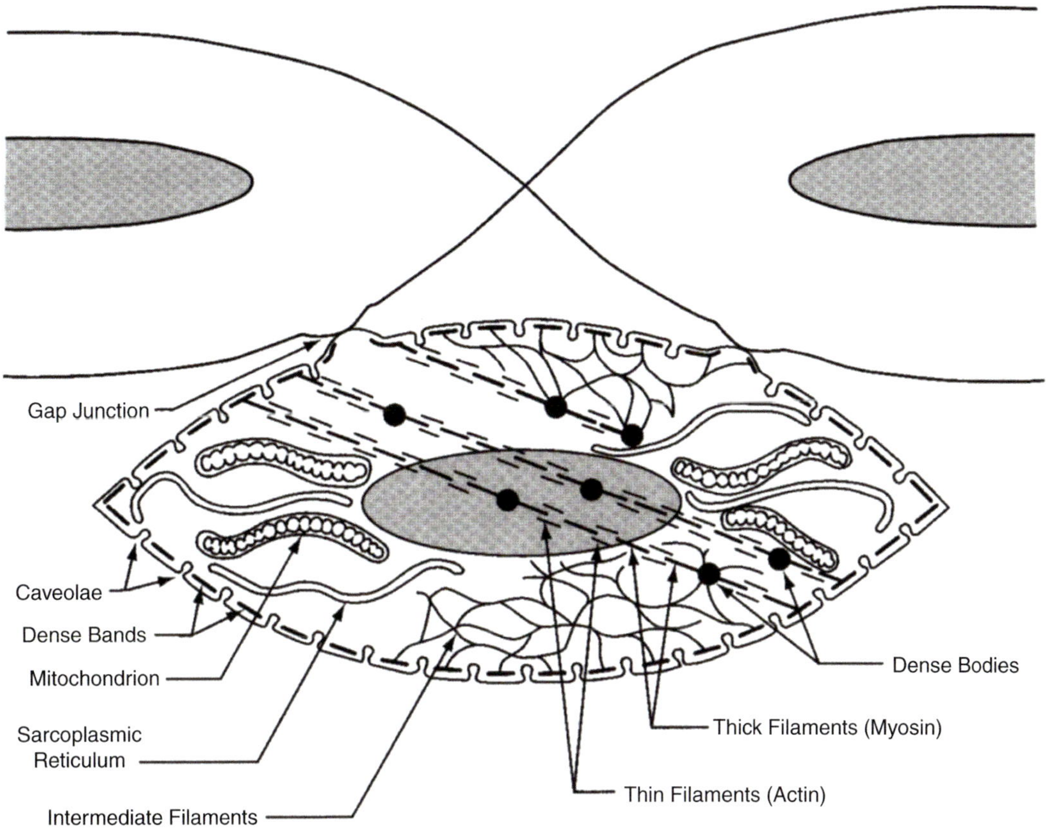

Fig. 4.4 Diagram of a smooth muscle cell to show the ultrastructure

70 μm in diameter and 120 μm deep, opening to the surface through narrow necks. The caveolae increase the cell surface by 50–70%. More than one-third of the surface area of a cell enters into the formation of caveolae. The basal lamina, an amorphous layer that covers the outer surface of a muscle cell, does not enter the caveolae. Elements of the smooth sarcoplasmic reticulum lie just beneath the caveolae. This juxtaposition supports the concept that the caveolae function like the t-tubules of skeletal muscle in facilitating transmembrane calcium flux to activate contraction.

Dense bands, aggregates of amorphous material, cover the inside of the cell membrane between the caveolae. These dense bands anchor the contractile and structural filaments of the sarcoplasm to the cell membrane. Both the abundant contractile filaments, actin and myosin, and the less abundant structural filaments, desmin, also attach to *dense bodies*, aggregates of amorphous material scattered throughout the sarcoplasm that resemble the membrane-associated dense bands. The dense bands and the dense bodies, providing points for the union of contractile and structural filaments both throughout the sarcoplasm and all along the cell membrane, assure the uniform distribution of forces throughout the cell.

Cell-to-cell junctions between adjacent smooth muscle cells provide linkages that assure the integration of muscle cell movements. Anatomists describe *intermediate junctions* as structures that possess features suggesting a role as mechanical linkages. The *gap junctions* provide for a physiological linkage through the cell-to-cell transmission of electrical currents and small molecules.

4.2.3 The Nerves of the Large Intestine

The motor functions of the large intestine result from an interplay between intrinsic and extrinsic nervous signalling. In other words, the movement and function of the colon depend on both the myogenic activity within the muscular layers of the colon and the signals to, from, and between the extensive nerve plexuses.

4.2.3.1 The Extrinsic Nerves

The large intestine receives its extrinsic nerve supply through the *vagus nerves,* from the *pelvic nerves* and from the *mesenteric nerves* (Fig. 4.5) [6–8]. The *vagus nerve branches* provide parasympathetic innervation, the cranial part of the craniosacral outflow, to the whole gastrointestinal tract and to the rostral end of the large intestine. The *pelvic nerves,* arising from the sacral cord, also distribute parasympathetic fibers, the sacral component of the craniosacral outflow, to the whole of the large intestine. The *mesenteric nerves* emerge from the prevertebral ganglia. The three prevertebral ganglia send branches alongside the corresponding three arteries to the gut. These are sympathetic nerves, elements of the thoracolumbar outflow from the central nervous system.

The magnitude of the mass of the large intestine relative to the small number of the extrinsic nerves makes it difficult to trace the distributions the branches of those nerves within the organ. Both physiological and anatomical observations suggest that vagal branches extend no farther than about the middle of the transverse colon, from which the pelvic nerves distribute fibers through the pelvic plexus to the remainder of the large intestine. It is likely that the pelvic nerves overlap to an unknown degree with the vagal nerves. The pelvic nerves distribute nerve fibers through the pelvic plexus to the remainder of the large intestine. The colonic branches from the pelvic plexus pierce the longitudinal muscle layers around the rectosigmoid junction and then ramify in the intermuscular space through the rectum [9–11]. Additional branches of these colonic nerves extend rostrally in the myenteric plexus as far as the transverse colon. Although the branches of nerves, referred to as *the ascending nerves of the colon* (Fig. 4.6), lie within the myenteric plexus which is avascular and does not have a perineurium, each branch resembles their origin extrinsic nerves in that they possess their own perineurium and blood supplies. Nerve fibers depart from these ascending nerves to enter into the surrounding myenteric plexus.

4.2.3.2 The Intrinsic Nerves

The *myenteric plexus,* the major intrinsic innervation of the large intestine, occupies the intermuscular space between the two muscle layers of the muscularis propria. The ganglia, nodes of closely apposed nerve cell bodies and enteroglial cells, lie in this plane with a regular and uniform distribution, joined by interganglionic fascicles. The mesh formed by the ganglia and the interganglionic fascicles, the *primary plexus*, delineates irregular polygonal spaces which themselves contain a *secondary plexus* composed of smaller fascicles that branch from the primary plexus. Still smaller bundles of nerve fibers form a tertiary plexus within the spaces of the secondary plexus. The size and density of distribution of ganglia and nerve cell bodies in the myenteric plexus decreases along the large intestine [12]. Thus, the nerve cell body density in the rectal myenteric plexus is lower than in any other part of the gastrointestinal system with the exception of the lower esophageal sphincter.

The plane of the myenteric plexus in the large intestine also contains interstitial cells of Cajal. These cells lie in the polygonal interstices of the plexus rather than in the substance of the ganglia and fascicles. The ganglia of the submucosa form a plexus that differs from the myenteric plexus in gross appearance [13]. The submucosal plexus ganglia are smaller, farther apart and less regularly distributed. The ganglia and fascicles of the submucosal plexus do not form a regular polygonal pattern, and there is no subdivision into secondary and tertiary plexuses. The submucosal and myenteric plexuses are similar however in the sense that the density of the submucosal plexus also tapers down as it approaches the anus.

The submucosal plexus in the large intestine contains two layers of ganglia and interconnecting nerve fascicles. One layer of ganglia, called *Meissner's plexus,* lies just beneath the muscularis mucosae. The other, *Henle's plexus*, lies close to the surface of the circular muscle layer. The two layers of the plexus, though distinct morphologically, are joined together by inter-ganglionic fascicles and thus should not be considered to be separate structures (see also Chap. 17). Henle's plexus in the submucosa gives off bundles of nerve fibers which descend to the underlying surface of the circular muscle layer and ramify

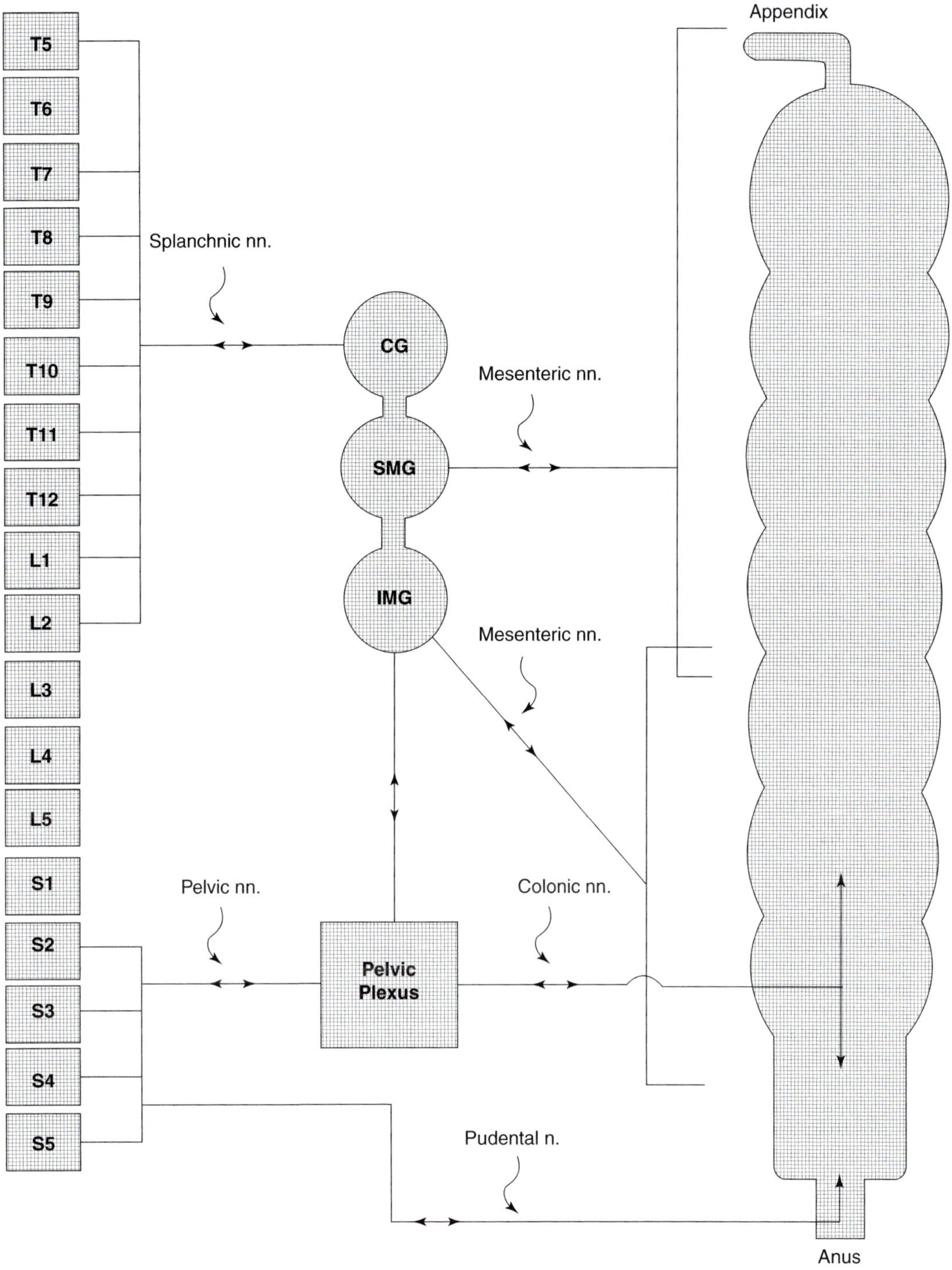

Fig. 4.5 The extrinsic innervation of the large intestine (*CG SMG IMG* three prevertebral ganglia). The blocks at the left represent the levels of the spinal cord

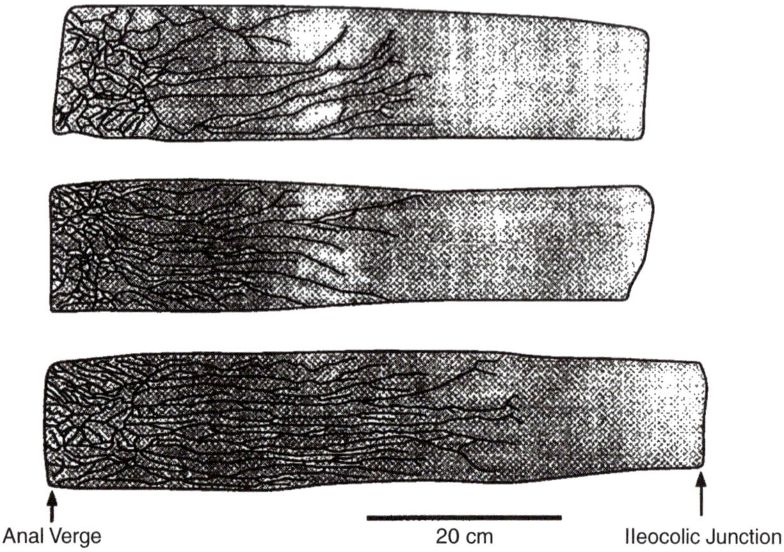

Fig. 4.6 Drawings of the ascending nerves of the colon in three cat colons

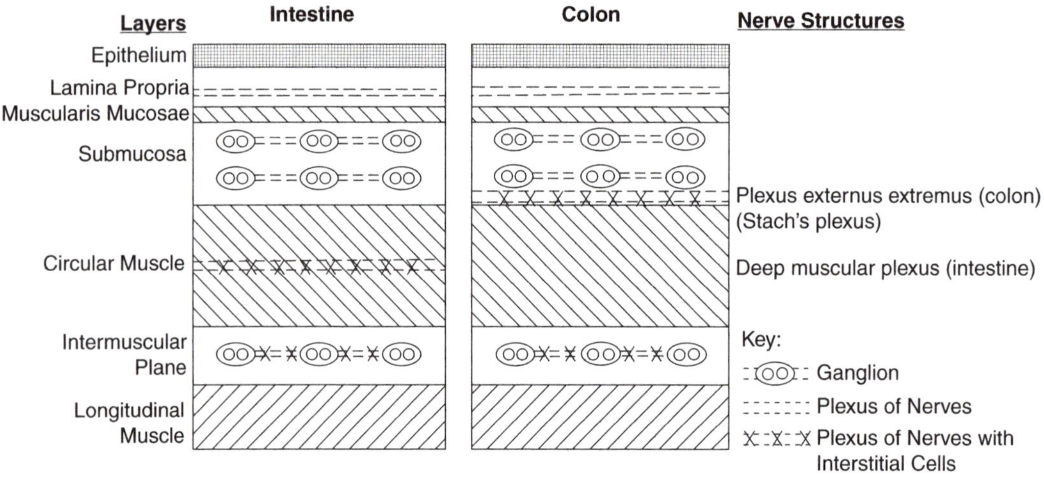

Fig. 4.7 Diagrammatic cross-sections of the wall of the small intestine and the large intestine

there. The branching continues to the point where bundles of nerve processes may contain only one or two nerve fibers. These tiny bundles do not lie directly on the surface of the circular muscle layer but instead lie on an intervening monolayer of *interstitial cells of Cajal.* These cells give off long branching processes which intersect abundantly to form a mat interposed closely to and between the nerve fibers and the smooth muscle cells, known more commonly as Stach's plexus and less commonly as the plexus externus extremus or the plexus submucosus extremus (Figs. 4.7 and 4.8) [14, 15].

4.3 Motor Functions of the Large Intestine

4.3.1 Component Processes of Motor Functions

"Motility" and "motor function," terms widely used to describe the actions of the visceral muscle of the gut, can mean several different things according to context. The terms can refer to any or all of three processes: (a) the flow of luminal contents in the gut; (b) the contractions and relaxations of the muscular walls of the gut that create

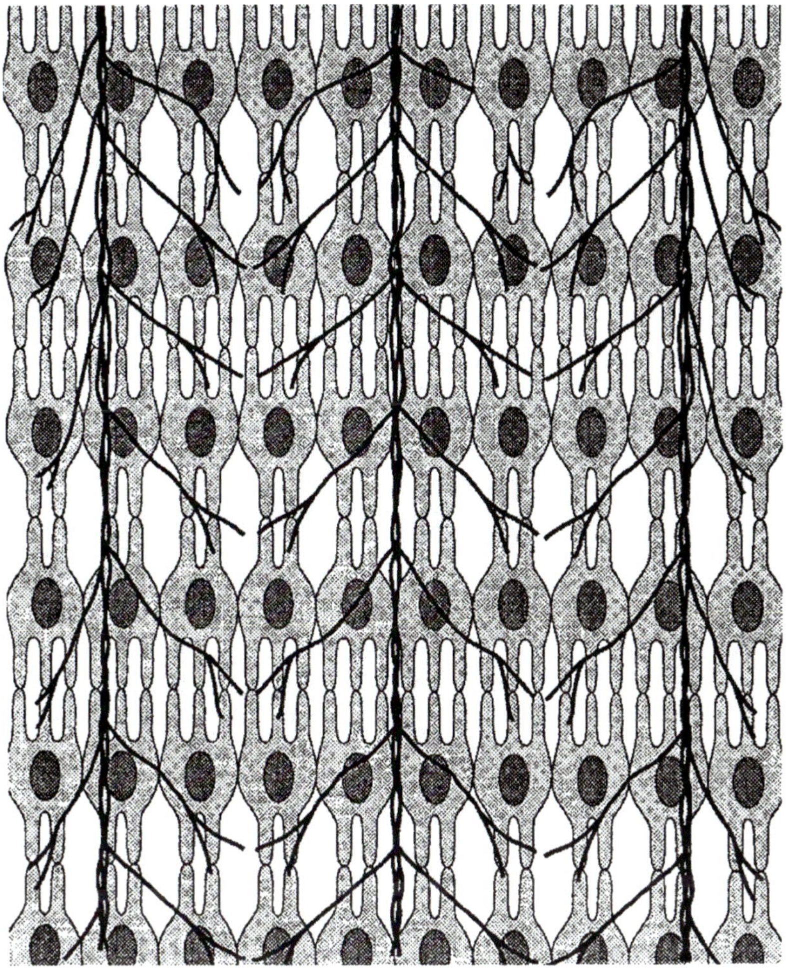

Fig. 4.8 Diagram of Stach's plexus (the plexus *submucosus extremus*) showing the mat of interstitial cells with overlying nerve fibers

these flows; and (c) the physiologic functions that control the force of contractions and their distribution in time and in space.

All three processes—flows, contractions, and controlling functions—constitute complex categories of events. For example, gas, mucus, chyme, and stool certainly all flow, but they must flow differently because they are non-Newtonian fluids with different physical characteristics. These different materials will cause slightly different patterns of colonic wall distension and thus likely have unique signals to the intrinsic neuromuscular pathways within the colon wall as well as the subsequent downstream processes [16]. Contractions can involve any or all of the three muscle layers of the large intestine with an enormous range in possible forces and spatiotemporal distributions. The functions of the muscular layers are influenced in varying degrees by hormonal, neuronal, and intrinsic muscular forces.

Colonic motility is a complicated process that remains to be better understood. Fortunately, the development of colonic manometry has facilitated numerous ongoing studies into better characterizing the components and factors that contribute to the complex nature of large intestine motility [17].

4.3.2 Gross Patterns of Contraction and Flow in the Large Intestine

4.3.2.1 The Functional Parts of the Large Intestine in Animals and Humans

The large intestine constitutes three functionally distinct units arranged in series. It resembles the stomach in this respect where the difference in behavior of the proximal and distal parts is well known. The functional differentiation of the colon into parts was first observed nearly a century ago.

In studies of animals, by radiography and by inspection of the organ exposed at laparotomy, both American and British investigators, at about the same time, saw different patterns of contractions and flow in the different parts of the large intestine [18, 19]. From their descriptions, one can discern three regions: the right colon, the mid colon, and the distal colon. These three segments are not sharply delineated but merge gradually into one another. Nonetheless, their patterns of contraction and flow seem to be quite distinct.

4.3.2.2 The Right Colon

"The usual movement of the transverse and ascending colon is antiperistalsis," wrote Cannon. By "antiperistalsis," he meant a pattern in which ring contractions of the circular muscle layer move retrograde, toward the cecum, rather than caudad like those of the stomach and small intestine. Cannon observed the large intestine of cats radiographically. Elliott and Barclay-Smith studied a variety of small mammals—cats, rats, guinea pigs, rabbits, dogs, ferrets, and hedgehogs—by direct observation of the colon exposed at laparotomy and also described antiperistalsis as the dominant pattern of contraction in the ascending colon. How commonly antiperistalsis occurs in humans remains to be discovered. Antiperistalsis is not obvious clinically under the conditions of the barium enema examination, and this may explain the fact that its very existence in humans is not currently acknowledged.

4.3.2.3 The Mid Colon

Both Cannon and Elliott and Barclay-Smith described contractions beyond the level of the hepatic flexure as coordinated antegrade peristalsis, contraction rings of the circular muscle layer moving caudad. This pattern occurred elsewhere, too, but if dominated in the mid colon. Antegrade peristalsis increased with colonic distension.

4.3.2.4 The Distal Colon

A still more caudal part of the colon shows very little spontaneous activity, but it responds much better than other parts of the colon to stimulation of the pelvic nerves. Such stimulation excites powerful occlusive ring contractions moving caudad.

4.3.2.5 Colonic Motility in Humans and the Mass Movement

The antegrade orientation of ring contractions in the middle parts of the large intestine seen at x-ray in humans agrees with the orientation of contractions seen in animals. One major manifestation of such antegrade contraction is the *mass movement*, first described over a century ago [20] and widely confirmed since. The mass movement appears to be a powerful lumen-occluding contraction ring that develops in the middle or distal parts of the colon after a short period of inhibition. It involves only a relatively short segment of the large intestine. First, haustral indentations disappear. Then, the powerful contraction ring sweeps the segment carrying its contents forward. Then, the haustral indentations reappear. This phenomenon occurs only a few times daily and seems to be precipitated especially by eating.

4.3.2.6 Feeding, Fasting, and Sleep

Feeding, fasting, and sleep all affect colonic motility, and the magnitude of the effect seems to be considerable. Colonic motility diminishes greatly during sleep compared to that seen in the awake state. Most observers imply or assume that this pattern is neurally mediated, but, in fact, no one has investigated the possibility that it is not.

Feeding considerably increases motility in the large intestine after a short delay, an effect which is often inaccurately called the gastro-colic reflex. It is a transient effect but one which produces considerable antegrade propulsion of stool.

Fasting also affects motility in the large intestine. The pronounced cycling of contractions in the small intestine that occurs in fasting has received a great deal of study. A somewhat similar cycling occurs in contractions in the large intestine, but the period of the cycle differs from that found in the small intestine. The purpose and the mechanism behind this cycling activity remain unclear.

4.3.2.7 The Anorectum

It now seems clear from studies done mainly in humans that the motility of the anorectum differs greatly from that of the rest of the large intestine. The rectum is inactive and empty for most of the time. After its evacuation in defecation, the rectum fills very slowly with feces that are delivered presumably by mass movements. The rectal retention of this fecal mass is facilitated by the receptive relaxation of the rectum and contraction of the anal sphincters. The internal anal sphincter remains contracted involuntarily as the rectum fills. The rectum exhibits brief powerful contractions at long intervals as it fills, especially at night, independent of contractions of the colon and not evacuative. When the degree of rectal filling is sufficient, the internal anal sphincters relax as the result of activation of the rectoanal reflex and a powerful and evacuating peristaltic contraction sweeps the rectum. This is the defecation reflex. As described above, the pan-colonic pressurization motor pattern of the colon is believed to be related to relaxation of the anal sphincter, particularly when motility is activated by meals; however, the mechanism is poorly understood [21].

4.3.2.8 A Summary of Contractions and Flow in the Large Intestine

Material entering the large intestine from the ileum tends to pool and to remain in the area of the cecum and ascending colon where there seems to be recirculation and mixing. This is, in part, the result of retrograde peristaltic contractions (antiperistalsis) in this proximal region of the large intestine. Antegrade flow is accomplished in part by the rhythmic peristaltic contractions which predominate in the middle regions of the organ. These antegrade peristaltic movements may be quite infrequent as they occur during the special phenomenon called the mass movement. This mass movement is a complex motor event occurring at long intervals of time, occupying only a part of the colon and involving inhibition of the muscle first, and then peristalsis. This complex event is the principal means for the antegrade flow of luminal contents in the large intestine. The rectum exhibits little activity at rest but simply expands to accommodate the fecal mass delivered to it by successive mass movements. In recent years, high-resolution manometry has led to identifying a concept of pan-colonic pressurization which may represent the main motor pattern of the colon. Pan-colonic pressurizations seem to occur in reaction to even mild distension of the colon and may serve to allow effective absorption, mixing, and propulsion of bowel contents. Furthermore, this pressurization pattern has been proposed to be, by mechanisms unknown at the present time, coordinated with simultaneous relaxation of the anal sphincter [21].

4.3.3 The Pacemaking System in the Large Intestine

4.3.3.1 The Electrical Slow Waves of the Large Intestine

The musculature of the large intestine wall generates pacemaking electrical signals that resemble those of the heart, both in form and function [22]. Similar signals arise in the musculature of the gastric antrum, as well as in that of the small intestine. Although the electrical signals generated by the large intestine differ from those of the other gastrointestinal viscera in some details, the processes in signal generation and function of the signals seem to be fundamentally the same. The unique features of the electromyogram of the large intestine relate to the directional pattern of the pacemaking electrical signals and to the precise layers in the wall that generate them. The pacemaking signals spread retrograde in the proximal large intestine. Contrarily, the pacemaking signals in the stomach and small intestine spread antegrade. Additionally, these electric signals tend to originate from the outer longitudinal muscle layer in the stomach and small intestine, whereas in the colon, they arise from the circular muscle layer in the large intestine.

4.3.3.2 The Function of Electrical Slow Waves

When electrical events and mechanical events are recorded simultaneously from a single point in the large intestine (or one in the small intestine or gastric antrum), one can see an electrical transient that recurs continuously with a fixed configuration. From baseline, a relatively rapid depolarization occurs, followed by a plateau which ultimately transitions into a slower depolarization. Such signals recur at a highly constant frequency that is characteristic for the locus of the recording. This electrical transient, called the *electrical slow wave* (or, formerly, the *basic electrical rhythm* or *electrical control activity*), continues regardless of whether the muscle at the recording site is contracting. When a contraction of the musculature occurs, the onset of that contraction is signaled by the appearance of one or more much more rapid electrical transients during the plateau of the electrical slow wave. That is, the beginning of a transient or phasic contraction can only occur during an interval of time which is governed by the period of the cycle of the electrical slow wave. The slow wave paces or governs the timing of rhythmic contractions.

When an electromyogram is recorded simultaneously from a series of electrodes aligned along the long axis of the large intestine (or small intestine or gastric antrum), the slow waves can be seen to spread from one end of the electrode array to another, propagating in a single direction at a fixed velocity. Since the initiation of a contraction is phase-locked to the electrical slow wave, this relationship means that the electrical slow wave governs the location of rhythmic contractions. *Thus, the electrical slow waves dictate the frequency, velocity, and direction of spread of rhythmic peristalsis.*

4.3.3.3 The Origin of the Electrical Slow Waves of the Large Intestine

For a long time, investigators interpreted the experimental evidence as indicating that the electrical slow waves originate in the smooth muscle of the gut, specifically in the longitudinal muscle layer in the small intestine and gastric antrum and in the circular muscle layer in the colon. It is now well established that the electrical slow waves arise in interstitial cells of Cajal [23]. In all species studied, the evidence from the large intestine is the strongest [24, 25], but it seems most likely that these cells are involved in the generation of pacemaker signals in the remainder of the gastrointestinal tract as well.

Two unique electrical slow wave types have been identified in the colon [26, 27]. One type arises in Stach's plexus in the inner surface of the circular muscle layer, whereas the other, also referred to as sinusoidal oscillations, arise near the myenteric plexus. There is little doubt that both wave types are generated by the interstitial cells of Cajal. The interstitial cells that lie in Stach's plexus generate a major set of the electrical slow waves, although it is not yet clear how the abundant nerve fibers in that plexus may also participate, possibly involved in signal regulation, controlling frequency, and amplitude [16]. The involvement of the circular muscle layer in the signal generation process is still actively being researched; however, it has been determined that sensory elements in the circular muscle layer are critical in activating stretch-induced polarized reflexes. It is likely that the abundant array of nerves regulate the signals, controlling their frequency and amplitude [16]. Undoubtedly, the circular muscle layer receives the aforementioned signals, transmitted through specialized gap junctions between the interstitial cells and the muscle cells.

4.3.3.4 The Spread of the Electrical Slow Waves

The first studies of the electrical slow waves of the large intestine were undertaken in the cat. These studies revealed a pattern of spread or migration that was consistent with the previously observed pattern of retrograde peristalsis in the proximal colon in that species. The site of the dominant pacemaker along the large intestine varied in position from time to time, but it was almost always located in a place such that slow waves spread retrograde in the proximal part of the organ and antegrade in the more distal sites. The location of the dominant pacemaker varied along the colon so that signal migration may fluctuate from retrograde to antegrade in the right colon, but the factors that govern its position remain unknown.

4.3.3.5 The Sinusoidal Oscillations

The colonic electromyogram also contains another set of electrical signals besides the electrical slow waves, a sinusoidal oscillation that occurs intermittently rather than continuously. The oscillation is much more rapid than the slow waves. These signals are associated with contractions of the circular muscle layer, contractions that can span the duration of several slow wave cycles. It appears that these rapid sinusoidal oscillations arise in the plane of the myenteric plexus, from the interstitial cells of Cajal that are located there. This specific electric signal correlates to the initiation and termination of a contraction. The sinusoidal oscillations relationship to the contractions are referred to as mass movements when they occur in the organ in situ. Hence, they seem likely to be both excited and inhibited by intrinsic nerves in the large intestine.

4.4 Neurogenic Factors in Large Intestinal Motility

4.4.1 The Nervous System of the Colon and Cell Types

There is no reason to suppose that the colonic innervation differs substantially from that of the small intestine with respect to the types of intrinsic nerves present. Adrenergic nerve fibers, mainly identified by catecholamine fluorescence staining, end chiefly in relation to ganglion cells of the myenteric plexus in the colon, with very few entering the muscle layers. Cholinergic nerve fibers, also largely identified by histochemistry, vary somewhat in staining intensity and seem to be the principal excitatory nerve fibers present. Nerve fibers also contain various peptides and other potential neurotransmitters, including VIP, GABA, somatostatin, serotonin, and nitric oxide. Both the classification of neurons on the basis of the co-localization of such substances and the mapping of nerve fibers classified in that way have not been done so carefully in the large intestine as it has been done in the guinea pig small intestine model. Likewise, comparisons between the myenteric and submucosal plexuses remain to be made. In terms of function, the principal excitatory motor nerves in the colonic musculature act by the release of acetylcholine and the principal inhibitory motor nerves act by the release of nitric oxide.

4.4.2 Intrinsic Reflexes in the Large Intestine

The existence of a peristaltic reflex in the colon was claimed by Bayliss and Starling [28], a response like that which they had seen in the small intestine. They discovered ascending excitation and descending inhibition in response to mucosal stimulation. This reflex was more readily evoked in some species than in others. Other investigators subsequently reported difficulty in demonstrating the reflex as initially reported [29, 30]. Hence, there are doubts about its universality, as well as about some of the details of its nature. It is not definitive that the intestinal peristaltic reflex can be invoked at all to explain the complex motor functions of the large intestine.

One reflex, however, is clearly demonstrated and clinically useful, the rectoanal inhibitory reflex [31], characterized by the relaxation of the internal anal sphincter in response to rectal distension. The distension of a balloon in the sigmoid colon or rectum induces relaxation of the internal anal sphincter by extrinsic pathways. The reflex is part of the defecation reflex. The effect is likely mediated through mechanoreceptors that sense mechanical stretch; however, the precise molecular structure of the receptor has not been elucidated. Moreover, inhibitory nerves utilizing the release of nitric oxide serve the efferent limb of this reflex arc.

4.4.3 Extrinsic Nervous Control of Large Intestinal Motility

The large intestine resembles the rest of the gut with respect to the effects of stimulation by the extrinsic nerves. Thus, the lumbar sympathetic nerves carry both excitatory and inhibitory fibers to all parts of the large intestine. The splanchnic nerves are primarily inhibitory. The vagi are excitatory mainly in the proximal colon. The pelvic nerves are excitatory through cholinergic and other mechanisms. It is clear that voluntary defecation is controlled by the cerebral cortex, by which the autonomic and somatic pathways are activated. The autonomic pathway initiates the propulsive activity of the smooth muscle of the colorectum and relaxation of the internal anal sphincter, whereas the somatic pathway leads to relaxation of the striated muscle of the external anal sphincter. Of note, the brain stem focus for control of the smooth muscle of the colorectum and internal anal sphincter is Barrington's nucleus, which lies in the floor of the fourth ventricle near the locus coeruleus [32].

The extrinsic nerves can mediate the effects of stimulation in the central nervous system. The stimulation of the hypothalamus and mesencephalon both alter colonic motor function. The existence of such effects, however, does not clearly establish the physiological importance of such central nervous controls. Certainly, the initiation of defecation seems always to be partly voluntary, and this implies some importance of the extrinsic nerves as discussed above. This voluntary control involves, however, the anorectum and pelvic floor more than the whole large intestine. The delineation of voluntary and involuntary control remains obscure. The borderline between voluntary and involuntary functions is even more mysterious at the caudal end of the gastrointestinal tract than it is at the rostral end in the oropharynx.

4.5 Myogenic Factors in the Motility of the Large Intestine

Clearly, tonic contraction is an important component in large intestinal motility. Tone, a stable or sustained contraction, is much more difficult to assess both in vivo and in vitro than rhythmic or periodic contractions. Still, tone can be seen to exist when circumstances temporarily abolish it. Thus, the tonic contraction of the internal anal sphincter disappears with the excitation of mucosal mechanoreceptors in the rectoanal inhibitory reflex [33]. The other major manifestation of tone in the large intestine is the haustral indentations. These narrow rings indent the lumen of the large intestine at rest at fairly regular intervals to produce the sacculated appearance of the herbivore colon. They were once considered to be fixed and fibrous structures, septa. Their disappearance as a part of the change that occurs during a mass movement, however, indicates that they must be, at least in large part, involved in tonic contractions.

The origin of tone in muscle is certainly not the same in all cases. Tone can reflect the tonic excitation of the muscle by excitatory motor nerves, which is the cause in the somatically innervated striated muscle. Tone could also be the result of hormonal factors. Or, it could represent some special property of the muscle itself. The origin of tone in much of the smooth muscle of the gut has not been investigated carefully. However, it has been extensively studied in the lower esophageal sphincter. Here, tone persists when that sphincter muscle is isolated in vitro, and after it is treated with tetrodotoxin. This and other evidence indicate that tone in the lower esophageal sphincter is partly, if not largely, myogenic. There is no reason to assume that tone in the large intestine has a different origin. In fact, tone in the internal anal sphincter is very much like that in the lower esophageal sphincter. Still, experiments to establish this point about tone convincingly for the bulk of the large intestine remain to be done. Of course, tonic contraction in the visceral musculature may have more than one origin.

4.6 Some Integrated Motor Functions

4.6.1 Continence

Clearly, the capacity to retain feces in the rectum is important, as most mammals possess that capacity and use it most of the time. Many of the nerve conduction studies of colorectal function have involved rats and other laboratory animals. Interestingly, rats being tetrapedal do not stop regular activity to defecate, and they do not utilize a defecatory posture, hence displaying a different defecatory behavior than humans. Humans being bipedal utilize an upright posture and have an inherent difference in structure and functional characteristics of the pelvic floor when compared to tetrapods. Moreover, the human capacity for continence involves mainly the anorectum. It involves two distinguishable functions, the reservoir function of the rectum and the closure of the anal canal. The voluntary control of defecation seems to be exerted primarily at the level of the external anal sphincter.

The reservoir function of the rectum is sometimes said to resemble that of the proximal stomach; however, there are several notable differences. The process of rectal filling is slower and more continuous. There is a continuous concentration of rectal contents rather than continuous dilution as occurs in the stomach. The stomach empties slowly and incompletely, but the emptying of the rectum is abrupt and complete. Still, the rectum seems to share with the gastric fundus some capacity for accommodation or receptive relaxation.

Continence appears to depend far more upon the closure of the anal canal provided by the two anal sphincters than upon the receptive relaxation of the rectum. The two sphincters, internal and external, operate in quite different ways. The internal anal sphincter, a thickening of the circular layer of visceral muscle at the end of the rectum, maintains its tone constantly except at times when the rectum has become full, at which point the rectoanal inhibitory reflex (RAIR) is initiated. The contraction of the internal anal sphincter contributes to most of the anal canal pressure that is measured at rest. That is, the internal anal sphincter is the primary determinant of continence at rest. The external anal sphincter, a striated musculature derived from the striated muscle of the pelvic floor and sharing the same somatic innervation, is important in continence mainly when sudden rectal distension has abolished the tonic contraction of the internal anal sphincter. The external anal sphincter exhibits a fairly constant resting tone. It can be further contracted by volition. This aforementioned increase in contraction serves to abort defecation when a rise in rectal pressure and a relaxation of the internal anal sphincter have occurred as the first steps in the sequence of events that lead to defecation. Thus, the external anal sphincter maintains continence mainly when defecation is imminent. Contraction of the external anal sphincter is not wholly volitional. Involuntary contractions of that sphincter can occur with sudden rectal distension and in response to stimulation of the perianal skin. Continence attributable to the external anal sphincter also requires normal anal and rectal sensation. Both hypersensitivity of the anorectal area and hyposensitivity can lead to incontinence, the former because of exaggerated reflexes and the latter because of the imperception of the imminence of rectal evacuation.

4.6.2 Defecation

Many different actions take place in a close temporal sequence during the process of defecation, indicating that the central nervous system clearly participates. Some of the voluntary actions are necessary to raise the intra-abdominal pressure. They include the closure of the airway, the descent of the diaphragm, and the contraction of the abdominal muscles, otherwise known as the Valsalva maneuver. The involuntary actions include the relaxation of the internal anal sphincter and the peristaltic contraction that empties the rectum.

The process of defecation begins firstly with sensory excitation and reflex mechanisms in the anorectum. The anorectal receptors are excited by mechanical stimulation of the rectum. Their exact location remains unknown, but much evidence suggests that they may be located in the mucosa very near to the squamocolumnar mucosal junction. In fact, this region contains an abundance of sensory nerve endings. It seems likely that various mechanical and chemical stimuli can excite these receptors to induce the urge to defecate. Secondly, the reflex relaxation of the internal anal sphincter follows. A third reflex function follows a little later. This is the powerful peristaltic contraction that evacuates the anorectum. It may involve much of the left colon, even up as far as the splenic flexure. The aforementioned phenomenon is also referred to as giant migrating contractions (GMCs). Studied extensively in the canine model, GMCs are characterized by daily forceful contractions, with the mean amplitude approximately three times larger than the mean peak amplitude of colonic phasic contractions. Additionally, rectal relaxation is synchronous with the initiation of these GMCs. Enteric nerves have been demonstrated to be integral for the initiation of GMCs and rectal relaxation. Moreover, the determinants of its location, velocity, and force continue to be investigated [34].

4.6.3 The Response of the Large Intestine to Eating

The *gastrocolic reflex*, a term that has broad currency, refers to the association of defecation with eating. The term is in error as the stimulus is not confined to the stomach or the colon. Additionally, the mechanism is not clearly established to truly be a reflex, either.

However, the general nature of the effect is clear. Eating increases the frequency and amplitude of contractions in both the right and left colon (and in the ileum), and this increase may be followed by defecation. The effect takes a little time to start, 20 minutes or more, and it lasts about 20–30 minutes.

Various studies have sought to define the nature of the effective stimulus. Efforts to demonstrate a "cephalic" mechanism, in which the sight, smell, or thought of food excites the effect, have failed to produce convincing evidence. Likewise, attempts to establish that the stomach is the sole source of the effect have failed. The entry of nutrients into the duodenum, however, seems to be a highly effective stimulus, and the response has been found to be mediated by chemoreceptors in the duodenal mucosa.

Although nervous mechanisms in the gut seem likely to participate to some extent in the effect, the pathways remain obscure. Even the nature of the motor nerves mediating the response is obscure, whether they are adrenergic, cholinergic, or nitrergic. Some evidence suggests that the effect is mediated in part by hormone release from the upper gastrointestinal tract triggered by nutrients. There are many such hormones to investigate, including gastrin, cholecystokinin, and motilin. It may be pointless to try to choose between neural and hormonal mechanisms for the effect because several mechanisms may be involved.

4.6.4 The Gut-Brain Axis: The Connection Between Emotions and Motility in the Large Intestine

For centuries, the association between human emotional psychology and the gastrointestinal tract function has been described. One example is the high rates of irritable bowel syndrome (IBS) symptoms in individuals with anxiety or depressive disorders [35]. Over the past few decades, several studies have recognized the specific interactions between the brain and the GI tract. These interactions are multifactorial and include bidirectional neuronal pathways of the parasympathetic and sympathetic nervous system, hormonal pathway involving the hypothalamic pituitary adrenal (HPA) axis, corticotrophin releasing factor (CRF) pathway, as well as gut microbiota and immunity [36]. Increasing evidence suggests that the enteric microbiome greatly impacts on gut-brain communication leading to the concept of a microbiome-gut-brain axis [37].

For example, IBS, which is associated with several psychological comorbidities including anxiety, has demonstrated the importance of the emotional stress-induced CRF pathway. Experimental studies have revealed that the activation of CRF pathways in healthy subjects reproduced the diarrheal characteristic features of IBS (colonic mast cell activation, visceral hyperalgesia, serotonin release, stimulation of colonic propulsive motor function, and watery diarrhea) [36]. Moreover, a great deal of effort continues to be directed to further elucidate the specific intimate bidirectional pathways between the GI tract and the brain.

References

1. Christensen J, editor. Gross and microscopic anatomy of the large intestine. New York: Raven Press; 1991.
2. Stevens CE. Comparative physiology of the vertebrate digestive system. Cambridge, New York, New

Rochelle, Melbourne, Sydney: Cambridge University Press; 1988.
3. Hume ID. Digestive physiology and nutrition of marsupials. Monographs on marsupial biology. Cambridge, UK: Cambridge University Press; 1982. p. 27–109.
4. Khashab MA, Pickhardt PJ, Kim DH, Rex DK. Colorectal anatomy in adults at computed tomography colonography: normal distribution and the effect of age, sex, and body mass index. Endoscopy. 2009;41(8):674–8.
5. Gabella G, editor. Structure of muscles and nerves in the gastrointestinal tract. 3rd ed. New York: Raven Press; 1994.
6. Furness JB, Costa M. The enteric nervous system. Edinburgh, London, Melbourne, New York: Churchill Livingstone; 1987.
7. Gabella G. Structure of the autonomic nervous system. London: Chapman and Hall; 1976.
8. Gabella G. Innervation of the gastrointestinal tract. Int Rev Cytol. 1979;59:129–93.
9. Christensen J, Rick GA. Distribution of myelinated nerves in ascending nerves and myenteric plexus of cat colon. Am J Anat. 1987;178(3):250–8.
10. Christensen J, Stiles MJ, Rick GA, Sutherland J. Comparative anatomy of the myenteric plexus of the distal colon in eight mammals. Gastroenterology. 1984;86(4):706–13.
11. Stach W. Ascending nerves of the plexus pelvinus of the wall of the large intestine and the limits of vagal and sacral parasympathetic innervation. Z Mikrosk Anat Forsch. 1971;84(1):65–90.
12. Christensen J, Rick GA, Robison BA, Stiles MJ, Wix MA. Arrangement of the myenteric plexus throughout the gastrointestinal tract of the opossum. Gastroenterology. 1983;85(4):890–9.
13. Christensen J, Rick GA. Nerve cell density in submucous plexus throughout the gut of cat and opossum. Gastroenterology. 1985;89(5):1064–9.
14. Christensen J, Rick GA. Intrinsic nerves in the mammalian colon: confirmation of a plexus at the circular muscle-submucosal interface. J Auton Nerv Syst. 1987;21(2–3):223–31.
15. Stach W. The extreme enteric plexus of the large intestine and its relation to the interstitial cells (Cajal). Z Mikrosk Anat Forsch. 1972;85(2):245–72.
16. Spencer NJ, Dinning PG, Brookes SJ, Costa M. Insights into the mechanisms underlying colonic motor patterns. J Physiol. 2016;594(15):4099–116.
17. Bharucha AE. High amplitude propagated contractions. Neurogastroenterol Motil. 2012;24(11):977–82.
18. Cannon WB. The movements of the intestines studied by means of the Rontgen rays. J Med Res. 1902;7(1):72–5.
19. Elliott TR. Antiperistalsis and other muscular activities of the colon. J Physiol. 1904;31(3–4):272–304.
20. Holzknecht G. Die normale Peristaltik des Colons. München Med Wschr. 1909;56:2401–3.
21. Corsetti M, Pagliaro G, Demedts I, Deloose E, Gevers A, Scheerens C, et al. Pan-colonic pressurizations associated with relaxation of the anal sphincter in health and disease: a new colonic motor pattern identified using high-resolution manometry. Am J Gastroenterol. 2017;112(3):479–89.
22. Christensen J, Caprilli R, Lund GF. Electric slow waves in circular muscle of cat colon. Am J Physiol. 1969;217(3):771–6.
23. Christensen J. A commentary on the morphological identification of interstitial cells of Cajal in the gut. J Auton Nerv Syst. 1992;37(2):75–88.
24. Conklin JL, Du C. Pathways of slow-wave propagation in proximal colon of cats. Am J Physiol. 1990;258(6 Pt 1):G894–903.
25. Du CA, Conklin JL. Origin of slow waves in the isolated proximal colon of the cat. J Auton Nerv Syst. 1989;28(2):167–77.
26. Smith TK, Reed JB, Sanders KM. Origin and propagation of electrical slow waves in circular muscle of canine proximal colon. Am J Physiol. 1987;252(2. Pt 1):C215–24.
27. Smith TK, Reed JB, Sanders KM. Interaction of two electrical pacemakers in muscularis of canine proximal colon. Am J Physiol. 1987;252(3. Pt 1):C290–9.
28. Bayliss WM, Starling EH. The movements and the innervation of the large intestine. J Physiol. 1900;26(1–2):107–18.
29. Hukuhara T, Miyake T. The intrinsic reflexes in the colon. Jpn J Physiol. 1959;9(1):49–55.
30. Raiford T, Mulinos MG. The myenteric reflex as exhibited by the exteriorized colon of the dog. Am J Physiol. 1934;110:129–36.
31. Schuster MM, Hendrix TR, Mendeloff AI. The internal anal sphincter response: manometric studies on its normal physiology, neural pathways, and alteration in bowel disorders. J Clin Invest. 1963;42:196–207.
32. Callaghan B, Furness JB, Pustovit RV. Neural pathways for colorectal control, relevance to spinal cord injury and treatment: a narrative review. Spinal Cord. 2018;56(3):199–205.
33. Garrett JR, Howard ER, Jones W. The internal anal sphincter in the cat: a study of nervous mechanisms affecting tone and reflex activity. J Physiol. 1974;243(1):153–66.
34. Tabe Y, Mochiki E, Yanai M, Toyomasu Y, Ando H, Ohno T, et al. Characterization of special propulsive contractions during rectal evacuation in a canine model of intestinal extrinsic denervation and rectal transection. Int J Colorectal Dis. 2010;25(1):53–61.
35. Gros DF, Antony MM, McCabe RE, Swinson RP. Frequency and severity of the symptoms of irritable bowel syndrome across the anxiety disorders and depression. J Anxiety Disord. 2009;23(2): 290–6.
36. Tache Y, Million M. Role of corticotropin-releasing factor signaling in stress-related alterations of colonic motility and hyperalgesia. J Neurogastroenterol Motil. 2015;21(1):8–24.
37. Cryan JF, O'Mahony SM. The microbiome-gut-brain axis: from bowel to behavior. Neurogastroenterol Motil. 2011;23(3):187–92.

Animal Models of Aganglionosis

5

Julia Brendel and Prem Puri

Contents

5.1 Introduction

Humans are not the only mammals suffering from aganglionosis, as aganglionosis and megacolon have also been described in different animal types like mice, rats, dogs or horses [1]. Especially by using rodents as experimental models for the human Hirschsprung's disease (HSCR), remarkable advances in understanding the genetics and cell biology of the developing enteric nervous system (ENS) as well as the pathology of HSCR had been achieved over the last few decades.

This chapter deals with the characteristics of aganglionosis in different animal models with special focus on rodents. Broadly speaking, there are four main types of animal models in use for the investigation of HSCR today [1]: firstly, natural occurring models, which are obviously the most ideal ones, as there is little or no interference to the animal prior to the study; secondly, transgenic animals, which allow researchers to mimic the natural occurrence of the condition and also identify specific genes involved in the regulation of the disease; and thirdly, teratogen-induced models, which have the drawback of exposure to a generalized noxa, which could lead to widespread detriments rather than simply targeting a specific organ system. Finally, surgically created models can closely simulate manlike conditions and surgical procedures.

In the recent years, HSCR animal models have been of particular importance for stem cell transplantation studies as replacement therapy and therapeutic targets for HSCR [2].

5.2 Natural Mutants

Aganglionic megacolon not only occurs in humans but also in other mammalians like mice, rats, cats, pigs, and horses [3–11]. These muta-

J. Brendel (✉)
Department of Pediatric Surgery, Hannover Medical School, Hannover, Germany
e-mail: Brendel.Julia@mh-hannover.de

P. Puri
National Children's Research Centre, Our Lady's Childrens Hospital, University College Dublin, Dublin, Ireland

School of Medicine and Medical Science and Conway Institute of Biomedical Research, University College Dublin, Dublin, Ireland
e-mail: prem.puri@ucd.ie

P. Puri (ed.), *Hirschsprung's Disease and Allied Disorders*,
https://doi.org/10.1007/978-3-030-15647-3_5

tions not only involve the intestine but also another neural crest derivative, the melanocytes, since the animals often have major areas of unpigmented skin and hair. First, aganglionosis was described in mice by Derrick and St. George-Grambauer in 1957 [12], who found that approximately 3.2 per 1000 individuals of their colony developed aganglionosis. The aganglionosis had an average length of 15–20 mm with no association of disruption in pigmentation of the color coat. Bielschowsky and Schofield described a colony in 1962, where 10% of the offspring were affected by aganglionosis with a high incidence of mammary cancer and pituitary adenomas, but no association to a white-colored coat [13]. Outbreeding experiments suggested an autosomal recessive inheritance with modification of the trait by other genetic factors.

In 1966, Lane investigated two strains of mice, the lethal spotting (*ls*) mice and the piebald spotting mice (s^l), both with aganglionosis as an autosomal recessive condition [3]. Lethal spotting mice present with an aganglionic segment of approximately 2 mm and a patched coat, whereas the piebald-lethal mice have approximately 10 mm of aganglionosis. Later, the defect was linked to chromosomes 2 and 14 [1]. Fujmoto et al. [14, 15] investigated extensively enterocolitis in piebald-lethal mice and identified two clinical types of enterocolitis in this mouse model. Two thirds of the cases with megacolon died within 3–4 weeks of age due to severe enterocolitis. The others developed besides megacolon a massive abdominal distension and died at 9–11 weeks of age. Dembowski et al. found enterocolitis in less than 50% of the mutants of the lethal spotting model; additionally the majority of these mice only presented with mild signs of inflammation [16]. Autosomal recessive inherited aganglionic rats, whereby 80–90% had total colonic aganglionosis and the rest was located in the mid-colon, were described by Ikadai et al. in 1979 [7]. The rodents had a white-colored coat and a high mortality rate with a survival length of 3–4 weeks due to enterocolitis and bowel obstruction. The so-called dominant megacolon (*dom*) mouse with distal colonic aganglionosis and a long hypoganglionic transition zone was examined by Lane and Liu in 1984 [6]. Occasionally, the entire large intestine is aganglionic. The dominant inherited allele for the mutation was found on chromosome 15 [1].

Histological studies in all these rodent models using acetylcholinesterase whole-mounts revealed that their histological structure is identical to the human, with increased nerve trunks in the distal aganglionosis, an often asymmetrical transition zone of variable length, and, more proximally, a normal plexus [17]. Numerous electrophysiological studies demonstrated abnormal discharges of myogenic action potentials in the aganglionic segments associated with tonic constriction and a reduction in the luminal diameter [18] and that the aganglionic bowel has no inhibitory junction potentials, which leads it to result in an uncontrolled manner contraction [1]. HSCR models have also provided insights into the physiology and embryology of the disease. Cass et al. [19] investigated neural crest cell (NCC) migration in the intestine of the natural mutants of lethal spotting mouse, piebald mouse and spotting lethal rat. They found a delayed migration in NCCs derived from the vagal neural crest and that some enteric precursors in the aganglionic distal hindgut derived from the sacral neural crest did not vary in quantity compared to normal embryos. Although they demonstrated that there is sacral neural crest contribution into the ENS, this contribution was shown to be functionally insignificant.

The English spotting coat color locus, also called dominant-white spotting locus in Checkered Giant rabbits, is triggered by an incompletely dominant allele (*En*). Homozygous *En/En* animals are almost completely white and subvital because of an underlying megacolon. Self-colored homozygous recessive wild-type rabbits (*en/en*) and normally spotted heterozygous *En/en* rabbits appear to be vital [20–22]. Fontanesi and colleagues found in *En/En* rabbits reduced and altered c-kit immunolabeled interstitial cells of Cajal (ICC) compared to *en/en* controls [23]. Electron microscopy analysis of the *En/En* rabbit tissue revealed neuro-ICC abnormalities reminiscent of the human non-aganglionic megacolon.

5.3 Knockout Models

Transgenic technology, provides a powerful tool with which to produce animal models to determine the functions of genes associated with human-inherited diseases. With advances in knockout and transgenic technology, various molecules, genes, and signaling pathways have been identified as crucial in the development of the enteric nervous system and the pathogenesis of (syndromic) HSCR and associated disorders.

We will focus here mainly on the animal studies which have led to a better understanding of the molecular genetics of HSCR. For further details on the genetics of human HCSR, see Chaps. 7 and 11

5.3.1 Knockout Mouse Models

Mice are of particular value for research in human diseases as they are biologically and genetically very similar to humans. Mice are highly reproductive, mature quickly, and have a short life span. Furthermore, the mouse genome is similar to the human genome, with both species sharing about 99% of the same genes [24]. The 16 most relevant HSCR knockout mouse models are illustrated in Table 5.1 and described hereafter [25]. Due to the deletion of a specific gene, the phenotypes of these knockout models are diverse and range from small bowel dilatation and muscular hypertrophy to total intestinal aganglionosis.

Table 5.1 Knockout models of Hirschsprung's disease and allied disorders and their human occurrence

Knockout mice	Gene	Function	Phenotype	Human locus	Percent in human HSC
Ret −/−	RET	Tyrosine kinase receptor	Total intestinal aganglionosis	10q11.2	70–80% long segment 50% familial 15–20% sporadic
Gdnf −/−	GDNF	Glia cell-derived neurotrophic factor	Total intestinal aganglionosis	5p12–13.1	<10%
Gfrα1 −/−	GFRα1	GDNF family receptor alpha 1	Total intestinal aganglionosis	10q26	–
Gfrα2 −/−	GFRα2	GDNF family receptor alpha 2	Hypoganglionosis	8p21	–
Ntn−/−	NTN	Neurturin, RET ligand	Hypoganglionosis	19p13	< 1%
Etr3 −/−, lethal spotted	Edn3	Endothelin-3	Distal hindgut aganglionosis	20q13	<5%
Ednrb −/−, piebald lethal	EDNRB	Endothelin-B receptor	Distal hindgut aganglionosis	13q22	<10%
Ece1 −/−	ECE-1	Endothelin-converting enzyme 1	Distal hindgut aganglionosis	1p36	< 1%
Sox10Dom, DOM	Sox10	Sry/HMG box transcription factor	Complete intestinal aganglionosis	22q13.1	< 1%
Phox2b −/−	Phox2b	Paired like homeobox 2	Complete intestinal aganglionosis	4p12–13	< 1%
Pax3 −/−	PAX3	Paired box gene 3	Total intestinal aganglionosis	2q35–36	–
Ncx−/−	Hox11L1	Homeobox 2	INDB-like condition	2p13.1	–
VIP−/−	VIP	Neuropeptide	Small bowel dilatation, muscular hypertrophy, hypoperistalsis	6q25	–
Ihh −/−	IHH	Indian hedgehog	Skip intestinal aganglionosis	2q33–35	–
Shh−/−	SHH	Sonic hedgehog	Ectopic mucosal neurons	7q36	–
Zfhx1b	ZFHX1B	Zinc finger/ homeodomain protein	Mowat-Wilson syndrome	2q22	–

Taken from [25], adapted from [17, 28, 41, 60, 97, 184, 185]

5.3.1.1 Ret/Gdnf/Gfrα1 and Ret/Ntn/Gfrα2

Initially, the R*et* gene was isolated in a tumor cell line. Astonishingly, a targeted gene deletion led to an aganglionosis-like phenotype, and, hence, the first targeted gene deletion knockout model was created [26]. In further studies, a total aganglionosis throughout the gut as well as associated renal anomalies could be confirmed in these animal models [27].

The *Ret* gene encodes a receptor tyrosine kinase with four ligands: glial cell line-derived growth factor (*Gdnf*), neurturin (*Ntn*), artemin (*Atm*), and persephin (*Psp*) [28]. The complete receptor complex includes not only the *Ret* receptor tyrosine kinase but also a glycosylphosphatidylinositol-anchored binding component (Gfrα1, Gfrα2, Gfrα3, and Gfrα4), acting as specific binding components: *Ret/Gfrα1* binds *Gdnf*, *Ret/Gfrα2* binds *Ntn*, *Ret/Gfrα3* binds *Atm*, and *Ret/Gfrα4* binds *Psp*. The compound functions as an adhesion molecule, which is required for NCC migration, and it is reported that it has a role in the survival or differentiation of NCCs which have stopped migrating [29, 30]. Disruptions in NCC colonization and reduced exhibition of neurons and glia in the gastric cardia and esophagus were detected in $Ret^{-/-}$ mice [31, 32]. Attributed to the abovementioned animal models, the *Ret* gene could be identified as the first gene responsible for HSCR, located in an area previously described as deleted on human chromosome 10 [33–38]. It is now well recognized that mutations in the *Ret* gene account for 50% of familial and 15–20% of sporadic cases of HSCR [36, 38–40]. The mechanisms of *Ret* mutations in HSCR may not only consist of abnormal cell signal transduction leading to the abnormal NCC colonization in the intestine, but also a negative regulation of signal induction of the *Ret* ligand *Gdnf* gene for promoting apoptosis of neural crest progenitor cells is reported. Pan and Li [41] discussed in their Hirschsprung's review extensively the role of *Ret* in facilitating apoptosis: *Ret* can stimulate cell development and survival in its ligands' presence, whereas *Ret* promotes apoptosis in the ligands' absence, as shown by Mehlen and Bredesen [42]. Triggering of apoptosis in 293T cells with inhibition of this effect in the presence of *Gdnf* was described by Bordeaux et al. [43]. It has been proposed that HSCR can also result from apoptosis of *Ret*-expressing enteric neuroblasts, generated by site-directed mutagenesis. Cells were transfected to investigate potential effects on *Gdnf* control of *Ret*-induced apoptosis. Independently of the extent of *Gdnf*, apoptosis was seen in most transfected cells with the gene mutation. Uesaka et al. [44] created a mouse model for HSCR by diminishing *Ret* expression levels, mimicking the features of HSCR with impaired migration and neuronal death causing colonic aganglionosis. They showed that reduced *Ret* expression directly affected the survival of colonic neurons via reduction of *Ret* expression after the period of enteric NCC migration and concluded that enteric neuronal survival is sensitive to *Ret* dosage and cell death may be involved in the causation of HSCR [44].

Gdnf is supposed to stimulate survival and proliferation of neural crest-derived precursor cells in the embryonic gut via its interaction with the *Ret* receptor [45–48]. $Gdnf^{-/-}$ and $Gfr\alpha 1^{-/-}$ mice present with almost identical phenotypes to $Ret^{-/-}$ mice, characterized by developmental disturbances of the ENS distal to the esophagus and absent kidneys [27, 49–53].

$Ret^{-/-}$ and $Gdnf^{-/-}$ mice have the absence of enteric neurons and die at birth [27, 49–51, 54]. $Ret^{+/-}$ and $Gdnf^{+/-}$ mice instead are viable and fertile. $Ret^{+/-}$ mice constitute normal numbers of enteric neurons, whereas $Gdnf^{+/-}$ mice exhibit hypoganglionosis with about a 50% reduction of enteric neurons [55, 56]. To our knowledge, a few *Gdnf* mutations but no *GFRα1* mutation have been identified in humans with HSCR [41, 45, 57–59].

The absence of *Ntn/Gfrα2*-mediated signaling leads to subtle abnormalities in ENS development [60]. $Ntn^{-/-}$ and $Gfr\alpha 2^{-/-}$ mice are viable and fertile with a decrease in the renal density of cholinergic neurons in the ENS [61, 62]. *Ntn*-deficient mice exhibit diminished nerve fiber density in the ENS and abnormalities in neurotransmitter release and gastrointestinal motility [56, 61]. *Ntn* seems to play a supportive role for maintenance of enteric neurons, ganglia, and cell size and can encourage the ENS precursor proliferation as well as neuronal differentiation [61, 63]. *Ntn* mutation alone is not assumed to result in HSCR, but could contribute to the severity of the disease [64]. *Ntn* mutations have been documented only in a few cases of human HSCR, presenting occasional mutations in *Ret* or another HSCR gene. This points toward a modifier role of *Ntn* in the etiology of HSCR [45, 57, 64–68].

5.3.1.2 Endothelins and Ednrb/Edn3/Ece1

Endothelins have been discovered randomly while investigating pig aortas for contractile substances [69]. They are intercellular local messengers with four members (endothelin-1 (*Edn1*), endothelin-2 (*Edn2*), endothelin-3 (*Edn3*) and vasoactive intestinal peptide (*VIP*)) and interact with two cell surface transmembrane receptors (endothelin-receptor A (*Ednra*) and endothelin-receptor B (*Ednrb*)) [28]. *Ednra* is linked to *Edn1*, but does not bind *Edn3* at physiologic concentrations, whereas *Ednrb* binds all ligands with high affinity [60].

Gene deletion knockout experiments have brought attention to the features of endothelins in neural crest development. Proendothelin is the precursor of endothelin and needs to be activated by a specific enzyme, the so called endothelin-converting enzyme (*Ece*). There are two types: *Ece1* and *Ece2* [28]. *Ece1* knockout mice present craniofacial and cardiac anomalies in addition to aganglionosis of the colon [70]. Hofstra et al. identified a patient with a heterozygous *Ece1* mutation, who, similar to the mouse models, exhibited HSCR and cardiac and craniofacial defects [71].

In further studies, *Edn3* and *Ednrb* have been recognized as the causes for the natural mutants of lethal spotting mice and piebald-lethal mice [72, 73] (Fig. 5.1). In the lethal spotting mice, a point mutation in the *Proendothelial-3* gene resulting in no *Edn3* was found, while a complete deletion of *Ednrb* was identified in the piebald-lethal mouse [72–75]. The other endothelins (*Edn1*, *Edn2*) seem to be responsible for the shorter length of aganglionosis in the lethal spotting mouse compared to piebald-lethal mouse due to partial interaction with *Ednrb*, which may generate a milder form of aganglionosis. ENS anomalies of heterozygous *Ednrb*-deficient spotting lethal rats mimic the abnormalities of human intestinal neuronal dysplasia B (INDB) [76], a condition in which malformation of the submucosal plexus leads to an increased proportion of oversized ganglia and, thus, results in chronic constipation. A 50–60% reduction in myenteric neurons in the ganglionic region of *Edn3*$^{-/-}$ mice with an absent colonic migrating motor complexes was found in this area [77].

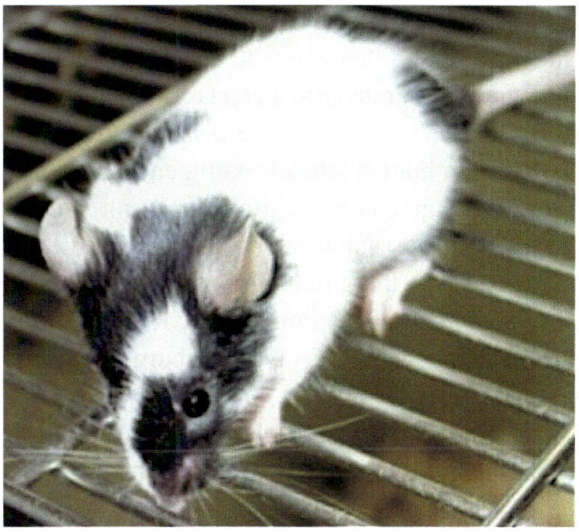

Fig. 5.1 Piebald-lethal mouse. (Courtesy as Dr. Nana Nakazawa-Tanaka, Tokyo, Japan)

Cheng et al. [78] noticed that *Ednrb*$^{-/-}$ mice develop enterocolitis similar to Hirschsprung-associated enterocolitis in humans. In a further study, they found that these mice also exhibit a profoundly abnormal immunophenotype characterized by small spleens, B and T cell splenic lymphopenia, and disordered splenic microarchitecture [79]. Zaitoun et al. investigated mice with NCC deletion of *Ednrb* to evaluate neuronal density and neurotransmitter expression in ganglia [80]. They found an inverse correlation between the neuronal density and expression of neuronal nitric oxide synthase (nNOS) and VIP, with progressive changes from the proximal to the distal intestine. Zaitoun et al. reported that the increase in nNOS expression correlating with a decrease in choline acetyltransferase (ChAT) expression may be responsible for the dysmotility seen in patients with HSCR [80].

All these animal model experiments led the way to the detection of the same genes in humans and gradually, defects in *Ednrb* [81–85] and *Edn3* [65, 86] have been discovered in humans. In human fetuses, both genes have been expressed on enteric neurons and gut mesenchyme cells, essential for normal migration [72, 73]. However, these mutations were identified in less than 10% of the human HSCR cases, especially in patients with Waardenburg-Shah syndrome [1, 39, 85–87].

Altered intestinal morphology in *VIP*$^{-/-}$ mice was shown by Lelievre et al. [88]. The knockout mice present a decrease in the length of the bowel compared to wild-type controls, small bowel dilatation, muscular hypertrophy, hypoperistalsis, and higher abundance of goblet cells. Most of these VIP$^{-/-}$ mice die during the first year of life with stenosis of the gut.

Recently, stem cell therapy has been established as a promising approach for the treatment of HSCR, and knockout mouse models are being used regularly to investigate the success of this new method. Fattahi and colleagues demonstrated that in vivo engraftment and migration of human pluripotent stem cell-derived ENS precursors rescued disease-related mortality in *Ednrb* mice [89]. Zhou et al. transplanted amniotic fluid-derived enteric neural stem cells in *Ednrb* knockout mice, resulting in decreased apoptosis, improved colonic motility, and increased survival of transplanted mice [90].

5.3.1.3 Sox10

Pusch et al. [91] discovered *Sox10*, a member of the sry-related family of transcription factors [92], during a comparative study of human/mouse sequences. *Sox10* encodes a transcription factor preserving the potency of enteric neural crest-derived progenitors and the differentiation of glial cells [93, 94]. In the natural Dom mouse HSCR model, failure of the *Sox10* gene due to early NCC death has been demonstrated to trigger intestinal aganglionosis [95, 96] and also disrupts normal neuron proportions in ganglionated small intestine, leading to deficits in intestinal transit [97, 98]. Homozygous and heterozygous rodents develop an unviable HSCR-phenotype [99]. Homozygous mutants die within 2 weeks of life, with the total absence of enteric NCC even within the esophagus [97]. Furthermore, Sox10 also controls cell migration and regulates Ret expression in combination with Pax3 [97, 100, 101]. In humans, *Sox10* mutations were detected in patients with Waardenburg-Shah syndrome [102].

Sox10 function is mediated by several regulatory elements such as *Ret*, *Edn3/Ednrb*, *L1cam*, *Sox8*, *SUFU*, *β1-integrins*, or *Zfhx1b* [103]. *Sox8* has been identified as a modifier gene in a mouse model of HSCR, assuming that *Sox8* and *Sox10* are jointly required for the preservation of vagal NCCs [104]. Loss of *Sox8* alleles in *Sox10* heterozygous mice reduced colonization of enteric NCCs [104].

5.3.1.4 Phox2B

Phox2B is a homeodomain-containing transcription factor regulating the *Ret* expression and therefore the development in the ENS [60, 105, 106]. Similar to the phenotype of the *Ret* knockout mouse, disruption of the *Phox2B* gene leads to a complete absence of ENS in mice [60]. *Phox2B* is the first gene for which a germline mutation predisposes to neuroblastoma [107, 108] and is the major locus for congenital central hypoventilation syndrome [97, 109–111]. Both conditions are frequently associated with HSCR [112–114].

5.3.1.5 Pax3

Neural cell precursors giving rise to enteric ganglia express *Pax3*, a member of the paired-box-containing family of nuclear transcription factors [115], activating an enhancer in the *Ret* gene in combination with *Sox10* [97, 101]. The heterozygous state of *Pax3* leads to a white belly spot and deficient enteric ganglia in mice; homozygous deficient embryos died during midgestation due to cardiac and neural tube defects [101, 116–118]. *Pax3* mutations have been identified in patients with Waardenburg-Shah syndrome without HSCR; however, *Pax3* mutations have not been detected in patients with isolated HSCR so far [119].

5.3.1.6 Homeobox Genes

Homeobox genes (*Hox*) are highly conserved genes of a network of transcription factors, which turn on cascades of other genes [120]. *Hox* genes are controlled in the form of a code (the enteric *Hox* code), which is essential for the correct morphogenesis and defines the different spatial, temporal, and combinatorial *Hox* expression patterns in the gut [121]. They play a key role in the development of the enteric plexus as revealed by studies in mouse and humans [121, 122]. *Hox* mutations in human HSCR have been described in several studies [123, 124].

Hox11L1

Hox11L1 (also known as Tlx2) is a homeobox transcription factor assumed to take part in NCC proliferation [125]. As *Hox11L1*$^{-/-}$ mice exhibit a condition similar to INDB; with partial death of enteric neurons, the *Hox11L1*$^{-/-}$ mouse model has been proposed as an eligible model for INDB. Homozygous mice are viable, but megacolon evolves at 3–5 weeks of age. Like in IND-phenotype, histological analyses revealed hyperplasia of myenteric ganglia in *Hox11L1*$^{-/-}$ mice [125, 126].

Hoxb5

Homeobox gene *Hoxb5* is a transcriptional activator in humans and mice and is expressed by vagal NCCs. Lui et al. [127] used transgenic mice to investigate the function of *Hoxb5* and its downstream target *Ret* in ENS development. They found that perturbation of *Hoxb5* led to *Ret* haploinsufficiency, constrained NCC migration, hypoganglionosis, and aganglionosis, respectively, assuming that *Hoxb5* may participate in the etiology of HSCR.

Hoxa

Homeobox transcription factor *Hoxa4* is expressed during embryonic development in the gut mesoderm. Transgenic mice with overexpression of *Hoxa4* exhibit megacolon with a mutable phenotype depending on the transgenic line and the time and severity of onset. The most heavily affected mice line die soon postnatal due to intestinal obstruction, whereas the least severely affected mice develop megacolon only rarely as adults [128]. Transgenic neonatal *Hoxa4* mice present hypoganglionosis in a short segment of the terminal colon with abnormally located ganglia [128, 129].

Doodnath et al. [130] ascertained that *Hoxa9* and *Hoxa13* are involved in the development of the zebrafish ENS as they found both of them migrating from the fore- and hindbrain down to the gut until *Hoxa9*- and *Hoxa13*-positive cells could be seen along the complete length of the intestine. Both transcription factors have been found in the developing gut of other animal models as well. Yokouchi et al. showed the expression of *Hoxa9* in the posterior part of small intestine and cecum of chick embryos [131]. The chick model was also used to demonstrate the expression of *Hoxa13* in the endoderm of the hindgut and cloaca in the early gut development. Its overexpression led to a failure to form a tail or gut phenotype [132, 133]. Warot et al. reported that *Hoxa13* is expressed in the terminal fraction of the gastrointestinal and urogenital tract during murine embryogenesis [123]. Both *Hox* genes, *Hoxa9*, and *Hoxa13*, were also identified in patients with HSCR. *Hoxa9* is in humans normally expressed in the kidney as well as in ileal and colonic mesenchyme. Méchine-Neuville et al. found increased expression of *Hox9* in the colon of HSCR patients compared to normal controls [124]. Garcia-Barcelo et al. [134] investigated *Hox* single nucleotide polymorphisms in Hirschsprung's patients in the Chinese population. They reported that these *Hox* SNPs, sharing intergenic and flanking regulatory regions, may affect the expression of genes in the cluster, especially an upstream of *Hoxa13*.

5.3.1.7 Hedgehog Genes

Sonic hedgehog (*Shh*) and Indian hedgehog (*Ihh*) genes potentially influence the survival and differentiation of NCCs [135]. Depletion of hedgehog results in partial intestinal aganglionosis together with megacolon or ectopic ganglia in mice [136]. *Ihh*$^{-/-}$ and *Shh*$^{-/-}$ mice die during early embryogenesis. Ramalho-Santos et al. found that late fetal *Ihh*$^{+/-}$ mice develop a dilated colonic region due to the absence of enteric neurons in the dilated intestinal region and parts of the small intestine, whereas in *Shh*$^{+/-}$ mice, nerve cell bodies are exhibited within the gut mucosa [137].

Gli1, *Gli2*, and *Gli3* are transcription factors for mediating hedgehog signaling in mammals [136]. Ectopic expression of *Gli1* results in hypoganglionosis, an effect similar to the loss of Ihh [97, 135]. Overexpression of human *Gli1* in transgenic mice leads to an HSCR-like phenotype, with correlating severity of the ENS phenotype depending on the expression level of the *Gli1* transgene [135, 136]. Missense mutations of *Gli1*, *Gli2*, and *Gli3* have been found in patients presenting with HSCR [136]. Suppressor of fused (*Sufu*) is a negative regulator of *Gli* transcription. Mice lacking *Sufu* in NCC die before the gut is completely colonized by enteric NCCs [97, 136]. *Sox10* has been shown to promote glial differentiation of central nervous system progenitors by downregulating *Sufu* expression [136, 138].

5.3.1.8 ZFHX1B Gene

The *ZFHX1B* gene (also known as *ZEB2, SIP1*) is an evolutionarily conserved gene, which is widely expressed in embryological development and encodes zinc finger and homeodomain-like sequence-containing transcription factor [139, 140]. NCC-deleted *ZFHX1B* mice exhibit defects in the peripheral nervous system of the digestive tract, loss of vagal NCCs, and anomalies in melanocyte development [141]. Nonsense mutations of the *ZFHX1B* gene have been found in patients with Mowat-Wilson syndrome, a congenital syndrome with diverse facial irregularities, intellectual disability, and epilepsy, which is occasionally associated with HSCR [142]. Because no *ZFHX1B* mutations have been reported in patients with isolated HSCR so far, the *ZFHX1B* gene may be a vulnerability gene for syndromic HSCR [41, 143].

5.3.1.9 Other Knockout Models

Recently, mouse models of HSCR and other developmental disorders of the ENS were reviewed by Bondurand and Southard-Smith [97]. The roles of cell surface molecules, cell adhesion molecules as well as transcription factors such as Foxd3, Hand2, Ascl1 (formerly known as Mash1), Hlx1, Dlx2, and their corresponding mouse models are described there extensively.

Model Created by Insertional Mutation or N-Ethyl-N-Nitrosourea Screens

Sox10Hry mutants are a model for Waardenburg-Shah syndrome and exhibit distal intestinal aganglionosis and hypopigmentation due to a 16 kb deletion upstream of the Sox10 gene, confirming the importance of distant *Sox10* regulatory elements [97, 144].

Loss of repression of the *Fam162b* gene in enteric NCCs leads to a transgenic line called *TashT* model, resulting in delayed enteric NCC migration and a partially penetrant aganglionic megacolon [97, 145].

Altered expression of the *Col6a4* gene (excess collagen VI) results in a HSCR-like disease model named *Holstein*, presenting with delayed enteric NCC colonization of the fetal bowel due to slower cell migration [97, 146].

β1 Integrins

Breau et al. [147] investigated the role of *β1 integrins* in ENS development. They deleted *β1 integrins* in the NCC of mice, which led to a failure of gut colonization and, thus, led to aganglionosis of the descending colon, similar to human HSCR. These *β1*-null enteric NCCs showed impaired adhesion on the extracellular matrix as well as severe modification of the ganglia network due to abnormal aggregates in the gut wall. Furthermore, the study demonstrated that *β1 integrins* are necessary for the maintenance of villi innervation in the small intestine. Additionally, Nagy et al. showed that endothelial cells support the migration of enteric NCCs via interaction of NCC surface-*β1 integrins* and extracellular matrix proteins expressed by the intestinal vasculature [148]. However, the participation of *β1 integrins* in the deficient migration of ganglion cells occurring in human HSCR was not verified [149].

Ercc1 Gene

The *Ercc1* gene is important for nucleotide excision repair, recombination repair, and the reparation of interstrand cross-links. Accidentally, Selfridge et al. [150] created a mouse model with intestinal obstruction as they originally planned to create a model for UV-induced melanoma by producing *Ercc1*-deficient melanocytes in mice. Expression of a regulating tyrosinase promoter was found in neural crest-derived lineages, which include the progenitors of the parasympathetic nervous system responsible for the innervation of the digestive tract. Initially, these rodents developed normally but died at the age of 4–6 months because of severe colonic obstruction due to a degenerated ENS. The authors assumed that accumulated unrepaired DNA damage in the *Ercc1*-deficient colonic ganglia leads to a colonic obstruction which is comparable to human late-onset HSCR.

5.4 Surgically Created HSCR

Chick embryos are the most widely used surgically created HSCR model, because they are easily available and the development of their ENS has been examined in numerous studies [1]. Surgical ablation of the premigratory neural crest leading to aganglionosis [151] can be used to investigate treatment strategies for the disease. Aganglionic bowel was shown to be recolonized with NCCs by transplanting tissue gained from the dorsal neural tube [152–154]. Additionally, early differentiated neurons from more proximal gut regions are able to recolonize the distal bowel and form enteric ganglia [154, 155]. There are variants of this HSCR in which ganglion cells are actually present, but gut dysmotility still results. One of such variants of HSCR is "hypoganglionosis," which is defined by scarce ganglionic nerve cells and a reduction in parasympathetic nerves in the intestinal wall [156] giving rise to megacolon similar to that proximal to the aganglionic segment in HSCR. O'Donnell and Puri found that the cholinergic nerve activity is decreased as a result of a reduction in nerve cell numbers in the chick embryo colorectum [157]. These results suggest that the cholinergic activity in the hypoganglionic chick model resembles that of human hypoganglionosis.

For transplantation of stem cells as an approach for HSCR therapy, the cells are usually injected into the diseased gut after laparotomy [2, 158]. Colonoscopic stem cell injection has also been proven to be successful [159].

5.5 Chemical Models of HSCR

The first chemical model of HSCR was described by Sato et al. in 1978 [160], who applied benzalkonium chloride (BAC) on rat colon and rectum generating segmental aganglionosis thereby. The treated part results in a narrow segment with a rescinded rectoanal reflex [160]. Later, this technique has been reproduced in studies with mice and guinea pigs [161, 162]. The BAC model has been further developed by using BAC in transgenic mice [163] or new application methods such as the colonoscopic route [164].

BAC is a cationic surface-acting agent that attaches and injures the cell membrane leading to cell damage and cell death due to irreversible depolarization. In this chemical HSCR model, BAC induces neuronal ablation in the gut wall [162], resulting in a loss of almost all myenteric neurons and glia in the treated sections. Compared to other HSCR models, the application of BAC is a cheap and easily feasible procedure with a longer survival rate of the animals. Therefore, the BAC model has been used regularly to investigate functional and structural changes of the neuronal eliminated intestine and to evaluate different surgical treatment strategies [165–171].

Furthermore, transplantation experiments for cellular therapy are performed regularly in the BAC model [2, 158, 172–175]. Several cell types and genes have been used for stem cell transplantation studies. For example, Shu et al. created a recombinant adenovirus enclosing *Gdnf* and *Ednrb* genes and transfected neural stem cells in primary culture [173]. After transplantation into murine colon wall of a BAC-induced aganglionic megacolon, these neural stem cells differentiated into neurons and neural glial cells, repaired the myenteric nerve plexuses, and restored the bowel function in part. Wagner et al. induced permanent aganglionosis only in an isolated gut segment, the jejunum [176]. Skin-derived precursor cells migrated to the intermuscular layer of the aganglionic segment, enabling enteric neuroglial differentiation [175]. They were later successful in segmental colonic isolation [177]. Liu et al. (2018) transplanted enteric neural stem cells engineered with *insulin-like growth factor 1* and observed improved colonic motility with a reduction of colonic bead expulsion time and recovery of electrical field stimulation-induced relaxation [2].

As further chemical model, the exposure to the antiemetic drug trimethobenzamide in utero leads to severe fetal damage with growth retardation, tardive dyskinesia, and development of megacolon in neonatal rats [178].

Certain metabolites of common medicines might increase the risk for HSCR [97]. Retinoic acid modulates mouse enteric NCC proliferation and differentiation in vitro [179] and retinol-binding protein 4 (*Rbp4*$^{-/-}$) mutants depleted of vitamin A were shown to present with colorectal aganglionosis due to impaired lamellipodia formation and reduced enteric NCC migration in response to *Gdnf* [97]. Therefore, it has been speculated that vitamin A deficiency may be a nongenetic risk factor that increases HSCR penetrance and expressivity [97, 180]. Additionally, ibuprofen has recently been shown to slow migration and inhibits bowel colonization by ENS precursors in zebrafish, chick, and mouse [181]. Mycophenolate treatment, an inhibitor of de novo guanine nucleotide biosynthesis, diminished ENS precursor proliferation, decelerated precursor migration, and induced intestinal aganglionosis in mice [182]. Addition of mycophenolate in HSCR mouse models caused increased penetrance and severity of the HSCR-like pathology. Furthermore, mycophenolate treatment decreased lamellipodia formation and proliferation in cultured enteric NCCs. Reduced ENS precursor proliferation led to mycophenolate-triggered migration defects and aganglionosis. Deletion of inosine-5′-monophosphate dehydrogenase (*Impdh2*) resulted in defects in multiple neural crest derivatives, including intestinal aganglionosis, agenesis of the craniofacial skeleton, and cardiac outflow tract with great vessel malformations [97, 183]. All these findings suggest a crucial role for de novo guanine nucleotide biosynthesis in ENS development and HSCR manifestation, proposing that some cases of HSCR may be preventable through dietary supplementation [97].

5.6 Conclusion and Future Directions

Animal models of aganglionosis have been essential in the discovery of genes, molecules, and pathways related to HSCR. Especially with advances in knockout and transgenic technology, substantial progress was achieved in understanding the molecular genetics of HSCR. Stem cell transplantation is a promising approach for potential treatment of HSCR. In the future, animal models of aganglionosis will continue to play a key role in the anatomic, physiologic, and pharmacologic understanding of HSCR.

Cross-References

- Development of the Enteric Nervous System
- Functional Anatomy of the Enteric Nervous System
- The Molecular Genetics of Hirschsprung's Disease
- Congenital Anomalies and Genetic Associations in Hirschsprung's Disease
- Histopathological Diagnosis and Differential Diagnosis of Hirschsprung's Disease

References

1. Mortell A, Montedonico S, Puri P. Animal models in pediatric surgery. Pediatr Surg Int. 2006;22(2):111–28. https://doi.org/10.1007/s00383-005-1593-4.
2. Liu W, Zhang L, Wu R. Enteric neural stem cells expressing insulin-like growth factor 1: a novel cellular therapy for Hirschsprung's disease in mouse model. DNA Cell Biol. 2018;37(7):642–8. https://doi.org/10.1089/dna.2017.4060.
3. Lane PW. Association of megacolon with two recessive spotting genes in the mouse. J Hered. 1966;57(1):29–31.
4. Dietzmann U. Über das Vorkommen des kongenitalen Megakolons (Hirschsprungsches Megakolon) bei der Katz: Occurrence of the congenital mega-

colon (Hirschsprung's mega-colon) in cats (Uber das Vorkommen des kongenitalen Megakolons (Hirschsprungsches Megakolon) bei der Katze). Monatsh Veterinarmed. 1968;23(9):349–52.
5. Osborne JC, Davis JW, Farley H. Hirschsprung's disease. A review and report of the entity in a Virginia swine herd. Vet Med Small Anim Clin. 1968;63(5):451–3.
6. Lane PW, Liu HM. Association of megacolon with a new dominant spotting gene (Dom) in the mouse. J Hered. 1984;75(6):435–9.
7. Ikadai H, Fujita H, Agematsu Y, et al. Observation of congenital aganglionosis rat (Hirschsprung's disease rat) and its genetical analysis. Congenit Anom (Kyoto). 1979;19:31–6.
8. Hultgren BD. Ileocolonic aganglionosis in white progeny of overo spotted horses. J Am Vet Med Assoc. 1982;180(3):289–92.
9. McCabe L, Griffin LD, Kinzer A, et al. Overo lethal white foal syndrome: equine model of aganglionic megacolon (Hirschsprung disease). Am J Med Genet. 1990;36(3):336–40. https://doi.org/10.1002/ajmg.1320360319.
10. Kernkamp HCH, Kanning HH. Primary megacolon (Hirschsprung's disease) in swine. N Am Vet. 1955;63:642–3.
11. Yang GC, Croaker D, Zhang AL, et al. A dinucleotide mutation in the endothelin-B receptor gene is associated with lethal white foal syndrome (LWFS); a horse variant of Hirschsprung disease. Hum Mol Genet. 1998;7(6):1047–52.
12. Derrick EH, George-Grambauer BMS. Megacolon in mice. J Pathol. 1957;73(2):569–71. https://doi.org/10.1002/path.1700730228.
13. Bielschowsky M, Schofield GC. Studies on megacolon in piebald mice. Aust J Exp Biol Med Sci. 1962;40:395–403.
14. Fujimoto T. Natural history and pathophysiology of enterocolitis in the piebald lethal mouse model of Hirschsprung's disease. J Pediatr Surg. 1988;23(3):237–42.
15. Fujimoto T, Reen DJ, Puri P. Inflammatory response in enterocolitis in the piebald lethal mouse model of Hirschsprung'sdisease. PediatrRes. 1988;24(2):152–5. https://doi.org/10.1203/00006450-198808000-00002.
16. Dembowski C, Hofmann P, Koch T, et al. Phenotype, intestinal morphology, and survival of homozygous and heterozygous endothelin B receptor--deficient (spotting lethal) rats. J Pediatr Surg. 2000;35(3):480–8.
17. Alzahem AM, Cass DT. Animal models of aganglionosis. In: Holschneider AM, Puri P, editors. Hirschsprung's disease and allied disorders: with 49 tables. 3rd ed. Berlin, Heidelberg: Springer; 2008. p. 51–62.
18. Wood JD. Electrical activity of the intestine of mice with hereditary megacolon and absence of enteric ganglion cells. Am J Dig Dis. 1973;18(6): 477–88.
19. Cass DT, Zhang AL, Morthorpe J. Aganglionosis in rodents. J Pediatr Surg. 1992;27(3):351.
20. Robinson R. Genetic studies of the rabbit. Hague: M. Nijhoff; 1958.
21. Bodeker D, Turck O, Loven E, et al. Pathophysiological and functional aspects of the megacolon-syndrome of homozygous spotted rabbits. Zentralbl Veterinarmed A. 1995;42(9):549–59.
22. Wleberneit D, Wegner W. Albino rabbits can suffer from megacolon-syndrome when they are homozygous for the English Spot\"\" gene (EnEn)\"\". World Rabbit Sci. 1995;3(1) https://doi.org/10.4995/wrs.1995.236.
23. Fontanesi L, Vargiolu M, Scotti E, et al. Endothelin receptor B (EDNRB) is not the causative gene of the English spotting locus in the domestic rabbit (*Oryctolagus cuniculus*). Anim Genet. 2010;41 (6):669–70. https://doi.org/10.1111/j.1365-2052.2010.02084.x.
24. Capecchi MR. Targeted gene replacement. Sci Am. 1994;270(3):52–9.
25. Zimmer J, Puri P. Knockout mouse models of Hirschsprung's disease. Pediatr Surg Int. 2015;31(9):787–94. https://doi.org/10.1007/s00383-015-3747-3.
26. Takahashi M, Buma Y, Iwamoto T, et al. Cloning and expression of the ret proto-oncogene encoding a tyrosine kinase with two potential transmembrane domains. Oncogene. 1988;3(5):571–8.
27. Schuchardt A, D'Agati V, Larsson-Blomberg L, et al. Defects in the kidney and enteric nervous system of mice lacking the tyrosine kinase receptor Ret. Nature. 1994;367(6461):380–3. https://doi.org/10.1038/367380a0.
28. Puri P, Shinkai T. Pathogenesis of Hirschsprung's disease and its variants: recent progress. Semin Pediatr Surg. 2004;13(1):18–24.
29. Robertson K, Mason I. Expression of ret in the chicken embryo suggests roles in regionalisation of the vagal neural tube and somites and in development of multiple neural crest and placodal lineages. Mech Dev. 1995;53(3):329–44.
30. Pouliot Y. Phylogenetic analysis of the cadherin superfamily. Bioessays. 1992;14(11):743–8. https://doi.org/10.1002/bies.950141104.
31. Durbec PL, Larsson-Blomberg LB, Schuchardt A, et al. Common origin and developmental dependence on c-ret of subsets of enteric and sympathetic neuroblasts. Development. 1996;122(1):349–58.
32. Taraviras S, Marcos-Gutierrez CV, Durbec P, et al. Signalling by the RET receptor tyrosine kinase and its role in the development of the mammalian enteric nervous system. Development. 1999;126(12):2785–97.
33. Martucciello G, Bicocchi MP, Dodero P, et al. Total colonic aganglionosis associated with interstitial deletion of the long arm of chromosome 10. Pediatr Surg Int. 1992;7(4) https://doi.org/10.1007/BF00183991.
34. Angrist M, Kauffman E, Slaugenhaupt SA, et al. A gene for Hirschsprung disease (megacolon) in the pericentromeric region of human chromosome 10. Nat Genet. 1993;4(4):351–6. https://doi.org/10.1038/ng0893-351.

35. Lyonnet S, Bolino A, Pelet A, et al. A gene for Hirschsprung disease maps to the proximal long arm of chromosome 10. Nat Genet. 1993;4(4):346–50. https://doi.org/10.1038/ng0893-346.
36. Romeo G, Ronchetto P, Luo Y, et al. Point mutations affecting the tyrosine kinase domain of the RET proto-oncogene in Hirschsprung's disease. Nature. 1994;367(6461):377–8. https://doi.org/10.1038/367377a0.
37. Lo L, Anderson DJ. Postmigratory neural crest cells expressing c-RET display restricted developmental and proliferative capacities. Neuron. 1995;15(3):527–39.
38. Edery P, Lyonnet S, Mulligan LM, et al. Mutations of the RET proto-oncogene in Hirschsprung's disease. Nature. 1994;367(6461):378–80. https://doi.org/10.1038/367378a0.
39. Kusafuka T, Puri P. Altered RET gene mRNA expression in Hirschsprung's disease. J Pediatr Surg. 1997;32(4):600–4.
40. Martucciello G, Ceccherini I, Lerone M, et al. Pathogenesis of Hirschsprung's disease. J Pediatr Surg. 2000;35(7):1017–25.
41. Pan Z-W, Li J-C. Advances in molecular genetics of Hirschsprung's disease. Anat Rec (Hoboken). 2012;295(10):1628–38. https://doi.org/10.1002/ar.22538.
42. Mehlen P, Bredesen DE. The dependence receptor hypothesis. Apoptosis. 2004;9(1):37–49. https://doi.org/10.1023/B:APPT.0000012120.66221.b2.
43. Bordeaux MC, Forcet C, Granger L, et al. The RET proto-oncogene induces apoptosis: a novel mechanism for Hirschsprung disease. EMBO J. 2000;19(15):4056–63. https://doi.org/10.1093/emboj/19.15.4056.
44. Uesaka T, Nagashimada M, Yonemura S, et al. Diminished Ret expression compromises neuronal survival in the colon and causes intestinal aganglionosis in mice. J Clin Invest. 2008;118(5):1890–8. https://doi.org/10.1172/JCI34425.
45. Angrist M, Bolk S, Halushka M, et al. Germline mutations in glial cell line-derived neurotrophic factor (GDNF) and RET in a Hirschsprung disease patient. Nat Genet. 1996;14(3):341–4. https://doi.org/10.1038/ng1196-341.
46. Worley DS, Pisano JM, Choi ED, et al. Developmental regulation of GDNF response and receptor expression in the enteric nervous system. Development. 2000;127(20):4383–93.
47. Amiel J, Lyonnet S. Hirschsprung disease, associated syndromes, and genetics: a review. J Med Genet. 2001;38(11):729–39.
48. Young HM, Hearn CJ, Farlie PG, et al. GDNF is a chemoattractant for enteric neural cells. Dev Biol. 2001;229(2):503–16. https://doi.org/10.1006/dbio.2000.0100.
49. Sanchez MP, Silos-Santiago I, Frisen J, et al. Renal agenesis and the absence of enteric neurons in mice lacking GDNF. Nature. 1996;382(6586):70–3. https://doi.org/10.1038/382070a0.
50. Pichel JG, Shen L, Sheng HZ, et al. Defects in enteric innervation and kidney development in mice lacking GDNF. Nature. 1996;382(6586):73–6. https://doi.org/10.1038/382073a0.
51. Moore MW, Klein RD, Farinas I, et al. Renal and neuronal abnormalities in mice lacking GDNF. Nature. 1996;382(6586):76–9. https://doi.org/10.1038/382076a0.
52. Cacalano G, Farinas I, Wang LC, et al. GFRalpha1 is an essential receptor component for GDNF in the developing nervous system and kidney. Neuron. 1998;21(1):53–62.
53. Enomoto H, Araki T, Jackman A, et al. GFR alpha1-deficient mice have deficits in the enteric nervous system and kidneys. Neuron. 1998;21(2):317–24.
54. Durbec P, Marcos-Gutierrez CV, Kilkenny C, et al. GDNF signalling through the Ret receptor tyrosine kinase. Nature. 1996;381(6585):789–93. https://doi.org/10.1038/381789a0.
55. Shen L, Pichel JG, Mayeli T, et al. Gdnf haploinsufficiency causes Hirschsprung-like intestinal obstruction and early-onset lethality in mice. Am J Hum Genet. 2002;70(2):435–47. https://doi.org/10.1086/338712.
56. Gianino S, Grider JR, Cresswell J, et al. GDNF availability determines enteric neuron number by controlling precursor proliferation. Development. 2003;130(10):2187–98.
57. Ivanchuk SM, Myers SM, Eng C, et al. De novo mutation of GDNF, ligand for the RET/GDNFR-alpha receptor complex, in Hirschsprung disease. Hum Mol Genet. 1996;5(12):2023–6.
58. Martucciello G, Thompson H, Mazzola C, et al. GDNF deficit in Hirschsprung's disease. J Pediatr Surg. 1998;33(1):99–102.
59. Borrego S, Fernandez RM, Dziema H, et al. Investigation of germline GFRA4 mutations and evaluation of the involvement of GFRA1, GFRA2, GFRA3, and GFRA4 sequence variants in Hirschsprung disease. J Med Genet. 2003;40(3):e18.
60. Gariepy CE. Intestinal motility disorders and development of the enteric nervous system. Pediatr Res. 2001;49(5):605–13. https://doi.org/10.1203/00006450-200105000-00001.
61. Heuckeroth RO, Enomoto H, Grider JR, et al. Gene targeting reveals a critical role for neurturin in the development and maintenance of enteric, sensory, and parasympathetic neurons. Neuron. 1999;22(2):253–63.
62. Rossi J, Luukko K, Poteryaev D, et al. Retarded growth and deficits in the enteric and parasympathetic nervous system in mice lacking GFR alpha2, a functional neurturin receptor. Neuron. 1999;22(2):243–52.
63. Heuckeroth RO, Lampe PA, Johnson EM, et al. Neurturin and GDNF promote proliferation and survival of enteric neuron and glial progenitors in vitro. Dev Biol. 1998;200(1):116–29. https://doi.org/10.1006/dbio.1998.8955.
64. Doray B, Salomon R, Amiel J, et al. Mutation of the RET ligand, neurturin, supports multigenic inheritance in Hirschsprung disease. Hum Mol Genet. 1998;7(9):1449–52.

65. Hofstra RM, Osinga J, Tan-Sindhunata G, et al. A homozygous mutation in the endothelin-3 gene associated with a combined Waardenburg type 2 and Hirschsprung phenotype (Shah-Waardenburg syndrome). Nat Genet. 1996;12(4):445–7. https://doi.org/10.1038/ng0496-445.
66. Salomon R, Attie T, Pelet A, et al. Germline mutations of the RET ligand GDNF are not sufficient to cause Hirschsprung disease. Nat Genet. 1996;14(3):345–7. https://doi.org/10.1038/ng1196-345.
67. Parisi MA, Kapur RP. Genetics of Hirschsprung disease. Curr Opin Pediatr. 2000;12(6):610–7.
68. Eketjall S, Ibanez CF. Functional characterization of mutations in the GDNF gene of patients with Hirschsprung disease. Hum Mol Genet. 2002;11(3):325–9.
69. Sakurai T, Yanagisawa M, Masaki T. Molecular characterization of endothelin receptors. Trends Pharmacol Sci. 1992;13(3):103–8.
70. Yanagisawa H, Yanagisawa M, Kapur RP, et al. Dual genetic pathways of endothelin-mediated intercellular signaling revealed by targeted disruption of endothelin converting enzyme-1 gene. Development. 1998;125(5):825–36.
71. Hofstra RM, Valdenaire O, Arch E, et al. A loss-of-function mutation in the endothelin-converting enzyme 1 (ECE-1) associated with Hirschsprung disease, cardiac defects, and autonomic dysfunction. Am J Hum Genet. 1999;64(1):304–8. https://doi.org/10.1086/302184.
72. Hosoda K, Hammer RE, Richardson JA, et al. Targeted and natural (piebald-lethal) mutations of endothelin-B receptor gene produce megacolon associated with spotted coat color in mice. Cell. 1994;79(7): 1267–76.
73. Baynash AG, Hosoda K, Giaid A, et al. Interaction of endothelin-3 with endothelin-B receptor is essential for development of epidermal melanocytes and enteric neurons. Cell. 1994;79(7):1277–85.
74. Rice J, Doggett B, Sweetser DA, et al. Transgenic rescue of aganglionosis and piebaldism in lethal spotted mice. Dev Dyn. 2000;217(1):120–32. https://doi.org/10.1002/(SICI)1097-0177(200001)217:1<120:AID-DVDY11>3.0.CO;2-U.
75. Leibl MA, Ota T, Woodward MN, et al. Expression of endothelin 3 by mesenchymal cells of embryonic mouse caecum. Gut. 1999;44(2):246–52.
76. von Boyen GBT, Krammer H-J, Suss A, et al. Abnormalities of the enteric nervous system in heterozygous endothelin B receptor deficient (spotting lethal) rats resembling intestinal neuronal dysplasia. Gut. 2002;51(3):414–9.
77. Roberts RR, Bornstein JC, Bergner AJ, et al. Disturbances of colonic motility in mouse models of Hirschsprung's disease. Am J Physiol Gastrointest Liver Physiol. 2008;294(4):G996–G1008. https://doi.org/10.1152/ajpgi.00558.2007.
78. Cheng Z, Dhall D, Zhao L, et al. Murine model of Hirschsprung-associated enterocolitis. I: phenotypic characterization with development of a histopathologic grading system. J Pediatr Surg. 2010;45(3):475–82. https://doi.org/10.1016/j.jpedsurg.2009.06.009.
79. Cheng Z, Wang X, Dhall D, et al. Splenic lymphopenia in the endothelin receptor B-null mouse: implications for Hirschsprung associated enterocolitis. Pediatr Surg Int. 2011;27(2):145–50. https://doi.org/10.1007/s00383-010-2787-y.
80. Zaitoun I, Erickson CS, Barlow AJ, et al. Altered neuronal density and neurotransmitter expression in the ganglionated region of Ednrb null mice: implications for Hirschsprung's disease. Neurogastroenterol Motil. 2013;25(3):44. https://doi.org/10.1111/nmo.12083.
81. Puffenberger EG, Hosoda K, Washington SS, et al. A missense mutation of the endothelin-B receptor gene in multigenic Hirschsprung's disease. Cell. 1994;79(7):1257–66.
82. Attie T, Till M, Pelet A, et al. Mutation of the endothelin-receptor B gene in Waardenburg-Hirschsprung disease. Hum Mol Genet. 1995;4(12):2407–9.
83. Amiel J, Attie T, Jan D, et al. Heterozygous endothelin receptor B (EDNRB) mutations in isolated Hirschsprung disease. Hum Mol Genet. 1996;5(3):355–7.
84. Auricchio A, Casari G, Staiano A, et al. Endothelin-B receptor mutations in patients with isolated Hirschsprung disease from a non-inbred population. Hum Mol Genet. 1996;5(3):351–4.
85. Kusafuka T, Wang Y, Puri P. Novel mutations of the endothelin-B receptor gene in isolated patients with Hirschsprung's disease. Hum Mol Genet. 1996;5(3):347–9.
86. Edery P, Attie T, Amiel J, et al. Mutation of the endothelin-3 gene in the Waardenburg-Hirschsprung disease (Shah-Waardenburg syndrome). Nat Genet. 1996;12(4):442–4. https://doi.org/10.1038/ng0496-442.
87. Kusafuka T, Wang Y, Puri P. Mutation analysis of the RET, the endothelin-B receptor, and the endothelin-3 genes in sporadic cases of Hirschsprung's disease. J Pediatr Surg. 1997;32(3):501–4.
88. Lelievre V, Favrais G, Abad C, et al. Gastrointestinal dysfunction in mice with a targeted mutation in the gene encoding vasoactive intestinal polypeptide: a model for the study of intestinal ileus and Hirschsprung's disease. Peptides. 2007;28(9):1688–99. https://doi.org/10.1016/j.peptides.2007.05.006.
89. Fattahi F, Steinbeck JA, Kriks S, et al. Deriving human ENS lineages for cell therapy and drug discovery in Hirschsprung disease. Nature. 2016;531(7592):105–9. https://doi.org/10.1038/nature16951.
90. Zhou Y, Besner G. Transplantation of amniotic fluid-derived neural stem cells as a potential novel therapy for Hirschsprung's disease. J Pediatr Surg. 2016;51(1):87–91. https://doi.org/10.1016/j.jpedsurg.2015.10.016.
91. Pusch C, Hustert E, Pfeifer D, et al. The SOX10/Sox10 gene from human and mouse: sequence, expression, and transactivation by the encoded HMG domain transcription factor. Hum Genet. 1998;103(2): 115–23.

92. Kuhlbrodt K, Herbarth B, Sock E, et al. Sox10, a novel transcriptional modulator in glial cells. J Neurosci. 1998;18(1):237–50.
93. Paratore C, Goerich DE, Suter U, et al. Survival and glial fate acquisition of neural crest cells are regulated by an interplay between the transcription factor Sox10 and extrinsic combinatorial signaling. Development. 2001;128(20):3949–61.
94. Kim J, Lo L, Dormand E, et al. SOX10 maintains multipotency and inhibits neuronal differentiation of neural crest stem cells. Neuron. 2003;38(1):17–31.
95. Southard-Smith EM, Kos L, Pavan WJ. Sox10 mutation disrupts neural crest development in Dom Hirschsprung mouse model. Nat Genet. 1998;18(1):60–4. https://doi.org/10.1038/ng0198-60.
96. Herbarth B, Pingault V, Bondurand N, et al. Mutation of the Sry-related Sox10 gene in Dominant megacolon, a mouse model for human Hirschsprung disease. Proc Natl Acad Sci U S A. 1998;95(9):5161–5.
97. Bondurand N, Southard-Smith EM. Mouse models of Hirschsprung disease and other developmental disorders of the enteric nervous system: old and new players. Dev Biol. 2016;417(2):139–57. https://doi.org/10.1016/j.ydbio.2016.06.042.
98. Musser MA, Correa H, Southard-Smith EM. Enteric neuron imbalance and proximal dysmotility in ganglionated intestine of the Sox10(Dom/+) Hirschsprung mouse model. Cell Mol Gastroenterol Hepatol. 2015;1(1):87–101. https://doi.org/10.1016/j.jcmgh.2014.08.002.
99. Kapur RP. Hirschsprung disease and other enteric dysganglionoses. Crit Rev Clin Lab Sci. 1999;36(3):225–73. https://doi.org/10.1080/10408369991239204.
100. Corpening JC, Deal KK, Cantrell VA, et al. Isolation and live imaging of enteric progenitors based on Sox10-Histone2BVenus transgene expression. Genesis. 2011;49(7):599–618. https://doi.org/10.1002/dvg.20748.
101. Lang D, Chen F, Milewski R, et al. Pax3 is required for enteric ganglia formation and functions with Sox10 to modulate expression of c-ret. J Clin Invest. 2000;106(8):963–71. https://doi.org/10.1172/JCI10828.
102. Kuhlbrodt K, Schmidt C, Sock E, et al. Functional analysis of Sox10 mutations found in human Waardenburg-Hirschsprung patients. J Biol Chem. 1998;273(36):23033–8.
103. Watanabe Y, Broders-Bondon F, Baral V, et al. Sox10 and Itgb1 interaction in enteric neural crest cell migration. Dev Biol. 2013;379(1):92–106. https://doi.org/10.1016/j.ydbio.2013.04.013.
104. Maka M, Stolt CC, Wegner M. Identification of Sox8 as a modifier gene in a mouse model of Hirschsprung disease reveals underlying molecular defect. Dev Biol. 2005;277(1):155–69. https://doi.org/10.1016/j.ydbio.2004.09.014.
105. Pattyn A, Morin X, Cremer H, et al. Expression and interactions of the two closely related homeobox genes Phox2a and Phox2b during neurogenesis. Development. 1997;124(20):4065–75.
106. Pattyn A, Morin X, Cremer H, et al. The homeobox gene Phox2b is essential for the development of autonomic neural crest derivatives. Nature. 1999;399(6734):366–70. https://doi.org/10.1038/20700.
107. Perri P, Bachetti T, Longo L, et al. PHOX2B mutations and genetic predisposition to neuroblastoma. Oncogene. 2005;24(18):3050–3. https://doi.org/10.1038/sj.onc.1208532.
108. Trochet D, Bourdeaut F, Janoueix-Lerosey I, et al. Germline mutations of the paired-like homeobox 2B (PHOX2B) gene in neuroblastoma. Am J Hum Genet. 2004;74(4):761–4. https://doi.org/10.1086/383253.
109. Bachetti T, Matera I, Borghini S, et al. Distinct pathogenetic mechanisms for PHOX2B associated polyalanine expansions and frameshift mutations in congenital central hypoventilation syndrome. Hum Mol Genet. 2005;14(13):1815–24. https://doi.org/10.1093/hmg/ddi188.
110. Amiel J, Laudier B, Attié-Bitach T, et al. Polyalanine expansion and frameshift mutations of the paired-like homeobox gene PHOX2B in congenital central hypoventilation syndrome. Nat Genet. 2003;33(4):459–61. https://doi.org/10.1038/ng1130.
111. Garcia-Barcelo M, Sham MH, Lui VCH, et al. Association study of PHOX2B as a candidate gene for Hirschsprung's disease. Gut. 2003;52(4):563–7.
112. Fitze G, Konig IR, Paditz E, et al. Compound effect of PHOX2B and RET gene variants in congenital central hypoventilation syndrome combined with Hirschsprung disease. Am J Med Genet A. 2008;146A(11):1486–9. https://doi.org/10.1002/ajmg.a.32300.
113. Lai D, Schroer B. Haddad syndrome: a case of an infant with central congenital hypoventilation syndrome and Hirschsprung disease. J Child Neurol. 2008;23(3):341–3. https://doi.org/10.1177/0883073807309242.
114. Amiel J, Sproat-Emison E, Garcia-Barcelo M, et al. Hirschsprung disease, associated syndromes and genetics: a review. J Med Genet. 2008;45(1):1–14. https://doi.org/10.1136/jmg.2007.053959.
115. Goulding MD, Chalepakis G, Deutsch U, et al. Pax-3, a novel murine DNA binding protein expressed during early neurogenesis. EMBO J. 1991;10(5):1135–47.
116. Auerbach R. Analysis of the developmental effects of a lethal mutation in the house mouse. J Exp Zool. 1954;127(2):305–29. https://doi.org/10.1002/jez.1401270206.
117. Epstein DJ, Vekemans M, Gros P. Splotch (Sp2H), a mutation affecting development of the mouse neural tube, shows a deletion within the paired homeodomain of Pax-3. Cell. 1991;67(4):767–74.
118. Epstein DJ, Vogan KJ, Trasler DG, et al. A mutation within intron 3 of the Pax-3 gene produces aberrantly spliced mRNA transcripts in the splotch

(Sp) mouse mutant. Proc Natl Acad Sci U S A. 1993;90(2):532–6.
119. Tassabehji M, Read AP, Newton VE, et al. Waardenburg's syndrome patients have mutations in the human homologue of the Pax-3 paired box gene. Nature. 1992;355(6361):635–6. https://doi.org/10.1038/355635a0.
120. Rings E, van den Berg M, Stokkers P. Expression of homeobox genes in the gastrointestinal tract. J Pediatr Gastroenterol Nutr. 1998;27(1):122–3.
121. Pitera JE, Smith VV, Thorogood P, et al. Coordinated expression of 3′ hox genes during murine embryonal gut development: an enteric Hox code. Gastroenterology. 1999;117(6):1339–51.
122. Fu M, VCH L, Sham MH, et al. Sonic hedgehog regulates the proliferation, differentiation, and migration of enteric neural crest cells in gut. J Cell Biol. 2004;166(5):673–84. https://doi.org/10.1083/jcb.200401077.
123. Warot X, Fromental-Ramain C, Fraulob V, et al. Gene dosage-dependent effects of the Hoxa-13 and Hoxd-13 mutations on morphogenesis of the terminal parts of the digestive and urogenital tracts. Development. 1997;124(23):4781–91.
124. Mechine-Neuville A, Lefebvre O, Bellocq J-P, et al. Increased expression of HOXA9 gene in Hirschsprung disease (Augmentation de l'expression du gene HOXA9 dans la maladie de Hirschsprung). Gastroenterol Clin Biol. 2002;26(12):1110–7.
125. Shirasawa S, Yunker AM, Roth KA, et al. Enx (Hox11L1)-deficient mice develop myenteric neuronal hyperplasia and megacolon. Nat Med. 1997;3(6):646–50.
126. Hatano M, Aoki T, Dezawa M, et al. A novel pathogenesis of megacolon in Ncx/Hox11L.1 deficient mice. J Clin Invest. 1997;100(4):795–801. https://doi.org/10.1172/JCI119593.
127. Lui VCH, Cheng WWC, Leon TYY, et al. Perturbation of hoxb5 signaling in vagal neural crests down-regulates ret leading to intestinal hypoganglionosis in mice. Gastroenterology. 2008;134(4):1104–15. https://doi.org/10.1053/j.gastro.2008.01.028.
128. Tennyson VM, Gershon MD, Sherman DL, et al. Structural abnormalities associated with congenital megacolon in transgenic mice that overexpress the Hoxa-4 gene. Dev Dyn. 1993;198(1):28–53. https://doi.org/10.1002/aja.1001980105.
129. Tennyson VM, Gershon MD, Wade PR, et al. Fetal development of the enteric nervous system of transgenic mice that overexpress the Hoxa-4 gene. Dev Dyn. 1998;211(3):269–91. https://doi.org/10.1002/(SICI)1097-0177(199803)211:3<269:AID-AJA8>3.0.CO;2-F.
130. Doodnath R, Wride M, Puri P. The spatio-temporal patterning of Hoxa9 and Hoxa13 in the developing zebrafish enteric nervous system. Pediatr Surg Int. 2012;28(2):115–21. https://doi.org/10.1007/s00383-011-2992-3.
131. Yokouchi Y, Sakiyama J, Kuroiwa A. Coordinated expression of Abd-B subfamily genes of the HoxA cluster in the developing digestive tract of chick embryo. Dev Biol. 1995;169(1):76–89.
132. Roberts DJ, Johnson RL, Burke AC, et al. Sonic hedgehog is an endodermal signal inducing Bmp-4 and Hox genes during induction and regionalization of the chick hindgut. Development. 1995;121(10):3163–74.
133. de Santa Barbara P, Roberts DJ. Tail gut endoderm and gut/genitourinary/tail development: a new tissue-specific role for Hoxa13. Development. 2002;129(3):551–61.
134. Garcia-Barcelo MM, Miao X, Lui VCH, et al. Correlation between genetic variations in Hox clusters and Hirschsprung's disease. Ann Hum Genet. 2007;71(Pt 4):526–36. https://doi.org/10.1111/j.1469-1809.2007.00347.x.
135. Yang JT, Liu CZ, Villavicencio EH, et al. Expression of human GLI in mice results in failure to thrive, early death, and patchy Hirschsprung-like gastrointestinal dilatation. Mol Med. 1997;3(12):826–35.
136. Liu JA-J, Lai FP-L, Gui H-S, et al. Identification of GLI mutations in patients with Hirschsprung disease that disrupt enteric nervous system development in mice. Gastroenterology. 2015;149(7):1837–1848.e5. https://doi.org/10.1053/j.gastro.2015.07.060.
137. Ramalho-Santos M, Melton DA, McMahon AP. Hedgehog signals regulate multiple aspects of gastrointestinal development. Development. 2000;127(12):2763–72.
138. Pozniak CD, Langseth AJ, Dijkgraaf GJP, et al. Sox10 directs neural stem cells toward the oligodendrocyte lineage by decreasing Suppressor of Fused expression. Proc Natl Acad Sci U S A. 2010;107(50):21795–800. https://doi.org/10.1073/pnas.1016485107.
139. Dastot-Le Moal F, Wilson M, Mowat D, et al. ZFHX1B mutations in patients with Mowat-Wilson syndrome. Hum Mutat. 2007;28(4):313–21. https://doi.org/10.1002/humu.20452.
140. Takagi T, Nishizaki Y, Matsui F, et al. De novo inbred heterozygous Zeb2/Sip1 mutant mice uniquely generated by germ-line conditional knockout exhibit craniofacial, callosal and behavioral defects associated with Mowat-Wilson syndrome. Hum Mol Genet. 2015;24(22):6390–402. https://doi.org/10.1093/hmg/ddv350.
141. de Putte V, Tom FA, Nelles L, et al. Neural crest-specific removal of Zfhx1b in mouse leads to a wide range of neurocristopathies reminiscent of Mowat-Wilson syndrome. Hum Mol Genet. 2007;16(12):1423–36. https://doi.org/10.1093/hmg/ddm093.
142. Wakamatsu N, Yamada Y, Yamada K, et al. Mutations in SIP1, encoding Smad interacting protein-1, cause a form of Hirschsprung disease. Nat Genet. 2001;27(4):369–70. https://doi.org/10.1038/86860.

143. Amiel J, Espinosa-Parrilla Y, Steffann J, et al. Large-scale deletions and SMADIP1 truncating mutations in syndromic Hirschsprung disease with involvement of midline structures. Am J Hum Genet. 2001;69(6):1370–7. https://doi.org/10.1086/324342.
144. Antonellis A, Bennett WR, Menheniott TR, et al. Deletion of long-range sequences at Sox10 compromises developmental expression in a mouse model of Waardenburg-Shah (WS4) syndrome. Hum Mol Genet. 2006;15(2):259–71. https://doi.org/10.1093/hmg/ddi442.
145. Bergeron K-F, Cardinal T, Toure AM, et al. Male-biased aganglionic megacolon in the TashT mouse line due to perturbation of silencer elements in a large gene desert of chromosome 10. PLoS Genet. 2015;11(3):e1005093. https://doi.org/10.1371/journal.pgen.1005093.
146. Soret R, Mennetrey M, Bergeron KF, et al. A collagen VI-dependent pathogenic mechanism for Hirschsprung's disease. J Clin Invest. 2015;125(12):4483–96. https://doi.org/10.1172/JCI83178.
147. Breau MA, Pietri T, Eder O, et al. Lack of beta1 integrins in enteric neural crest cells leads to a Hirschsprung-like phenotype. Development. 2006;133(9):1725–34. https://doi.org/10.1242/dev.02346.
148. Nagy N, Mwizerwa O, Yaniv K, et al. Endothelial cells promote migration and proliferation of enteric neural crest cells via beta1 integrin signaling. Dev Biol. 2009;330(2):263–72. https://doi.org/10.1016/j.ydbio.2009.03.025.
149. Tanyel FC, Muftuoglu SF, Dagdeviren A, et al. Expression of beta-1 integrins in ganglionic and aganglionic segments of patients with Hirschsprung's disease. Eur J Pediatr Surg. 1997;7(1):16–20. https://doi.org/10.1055/s-2008-1071042.
150. Selfridge J, Song L, Brownstein DG, et al. Mice with DNA repair gene Ercc1 deficiency in a neural crest lineage are a model for late-onset Hirschsprung disease. DNA Repair (Amst). 2010;9(6):653–60. https://doi.org/10.1016/j.dnarep.2010.02.018.
151. Meijers JH, Tibboel D, van der Kamp AW, et al. A model for aganglionosis in the chicken embryo. J Pediatr Surg. 1989;24(6):557–61.
152. Payette RF, Tennyson VM, Pomeranz HD, et al. Accumulation of components of basal laminae: association with the failure of neural crest cells to colonize the presumptive aganglionic bowel of ls/ls mutant mice. Dev Biol. 1988;125(2):341–60.
153. Gershon MD, Chalazonitis A, Rothman TP. From neural crest to bowel: development of the enteric nervous system. J Neurobiol. 1993;24(2):199–214. https://doi.org/10.1002/neu.480240207.
154. Rothman TP, Le Douarin NM, Fontaine-Perus JC, et al. Developmental potential of neural crest-derived cells migrating from segments of developing quail bowel back-grafted into younger chick host embryos. Development. 1990;109(2):411–23.
155. Thiery JP, Duband JL, Delouvee A. Pathways and mechanisms of avian trunk neural crest cell migration and localization. Dev Biol. 1982;93(2):324–43.
156. Natsikas NB, Sbarounis CN. Adult Hirschsprung's disease. An experience with the Duhamel-Martin procedure with special reference to obstructed patients. Dis Colon Rectum. 1987;30(3):204–6.
157. O'Donnell A-M, Puri P. Hypoganglionic colorectum in the chick embryo: a model of human hypoganglionosis. Pediatr Surg Int. 2009;25(10):885–8. https://doi.org/10.1007/s00383-009-2444-5.
158. Zhou CB, Peng CH, Pang WB, et al. Treating congenital megacolon by transplanting GDNF and GFRα-1 double genetically modified rat bone marrow mesenchymal stem cells. Genet Mol Res. 2015;14(3):9441–51. https://doi.org/10.4238/2015.August.14.8.
159. Cheng LS, Hotta R, Graham HK, et al. Endoscopic delivery of enteric neural stem cells to treat Hirschsprung disease. Neurogastroenterol Motil. 2015;27(10):1509–14. https://doi.org/10.1111/nmo.12635.
160. Sato A, Yamamoto M, Imamura K, et al. Pathophysiology of aganglionic colon and anorectum: an experimental study on aganglionosis produced by a new method in the rat. J Pediatr Surg. 1978;13(4):399–435.
161. Parr EJ, Sharkey KA. Multiple mechanisms contribute to myenteric plexus ablation induced by benzalkonium chloride in the guinea-pig ileum. Cell Tissue Res. 1997;289(2):253–64.
162. Yoneda A, Shima H, Nemeth L, et al. Selective chemical ablation of the enteric plexus in mice. Pediatr Surg Int. 2002;18(4):234–7. https://doi.org/10.1007/s003830100681.
163. Fujimura T, Shibata S, Shimojima N, et al. Fluorescence visualization of the enteric nervous network in a chemically induced aganglionosis model. PLoS One. 2016;11(3):e0150579. https://doi.org/10.1371/journal.pone.0150579.
164. Khalil HA, Kobayashi M, Rana P, et al. Mouse model of endoscopically ablated enteric nervous system. J Surg Res. 2016;200(1):117–21. https://doi.org/10.1016/j.jss.2015.07.034.
165. Dahl JL, Bloom DD, Epstein ML, et al. Effect of chemical ablation of myenteric neurons on neurotransmitter levels in the rat jejunum. Gastroenterology. 1987;92(2):338–44.
166. See NA, Epstein ML, Dahl JL, et al. The myenteric plexus regulates cell growth in rat jejunum. J Auton Nerv Syst. 1990;31(3):219–29.
167. See NA, Epstein ML, Schultz E, et al. Hyperplasia of jejunal smooth muscle in the myenterically denervated rat. Cell Tissue Res. 1988;253(3):609–17.
168. See NA, Greenwood B, Bass P. Submucosal plexus alone integrates motor activity and epithelial transport in rat jejunum. Am J Physiol. 1990;259(4 Pt 1):8.
169. Luck MS, Dahl JL, Boyeson MG, et al. Neuroplasticity in the smooth muscle of the myen-

terically and extrinsically denervated rat jejunum. Cell Tissue Res. 1993;271(2):363–74.
170. Holle GE. Changes in the structure and regeneration mode of the rat small intestinal mucosa following benzalkonium chloride treatment. Gastroenterology. 1991;101(5):1264–73.
171. Holle GE, Forth W. Myoelectric activity of small intestine after chemical ablation of myenteric neurons. Am J Physiol. 1990;258(4 Pt 1):26.
172. Dong YL, Liu W, Gao YM, et al. Neural stem cell transplantation rescues rectum function in the aganglionic rat. Transplant Proc. 2008;40(10):3646–52. https://doi.org/10.1016/j.transproceed.2008.06.107.
173. Shu X, Meng Q, Jin H, et al. Treatment of aganglionic megacolon mice via neural stem cell transplantation. Mol Neurobiol. 2013;48(3):429–37. https://doi.org/10.1007/s12035-013-8430-x.
174. Zhang L, Zhao B, Liu W, et al. Cotransplantation of neuroepithelial stem cells with interstitial cells of Cajal improves neuronal differentiation in a rat aganglionic model. J Pediatr Surg. 2017;52(7):1188–95. https://doi.org/10.1016/j.jpedsurg.2017.01.065.
175. Wagner JP, Sullins VF, Dunn JCY. Skin-derived precursors generate enteric-type neurons in aganglionic jejunum. J Pediatr Surg. 2014;49(12):1809–14. https://doi.org/10.1016/j.jpedsurg.2014.09.023.
176. Wagner JP, Sullins VF, Dunn JCY. A novel in vivo model of permanent intestinal aganglionosis. J Surg Res. 2014;192(1):27–33. https://doi.org/10.1016/j.jss.2014.06.010.
177. Wagner JP, Sullins VF, Khalil HA, et al. A durable model of Hirschsprung's colon. J Pediatr Surg. 2014;49(12):1804–8. https://doi.org/10.1016/j.jpedsurg.2014.09.024.
178. Erol G, Yasemin A, Gokcimen A, Ozdemir O. Growth failure, tardive dyskinesia, megacolon development, and hepatic damage in neonatal rats following exposure to trimethobenzamide in utero. J Matern Fetal Neonatal Med. 2011;24(9):1176–80. https://doi.org/10.3109/14767058.2010.536867.
179. Sato Y, Heuckeroth RO. Retinoic acid regulates murine enteric nervous system precursor proliferation, enhances neuronal precursor differentiation, and reduces neurite growth in vitro. Dev Biol. 2008;320(1):185–98. https://doi.org/10.1016/j.ydbio.2008.05.524.
180. Fu M, Sato Y, Lyons-Warren A, et al. Vitamin A facilitates enteric nervous system precursor migration by reducing Pten accumulation. Development. 2010;137(4):631–40. https://doi.org/10.1242/dev.040550.
181. Schill EM, Lake JI, Tusheva OA, et al. Ibuprofen slows migration and inhibits bowel colonization by enteric nervous system precursors in zebrafish, chick and mouse. Dev Biol. 2016;409(2):473–88. https://doi.org/10.1016/j.ydbio.2015.09.023.
182. Lake JI, Tusheva OA, Graham BL, et al. Hirschsprung-like disease is exacerbated by reduced de novo GMP synthesis. J Clin Invest. 2013;123(11):4875–87. https://doi.org/10.1172/JCI69781.
183. Lake JI, Avetisyan M, Zimmermann AG, et al. Neural crest requires Impdh2 for development of the enteric nervous system, great vessels, and craniofacial skeleton. Dev Biol. 2016;409(1):152–65. https://doi.org/10.1016/j.ydbio.2015.11.004.
184. Tam PKH, Garcia-Barceló M. Genetic basis of Hirschsprung's disease. Pediatr Surg Int. 2009;25(7):543–58. https://doi.org/10.1007/s00383-009-2402-2.
185. Newgreen D, Young HM. Enteric nervous system: development and developmental disturbances--part 2. Pediatr Dev Pathol. 2002;5(4):329–49. https://doi.org/10.1007/s10024-002-0002-4.

Familial Hirschsprung's Disease

6

Prem Puri and Hiroki Nakamura

Contents

6.1 Introduction

Hirschsprung's disease (HSCR) is a congenital disorder of the enteric nervous system, characterized by the absence of enteric ganglia in variable lengths of the distal bowel. The absence of ganglion cells in HSCR is attributed to a genetically determined aberrant development of the enteric nervous system, resulting in the failure of the enteric neural crest cells to colonize the distal bowel. Although the majority of cases of HSCR are sporadic, HSCR is known to occur in families. The reported incidence of familial cases varies from 3.6% to 7.8% in different series [2, 3, 20, 26]. A familial incidence of 15–22% has been reported in total colonic aganglionosis and 50% in the rare total intestinal aganglionosis [2, 3, 20, 26]. The mode of inheritance may vary from dominant with reduced penetrance, mostly found in nonsyndromic familial HSCR patients, to recessive in families with syndromic HSCR [17]. Most HSCR cases are sporadic and are believed to be multifactorial and polygenic in nature.

P. Puri (✉)
University College Dublin, Dublin, Ireland

National Children's Research Centre, Our Lady's Children's Hospital Crumlin, Dublin, Ireland
e-mail: prem.puri@ncrc.ie

H. Nakamura
National Children's Research Centre, Our Lady's Children's Hospital Crumlin, Dublin, Ireland
e-mail: hinakamu@juntendo.ac.jp

6.2 Recurrence Risk in Siblings

Badner et al. [4] demonstrated that the recurrence risk to siblings is dependent upon the sex of the person affected and the extent of the aganglionosis. If the index patient is female, the proportion of affected siblings is higher. The recurrence risk to siblings also increases as the aganglionosis becomes more extensive (Table 6.1) [4]. Risk of recurrence of the disease is greater in relatives of an affected female than an affected male. Risk of recurrence is also greater in relatives of a patient with long-segment compared to short-segment disease. For example, the recurrence risk in a sibling of a female with long-segment HSCR is 33% for a male and 9% for a female, whereas the recurrence risk in a sibling of a male with long-

P. Puri (ed.), *Hirschsprung's Disease and Allied Disorders*,
https://doi.org/10.1007/978-3-030-15647-3_6

Table 6.1 Recurrence risk to siblings in Hirschsprung's disease

Segment affected	Sex of index patient	Sex of sibling	Recurrence risk (%)
Rectosigmoid HSCR	Male	Male	5
	Male	Female	1
	Female	Male	5
	Female	Female	3
Long-segment HSCR	Male	Male	17
	Male	Female	13
	Female	Male	33
	Female	Female	9

segment HSCR is 17% for a male and 13% for a female. These risks fall to 5% and below for siblings of a patient with rectosigmoid HSCR (Table 6.1).

The long-segment HSCR, total colonic aganglionosis, and total intestinal aganglionosis show a strong trend toward a significant familial association. Mc Laughlin and Puri [13], in a systematic review, analyzed the patterns of HSCR in the published literature. They found 330 cases of familial HSCR among 4331 index cases of HSCR, giving an overall rate of 7.6% for familial recurrence (Table 6.2). In children with total aganglionosis (n = 525), 20% of cases were reported to have familial recurrence (Table 6.3). Recurrence of HSCR within the families predominantly occurred in siblings (62%) and was reported between parent and child in 22% and in other relatives in 16%. The authors observed a high variability in rates of familial HSCR between different centers (Table 6.2). They believed that the systematic review most likely underestimated the rate of familial recurrence of HSCR because studies included in their review were not specifically designed to report comprehensive familial data.

Mc Laughlin and Puri [13] reported that HSCR recurred at a higher rate in families of patients with total colonic aganglionosis (TCA) (1 in every 5 cases). These findings are consistent with reports suggesting that TCA represents a distinct entity in terms of etiology, displaying increased penetrance and dominant inheritance in families of affected patients rather that the multifactorial or recessive patterns of inheritance in other HSCR cases.

Table 6.2 Familial recurrence in Hirschsprung's disease

Author	Year	HSCR cases (n)	Familial cases (n)
Carter	1981	207	21
Orr	1983	103	5
Klein	1984	26	3
Badner	1990	218	8
Moore	1991	370	28
Ryan	1992	179	13
Engum	1993	260	20
Cilley	1994	15	3
Russell	1994	224	11
Shono	1994	110	14
Jung	1995	137	4
Marty	1995	135	23
Fortuna	1996	82	6
Reding	1997	59	4
Sarioglu	1997	302	6
Bjornland	1998	48	4
Svensson	1998	69	7
Weber	1999	107	8
Yanchar	1999	107	14
Mir	2001	10	1
Fitze	2003	76	5
Murthi	2003	63	2
De Lagauise	2004	55	2
Wang	2004	147	5
Luis	2006	100	12
Ziad	2006	102	3
Koh	2008	14	2
Pini Prato	2008	112	9
Shinall	2008	60	2
Moore	2010	118	18
Ruiz-Ferrer	2011	217	27
Lee	2012	44	0
Nah	2012	76	3
Levitt	2013	67	2
Virtanen	2013	91	15
More	2014	54	2
Jakobson-Setton	2015	21	3
Neuvonen	2015	146	15
	Total	4331	330

Most studies investigating familial recurrence in HSCR have been conducted on selected patients without complete genealogical information and thus resulting in some bias. Teerlink et al. [25] recently described familial clustering of HSCR cases using the well-established unbiased familial aggregation techniques within the

Table 6.3 Familial recurrence in total colonic aganglionosis

Author	Year	TCA cases (*n*)	Familial (*n*)
N-fekete	1986	27	5
Cass	1987	32	5
Galifer	1987	6	1
Dykes	1989	9	1
Festen	1989	11	4
Moore	1991	30	11
Bickler	1992	21	7
Marty	1995	12	6
Azzis	1996	16	2
Emslie	1997	5	1
Hoehner	1998	29	4
Tsuji	1999	48	10
Hernadez	2003	15	3
Escobar	2005	36	10
Anupuma	2007	25	0
Barrena	2008	41	12
Choe	2008	17	4
Menezes	2008	58	5
Raboei	2008	12	4
Shen	2009	29	4
Moore	2010	22	7
Travassos	2011	15	2
Yeh	2014	9	2
	Total	525	110

context of a population genealogy. They investigated the relative risk (RR) in relatives which is defined as the ratio of observed number of affected relatives of cases to the expected number of affected relatives of cases. They found that the estimated RRs among all first-degree relatives of cases, and in selected sets of first-degree relatives, are significantly elevated, as were RRs for second- and fourth-degree relatives. The authors concluded that the population-based genealogy methodology provides unbiased risk estimates and may have clinical value in predicting recurrence in HSCR.

6.3 Syndromic Hirschsprung's Disease

In the majority of patients, HSCR occurs as an isolated anomaly. In the European surveillance, Best et al., [5] reported that of the 1322 singleton cases of HSCR, 1039 (78.6%) were isolated cases, 146 (11%) had associated chromosomal anomalies or genetic syndromes, and 137 (10.3%) had other associated structural anomalies. Down's syndrome is the most common chromosomal anomaly and has been reported in 4.5% to 16% of patients with HSCR [5, 14, 16]. Other chromosomal abnormalities that have been described in association with HSCR include interstitial deletion of distal 13q, partial deletion of 2p, reciprocal translation and trisomy 18 mosaic. A number of unusual hereditary syndromes have been reported in patients with HSCR. These include Shah-Waardenburg syndrome, multiple endocrine neoplasia (MEN) type 2 syndrome, congenital central hypoventilation syndrome (Ondine's curse), Goldberg-Shprintzen syndrome, Kaufman-McKusick syndrome, Bardet-Biedl syndrome, Smith-Lemli-Opitz syndrome, cartilage-hair hypoplasia syndrome, and syndromes with HSCR and distal limb anomalies [1, 8, 22].

The recurrence risk and prognosis of syndromic HSCR and HSCR associated with chromosomal anomalies depends on the recurrence of the associated syndrome rather than on the HSCR [1, 8, 24]. Cases of familial recurrence of syndromic HSCR are predominantly limited to RET mutation together with MEN2A or EDNRB mutation together with Shah-Waardenburg syndrome. Other syndromic associations recur within families very rarely.

6.4 Hirschsprung's Disease in Twins

HSCR in twins is extremely rare. Monozygotic twins concordant for disease expression have previously been reported in the literature, supporting the genetic etiology and pathogenesis of disease penetrance [7, 15]. On the other hand, multiple other case studies reported discordant disease in monozygotic twins, discussing the role of genetic and environmental factors [9, 18, 19, 23].

Henderson et al. [11] performed a systematic review to analyze the patterns of HSCR in twins published in the literature. Their analysis found 18 twin pairs, and HSCR was present in two-thirds of the twin subjects. Of the 36 individuals, there were 24 confirmed cases of HSCR (67%), of which the majority were male (83%), with a ratio of affected males to females of 5:1. Of the 18 twin pairs, 12 pairs were monozygotic twins, 4 pairs were dizygotic twins, and in 2 pairs zygosity was not reported. Rectosigmoid HSCR was reported in 71% of the affected patients, long-segment disease was reported in 21%, and 8% presented with total colonic aganglionosis. Three twin pairs (17%) had at least one family member affected by HSCR. The authors concluded that the inheritance pattern in twins with HSCR is most likely a multi factorial inheritance with a variable penetrance. In future, conclusive genetic testing in HSCR twins may provide the crucial element to deciphering HSCR transmission.

6.5 Consanguinity and Hirschsprung's Disease

The practice of consanguineous marriage or marriage between close biological relatives is very heterogeneous across the world ranging from less than 1% in North American and most European to over 50% in some regions in Asia and Middle Eastern countries [6, 10, 12]. Even though consanguinity between parents is common in the Middle East and some countries in Asia, the occurrence of HSCR in the offspring of consanguineous parents has not been well documented from these regions. A study analyzing HSCR in Oman reported a consanguinity rate of 75% among parents of HSCR patients compared to a consanguinity rate of 33% in the general population [21]. A more recent study from Bangladesh reported that the rate of consanguinity among parents of HSCR babies was 16% compared to 10% in the general population [12].

6.6 Conclusion

Familial recurrence of HSCR is frequent and should be discussed with families of index patients. Genetic counseling should be offered to these families and in particular for those patients with long-segment and total colonic aganglionosis.

References

1. Amiel J, Lyonnet S. Hirschsprung disease, associated syndromes, and genetics: a review. J Med Genet. 2001;38(11):729–39.
2. Angrist M, Bolk S, Thiel B, Puffenberger EG, Hofstra RM, Buys CH, et al. Mutation analysis of the RET receptor tyrosine kinase in Hirschsprung disease. Hum Mol Genet. 1995;4(5):821–30.
3. Attie T, Pelet A, Edery P, Eng C, Mulligan LM, Amiel J, et al. Diversity of RET proto-oncogene mutations in familial and sporadic Hirschsprung disease. Hum Mol Genet. 1995;4(8):1381–6.
4. Badner JA, Sieber WK, Garver KL, Chakravarti A. A genetic study of Hirschsprung disease. Am J Hum Genet. 1990;46(3):568–80.
5. Best KE, Addor MC, Arriola L, Balku E, Barisic I, Bianchi F, et al. Hirschsprung's disease prevalence in Europe: a register based study. Birth Defects Res A Clin Mol Teratol. 2014;100(9):695–702.
6. Bittles A. Consanguinity and its relevance to clinical genetics. Clin Genet. 2001;60(2):89–98.
7. Bodian M, Carter CO, Ward BC. Hirschsprung's disease. Lancet. 1951;1(6650):302–9.
8. Gariepy CE. Genetic basis of Hirschsprung disease: implications in clinical practice. Mol Genet Metab. 2003;80(1–2):66–73.
9. Hannon RJ, Boston VE. Discordant Hirschsprung's disease in monozygotic twins: a clue to pathogenesis? J Pediatr Surg. 1988;23(11):1034–5.
10. Hashmi MA. Frequency of consanguinity and its effect on congenital malformation – a hospital based study. J Pak Med Assoc. 1997;47(3):75–8.
11. Henderson D, Zimmer J, Nakamura H, Puri P. Hirschsprung's disease in twins: a systematic review and meta-analysis. Pediatr Surg Int. 2017;33(8):855–9.
12. Karim A, Akter M, Aziz TT, Hoque M, Chowdhury TK, Imam MS, et al. Epidemiological characteristics of Hirschsprung's disease (HSCR): results of a case series of fifty patients from Bangladesh. J Pediatr Surg. 2018;53(10):1955–9.
13. Mc Laughlin D, Puri P. Familial Hirschsprung's disease: a systematic review. Pediatr Surg Int. 2015;31(8):695–700.
14. Menezes M, Puri P. Long-term clinical outcome in patients with Hirschsprung's disease and associated Down's syndrome. J Pediatr Surg. 2005;40(5):810–2.
15. Mohammed AA, Gahukamble DB. Concordant expression of Hirschsprung's disease in monozygous twins. Saudi Med J. 2000;21(2):200–1.
16. Moore SW. Chromosomal and related Mendelian syndromes associated with Hirschsprung's disease. Pediatr Surg Int. 2012;28(11):1045–58.
17. Moore SW, Zaahl M. Clinical and genetic correlations of familial Hirschsprung's disease. J Pediatr Surg. 2015;50(2):285–8.
18. Moore TC, Landers DB, Lachman RS, Ament ME. Hirschsprung's disease discordant in monozygotic twins: a study of possible environmental factors

in the production of colonic aganglionosis. J Pediatr Surg. 1979;14(2):158–61.
19. Patel RV, Lawther S, McCallion WA. Discordant monozygotic total colonic Hirschsprung's disease presenting with neonatal isolated ileal perforation. BMJ Case Rep. 2013;2013. pii: bcr2013200743. https://doi.org/10.1136/bcr-2013-200743
20. Puri P, Tomuschat C. Hirschsprung's disease. In: Puri P, editor. Newborn surgery. 4th ed. Boca Raton: CRC Press; 2018. p. 667–83.
21. Rajab A, Freeman NV, Patton MA. Hirschsprung's disease in Oman. J Pediatr Surg. 1997;32(5):724–7.
22. Ryan ET, Ecker JL, Christakis NA, Folkman J. Hirschsprung's disease: associated abnormalities and demography. J Pediatr Surg. 1992;27(1):76–81.
23. Siplovich L, Carmi R, Bar-Ziv J, Karplus M, Mares AJ. Discordant Hirschsprung's disease in monozygotic twins. J Pediatr Surg. 1983;18(5):639–40.
24. Stewart DR, von Allmen D. The genetics of Hirschsprung disease. Gastroenterol Clin North Am. 2003;32(3):819–37, vi
25. Teerlink CC, Bernhisel R, Cannon-Albright LA, Rollins MD. A population-based description of familial clustering of Hirschsprung disease. J Pediatr Surg. 2018;53(7):1355–9.
26. Tomuschat C, Puri P. RET gene is a major risk factor for Hirschsprung's disease: a meta-analysis. Pediatr Surg Int. 2015;31(8):701–10.

Genetics of Hirschsprung's Disease

7

Paul K. H. Tam, Clara S. M. Tang, and Maria-Mercè Garcia-Barceló

Contents

P. K. H. Tam (✉) · C. S. M. Tang
M.-M. Garcia-Barceló
Department of Surgery, Li Ka Shing Faculty of Medicine, The University of Hong Kong, Hong Kong SAR China, Hong Kong SAR
e-mail: paultam@hku.hk; claratang@hku.hk; mmgarcia@hku.hk

P. Puri (ed.), *Hirschsprung's Disease and Allied Disorders*,
https://doi.org/10.1007/978-3-030-15647-3_7

Abbreviations

CDS	Coding sequences
ENS	Enteric nervous system
FMTC	Familiar medullary thyroid carcinoma
HSCR	Hirschsprung disease, Hirschsprung's disease, Congenital intestinal aganglionosis, Congenital megacolon
L-HSCR	Long segment aganglionosis
MEN	Multiple Endocrine Neoplasia
NCCs	Neural crest cells
NCDS	Non-coding regions
PTC	Papillary thyroid carcinoma
S-HSCR	Short segment aganglionosis
TCA	Total colonic aganglionosis

7.1 Introduction

Understanding how genes (DNA sequences that when expressed encode proteins) and regulatory sequences (DNA sequences that control the expression of genes) function together and interact among themselves and environmental factors is paramount to the discovery of the mechanisms involved in normal biological processes. Disruption of the normal processes contributes to the pathogenesis of many disorders. In this respect, the study of the genetics and molecular basis of Hirschsprung's disease (HSCR) has made, and it is making, a significant contribution to the understanding of heritable oligogenic disorders where genetic variants in more than one gene are necessary for the disease to manifest.

HSCR is a developmental disorder characterized by the absence of ganglion cells of the lower digestive tract. The incidence of HSCR varies across populations and is highest among Asians (2.8/10,000 live births). Aganglionosis is attributed to an abnormal development of the enteric nervous system (ENS) whereby ganglion cells fail to innervate the lower gastrointestinal tract. HSCR most commonly presents *sporadically* (80% of the patients are born to unaffected parents), although it can be *familial*, where the patient is born to an affected parent/s and/or has affected relatives. Thus, the inheritance pattern of HSCR is complex and also displays variability in the length of the aganglionic segment and the concomitance with other developmental disorders as HSCR can be an isolated clinical feature (*isolated HSCR*) or be part of a phenotypic spectrum of several syndromes (*syndromic HSCR;*), neurocristopathies and/or chromosome abnormalities [1–3]. The syndromic HSCR form may reflect gene pleiotropy (gene with effect on several traits) or the involvement of large chromosomal abnormalities whereby several genes affecting several traits are involved. Independent of whether HSCR is isolated or syndromic, patients are also classified according to the extent of the aganglionosis into short-segment aganglionosis (S-HSCR; 80% patients), long-segment (L-HSCR; 15%) and total colonic aganglionosis patients (TCA; 5%).

The genetic complexity observed in HSCR can be conceptually understood in the light of the molecular and cellular events that take place during the ENS development. The ganglion cells of the fully developed ENS are derived from vagal neural crest cells (NCCs) of the neural tube [4] which have to migrate and differentiate to populate the gut. During the colonization process, the NCCs have to adapt to a constantly changing intestinal environment that strongly influences their differentiation into enteric neurons. The entire process is regulated by specific molecular signals from both within the neural crest and intestinal environment so that the success of the colonization of the gut by enteric ganglion precursors depends on the synchronization and balance of the signalling network implicated. Conceivably, DNA alterations in the genes encoding the signalling molecules may interfere with the colonization process and consequently represent a primary aetiology for HSCR or other neurocristopathies. Since the range of interactions during ENS development is large, the HSCR phenotype and presentation (isolated/syndromic; sporadic/familial; aganglionosis length) are variable and may result from (i) a single severe DNA variant impairing the function of a crucial gene encoding a critical signalling molecule, (ii) the accumulation of variants with milder effects in several genes or (iii) the former and the latter combined. Indeed, the genetic background of an individual can exacerbate or mollify the effect of some major damaging genetic variants. Certainly, the existence of non-clinically affected individuals carrying mutations in major genes invokes a compensatory effect by other genes. Indeed, although L-HSCR/TCA is mostly transmitted in an autosomal dominant manner (familial HSCR), the penetrance of the culprit mutation can vary within family members leading to phenotypic unpredictability. On the other hand, S-HSCR follows a complex, non-Mendelian inheritance pattern subject to gender bias where more males are affected than females in a 4-to-1 ratio. These remarkable phenotypic differences among HSCR types or categories are underlain by a category-specific genetic architecture where the role of several genes and different types of genetic variants are amalgamated. Table 7.1 lists the main genes known to be involved in either syndromic or isolated HSCR.

HSCR has become a model for oligogenic and polygenic disorders in which the phenotypes and mode of transmission result from interactions between different genes.

Table 7.1 Main genes known to be involved in either syndromic or isolated HSCR

Gene	Phenotype[b]	No. isolated HSCR patients
RET[a]	HSCR (isolated)	≈50% familial 20% sporadic
	MEN2A with HSCR	
	MEN2B with HSCR	
	FMTC with HSCR	
GDNF	HSCR (isolated)	VR
GFRα1	HSCR (isolated)	VR
NTN	HSCR (isolated)	VR
PSPN	HSCR (isolated)	VR
EDNRB	HSCR (isolated)	R
	Waardenburg-Shah syndrome type 4	
EDN3	HSCR (isolated)	VR
	Waardenburg-Shah syndrome type 4	
ECE-1	HSCR (isolated)	VR
SOX10	HSCR (isolated)	VR (one patient reported)
	Waardenburg-Shah syndrome type 4	
PHOX2B[a]	Haddad syndrome	
	Neuroblastoma and HSCR	
ZFHX1B	Mowat-Wilson syndrome with HSCR	
L1CAM	X-linked hydrocephalus with HSCR	
KIAA1279	Goldberg-Shprintzen syndrome with HSCR	
NRG1[a]	HSCR (isolated)	R
NRG3	HSCR (isolated and syndromic)	VR/CNV
SEMA3C/3D[a]	HSCR (isolated)	R
GLI1	HSCR (isolated)	VR
GLI2	HSCR (isolated)	VR
GLI3	HSCR (isolated)	VR
	Pallister-Hall syndrome with HSCR	R
DENND3	HSCR (isolated)	VR
NCLN	HSCR (isolated)	VR
NUP98	HSCR (isolated)	VR
TBATA	HSCR (isolated)	VR
VCL	HSCR (isolated)	VR
BACE 2	HSCR (isolated)	R

[a]Gene with common variants associated with HSCR. Rare (R): gene mutations identified in less than 7% of the HSCR patients screened and reported. Very rare (VR): gene mutations identified in less than1% of the HSCR patients screened and reported

Table 7.1 (continued)

[b]Patients with isolated HSCR may have additional isolated anomalies without forming part of any genetic syndrome (no observable pattern of association thus far, i.e. Meckel's diverticulum)

CNV copy number variant

7.2 Mutations in HSCR Genes: *RET* Is the Major but not the Sole HSCR Gene

The genetic factors contributing to HSCR have been studied since the late 1980s/early 1990s when it became clear that around 80% of the patients with affected relatives (familial HSCR) had damaging variants in the *RET* (*RE*arranged during *T*ransfection) gene [5–7]. Incidentally, *RET* was first identified as the locus for Multiple Endocrine Neoplasia (MEN), papillary thyroid carcinoma (PTC) and familiar medullary thyroid carcinoma (FMTC) [1]. The co-occurrence of HSCR with multiple endocrine neoplasia type 2 (MEN2) prompted the search for a HSCR gene in that chromosomal region [7]. The *RET* damaging variants detected in HSCR patients were rare, that is, mainly privy to patients and relatives and hardly observed in the general population. For clarity sake, genetic variants with a damaging effect on the protein and whose frequency in the general population is less than 1% will be referred to as mutations thereon. Concurrent studies on the role of *RET* in the development of the ENS [8] together with the observation of colon aganglionosis in mice with a disrupted *Ret* gene [9] corroborated the significance of the findings in human patients. *RET* became the major HSCR gene. Mechanistically, it was shown that the RET protein is expressed on the cellular membrane of the ENS precursors functioning as a receptor for the Glial cell line-Derived Neurotrophic Factor (GDNF) family. Activation of the RET receptor by these neurotrophic factors was shown to be essential for the migration and differentiation of NCC into enteric neurons [10, 11]. Within this framework, it was established that the correct development of the ENS depends on the ability of these neurotrophic factors to activate RET, on the ability of the RET receptor to transduce the signal and on the competence of the intracellular machinery to elaborate a response.

The vast screening of HSCR patients for mutations in the coding sequences (CDS) of *RET* that took place during the late 1990s demonstrated that *RET* mutations were mainly found in *familial cases* and that there was no correlation between the type of variant/mutation and the phenotype, i.e. the same mutation could give rise to aganglionosis of different lengths in different individuals, even within the same family [12–14]. The fact that not all HSCR patients bore mutations in *RET* implied that mutations in other genes had to account for the rest of the HSCR patients or that mutations occurred in regions of the genome not being investigated, namely regulatory non-coding regions (NCDS).

The genes subsequently investigated for mutations in their CDS were those encoding the natural RET ligands, other interacting partners and signalling molecules known to be involved in the development of the ENS through studies of animal models, known interactions among relevant molecules and early human studies on common genetic variants (see below). During the late 1990s and early 2000s, Sanger sequencing of candidate genes led to the identification of mutations – *albeit at a much lower rate than those in RET* – in several genes including *GDNF*, *NRTN*, *PHOX2B*, *EDNRB*, *EDN3*, *ECE1*, *SOX10*, *DNMT3B*, *ZFHX1B*, *KIAA1279*, *SEMA3C/D* and *NRG1* [15–19]. Most of these genes encode protein members of important *interrelated signalling pathways* that are critical for the development of enteric ganglia including the GDNF/RET receptor tyrosine kinase, the endothelin type B receptor, the SOX10 mediated transcription as well as the ERNRB/NRG1 pathway. In fact, as new HSCR genes were being discovered through mutational analysis, studies on interactions between molecules, new pathways and mechanisms were concomitantly being revealed. For instance, interactions between neuregulin 1 and semaphorin 3D and RET were dissected and scrutinized, likewise with the other molecules encoded by putative candidate genes [17, 18, 20].

The revolution in sequencing technologies that took place in the last decade made the screening of the whole CDS (exome) and of the whole genome of HSCR patients feasible at a relatively affordable price. These technologies (whole exome sequencing (WES) and whole genome sequencing – WGS) permitted the discovery of new mutations in the ENS-relevant genes as well in genes whose role in the ENS was unknown. For instance, *GLI* genes, which had been known to be involved in ENS development and to interact with in ENS molecules were shown, for the first time, to lead to HSCR in humans [21]. On the other hand, "unsuspected genes" such as *DENND3, NCLN, NUP98, TBATA* and *VCL* were found to be relevant for the ENS development [22, 23]. A recent large-scale WGS analysis of short-segment patients and controls found that patients had a significant excess of rare protein-altering variants not only in genes previously associated with Hirschsprung disease but also in the β-secretase 2 gene (BACE2) [24]. BACE2 encodes an aspartyl protease that cleaves amyloid beta precursor protein preventing Aβ accumulation that damages neurons in Alzheimer disease. Functional study using human induced pluripotent stem cells (hiPSC) showed that BACE2 abolishes Aβ production and prevents the accumulation of amyloid to protect neurons from undergoing apoptosis, suggesting that the BACE1-APPBACE2 pathway would be another key pathway underlying HSCR pathogenesis [24].

7.3 HSCR Genes Can Also Be Mutated in Healthy Individuals

These powerful sequencing technologies have somehow opened a "Pandora's box", not only because of the fear of misusing personal genetic data but also the difficulties inherent to big data handling and interpretation. Indeed, we are now able to have a full picture of the whole exome and the whole genome of HSCR patients as well as of healthy individuals. Each patient may have mutations in more than one gene (known HSCR gene or otherwise) and the mutated genes differ among individuals. In this scenario, it has become terribly difficult to assess the involvement of a gene in HSCR or the pathogenicity of any genetic variant (as its effect may be mild on its own but can become extremely damaging in the presence of other variants in other genes). Being able to observe the whole exome or the whole genome of an individual has enlightened the concept of genetic "complexity" and phenotypic variability inherent to HSCR. As mentioned above, a mutation in a HSCR gene, *RET* for instance, may have different effects even within a family, where some members can be affected with L-HSCR, some with S-HSCR and some are unaffected even though they carry the culprit mutation. The variable effect of a mutation is due to the presence of other genetic variants (not necessarily damaging/mutations) in other genes of the individual's genome. Likewise, it is known that some mutations can be found in unaffected individuals of the general population who remain healthy because of the attenuation effect of other genetic variants in their genome. Therefore, phenomena such as epitasis (interaction among different genes) and gene regulation interference are the norm and account for the complexity observed, mainly in HSCR patients that appear sporadically or that do not transmit the disorder following the typical Mendelian pattern of inheritance.

WES and WGS studies [24–26] have demonstrated that the disorder is mainly oligogenic (more than one gene is to be mutated for the disease to manifest) and genetically heterogeneous, whereby different genes (alone or combined) can give rise to HSCR. WGS has also shown that mutations do occur in regions of the DNA that regulate gene expression. Indeed, a lack or reduced expression of an ENS protein can also be the cause of HSCR, as seen in patients who have a complete deletion of *RET* or other main HSCR genes [6] *(see copy number variants section below)*.

As the variants we are dealing with are rare, reside in any of the known/unknown ENS genes of both patients and healthy individuals, associating a gene or group of genes with HSCR is not straightforward. Thus, geneticists and statisticians have resorted to burden tests to statistically associate a gene or a pathway with HSCR. Basically, these tests aggregate information across several variant sites within a gene, a group of interacting genes or a pathway and compare the aggregate frequency of "qualifying variants" between patients and control subjects for each gene, group or pathway [27].

7.4 Role of Common Variants in HSCR and Variation of the Incidence of HSCR Across Populations

While screening the CDS of *RET* for mutations in HSCR patients, it became apparent that variants of little or no effect on the RET protein conformation were found at frequencies higher than 1% in both patients and control population [28]. The importance of this observation rested in the fact that the frequencies in which these variants were found in patients were statistically different from those in which the very same variants were found in controls. These common variants (ubiquitously found in the population) were non-randomly associated with HSCR and were rightly thought to contribute to HSCR. It took several studies at genetic and functional levels to understand the mechanics whereby such presumably innocuous and ubiquitous variants could have a role in a disease where mutations were thought to be the only cause of the disorder. Importantly, these early studies showed that the frequencies for the HSCR-associated *RET* SNP were much higher (in both patients and controls) in Chinese than in Caucasians, therefore accounting for the high incidence of HSCR in Chinese and explaining the population differences in the incidence of HSCR [29, 30]. Expanding the Sanger sequencing search for mutations beyond CDS of *RET* led to the discovery of a common variant (common single nucleotide polymorphism or SNP) in the intron 1 of *RET* [31] linked to those CDS SNPs initially detected. This *RET* non-coding common polymorphism, rs2435357, explains 10–20 times more genetic variance than rare *RET* mutations. Also, the genetic effect of the common HSCR-associated enhancer variant (rs2435357) is directly proportional to the subtype prevalence, i.e. a larger effect in male, S-HSCR. On the contrary, the frequency of the *RET* CDS mutations correlates positively with disease severity [31, 32]. Mechanistically, this genetic variant overlaps a transcription factor binding site, thus interfering with the correct expression of *RET* mRNA and, consequently, affecting the amount of RET receptor expressed in the NCCs. As this common SNP is also present in the control population, again, it is implicit that the genetic background of an individual is essential for the manifestation of the disorder. Additionally, the technological advances of the late 1990s and early 2000s allowed the search of the whole genome for common variants associated with the disorder. Thus far, four genome-wide association studies (GWAS; where the frequencies of the variants are compared between patients and controls to establish association of the variant with the disease) and one meta-analysis of GWAS have been carried out [17, 33–36]. In addition to *RET*, two novel genes whose common variants were associated with HSCR were discovered: semaphorin 3C/3D (*SEMA3*) and neuregulin-1 (*NRG1*). Of note, while the association of *NRG1* variants was universal, that of *SEMA3* was privy to Europeans. Again, these observations do account for the differences in HSCR incidences across populations. While the role of *RET* in ENS had long been established, these GWAS unravelled genes that although known to be players in the ENS development, their contribution to the HSCR in humans was unprecedented. Semaphorins 3C and 3D are involved in axon guidance and neuronal migration and neuregulin-1 in NCCs' survival and differentiation. Follow-up mutational scans of these two new genes revealed similar genetic properties to those reported for *RET*, whereby both common and rare variants underlie the genetic risk to HSCR [17, 18, 37, 38]. Unlike *RET*-associated common variants, the mechanisms by which these novel HSCR-associated variants influence genetic susceptibility remain largely unknown. These common variant association studies revealed that *NRG1* HSCR-associated variants increased risk to disease in the presence of the *RET* HSCR-associated variants which implies genetic and, most likely, functional interaction between these two genes [20, 34]. In fact, *NRG1* is a key gene for gliogenesis (non-neuronal glia generation) and *RET* to neurogenesis and the interaction between these two players indicates that a correct balance between neurogenesis and gliogenesis is critical for ENS development. Moreover, the interaction between these two genes and possibly many others not only involves common variants but also mutations or rare variants, which altogether adds to the complexity and current unpredictability of the disease.

7.5 From Chromosomal Abnormalities to Copy Number Variants in Hirschsprung's Disease Patients

Down described the trisomy 21 syndrome in 1866. Yet, the cause of this syndrome (extra copy of the entire chromosome 21) was discovered 90 years later. Since then, the number of conditions caused by variations in chromosome number, structure or content has increased due to technological advances which permit the screening of the whole genome for the detection of genomic copy number changes at a resolution of 50 base pairs. For clarity sake, here, we will deal with *C*opy *N*umber *V*ariations (CNVs) of at least 1Kb in size for which copy number differences have been observed in the comparison of two or more genomes. CNVs represent an important portion of missing heritability (proportion of phenotypic variation attributable to genetic variation) for human diseases and HSCR in particular. In fact, the two major HSCR genes, *RET* and *EDNRB*, are the perfect paradigm of how structural variations (chromosomal interstitial deletions of the chromosomal regions encompassing these genes) lead to the discovery of HSCR predisposing genes [6, 39]. As mentioned above, subsequent sequencing analysis of these genes in independent HSCR patients worldwide revealed a myriad of mutations in their coding regions. This clearly indicated that any gene harbouring a deleterious structural mutation could become a candidate gene to be screened by other methods for additional, presumably smaller, deleterious mutations in unrelated individuals.

The relevance of CNVs in HSCR is exacerbated by the fact that 30% of the HSCR patients present with additional syndromes, some caused by chromosome abnormalities and some uncharacterized. Indeed, chromosomal abnormalities appear in 12% of cases, with Down syndrome being the most common. Importantly, a wide spectrum of concomitant anomalies have been described among HSCR cases with an incidence varying from 5% to 30% [1]. Most of these patients have normal karyotypes and no CDS mutations in HSCR genes, thus likely to harbour structural variations involving several genes (missed by conventional karyotyping methods), hence the syndromic phenotype. Given the early impact of CNVs on gene discovery and the non-random association of HSCR with syndromes, it was thought that structural variations could also affect non-syndromic HSCR. The known HSCR genes were the first to be targeted for CNVs surveys [40, 41], which indeed revealed CNV changes affecting some ENS genes. These studies were followed by the genome-wide CNVs surveys [42, 43]. Both studies identified chromosomal regions affected only in patients; yet, the most relevant finding was perhaps the enrichment of a CNV encompassing *NRG3* in patients. Besides its statistical association with HSCR, this new HSCR gene, *NRG3*, encodes a protein similar to its paralog *NRG1* and both play important roles in the developing nervous system. In addition, a CNV deletion encompassing a NRG3/NRG1 receptor *ErbB4* was also observed uniquely in a syndromic HSCR patient. These findings established the contribution of the Neuregulin protein family to the disease. Overall, Tang's study [43] showed that compared to individuals of the general population, HSCR patients are enriched with CNVs that interfere with genes (deletion or duplication of genes or gene regions). Also, syndromic-HSCR patients carried significantly longer CNVs than the non-syndromic HSCR patients or controls. Yet, no differences in CNV distribution have ever been observed when HSCR patients are stratified according to the severity of the aganglionosis. Table 7.2 summarizes the CNVs >1megabase identified in HSCR patients.

Table 7.2 Chromosomal abnormalities and CNVs (>1 megabase) detected in isolated or syndromic patients [15, 43]

Chromosomal region	Phenotype
Del 2q22–23	Mowat-Wilson syndrome
Tri 8p21.2-p21.3	Isolated HSCR
Del 10q11	Mental retardation
Del 10q11 (not encompassing *RET*)	Mental retardation
Del 11q14.2-q23.2	Mental retardation; hydrocephalus, microcephaly, congenital hypotonia
Del 11q23.2-q25	Isolated HSCR
Del 13q22 (EDNRB)	Mental and growth retardation; dysmorphism
Del 15q11.2-q13.1	Isolated HSCR
Dup 16p11.2-p12.3	Mental retardation; epilepsy
Del /Dup 17q21	Mental retardation; multiple congenital anomalies
Tri 21	Down syndrome (>10% of HSCR patients)

Del deletion, *Dup* duplication, *Tri* trisomy. Except for Tri 21, the number of patients carrying these CNVs is lower than 1%

7.6 Genetic Counselling

Given the genetic complexity of HSCR, it is obvious that genetic counselling is not straightforward. Relative figures can be provided by taking into account the gender and aganglionosis length of the affected individual and the gender of the sibs [1]. Nonetheless, the reduced penetrance of the mutations and the oli–/multigenic nature of the disease make it difficult to rationally predict and assess the risk. Genetic testing for HSCR is only performed on a research basis, and due to the advances of the surgical management of HSCR, its utility is questionable.

Yet, as outlined earlier, mutations in *RET* also underlie inherited cancer syndromes MEN2A and MEN2B and FMTC. In HSCR patients, *RET* mutations are dispersed throughout the gene, while in MEN2A and FMTC patients, mutations are clustered in the cysteine codons of the *RET* extracellular domain (exons 10 and 11). Although HSCR and MEN2A are two different entities, occasionally they co-segregate in some families and affected individuals carry a single mutation in exon 10 or 11. Importantly, *RET* mutations identical to those found in MEN2A have been detected in HSCR patients with no clinical symptoms of MEN2A [44]. That means that some HSCR patients may be exposed to a highly increased risk of tumours. Where HSCR patients carry these tumour-specific mutations, exploration of the family history of MEN2A and periodic screening for tumours is advisable. In families segregating both MEN2A and HSCR, *RET* gene testing, tumour screening and prophylactic thyroidectomy are also warranted.

7.7 Conclusion and Future Directions: Making Sense of Genetic Data in HSCR

From all of the above, we have learnt that mutations, common variants and/or CNVs affecting both CDS and non-CDS regions of genes involved in the development of the ENS can contribute to HSCR to different extents. Also, although mutations in the main HSCR genes are more likely to be found in familial cases and in patients with severe aganglionosis, common variants of the very main gene or common and/or rare variants in other genes may "confer" to determine the manifestation of the phenotype. More often than not, HSCR patients have more than one gene mutated and these co-existing mutated genes tend to interact (Fig. 7.1). Importantly, members of a given protein family can be associated with the same phenotype, individually or together, as seen in the case of neuregulins, and the same is true for protein members of interrelated pathways as seen with RET, EDNRB and other pathways.

To illustrate such complexity, let us consider the role of *RET* HSCR-associated common variants. Their effect is to sensitize the genetic background by decreasing the levels of *RET* expression but not to critical levels (these SNPs are also in controls). Additional variants or mutations in such background may therefore lead to a critical situation whereby HSCR would manifest. While this is conceptually simple and understandable, expanding this concept to the large number of ENS genes, to the different effects of their mutations or variants, becomes daunting as many genes can exert their influence in ENS and each patient may have different genes conveying effects of different sizes and interacting among themselves. In addition, it should not be forgotten the possible contribution of epigenetic factors as well as the possibility of developmental mutations, that is, mutations that occur post-zygotically and affect only those lineages from which NCCs derive [45, 46]. These mutations would not be detected in blood DNA, the usual source for genetic studies.

As the successful colonization of the gut by the ENS precursors depends on a coordinated and balanced network of interacting molecules, there should exist a critical molecule or a group of molecules linking and coordinating the downstream molecules and ultimately determining the phenotype. The finding of these molecules would mean the finding of a therapeutic target applicable to all patients in spite of their diversity. This, together with the vast amount of information generated by genome-scale investigations, has stimulated a parallel development of new analytical frameworks and tools at bioinformatics, mathematic and functional level. Algorithms integrating genes into pathways, test where genes are grouped into sets and so on, are being developed to try to make sense of the data. Also, attempts are being made to generate biologically relevant representations of each individual. In HSCR, the genetic profile of each patient is generated using WES and WGS data [22, 24]. Given the uniqueness of each patient, and the heterogeneity of the disorder, pathway-based personalized analysis may be the way to go. Yet, the only way to fully assess the "leading" mutated gene is by deriving enteric-NCC from induced pluripotent stem cells (iPSC) from patients, editing/correcting the "mutation" or variant using clustered regularly interspaced short palindromic repeats/Cas9CRISPR/Cas9 and testing the ENCC-iPSC-induced migration

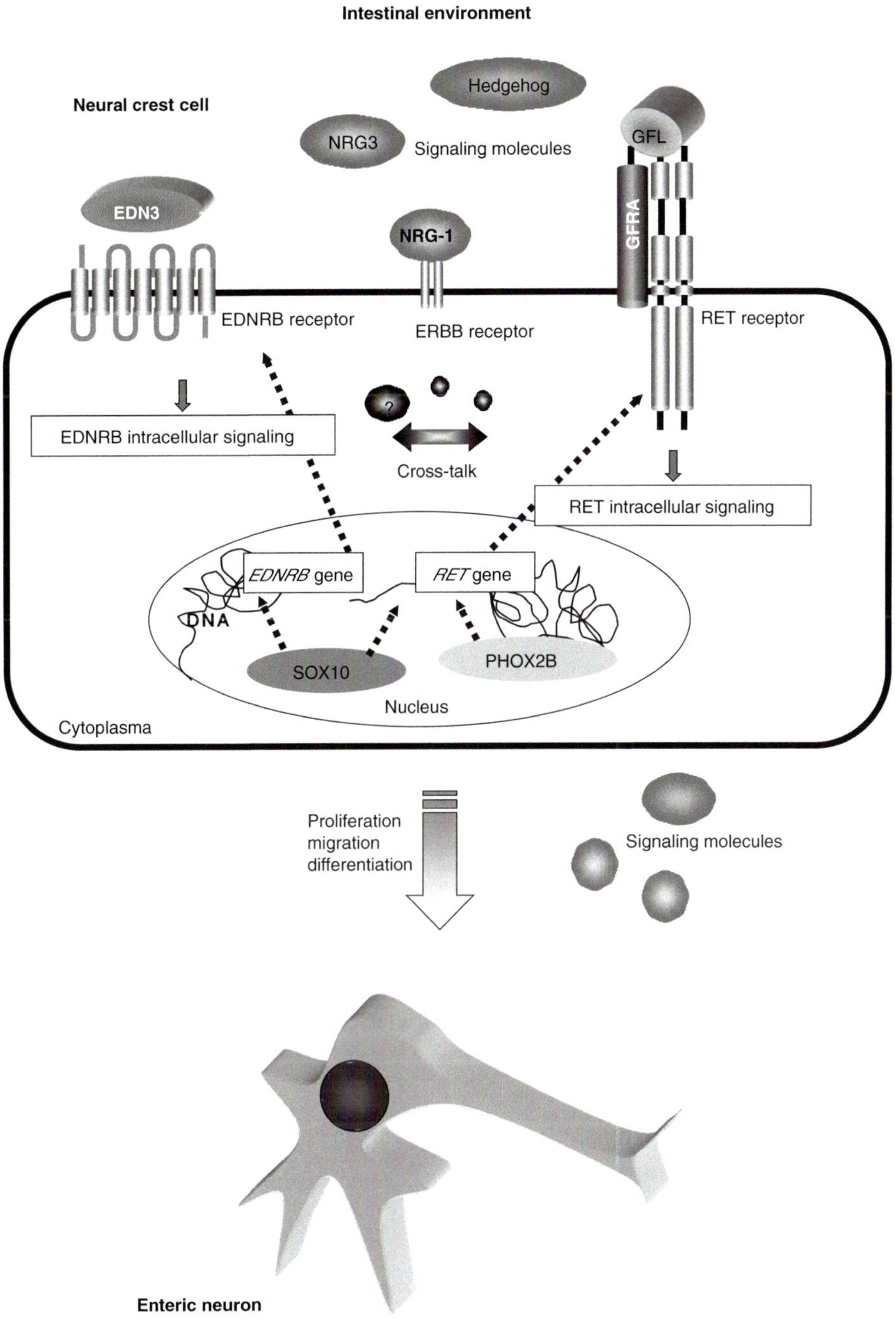

Fig. 7.1 Schematic representation of the network of interactions that govern the development of the enteric nervous system. (Adapted and updated from [3]). Expression of the *RET* gene (regulated by transcription factors) leads to the formation of the RET protein which functions as a receptor for the Glial cell line-Derived Neurotrophic Factor family (GFL) through co-receptors (GFRA). Activation of the RET receptor by these signalling molecules of the gut environment activates the intracellular machinery necessary for the migration, proliferation and differentiation of NCCs into enteric neurons. Similarly, the EDNRB receptor is activated by EDN3 and initiates a series of events that will also regulate the development of the enteric nervous system in conjunction with the RET pathway. The ERBB/NRGs1 pathway is also represented. Double head arrows indicated interrelation between pathways. Transcription factors involved in *RET* regulation are pictured in the nucleus. Question marks represent yet unidentified molecules that should be members of the network (see modifying genes and interaction between signalling pathways section in the text). Many molecules involved in ENS development are not represented in this figure for simplicity

and differentiation capacities before and after the correction of the mutation being assessed. This approach has been successful in several instances and, although tedious, is a prelude to personalized treatment of HSCR [23, 47].

Acknowledgements The authors would like to acknowledge the Theme Based Research (TBR) T12C-714/14-R1 grant to PT.

References

1. Amiel J, Sproat-Emison E, Garcia-Barcelo MM, Lantieri F, Burzynski G, Borrego S, et al. Hirschsprung disease, associated syndromes and genetics: a review. J Med Genet. 2008;45(1):1–14.
2. Tam PKH. Hirschsprung's disease: a bridge for science and surgery. J Pediatr Surg. 2016;51(1):18–22.
3. Tam PKH, Garcia-Barcelo MM. Genetic basis of Hirschsprung's disease. Pediatr Surg Int. 2009;25(7):543–58.
4. Burns AJ, Douarin NM. The sacral neural crest contributes neurons and glia to the post-umbilical gut: spatiotemporal analysis of the development of the enteric nervous system. Development. 1998;125(21):4335–47.
5. Edery P, Lyonnet S, Mulligan LM, Pelet A, Dow E, Abel L, et al. Mutations of the RET proto-oncogene in Hirschsprung's disease. Nature. 1994a;367(6461):378–80.
6. Fewtrell MS, Tam PKH, Thomson AH, Fitchett M, Currie J, Huson SM, et al. Hirschsprung's disease associated with a deletion of chromosome 10 (q11.2q21.2): a further link with the neurocristopathies? J Med Genet. 1994;31(4):325–7.
7. Lyonnet S, Bolino A, Pelet A, Abel L, Nihoul-Fekete C, Briard ML, et al. A gene for Hirschsprung disease maps to the proximal long arm of chromosome 10. Nat Genet. 1993;4(4):346–50.
8. Pachnis V, Durbec P, Taraviras S, Grigoriou M, Natarajan D III. Role Of the RET signal transduction pathway in development of the mammalian enteric nervous system. Am J Physiol. 1998;275(2 Pt 1):G183–6.
9. Schuchardt A, D'Agati V, Larsson-Blomberg L, Costantini F, Pachnis V. RET-deficient mice: an animal model for Hirschsprung's disease and renal agenesis. J Intern Med. 1995;238(4):327–32.
10. Pachnis V, Mankoo B, Costantini F. Expression of the c-ret proto-oncogene during mouse embryogenesis. Development. 1993;119(4):1005–17.
11. Taraviras S, Marcos-Gutierrez CV, Durbec P, Jani H, Grigoriou M, Sukumaran M, et al. Signalling by the RET receptor tyrosine kinase and its role in the development of the mammalian enteric nervous system. Development. 1999;126(12):2785–97.
12. Edery P, Pelet A, Mulligan LM, Abel L, Attie T, Dow E, et al. Long segment and short segment familial Hirschsprung's disease: variable clinical expression at the RET locus. J Med Genet. 1994b;31(8):602–6.
13. Sancandi M, Ceccherini I, Costa M, Fava M, Chen B, Wu Y, et al. Incidence of RET mutations in patients with Hirschsprung's disease. J Pediatr Surg. 2000;35(1):139–42.
14. Svensson PJ, Molander ML, Eng C, Anvret M, Nordenskjold A. Low frequency of RET mutations in Hirschsprung disease in Sweden. Clin Genet. 1998;54(1):39–44.
15. Alves MM, Sribudiani Y, Brouwer RW, Amiel J, Antinolo G, Borrego S, et al. Contribution of rare and common variants determine complex diseases-Hirschsprung disease as a model. Dev Biol. 2013;382(1):320–9.
16. Brooks AS, Bertoli-Avella AM, Burzynski GM, Breedveld GJ, Osinga J, Boven LG, et al. Homozygous nonsense mutations in KIAA1279 are associated with malformations of the central and enteric nervous systems. Am J Hum Genet. 2005;77(1):120–6.
17. Jiang Q, Arnold S, Heanue T, Kilambi KP, Doan B, Kapoor A, et al. Functional loss of semaphorin 3C and/or semaphorin 3D and their epistatic interaction with ret are critical to Hirschsprung disease liability. Am J Hum Genet. 2015;96(4):581–96.
18. Tang CS, Ngan ES, Tang WK, So MT, Cheng G, Miao XP, et al. Mutations in the NRG1 gene are associated with Hirschsprung disease. Hum Genet. 2012b;131(1):67–76.
19. Torroglosa A, Enguix-Riego MV, Fernandez RM, Roman-Rodriguez FJ, Moya-Jimenez MJ, de Agustin JC, et al. Involvement of DNMT3B in the pathogenesis of Hirschsprung disease and its possible role as a regulator of neurogenesis in the human enteric nervous system. Genet Med. 2014;16(9):703–10.
20. Gui H, Tang WK, So MT, Proitsi P, Sham PC, Tam PKH, et al. RET and NRG1 interplay in Hirschsprung disease. Hum Genet. 2013;132(5):591–600.
21. Liu JA, Lai FP, Gui HS, Sham MH, Tam PKH, Garcia-Barcelo MM, et al. Identification of GLI mutations in patients with Hirschsprung disease that disrupt enteric nervous system development in mice. Gastroenterology. 2015;149(7):1837–1848.e1835.
22. Gui H, Schriemer D, Cheng WW, Chauhan RK, Antinolo G, Berrios C, et al. Whole exome sequencing coupled with unbiased functional analysis reveals new Hirschsprung disease genes. Genome Biol. 2017;18(1):48.
23. Lai FP, Lau ST, Wong JK, Gui H, Wang RX, Zhou T, et al. Correction of Hirschsprung-associated mutations in human induced pluripotent stem cells via clustered regularly interspaced short palindromic repeats/Cas9, restores neural crest cell function. Gastroenterology. 2017;153(1):139–153.e138.
24. Tang CS, Zhuang X, Lam WY, Ngan ES, Hsu JS, Michelle YU, et al. Uncovering the genetic lesions underlying the most severe form of Hirschsprung dis-

ease by whole-genome sequencing. Eur J Hum Genet. 2018;26(6):818–26.
25. Luzon-Toro B, Gui H, Ruiz-Ferrer M, Tang CS, Fernandez RM, Sham PC, et al. Exome sequencing reveals a high genetic heterogeneity on familial Hirschsprung disease. Sci Rep. 2015;5:16473.
26. Tang CS, Li P, Lai FP, Fu AX, Lau ST, So MT, Lui KN, Li Z, Zhuang X, Yu M, Liu X, Ngo ND, Miao X, Zhang X, Yi B, Tang S, Sun X, Zhang F, Liu H, Liu Q, Zhang R, Wang H, Huang L, Dong X, Tou J, Cheah KS, Yang W, Yuan Z, Yip KY, Sham PC, Tam PKH, Garcia-Barcelo MM, Ngan ESW. Identification of genes associated with Hirschsprung disease, based on whole-genome sequence analysis, and potential effects on enteric nervous system development. Gastroenterology. 2018;155(6):1908–22.
27. Lee S, Abecasis GR, Boehnke M, Lin X. Rare-variant association analysis: study designs and statistical tests. Am J Hum Genet. 2014;95(1):5–23.
28. Borrego S, Saez ME, Ruiz A, Gimm O, Lopez-Alonso M, Antinolo G, et al. Specific polymorphisms in the RET proto-oncogene are over-represented in patients with Hirschsprung disease and may represent loci modifying phenotypic expression. J Med Genet. 1999;36(10):771–4.
29. Garcia-Barcelo MM, Ganster RW, Lui VC, Leon TY, So MT, Lau AM, et al. TTF-1 and RET promoter SNPs: regulation of RET transcription in Hirschsprung's disease. Hum Mol Genet. 2005;14(2):191–204.
30. Garcia-Barcelo MM, Sham MH, Lui VC, Chen BL, Song YQ, Lee WS, et al. Chinese patients with sporadic Hirschsprung's disease are predominantly represented by a single RET haplotype. J Med Genet. 2003;40(11):e122.
31. Emison ES, McCallion AS, Kashuk CS, Bush RT, Grice E, Lin S, et al. A common sex-dependent mutation in a RET enhancer underlies Hirschsprung disease risk. Nature. 2005;434(7035):857–63.
32. Emison ES, Garcia-Barcelo MM, Grice EA, Lantieri F, Amiel J, Burzynski G, et al. Differential contributions of rare and common, coding and noncoding Ret mutations to multifactorial Hirschsprung disease liability. Am J Hum Genet. 2010;87(1):60–74.
33. Fadista J, Lund M, Skotte L, Geller F, Nandakumar P, Chatterjee S, et al. Genome-wide association study of Hirschsprung disease detects a novel low-frequency variant at the RET locus. Eur J Hum Genet. 2018;26(4):561–9.
34. Garcia-Barcelo MM, Tang CS, Ngan ES, Lui VC, Chen Y, So MT, et al. Genome-wide association study identifies NRG1 as a susceptibility locus for Hirschsprung's disease. Proc Natl Acad Sci U S A. 2009;106(8):2694–9.
35. Kim JH, Cheong HS, Sul JH, Seo JM, Kim DY, Oh JT, et al. A genome-wide association study identifies potential susceptibility loci for Hirschsprung disease. PLoS One. 2014;9(10):e110292.
36. Tang CS, Gui H, Kapoor A, Kim JH, Luzon-Toro B, Pelet A, et al. Trans-ethnic meta-analysis of genome-wide association studies for Hirschsprung disease. Hum Mol Genet. 2016;25(23):5265–75.
37. Luzon-Toro B, Fernandez RM, Torroglosa A, de Agustin JC, Mendez-Vidal C, Segura DI, et al. Mutational spectrum of semaphorin 3A and semaphorin 3D genes in Spanish Hirschsprung patients. PLoS One. 2013;8(1):e54800.
38. Luzon-Toro B, Torroglosa A, Nunez-Torres R, Enguix-Riego MV, Fernandez RM, de Agustin JC, et al. Comprehensive analysis of NRG1 common and rare variants in Hirschsprung patients. PLoS One. 2012;7(5):e36524.
39. Puffenberger EG, Kauffman ER, Bolk S, Matise TC, Washington SS, Angrist M, et al. Identity-by-descent and association mapping of a recessive gene for Hirschsprung disease on human chromosome 13q22. Hum Mol Genet. 1994;3(8):1217–25.
40. Jiang Q, Ho YY, Hao L, Nichols Berrios C, Chakravarti A. Copy number variants in candidate genes are genetic modifiers of Hirschsprung disease. PLoS One. 2011;6(6):e21219.
41. Sanchez-Mejias A, Nunez-Torres R, Fernandez RM, Antinolo G, Borrego S. Novel MLPA procedure using self-designed probes allows comprehensive analysis for CNVs of the genes involved in Hirschsprung disease. BMC Med Genet. 2010;11:71.
42. Bae JS, Koh I, Cheong HS, Seo JM, Kim DY, Oh JT, et al. A genome-wide association analysis of chromosomal aberrations and Hirschsprung disease. Transl Res. 2016;177:31–40.e36.
43. Tang CS, Cheng G, So MT, Yip BH, Miao XP, Wong EH, et al. Genome-wide copy number analysis uncovers a new HSCR gene: NRG3. PLoS Genet. 2012a;8(5):e1002687.
44. Romeo G, Ceccherini I, Celli J, Priolo M, Betsos N, Bonardi G, et al. Association of multiple endocrine neoplasia type 2 and Hirschsprung disease. J Intern Med. 1998;243(6):515–20.
45. Brosens E, MacKenzie KC, Alves MM, Hofstra RMW. Do RET somatic mutations play a role in Hirschsprung disease? Genet Med. 2018; https://doi.org/10.1038/gim.2018.6.
46. Jiang Q, Liu F, Miao C, Li Q, Zhang Z, Xiao P, et al. RET somatic mutations are underrecognized in Hirschsprung disease. Genet Med. 2017; https://doi.org/10.1038/gim.2017.178.
47. Tam PKH, Chung PHY, St Peter SD, Gayer CP, Ford HR, Tam GCH, et al. Advances in paediatric gastroenterology. Lancet. 2017;390(10099):1072–82.

Stem Cell Therapy for Enteric Neuropathies

8

Conor J. McCann, Allan M. Goldstein, Ryo Hotta, Nikhil Thapar, Robert M. W. Hofstra, and Alan J. Burns

Contents

C. J. McCann · N. Thapar
Stem Cells and Regenerative Medicine, UCL Great Ormond Street Institute of Child Health, London, UK

A. M. Goldstein · R. Hotta
Department of Pediatric Surgery, Massachusetts General Hospital, Harvard Medical School, Boston, MA, USA

R. M. W. Hofstra
Department of Clinical Genetics, Erasmus University Medical Centre, Rotterdam, The Netherlands

A. J. Burns (✉)
Stem Cells and Regenerative Medicine, UCL Great Ormond Street Institute of Child Health, London, UK

Department of Clinical Genetics, Erasmus University Medical Centre, Rotterdam, The Netherlands

Takeda Pharmaceuticals International, Cambridge, MA, USA
e-mail: alan.burns@ucl.ac.uk

8.1 Introduction

Diseases and disorders of the enteric nervous system (ENS) of the gastrointestinal (GI) tract comprise a range of conditions where the ENS is absent or damaged, or has less well-defined defects that may include loss of neuronal subtypes, or possibly structural abnormalities such as neuronal wiring defects. These conditions can be life threatening when the ENS is absent in part of the gut, as in Hirschsprung disease (HSCR), or more chronic and lifelong in others (e.g., chronic intestinal pseudo-obstruction (CIPO)). A common feature of enteric neuropa-

P. Puri (ed.), *Hirschsprung's Disease and Allied Disorders*,
https://doi.org/10.1007/978-3-030-15647-3_8

thies is that there are no definitive cures, with symptomatic management as the current standard of care. These features highlight the need for novel therapies for enteric neuropathies. One appealing approach is to replace/repair the ENS by transplanting stem cells into diseased gut [13]. Although various stem cells types including neural, autologous, or pluripotent stem cells could potentially be used for therapy, the identification, isolation, and expansion of enteric neural stem cells (ENSCs) that reside within the gut have been extensively studied for the last 20 years or so, and these cells have been transplanted into animal models of enteric neuropathy where they have been shown to form the ENS (see Sect. 8.3; reviewed in [13, 14, 71]). When considering the development of a stem cell therapy for enteric neuropathies, the question of which disease to begin with is crucial. Factors to consider include clinical need, preclinical supporting data, which stem cells to use, how would they be administered to the gut, and what outcome measures would be assessed. Taking these factors into account, HSCR appears to be the ideal candidate for stem cell therapy for a number of reasons: (i) there is a high clinical need (the current treatment is surgical removal of the affected aganglionic gut region, with associated complications and morbidity); (ii) there is a well-defined phenotypic defect with an absence of neurons in a definitive segment of gut that would comprise the site for local stem cell transplantation; (iii) ENSCs could be harvested from the ganglionic segment of a patient's gut, expanded/optimized in vitro and transplanted into the aganglionic segment of gut of the same patient in an autologous manner, negating the need for immunosuppression; and (iv) there are extensive preclinical supporting data on ENSCs and on ENSC transplant into animal (mainly mouse) gut in vivo. Here, we delve deeper into these and other important factors to consider around stem cell therapy and outline how we are close to the point of developing such a therapy for enteric neuropathies in general and HSCR specifically.

8.2 Target Diseases

ENSC therapy has potential application for the treatment of any neurointestinal disease characterized by congenital absence or acquired loss of enteric neurons. Most of the research in this area has focused on the treatment of HSCR. ENSCs have been successfully isolated from the ganglionic and aganglionic bowel of patients with HSCR [16, 50, 59]. These HSCR-derived ENSCs have been successfully expanded in culture and transplanted into embryonic hindgut [16], postnatal mouse models of HSCR [16], and explanted human HSCR bowel [50, 59]. ENSCs have also been isolated from wild-type and HSCR mice and transplanted ex vivo into human aganglionic colon [44] or in vivo into aganglionic mouse colon [35]. These studies demonstrate that the grafted cells can survive, proliferate, migrate, and differentiate in the aganglionic host environment. Importantly, the ability to use donor cells derived from HSCR bowel supports the potential of autologous therapy in the future. However, whether the transplanted cells generate functioning neuronal networks capable of restoring gut motility in the aganglionic segment remains unclear. Recently, Fattahi et al. [23] directed human embryonic stem (ES) cells to an ENS lineage and transplanted those cells into the ceca of *Ednrb*$^{-/-}$mice. Unlike control mice, those that received ES cell-derived enteric neural crest progenitors had grafted cells throughout the colon and survived, suggesting that the cell therapy prevented the mortality typically seen in these mice. However, improved gut motility was not demonstrated, leaving the mechanism for the increased survival unclear. Nevertheless, while additional studies are certainly needed, these promising results offer hope for the clinical utility of cell therapy for treating HSCR.

While HSCR is an appealing disease target for cell-based therapy, it may be among the most challenging. Since the target tissue in HSCR is entirely devoid of an ENS, a complete neuroglial network needs to be established. This requires differentiation of all appropriate neuronal subtypes and establishment of the necessary connections between neurons and effector cells, including smooth muscle cells and other neurons. Additionally, the aganglionic area requiring repopulation can be extensive. Therefore, other neurointestinal diseases may offer alternative initial targets for restoration of gastrointestinal function.

Esophageal achalasia is due to loss of inhibitory myenteric neurons in the esophagus and lower esophageal sphincter (LES), leading to esophageal aperistalsis and LES non-relaxation. These neurons are lost due to autoimmune reactions that lead to inflammation and subsequently to neurodegeneration of these inhibitory cells in the myenteric plexus [27]. What makes esophageal achalasia a potentially attractive target disease for neuronal stem cell therapy is (i) our clear understanding of the neuronal deficit, (ii) the localized area of neuronal deficiency, and (iii) the ability to deliver cells to the target region endoscopically [13]. Stem cell therapy could thus restore the missing neuronal nitric oxide synthase (nNOS)- and vasoactive intestinal peptide (VIP)-expressing inhibitory neurons and thereby improve esophageal and LES function in patients with esophageal achalasia. This concept has been proposed [61], but not yet tested experimentally.

Other potential target diseases include idiopathic gastroparesis and diabetic gastroparesis, both of which are associated with a deficiency of nNOS-expressing cells in the stomach [30]. The use of stem cell therapy for delayed gastric emptying was tested by Micci et al. [51], who injected neuronal stem cells into the pylorus of nNOS-deficient mice and found an improvement in gastric emptying as early as 1 week after cell delivery. However, the etiology of gastroparesis is heterogeneous and can include alterations in the extrinsic neural supply to the stomach as well as abnormalities in the interstitial cells of Cajal (ICC). ENSC therapy is most likely to help patients with a neuropathic cause attributable to the ENS, and therefore an improved ability to diagnose the cause of gastroparesis in a given patient will likely be needed prior to deciding whether they are a candidate for neuronal stem cell therapy.

While there are other neurointestinal diseases, whether they will serve as feasible targets for ENSC therapy remains to be seen. Chronic intestinal pseudo-obstruction (CIPO), for example, can have a neurointestinal cause, typically characterized by an inflammatory neuropathy that can lead to neuronal degeneration [29]. CIPO typically affects the entire small intestine, and sometimes the stomach and colon as well. It is currently difficult to envision delivering cells to such an extensive part of the bowel, although future advances may identify ways to achieve massive expansion of ENSCs in vitro to generate the numbers of cells required and novel methods for delivering the cells to such a broad area. The field of ENSC transplantation is in its infancy, and extensive work is needed to address the many challenges that exist. Among these challenges is the importance of selecting the best target disease for initial first-in-human clinical trials. Targeting a localized region, as in esophageal achalasia or short-segment HSCR, is appealing. The absence of a specific neuronal subtype, as occurs in esophageal achalasia or gastroparesis, is also attractive. Demonstrating feasibility, safety, and efficacy in these diseases would serve as critical proof-of-concept and establish an important precedent for expanding the use of ENSC therapy to other enteric neuropathies.

8.3 Animal Models

As enteric neuropathies exist throughout the gastrointestinal (GI) tract, in multiple forms, a number of small animal models and model systems which recapitulate the myriad phenotypes observed in human disease have been utilized to investigate disease mechanisms and provide models for regenerative medicine studies. The archetypal disease model for regenerative medicine studies is HSCR, given the well-defined aganglionosis which results from disrupted neural crest cell colonization of variable lengths of the distal GI tract [15]. Due to the multigenic nature of HSCR [2], multiple murine models exist, based on HSCR-associated genes such as *Ret*, *GDNF*, *GFRa1*, *ET3*, *EdnrB*, and *Sox10,* some of which have been utilized for both developmental and cell therapy investigations [71]. Such models provide exciting avenues to study HSCR because of these shared gene defects. However, it is important to understand that critical differences exist in disease mechanisms which may prevent direct correlation of animal study findings to human disease.

Loss-of-function mutations in RET are the most common cause of HSCR in humans. Patients with familial RET mutations typically present with incomplete penetrance [5], whereas $Ret^{+/-}$mice (e.g., 129S/Sv-Ret^{tm1Cos}/J) do not display defects in ENS colonization and appear to be asymptomatic [4]. However, genetic manipulation and titration of Ret expression to 30% results in HSCR-like aganglionosis in mice [68]. Additionally, the genetic background of laboratory murine models has also been shown to have important effects on ENS development and HSCR phenotypes [20]. Hence, investigation of multiple models of disease has been required to build a body of evidence which is applicable to the human condition.

In terms of ENS cell replacement studies for HSCR, multiple model systems have been utilized to investigate the potential integration, functional development of neurons, and rescue of motility after stem cell transplantation. Ex vivo animal model studies have highlighted the ability of ENS stem cells to integrate in aneural avian, mouse, and human gut segments demonstrating the restorative potential of ENS stem cells [16, 43, 50, 59]. Indeed, organ culture investigations have provided critical evidence for the potential patient-specific isolation of ENS stem cells from ganglionated patient bowel and transplantation to autologous aganglionic gut segments [33]. Such ex vivo studies, while being valuable in demonstrating proof-of-principle evidence of ENS stem cell integration, have limited clinical relevance as they cannot, by definition, replicate the in vivo characteristics of enteric neuropathies or the recipient microenvironment.

To date, a number of in vivo proof-of-principle transplantation studies have shown the development of stem cell-derived neurons in ganglionated wild-type mouse colonic segments [18, 19, 24, 36]. More recently, progression of stem cell-based transplantation studies to pathophysiological models has shown integration of donor-derived cells in an $Ednrb^{-/-}$ HSCR-like mouse model [35], restoration of colonic motility within an $nNOS^{-/-}$ mouse model [48], and rescue of $Ednrb^{s-l/s-l}$(SSL/LEJ) mice which display a HSCR-like phenotype [23]. While these studies provide promising data suggesting that stem cell rescue of "lost" neurons in HSCR may be possible, differences in the disease phenotype in individual models prevent direct correlation to the human disease setting. The majority of stem cell studies, to date, have been performed on neonatal mice without previous intervention. Given that human HSCR patients typically require multiple medical interventions (e.g., decompression, stoma formation, or surgical removal of affected bowel) at very early stages, the direct comparison of murine studies is difficult. Moves toward larger animal models such as rat [65] or pig, where it may be possible to better replicate the clinical development of HSCR and scale of aganglionosis, may provide an alternative approach to examine stem cell transplantation for this devastating disease.

8.4 Sources of Stem Cells for Therapy

As outlined in the section above, a significant body of work, using ex vivo and in vivo animal models, supports the idea of using cell replacement therapy for enteric neuropathies. Although different stem cell types, obtained from different tissue sources, have been used experimentally, the optimal source of stem cells to repair/replace the ENS in the defective portion of bowel of patients with enteric neuropathies has yet to be established. The cell types that could be used for ENS cell therapy fall into two main categories: (enteric) neural stem cells and pluripotent stem cells.

8.4.1 Neural Stem Cells

8.4.1.1 Enteric Neural Stem Cells (ENSCs)

Work in rodents and with human tissue established that ENS neural stem/progenitor cells exist in the postnatal GI tract [11, 12, 40]. The existence of these resident enteric neural stem cells (ENSCs) within the gut offers the possibility of using patient-derived, autologous stem cells to treat disease. This is particularly appealing for HSCR, as ENSCs could be obtained from the ganglionated portion of a patient's bowel, expanded in culture, and then transplanted into the aganglionic segment, thus avoiding the need for immune suppression after transplantation [59]. Studies using both mouse and human ENSCs support the idea of using ENSCs as a therapy for enteric neuropathies. Following transplant, ENSCs have been shown to migrate, proliferate, differentiate, and functionally integrate with the ENS in normal mice and in aganglionic models of disease [18, 19, 23, 24, 35, 36, 48]. However, it has been reported that ENSCs have limited capacity for self-renewal [12, 40] and thus further optimization of these cells may be required. This topic is elaborated upon in Sect. 8.5. Other potential issues with using ENSCs for human therapy include scale-up and manufacture. The majority of preclinical studies using mouse and human ENSCs have involved the transplant of relatively small numbers of cells (as neurospheres) into mouse models in vivo. It remains to be seen whether cell manufacture methods can be developed to scale up production of ENSCs to provide sufficient cell numbers for ENS rescue in human gut. Finally, it remains unclear whether patient-derived ENSCs, which may possess disease-causing genetic mutations, are compromised in their ability to rescue/reform the ENS. For example, mutations in RET are the most prevalent in HSCR and although the ENS in the proximal bowel usually functions well in HSCR patients, it is unclear whether the therapeutic potential of ENSCs with pathogenic RET mutations would be diminished. Interestingly, this question was indirectly addressed in recent work by Lai et al. [42] using iPSC technology to generate enteric neurons harboring RET mutations. These studies showed that patient-derived cells and cells with engineered mutations had migration and differentiation defects that could be restored by CRISPR/Cas9 gene correction. Thus, gene correction may ultimately be required for autologous or iPSC cell therapy for HSCR and for other enteric neuropathies with a genetic component.

8.4.1.2 Central Nervous System (CNS) Neural Stem Cells

CNS-derived stem cells are a well-characterized population of cells with an extensive capacity for self-renewal. Following implantation to the brain and other structures, these cells have been shown to produce phenotypes that are appropriate for the environment into which they are transplanted. Based on this characteristic, a number of studies have investigated the ability of CNS-derived neural stem cells to repair the ENS and shown that they can survive and make contributions to functional improvements in gut motility disorders [41, 52, 53]. Further, Kulkarni et al. [41] showed that the gut microenvironment is capable of inducing CNS-derived stem cells to generate neurons that share some of the characteristics of enteric neurons, supporting their therapeutic use for enteric neuropathies. However, the use of CNS neural stem cells for the treatment of enteric neuropathies would be problematic. They are not readily accessible, since isolation from stem cell-rich regions of the brain involves highly invasive procedures, and studies have shown that ENS-derived progenitors have better migration, proliferation, and neuronal differentiation capability compared with CNS progenitors when transplanted into the colon [24].

8.4.2 Pluripotent Stem Cells

Pluripotent stem cells, that include human embryonic stem (ES) cells and induced pluripotent stem (iPS) cells, have the capacity to give rise to any cell of the body, thus making them an exciting therapeutic tool to treat a multitude of diseases, including enteric neuropathies. However, pluripotent stem cell technology is still relatively new to the ENS field, certainly in comparison with ENSC which were suggested for HSCR therapy as long ago as the late 1990s [56]. Nevertheless, a small number of studies have hinted at the tremendous potential of pluripotent stem cells for modeling enteric neuropathies and for therapy.

In pioneering studies, Studer and colleagues [23] used ES-derived cells (both human ES and iPS cell lines) that were induced to neural crest (NC) cells and then differentiated to enteric NC precursors that gave rise to functional enteric neurons. To assess the ability of human ES cell-derived enteric NC precursors to migrate within the colon, the authors injected labeled cells into immunodeficient mice. Two to four weeks after transplantation, the cells had migrated extensively and repopulated the host colon over its entire length forming ganglion-like clusters. These findings suggested that these cells have good therapeutic potential due to their ability to form an extensive ENS. As a next step, ES cell-derived ENC precursors were transplanted into the *Ednrb*$^{s\text{-}l/s\text{-}l}$ genetic mouse model of HSCR (these animals develop megacolon and show high mortality). These cells migrated within the HSCR colon and showed localization to the myenteric and submucosal regions. Remarkably, all injected animals survived. These studies not only demonstrated that human PS-cell-derived ENS precursors are capable of rescuing disease-related mortality in HSCR mice but also outlined an efficient strategy to generate enteric precursors from human ES cells that could potentially enable the large-scale production of enteric neurons for cell therapy on demand [23]. Similar work by Li et al. [43] directed human iPSCs to differentiate into neural crest stem cells that when co-cultured with gut smooth muscle differentiated into enteric neuronal subtypes with typical electrophysiological characteristics of functional neurons. When these cells were transplanted into aneural or aganglionic chick, mouse, or human gut tissues, the iPSC-derived cells showed extensive migration and differentiation, generating enteric neurons and glia further highlighting these cells as an ideal cell source for enteric neural cell therapy. In addition to this potential therapeutic role of iPSCs, other work has highlighted the use of these cells for modeling enteric neuropathy. For example, recent work in the lab of Prof. James Wells used a tissue engineering approach with ES and iPSC to generate human intestinal tissue containing a functional ENS to study human GI motility defects [70]. Studies by Lai et al. [42] have utilized iPSCs created from patients with different forms of HSCR (total colonic aganglionosis and short-segment HSCR), as well as RET$^{+/-}$ and RET$^{-/-}$ iPSCs with the aim of using the CRISPR/Cas9 gene editing system to determine how these mutations affect enteric NC cell function. The authors found that enteric NC cells that were derived from these iPSC lines had cell migration and differentiation defects. CRISPR/Cas9 correction of a RET mutation and of a mutation identified in the vinculin gene rescued the differentiation and migration defects and restored function in these cells. Such an experimental strategy, combining patient-specific iPSCs, the CRISPR/Cas9 system, and whole-exome sequencing can thus be used to identify mutations that functionally contribute to a complex disease such as HSCR.

Thus, in addition to representing a potentially ideal cell source, which can be genetically manipulated for ENS stem cell therapy, iPSCs are proving to be a powerful tool for identifying disease-associated mutations and determining how such mutations affect cell function and contribute to pathogenesis.

8.5 Methodology

8.5.1 Enteric Neural Stem Cell Harvesting, Selection, and Propagation

ENSCs reside within the ganglionated myenteric and submucous plexuses of the ENS within the gastrointestinal tract. These cells can be obtained in a stepwise process involving manual tissue dissection, enzymatic dissociation, cell sorting based on neural crest lineage, and culture in specialized conditions whereby the cells spontaneously form spherical structures termed “neurospheres”[56]. Practically, once gut has been obtained, either as full thickness gut or as submucosal biopsies, the mucosa is peeled away to exclude this layer, and then the tissue is enzymatically dissociated using dispase and collagenase. However, at this stage the cultures contain a mix of enteric neurons and glia, ENSCs, smooth muscle, ICC, fibroblasts, etc. that are present within the different gut layers. The heterogeneous nature of the cell population could affect transplant success, and a key question is what is the optimum cell "product" for ENS therapy: a mix of these various cell types that may provide paracrine factors that affect the ENS stem cells and/or the local gut environment following transplant or a purer population of stem cells with better potential for ENS rescue. The answer is currently unknown, and more transplants with various cell compositions will be required to address this. Nevertheless, numerous studies have opted to obtain purer populations of stem cells by using cell sorting based on the neural crest lineage of the ENS and ENSCs (reviewed in [13, 63]). Sorting by fluorescent-activated cell sorting (FACS) (with fluorescent markers driven by Wnt1, Sox2, or Nestin in transgenic mice; antibodies against HNK-1, NC-1, p75, alpha-4-integrin, or CD49) has been the preferred route, but magnetic beads linked to the neural crest marker p75 can also be used effectively to sort human cells. Following sorting, further cell culture, in media favoring neurogenesis and containing EGF and FGF, results in the formation of "neurospheres" in 1–2 weeks [10, 50, 63]. These neurospheres have typically been used as the therapeutic "cell package" for transplant into mouse gut in vivo, but it remains to be seen whether these cellular aggregates will be translated to human therapy and if so whether they can be produced on a scale sufficient to rescue the ENS in aganglionic human gut.

8.5.2 Enteric Neural Stem Cell Optimization/Priming Prior to and Following Transplant

Although many previous studies have shown that ENSCs can be isolated, expanded [1, 12, 39, 40, 56], and transplanted into animal models of HSCR [18, 25, 32, 33, 35, 44, 54, 67] or gut obtained from patients with HSCR [50, 59], the capacity of these cells to proliferate, migrate, and differentiate has been limited [9, 26, 39, 54]. It is also clear that large numbers of cells will need to be transplanted to colonize the entire aganglionic region and generate the extensive enteric neural network required to restore gut function [13, 14]. Therefore, it is necessary to scale up the number of ENSCs as well as to augment their capacity for migration and differentiation prior to transplantation.

A number of previous studies have demonstrated that proliferation of ENSCs is increased by additional growth factors, exogenous proteins, or agonists in culture medium such as glial cell line-derived neurotrophic factor (GDNF) [9, 12, 39, 49], retinoic acid [60], 5-HT_4 receptor agonist [34, 45], and inhibitor of glycogen synthase kinase 3 (GSK3) [59]. It has recently been shown that supplementation with GDNF or GSK3 inhibitor in the culture medium results in up to 12-fold increase in the number of ENSCs [49, 59]. The effect of priming ENSCs with GDNF also enhances their migration. GDNF-treated ENSCs migrate further to colonize a significantly larger area (twofold) of recipient gut while maintaining equivalent capacity to differentiate into neurons 4 weeks following transplantation into the wall of mice colon in vivo [49]. These results suggest that exogenous growth factors can be used to expand the pool of donor ENCCs in culture and, more interestingly, that priming of ENSCs during the culture period is sufficient for them to migrate further following transplantation in vivo.

Recent advances in genetic engineering have enabled researchers to deliver or modify the genes of interest to control cell fate or to augment cell capacity. Liu et al. have shown that overexpression of the anti-apoptotic gene, Bcl-2, significantly increased cell survival, neuronal differentiation, and colonic muscle relaxation 8 weeks after transplantation of neuroepithelial stem cells into denervated rat colon [46]. While this approach may enhance the survival of transplanted cells, there is significant concern regarding the delivery of genes commonly associated with human cancer. More recently, Lai et al. generated iPSCs from skin fibroblasts obtained from patients with HSCR (HSCR-iPSCs) [42]. Enteric neural crest cells (ENCCs) have been subsequently derived from this HSCR-iPSCs line and have been used as a stem cell-based disease model of HSCR in a dish. ENCCs derived from HSCR-iPSCs exhibit defects in migration and neuronal differentiation. Further investigation of HSCR-iPSCs-derived ENCCs using genetic and transcriptome analyses identified a novel genetic mutation that is functionally associated with pathogenesis of HSCR. More interestingly, correction of the genetic mutations in "diseased" iPSCs using CRISPR-Cas9 genome editing technologies successfully restored those defects in differentiation and migration [42]. This approach is extremely important, particularly for the use of patient-derived autologous cell transplantation. Although an autologous cell source has advantages over most of the other possible donor cells in their potential to bypass ethical and immunological difficulties, they might be defective in their proliferative or migratory ability due to the causative HSCR gene mutations [42, 63]. Nonetheless, further studies will be warranted to determine if "disease-corrected" HSCR-iPSCs-derived ENCCs behave normally and regenerate the ENS following transplantation into the aganglionic environment in vivo.

Co-delivery of exogenous protein or drug compounds with ENSCs to the recipient gut has also been demonstrated to improve cell survival and proliferation. Micci et al. injected neural stem cells with caspase-1 inhibitor to the pyloric wall of mice in vivo showing reduced apoptosis and increased proliferation of transplanted cells, resulting in better cell survival in vivo [53]. More recently, Hotta et al. loaded 5-HT_4 receptor agonist into liposomal nanoparticles and co-delivered them with ENSCs into the colonic wall of mice in vivo. This fabrication was designed to achieve slow release of this drug, and it was observed that neuronal differentiation and proliferation of ENSCs is significantly increased 2 weeks following co-transplantation [34]. Although this approach seems to be rather straightforward compared to the others, the impact of non-specific or off-target effects will need to be clarified before clinical application.

8.5.3 Cell Delivery

Successful transplant outcomes are likely to depend not only on selecting the most appropriate cell type, perhaps primed and in sufficient numbers to generate an ENS capable of effecting change, but also on the optimal delivery of such cells into the recipient gut. Such delivery would arguably need to be accurate and designed to specifically target diseased gut segments and retain cells within the recipient gastrointestinal tract. The particular challenge of the gastrointestinal tract is its enormity in terms of length as well as complex multilayered structure with a rich immune component and vascular supply. All of these present possible obstacles to the precision, sustainability, sufficiency, and ultimately success of engraftment necessary for effective rescue of severe enteric neuropathies such as HSCR. Conversely, perhaps one need not be too worried about this given evidence to date that suggests that even without precise delivery of the neural progenitors to ideal locations within the gut wall, the cells tested to date appear to ultimately locate themselves appropriately along the length of and within the wall of the gastrointestinal tract to effect functional change. McCann et al. transplanted three neurospheres into a small pocket in the tunica muscularis of the distal colon of postnatal day 14–17 *nNOS*$^{-/-}$ mice and showed that cells emigrating from the neurospheres were not only able to integrate within the endogenous ENS at the level of the myenteric plexus but migrate and colonize the entire length of the colon to effect functional rescue [48]. Fattahi et al. injected a cell suspension of human embryonic stem cell-derived enteric neural crest precursor cells in Matrigel into the cecum of *Ednrb*$^{s\text{-}l/s\text{-}l}$(HSCR mouse model) similarly targeting the muscle layer. One to two weeks after transplantation, the labeled transplanted donor cells had migrated extensively and repopulated the host colon over its entire length, incorporating themselves within the muscle wall, and survival of these mice was dramatically improved [23].

It should be noted that much of these experiments have been done within experimental small animal models or samples of human gut prepared and cultured in vitro. To date, a number of methods have been used for the delivery of therapeutic cells or neurospheres into the gastrointestinal tract including (i) direct injection into the gut wall, (ii) application onto its serosal surface, (iii) intraperitoneal injection, and (iv) intravascular delivery.

Direct injection of cells or neurospheres into the gut wall is arguably the most attractive form of delivery given the potential ability not only to target diseased segments of gut but also to deliver the cells closest to their target locations at the same time minimizing seeding of cells into ectopic locations. Direct injection of cells or neurospheres into the gut wall has been utilized in a number of animal studies with reported success [3, 23, 46, 48, 51, 55]. Cheng et al. [17] reported the use of colonoscopy to successfully deliver enteric neural stem/progenitor cells into the aganglionic distal colon of HSCR model mice (*Ednrb−/−*).

These preliminary studies utilizing small animals, however, carry inherent obstacles related to the limitations of being able to minimize the fluid volume the cells are suspended in and the size of the delivery "needles." Coupled with the hydrostatic forces generated by the injection, these factors may cause damage, even perforation of the intestinal wall, and backflow leakage through the injection site once the needle is withdrawn, as well as reduce the viability of cells themselves. Furthermore, the forced spread of cells within the gut wall may make it difficult to accurately deliver the cells into appropriate layers. Some of these problems may be reduced by modifying the protocols. Fattahi et al. utilized 70% Matrigel as a carrier for cell injection to ensure that the cells stayed in place following the injection and prevented backflow into the peritoneum [23]. Such biomaterials polymerize in situ and enhance retention. These could also be supplemented with factors such as GDNF, which have been shown to enhance migration of donor cells [49].

Issues related to the volume for injection and cell viability may be reduced by the use of whole neurospheres rather than dissociating into a near single-cell suspension. Indeed, a number of successful enteric neural cell transplantation studies have shown extensive proliferation, migration, and appropriate neuronal and glial differentiation following transplantation of enteric neurospheres into the distal colon of wild-type mice [10, 21, 36, 48]. McCann et al. implanted neurospheres into the distal colon of a mouse model of enteric neuropathy and showed that donor cells were capable of complete colonization of the colon as well as functional integration and, ultimately, rescue of the organ. The recipient disease model in this case was the NOS knockout, which although lacking NOS neurons has an otherwise robust ENS, which may support the transplanted cells [48]. It remains to be shown whether such significant colonization is possible within the aganglionic colon, with only Fattahi et al. describing colonization of the gut with ENSCs derived from human pluripotent stem cells (hPSCs) [23].

Actual injection into the gut wall, with its inherent problems, may not be necessary with serosal application of donor neural progenitor cells. Cooper et al. carried out in vivo ENSC transplants into wild-type mice by inserting donor neurospheres into small pockets in the serosa of recipient bowel [18]. They showed that although some spread occurred on the serosa, cells were able to migrate into the myenteric plexus and integrate with endogenous networks. Hetz et al. applied human enteric neural progenitor cells held within a biodegradable fibrin matrix onto the serosal surface of mouse intestine that had undergone chemical denervation [33]. They showed spread and integration of transplanted cells within the longitudinal muscle. Further studies are needed in order to understand the efficiency of cell spread, viability, and their ability to affect functional rescue.

Alternative methods to deliver cells, including intraperitoneal and vascular approaches, although attractive in theory, are not supported by any significant body of evidence to date. Following on from earlier work by Martucciello and colleagues, Tsai et al. transplanted neural crest cells that had been selected on the basis of their p75 and $\alpha 4$ integrin expression [47, 67]. Cells seeded into the peritoneal cavity appeared to preferentially target the small intestine, which may limit its utility for the purposes of conditions such as HSCR that predominantly affect the large intestine. Although studied in other organs, thus far, no study appears to have addressed the use of the intestine's vascular supply to deliver cells into the gastrointestinal tract. This remains a potential route for the delivery of cells.

Although there has been pleasing success in experimental models, it is not clear whether cell engraftment will be successful in human patients although a number of well-established techniques already exist by which treatments are delivered into the wall of the gastrointestinal tract, including by minimally invasive laparoscopic and endoscopic techniques enhanced by improved imaging such as ultrasound, which may help more accurate delivery of cells. Apart from small neonates, it is expected that "scaling up" to humans may reduce the magnitude of the potential problems purely given the presumed ability of the larger and stronger gut to withstand the injection volume and forces. Furthermore, techniques such as endoscopy would allow for the possibility of multiple injections and repeated delivery to maximize engraftment and coverage of the disease area.

8.5.4 Measuring Transplant Success

To date, a large number of technical approaches have been utilized to assess "success" of stem cell transplantation for enteric disease. The approaches used in these studies have tended to be dependent on the evaluation stage of a particular study, with early "proof-of-principle" studies adopting more qualitative approaches to assess integration. As studies have progressed along the preclinical evaluation pathway, refinement of such qualitative approaches and inclusion of more quantitative approaches assessing functional outcomes have allowed for a clearer picture of what "success" constitutes. Ultimately, "successful" transplantation of stem cells for HSCR will be defined by the ability of such cells to improve gut function. However, a series of anatomic, molecular, and neurochemical assessments are required in animal models to determine (i) stem cell engraftment, (ii) proliferative capacity, (iii) safety, (iv) directed differentiation, (v) functional integration, and (vi) functional modulation of motility prior to any clinical application.

8.5.4.1 Stem Cell Engraftment

Engraftment of stem cells after transplantation to the colon has been noted in a number of early preclinical studies of ENSC transplantation to the murine colon [18, 36]. Here transplanted embryonic or postnatal ENSC expressing fluorescent markers were found to engraft within the colon of wild-type mice and migrated from the presumptive site of transplantation to cover approximately 5–11 mm^2 by 4 weeks. Transplanted cells appeared to extend neural projections both longitudinally and radially and were found to migrate through the *muscularis* to form or contribute to ganglia-like structures within the myenteric plexus. More recently, McCann et al., using whole-organ confocal imaging techniques, have suggested that such migration may be an underestimation of the potential of ENSCs to colonize the colon [48]. Four weeks after transplantation of early postnatal murine ENSC to the distal colon of an *nNOS*$^{-/-}$ knockout model, donor-derived cells were observed up to a distance of 42 mm from the presumptive transplant site. Again, migration through the *muscularis* and integration within endogenous ganglia were observed.

8.5.4.2 Proliferative Capacity

A key component of any stem cell treatment is the ability to harness "stem-like" proliferative capacity to allow for donor cell expansion. It is critically important, however, that such proliferative capacity can be modulated, endogenously or exogenously, to prevent the formation of tumors. Incorporation of S-phase markers such as EDU or BrdU by graft-derived neurons after in vivo transplantation has been used to study the proliferative capacity of stem/progenitor cells [18, 36, 48]. Interestingly, there appears to be a time-dependent reduction in proliferative capacity, as incorporation of BrdU was observed when applied at early timepoints (day 1) but not at later timepoints (4 weeks) post-transplantation [18]. These results suggest endogenous modulation of transplanted cells acts to prevent uncontrolled proliferation.

8.5.4.3 Safety

The majority of in vivo murine studies performed, to date, have examined restricted donor cell engraftment within the organ of transplantation (i.e., colon) over relatively short periods >4 weeks [36, 48, 64]. However, in terms of therapeutic benefit, long-term survival of graft-derived cells will be critical for clinical translation. Cooper et al. [18] successfully assessed various safety parameters including off-target integration and long-term safety to show that engraftment of donor-derived cells appeared to be maintained up to 24 months post-transplantation and that there did not appear to be "off-target" engraftment in peripheral organs including the brain, lungs, heart, liver, spleen, kidneys, adrenal glands, and gut mesentery. Such results offer a promising safety profile for the use of autologous ENSC for the treatment of HSCR. This aspect is further elaborated on in Sect. 8.6.

8.5.4.4 Directed Differentiation

Crucial to the successful implementation of restorative cellular therapy is the ability of stem/progenitor cells to adopt the appropriate localization within the gut wall and undergo neuronal differentiation to give rise to a repertoire of enteric neurons, which will ultimately allow for corrective functional rescue when integrated with the endogenous ENS. Preliminary studies have provided such information, suggesting that after in vivo transplantation, stem/progenitor cells can undergo subtype-specific differentiation to form a variety of neural subtypes including ChAT, VAChT, nNOS, calretinin, calbindin, and VIP-expressing neurons [18, 36, 48, 64]. Interestingly, the underlying mechanisms which allow for such directed differentiation of donor stem/progenitor cells in vivo remain unclear. However, ongoing studies aimed at assessing the molecular pathways involved in the differentiation of pluripotent stem cells toward an enteric neural crest fate, and beyond, may provide an insight into these mechanisms [23, 31].

8.5.4.5 Functional Integration

Ex vivo assessment of transplanted colonic tissue has provided critical data supporting the functional integration of donor neurons within recipient bowel, after transplantation. Initial investigations via intracellular recordings demonstrated electrical activity within individual ENSC-derived neurons after transplantation to the wild-type colon [36]. Cooper et al. have subsequently demonstrated functional integration of both mouse and human donor-derived neurons with the endogenous ENS by calcium imaging [18, 19]. Furthermore, a recent study utilizing an optogenetic approach has successfully demonstrated that donor ENSC-derived neurons can mediate motor control with the presence of donor neuron-initiated excitatory and inhibitory junction potentials in colonic muscle cells [64]. Together, these studies demonstrate that transplanted stem cells have the ability to generate functional neurons in vivo, integrate with the endogenous ENS, and provide the necessary circuitry for motor control in a transplanted wild-type murine colonic microenvironment.

8.5.4.6 Functional Modulation of Motility

While the above studies demonstrate the promise for the functional integration of donor neurons within wild-type "normal" bowel, a key step in the progression of any cellular therapy for HSCR is the demonstration of rescue of gut pathophysiology. Stem cell application to aganglionic models has provided clear evidence that donor-derived cells have the ability to integrate within various "Hirschsprung-like" models [16, 33, 35, 59, 67]. Recent work on the neuronal nitric oxide knockout (*nNOS*$^{-/-}$) mouse model has shown that transplantation of enteric neural stem cells can restore function with the rescue of donor-derived nNOS^{+} neurons. This model displays slow colonic transit with the loss of nNOS neurons providing a mechanism to examine functional rescue, in vivo, at the whole-organ level. Interestingly after transplantation transit time was rescued toward wild-type levels, as assessed with ex vivo organ bath physiology and in vivo transit time assays [48]. Moreover, a study utilizing transplantation of pluripotent-derived enteric neural crest cells has shown rescue of HSCR phenotype with the remarkable survival of 100% of transplanted $Ednrb^{s-l/s-l}$ (SSL/LEJ) mice [23]. These studies taken together suggest that a cellular therapy for the treatment of HSCR may be achievable. However, future studies will be required to ascertain the most appropriate donor cell of choice, and ultimately "first-in-human" studies will be required to determine the safety profile of any chosen cell type before moving to small-scale clinical trials to determine the "success" of clinical application.

8.6 Safety Considerations

Pluripotent stem cells (PSCs) are becoming increasingly popular as a therapeutic tool and are currently being used in many clinical trials and for a number of conditions including macular degeneration, spinal cord injury, diabetes, heart disease, and Parkinson's disease [66], with many more forthcoming. However, before these trials can safely be turned into routine therapies, a better understanding of the behavior of these cells, and monitoring and understanding the possible genetic changes that might have occurred during processing, is required.

Safety discussions have focused mainly on the following topics: (i) the formation of teratocarcinomas from the transplanted hPSCs, (ii) the ectopic migration of the hPSCs outside the tissue of interest, and (iii) the occurrence of somatic mutations in hPSCs. To address these points in order, teratocarcinomas arise from undifferentiated stem cells with malignant potential. However, most likely the cell therapy will consist of administering progenitors or differentiated derivatives, and not undifferentiated stem cells. Therefore, the chance of teratocarcinomas is small. Still, one should avoid the accidental transplantation of undifferentiated cells. Another safety issue is the spread of the transplanted cells outside the tissue of interest. When cells end up in the wrong tissues, possibly in combination with (epi)genetic changes, this might have profound consequences. Monitoring the spread of cells is therefore crucial. What primarily needs our attention are the potential (epi)genetic changes that may have arisen while culturing PSCs. It is these somatic (epi)genetic changes that may have substantial impact on the behavior of the PSCs and may even lead to malignant transformation of the mutated cells [28]. Monitoring the PCSs for such genetic changes is therefore crucial. Discussions are still ongoing on how to screen cells, in other words with what resolution, and how to interpret the results, in order to evaluate their significance for the safety of therapeutic applications. It has been proposed that an international working group should evaluate the genetic and epigenetic changes observed in hPSC lines. A framework should be established for evaluating the risks that these changes may pose for clinical use. In the next section we discuss in more detail somatic genetic alterations and their possible consequences.

8.6.1 Somatic Genetic Alterations

The cells that will be used for therapy for enteric neuropathies could come from different sources. They could come from the patient (gut derived stem cells or iPSC derived) but they might also be derived from donors, iPSCs or ESC (pluripotent stem cells). A common feature of these cells is that they likely need to be expanded in number substantially before transplant as a therapeutic product. A disadvantage of the significant cell expansion needed to create large numbers of cells is the propensity of pluripotent stem cells in particular to acquire genetic and epigenetic changes upon long-term culture and expansion [8, 22, 38]. Such changes may reduce the efficacy of generating specific cell derivatives or could potentially compromise safety, for example, by promoting tumor growth.

Several studies have been performed to determine the genetic alterations that can occur in these stem cells. The methods used determine the limits of detection, both in size and frequency of the detectable rate. G-banding karyotyping has the lowest resolution as it detects differences of five to ten million base-pairs. Sequencing has the highest resolution as it can detect single base changes. The detectable rate (the frequency in which the genetic alteration is found) is low when karyotyping, depending on the number of metaphases one wants to karyotype. It is highest in (ultra-deep) Next generation sequencing, digital PCR or single cell sequencing.

Most studies have used standard cytogenetic techniques (G-band karyotyping). An ISCI survey of well over 100 hPSC lines [38] showed many chromosomal changes that seem to be nonrandom such as chromosomal alterations, gains of whole, or parts of, chromosomes 1, 12, 17, and 20, as well as losses of regions of chromosomes 10, 18, and 22, which are commonly found. Occasional karyotypic changes affecting almost all other chromosomes (except chromosome 4) have also been reported. However, the changes are sporadic and form no discernible pattern. These changes seem to provide a selective growth advantage to the mutated cells [58] and are readily detectable by standard cytogenetic techniques. However, they are often present in a small proportion of cells, in <10% of the cells in a PSC line [7].

Besides karyotyping the use of microarray or sequencing analysis of fluorescent in situ hybridization (FISH) has been introduced, increasing the resolution of the analysis enormously. By using SNP arrays small copy number variations (CNVs) have been discovered. For instance, it was shown that the BCL2L1 gene, a gene on chromosome 20, was often overrepresented in seemingly karyotypically normal diploid cells (22 out of 79 lines) [38]. The BCL2L1 gene is believed to drive the selective advantage of cells by limiting apoptosis of hPSCs during passaging. This gene is located on chromosome 20 which is often found overrepresented [6, 57]. Clearly, screening the hPSCs with high-resolution SNP arrays resulted in many genetic aberrations; however, other than the BCL2L1 gene, no recurrent events were found in these studies. It is likely that the combination of duplications and losses is responsible for the growth advantage seen in the cell lines analyzed.

8.6.2 Epigenetic Changes

Epigenetic changes occur in hPSCs, but repetitive changes have not been described. In the ISCI study, extensive changes in the DNA methylation of many genes was observed, but no consistent patterns were recognized [38].

Perhaps the most widely observed epigenetic change in hPSCs is the loss of X-inactivation. While the presence of two active X chromosomes may indicate a primitive or naïve state for hPSCs, many female hPSCs appear to have an inactive X chromosome [37]. Although these observations of genetic and epigenetic instability do raise safety concerns about the use of hPSC derivatives for regenerative medicine, their real significance remains unclear.

8.6.3 Possible Safety Mitigations

Due to the risks associated with significant cell expansion in vitro, one should opt for a limited number of passages before transplantation. Cells should be checked genetically preferably by SNP arrays or exome sequencing. As long as the effects of individual genetic variants on the PCSs or differentiated cell types are uncertain, or when we do not know whether the cells will spread throughout the body, one might consider introducing a conditional suicide gene to provide a fail-safe strategy for eliminating cells after transplantation if a problem were to arise.

8.7 First-in-Human Studies

It is clear that the last years have witnessed unprecedented progress in the march toward tangible stem cell therapies for conditions such as HSCR. The chapter thus far has detailed the significant advancement from the harvesting and propagation of therapeutic cells from the gastrointestinal tract or their derivation from pluripotent stem cells through to the functional rescue of established models of enteric neuropathies including HSCR along with robust data on the sustainability of engraftment and long-term safety. Although there remains much to do, including the optimization of protocols specifically related to human neural progenitor cells for therapy, there is now the real prospect for initial trials in human subjects. Only through such trials can we start to understand and address critical challenges regarding the true potential of such therapies.

8.7.1 Obtaining and Preparing Cells for Therapy

Although refinement is clearly needed, the harvesting of human-derived ENSCs for transplantation has already been established by a number of groups [1, 16, 19, 44, 50, 59]. These studies have mostly utilized tissue obtained at surgery but also include the use of endoscopic techniques [50], which also provide an attractive method for cell delivery. It is clear, however, that the harvesting and propagation of human cells are arduous and inefficient, reflected in the fact that the published literature to date, specifically related to the in vivo transplantation into small animal models, is sparse in terms of the testing of human adult stems cells. This of course will in part relate to immunological issues that limit engraftment, but in the collective experience of the co-authors, human cells have proved difficult to harvest or select for, to propagate in culture, and ultimately to transplant in sufficient quantities to effect functional change. If an autologous strategy is to be utilized, there may be challenges from the potential inherent dysfunction of neural progenitors harvested from the gut of patients suffering from diffuse or segmental enteric neuropathy or the suitability of the environment of such gut to receive or sustain transplanted therapeutic cells. Even if restoration of genetic normality is not possible, it is likely that some form of cellular manipulation will be needed to improve transplantation success by directing appropriate neural differentiation and enhancing engraftment of cells.

Work needs to be done to optimize protocols to harvest, propagate, manipulate, prime and transplant cells as well as to scale up the methodology. In part, the advent of human pluripotent stem cells, including iPSC from patients themselves has begun to address some of the challenges, including the robust generation of suitable cells for therapy [23, 62, 70]. Work will now need to address the control and long-term safety of these cells within the in vivo environment and the mechanisms related to their engraftment and effects including on neuromuscular function. Whether from the gut or human pluripotent cells, protocols for the generation of appropriate cells for therapy of enteric neuropathies will need to be adapted to satisfy regulatory bodies and approval as clinical-grade medicines, although these should be feasible given that a number of cellular therapies are already established in clinical practice.

8.7.2 In Whom Should Initial Human Trials Be Carried Out, and How Would Transplant Success Be Assessed?

Initial human trials of cell transplantation for therapy of enteric neuropathies could arguably be carried out in three possible scenarios:

(i) Into the unaffected non-neuropathic intestine of adult volunteers with terminal diseases such as cancers. In patients with terminal rectal or distal colonic cancers, colostomies may be formed to bypass more distal obstruction by the tumor. In such patients iPS cells could be generated from tissue (e.g., the skin) samples collected electively, or gut tissue cells could be harvested at the time of stoma surgery or by elective endoscopy. Following their selection, propagation, manipulation, and labeling (to enable tracing), ENSCs could then be transplanted back into the patients by endoscopy and the recipient transplanted intestine harvested once the patient is deceased to facilitate assessment of cell viability, spread, functional integration, and safety.

(ii) Into the affected neuropathic gut of pediatric patients whose enteric neuropathy is deemed severe and incurable, and currently available interventions such as resective or decompressive surgery, or that designed to minimize obstruction to flow through sphincter (e.g., myectomy), offer no real prospect of symptom improvement or are deemed to carry excessive risk. Arguably, these conditions could include esophageal achalasia and total intestinal aganglionic HSCR, where there appears to be complete destruction or congenital absence of the ENS, respectively [29]. In the former, the target tissue is restricted and more feasible to colonize, but challenges related to immune-mediated destruction of the transplanted neural cells may need to be addressed. In the latter the diseased segment may be too extensive although smaller segments of aganglionic gut could be targeted such as that proximal to a stoma placed higher up the gastrointestinal tract, e.g., jejunal or proximal ileum. Utilizing an autologous approach, cells again could be derived using iPSC strategies or harvested at the time of stoma formation or endoscopy. In such patients, it is likely that the transplanted intestine may not be easily available for study and assessment of functional improvement would provide the main measure of outcome. This may well be possible with the advent of improved tools for the physiological assessment of the gastrointestinal tract in patients such as high-resolution manometry. Ethical consideration, however, would need to be given to such trials of therapy given their success is unknown and the presence of life sustaining interventions such as parenteral nutrition and intestinal transplantation that have a profile of improving safety and outcomes.

(iii) Into the distal aganglionic segment (anal sphincter and rectum) that is necessarily retained in patients with HSCR following current pull-through surgery and as an adjunct to it. Not only would this strategy provide a more achievable target in terms of the size of diseased segment but it may also alleviate some of the long-term complications and challenges that are known to underlie the poor quality of life of such patients [69] including fecal incontinence and difficult defecation. Again, an autologous strategy such as that described above could be used to obtain cells for therapy. Assessing transplant success may rely on functional improvement utilizing investigations such as anorectal manometry (e.g., restitution of the recto-anal inhibitory reflex) or monitoring of symptoms.

With regard to other enteric neuropathies, there is no doubt that some disorders, such as those classed as chronic intestinal pseudo-obstruction (now referred to in children as pediatric intestinal pseudo-obstruction (PIPO)), carry considerable morbidity and mortality and would benefit from early human trials to start to address their abysmal outcomes. The biggest challenge, however, and arguably one that should be addressed before contemplation of trials remains the need for a better understanding of their precise nature to guide what elements of the ENS are dysfunctional or missing and therefore need to be rescued in these conditions. In addition, disorders such as PIPO generally affect the intestine diffusely, on occasion its entire length, making it even less amenable to cell therapy. For many such conditions, trials of cell therapy remain a more distant prospect, and palliative approaches such as surgery, provision of specialized (including parenteral) nutrition, and intestinal transplantation remain the mainstay of treatment.

8.7.3 Delivery of Cells and Posttransplant Considerations

Irrespective of whether adult ENSCs (harvested by endoscopy or at surgery) are used or pluripotent stem cells generated from patient cells (e.g., fibroblasts), the most attractive methodology would be autologous transplantation where the harvested cells are transplanted back into the patients endoscopically or at the time of elective surgery. Endoscopy is a well-established and effective technique for delivering therapy into the gut wall, and the precision of delivery of cells could further be guided using contemporary imaging techniques such as ultrasound. It also provides a means for the repeatable and reproducible delivery of cells meaning that engraftment of segments of diseased intestine by therapeutic cells could occur as staged procedures occurring over time rather than a one-hit strategy. Minimally invasive, including laparoscopic, surgery has also considerable potential for the delivery of cells although is less amenable to being used as a repetitive strategy.

The gut is a huge immune organ, and immunological rejection will no doubt provide an obstacle to cell transplantation. Autologous transplantation should obviate the need for immunosuppression, but should it be needed, there is significant clinical experience with its use to induce tolerance of grafts.

Overall, there is no doubt that we are at the cusp of trials in humans. The confidence in this statement comes less from the considerable work that still needs to be done but more from the fact that there is now a critical mass of researchers, both clinicians and scientists, collaborating to realize such a goal.

8.8 Conclusions

The field of enteric stem cell biology is at an exciting time where the possibility of treating enteric neuropathies with stem cell replacement therapy is approaching reality. Over two decades of preclinical work, mainly performed in mice, has demonstrated that enteric neural stem cells can be selectively isolated from the gut, expanded in number in vitro, and transplanted into gut where the cells migrate, proliferate, differentiate into appropriate neuronal and glial cell types, become functionally active, and are capable of restoring function. These studies support the idea that such an approach could rescue the absent ENS in HCSR. However, developing a therapeutic stem cell product for delivery to infants with HSCR is not a trivial undertaking and a number of questions need to be addressed before this can happen. What is the stem cell product? Heterogeneous neurospheres or purer populations of stem cells? Can cell production be scaled up under good manufacturing practice (GMP) conditions? How will stem cells be delivered to human gut? How can they be visualized and tracked after transplant? Are they safe? How will transplant success be ascertained? These and other issues are currently being addressed by a number of groups worldwide with the collective aim of developing a curative stem cell therapy for devastating diseases of the ENS such as HSCR.

References

1. Almond S, Lindley RM, Kenny SE, Connell MG, Edgar DH. Characterisation and transplantation of enteric nervous system progenitor cells. Gut. 2007;56:489–96.
2. Amiel J, Sproat-Emison E, Garcia-Barcelo M, Lantieri F, Burzynski G, Borrego S, Pelet A, Arnold S, Miao X, Griseri P, Brooks AS, Antinolo G, de Pontual L, Clement-Ziza M, Munnich A, Kashuk C, West K, Wong KK, Lyonnet S, Chakravarti A, Tam PK, Ceccherini I, Hofstra RM, Fernandez R, Hirschsprung Disease C. Hirschsprung disease, associated syndromes and genetics: a review. J Med Genet. 2008;45:1–14.
3. Anitha M, Joseph I, Ding X, Torre ER, Sawchuk MA, Mwangi S, Hochman S, Sitaraman SV, Anania F, Srinivasan S. Characterization of fetal and postnatal enteric neuronal cell lines with improvement in intestinal neural function. Gastroenterology. 2008;134:1424–35.
4. Asai N, Fukuda T, Wu Z, Enomoto A, Pachnis V, Takahashi M, Costantini F. Targeted mutation of serine 697 in the Ret tyrosine kinase causes migration defect of enteric neural crest cells. Development. 2006;133:4507–16.
5. Attie T, Pelet A, Edery P, Eng C, Mulligan LM, Amiel J, Boutrand L, Beldjord C, Nihoul-Fekete C, Munnich A, et al. Diversity of RET proto-oncogene mutations in familial and sporadic Hirschsprung disease. Hum Mol Genet. 1995;4:1381–6.
6. Avery S, Hirst AJ, Baker D, Lim CY, Alagaratnam S, Skotheim RI, Lothe RA, Pera MF, Colman A, Robson

P, Andrews PW, Knowles BB. BCL-XL mediates the strong selective advantage of a 20q11.21 amplification commonly found in human embryonic stem cell cultures. Stem Cell Reports. 2013;1:379–86.
7. Baker D, Hirst AJ, Gokhale PJ, Juarez MA, Williams S, Wheeler M, Bean K, Allison TF, Moore HD, Andrews PW, Barbaric I. Detecting genetic mosaicism in cultures of human pluripotent stem cells. Stem Cell Reports. 2016;7:998–1012.
8. Baker DE, Harrison NJ, Maltby E, Smith K, Moore HD, Shaw PJ, Heath PR, Holden H, Andrews PW. Adaptation to culture of human embryonic stem cells and oncogenesis in vivo. Nat Biotechnol. 2007;25:207–15.
9. Barlow A, de Graaff E, Pachnis V. Enteric nervous system progenitors are coordinately controlled by the G protein-coupled receptor EDNRB and the receptor tyrosine kinase RET. Neuron. 2003;40:905–16.
10. Binder E, Natarajan D, Cooper J, Kronfli R, Cananzi M, Delalande JM, McCann C, Burns AJ, Thapar N. Enteric neurospheres are not specific to neural crest cultures: implications for neural stem cell therapies. PLoS One. 2015;10:e0119467.
11. Bixby S, Kruger GM, Mosher JT, Joseph NM, Morrison SJ. Cell-intrinsic differences between stem cells from different regions of the peripheral nervous system regulate the generation of neural diversity. Neuron. 2002;35:643–56.
12. Bondurand N, Natarajan D, Thapar N, Atkins C, Pachnis V. Neuron and glia generating progenitors of the mammalian enteric nervous system isolated from foetal and postnatal gut cultures. Development. 2003;130:6387–400.
13. Burns AJ, Goldstein AM, Newgreen DF, Stamp L, Schafer KH, Metzger M, Hotta R, Young HM, Andrews PW, Thapar N, Belkind-Gerson J, Bondurand N, Bornstein JC, Chan WY, Cheah K, Gershon MD, Heuckeroth RO, Hofstra RM, Just L, Kapur RP, King SK, McCann CJ, Nagy N, Ngan E, Obermayr F, Pachnis V, Pasricha PJ, Sham MH, Tam P, Vanden Berghe P. White paper on guidelines concerning enteric nervous system stem cell therapy for enteric neuropathies. Dev Biol. 2016;417:229–51.
14. Burns AJ, Thapar N. Neural stem cell therapies for enteric nervous system disorders. Nat Rev Gastroenterol Hepatol. 2014;11:317–28.
15. Burzynski G, Shepherd IT, Enomoto H. Genetic model system studies of the development of the enteric nervous system, gut motility and Hirschsprung's disease. Neurogastroenterol Motil. 2009;21:113–27.
16. Cheng LS, Hotta R, Graham HK, Belkind-Gerson J, Nagy N, Goldstein AM. Postnatal human enteric neuronal progenitors can migrate, differentiate, and proliferate in embryonic and postnatal aganglionic gut environments. Pediatr Res. 2017;81:838–46.
17. Cheng LS, Hotta R, Graham HK, Nagy N, Goldstein AM, Belkind-Gerson J. Endoscopic delivery of enteric neural stem cells to treat Hirschsprung disease. Neurogastroenterol Motil. 2015;27:1509–14.
18. Cooper JE, McCann CJ, Natarajan D, Choudhury S, Boesmans W, Delalande JM, Vanden Berghe P, Burns AJ, Thapar N. In vivo transplantation of enteric neural crest cells into mouse gut; engraftment, functional integration and long-term safety. PLoS One. 2016;11:e0147989.
19. Cooper JE, Natarajan D, McCann CJ, Choudhury S, Godwin H, Burns AJ, Thapar N. In vivo transplantation of fetal human gut-derived enteric neural crest cells. Neurogastroenterol Motil. 2017;29(1) https://doi.org/10.1111/nmo.12900.
20. Dang R, Torigoe D, Suzuki S, Kikkawa Y, Moritoh K, Sasaki N, Agui T. Genetic background strongly modifies the severity of symptoms of Hirschsprung disease, but not hearing loss in rats carrying Ednrb(sl) mutations. PLoS One. 2011;6:e24086.
21. Dettmann HM, Zhang Y, Wronna N, Kraushaar U, Guenther E, Mohr R, Neckel PH, Mack A, Fuchs J, Just L, Obermayr F. Isolation, expansion and transplantation of postnatal murine progenitor cells of the enteric nervous system. PLoS One. 2014;9:e97792.
22. Draper JS, Smith K, Gokhale P, Moore HD, Maltby E, Johnson J, Meisner L, Zwaka TP, Thomson JA, Andrews PW. Recurrent gain of chromosomes 17q and 12 in cultured human embryonic stem cells. Nat Biotechnol. 2004;22:53–4.
23. Fattahi F, Steinbeck JA, Kriks S, Tchieu J, Zimmer B, Kishinevsky S, Zeltner N, Mica Y, El-Nachef W, Zhao H, de Stanchina E, Gershon MD, Grikscheit TC, Chen S, Studer L. Deriving human ENS lineages for cell therapy and drug discovery in Hirschsprung disease. Nature. 2016;531:105–9.
24. Findlay Q, Yap KK, Bergner AJ, Young HM, Stamp LA. Enteric neural progenitors are more efficient than brain-derived progenitors at generating neurons in the colon. Am J Physiol Gastrointest Liver Physiol. 2014;307:G741–8.
25. Fujimura T, Shibata S, Shimojima N, Morikawa Y, Okano H, Kuroda T. Fluorescence visualization of the enteric nervous network in a chemically induced aganglionosis model. PLoS One. 2016;11:e0150579.
26. Fujiwara N, Miyahara K, Nakazawa-Tanaka N, Akazawa C, Yamataka A. Altered differentiation of enteric neural crest-derived cells from endothelin receptor-B null mouse model of Hirschsprung's disease. Pediatr Surg Int. 2016;32:1095–101.
27. Furuzawa-Carballeda J, Torres-Landa S, Valdovinos MA, Coss-Adame E, Martin Del Campo LA, Torres-Villalobos G. New insights into the pathophysiology of achalasia and implications for future treatment. World J Gastroenterol. 2016;22:7892–907.
28. Goldring CE, Duffy PA, Benvenisty N, Andrews PW, Ben-David U, Eakins R, French N, Hanley NA, Kelly L, Kitteringham NR, Kurth J, Ladenheim D, Laverty H, McBlane J, Narayanan G, Patel S, Reinhardt J, Rossi A, Sharpe M, Park BK. Assessing the safety of stem cell therapeutics. Cell Stem Cell. 2011;8:618–28.
29. Goldstein AM, Thapar N, Karunaratne TB, De Giorgio R. Clinical aspects of neurointestinal disease:

pathophysiology, diagnosis, and treatment. Dev Biol. 2016;417:217–28.
30. Grover M, Farrugia G, Lurken MS, Bernard CE, Faussone-Pellegrini MS, Smyrk TC, Parkman HP, Abell TL, Snape WJ, Hasler WL, Unalp-Arida A, Nguyen L, Koch KL, Calles J, Lee L, Tonascia J, Hamilton FA, Pasricha PJ, Consortium NGCR. Cellular changes in diabetic and idiopathic gastroparesis. Gastroenterology. 2011;140(1575–1585):e1578.
31. Hackland JOS, Frith TJR, Thompson O, Marin Navarro A, Garcia-Castro MI, Unger C, Andrews PW. Top-down inhibition of BMP signaling enables robust induction of hPSCs into neural crest in fully defined, xeno-free conditions. Stem Cell Reports. 2017;9:1043–52.
32. Heanue TA, Pachnis V. Prospective identification and isolation of enteric nervous system progenitors using Sox2. Stem Cells. 2011;29:128–40.
33. Hetz S, Acikgoez A, Voss U, Nieber K, Holland H, Hegewald C, Till H, Metzger R, Metzger M. In vivo transplantation of neurosphere-like bodies derived from the human postnatal and adult enteric nervous system: a pilot study. PLoS One. 2014;9:e93605.
34. Hotta R, Cheng L, Graham HK, Nagy N, Belkind-Gerson J, Mattheolabakis G, Amiji MM, Goldstein AM. Delivery of enteric neural progenitors with 5-HT4 agonist-loaded nanoparticles and thermosensitive hydrogel enhances cell proliferation and differentiation following transplantation in vivo. Biomaterials. 2016a;88:1–11.
35. Hotta R, Cheng LS, Graham HK, Pan W, Nagy N, Belkind-Gerson J, Goldstein AM. Isogenic enteric neural progenitor cells can replace missing neurons and glia in mice with Hirschsprung disease. Neurogastroenterol Motil. 2016b;28:498–512.
36. Hotta R, Stamp LA, Foong JP, McConnell SN, Bergner AJ, Anderson RB, Enomoto H, Newgreen DF, Obermayr F, Furness JB, Young HM. Transplanted progenitors generate functional enteric neurons in the postnatal colon. J Clin Invest. 2013;123:1182–91.
37. International Stem Cell Initiative, Adewumi O, Aflatoonian B, Ahrlund-Richter L, Amit M, Andrews PW, Beighton G, Bello PA, Benvenisty N, Berry LS, Bevan S, Blum B, Brooking J, Chen KG, Choo AB, Churchill GA, Corbel M, Damjanov I, Draper JS, Dvorak P, Emanuelsson K, Fleck RA, Ford A, Gertow K, Gertsenstein M, Gokhale PJ, Hamilton RS, Hampl A, Healy LE, Hovatta O, Hyllner J, Imreh MP, Itskovitz-Eldor J, Jackson J, Johnson JL, Jones M, Kee K, King BL, Knowles BB, Lako M, Lebrin F, Mallon BS, Manning D, Mayshar Y, McKay RD, Michalska AE, Mikkola M, Mileikovsky M, Minger SL, Moore HD, Mummery CL, Nagy A, Nakatsuji N, O'Brien CM, Oh SK, Olsson C, Otonkoski T, Park KY, Passier R, Patel H, Patel M, Pedersen R, Pera MF, Piekarczyk MS, Pera RA, Reubinoff BE, Robins AJ, Rossant J, Rugg-Gunn P, Schulz TC, Semb H, Sherrer ES, Siemen H, Stacey GN, Stojkovic M, Suemori H, Szatkiewicz J, Turetsky T, Tuuri T, van den Brink S, Vintersten K, Vuoristo S, Ward D, Weaver TA, Young LA, Zhang W. Characterization of human embryonic stem cell lines by the International Stem Cell Initiative. Nat Biotechnol. 2007;25:803–16.
38. International Stem Cell Initiative, Amps K, Andrews PW, Anyfantis G, Armstrong L, Avery S, Baharvand H, Baker J, Baker D, Munoz MB, Beil S, Benvenisty N, Ben-Yosef D, Biancotti JC, Bosman A, Brena RM, Brison D, Caisander G, Camarasa MV, Chen J, Chiao E, Choi YM, Choo AB, Collins D, Colman A, Crook JM, Daley GQ, Dalton A, De Sousa PA, Denning C, Downie J, Dvorak P, Montgomery KD, Feki A, Ford A, Fox V, Fraga AM, Frumkin T, Ge L, Gokhale PJ, Golan-Lev T, Gourabi H, Gropp M, Lu G, Hampl A, Harron K, Healy L, Herath W, Holm F, Hovatta O, Hyllner J, Inamdar MS, Irwanto AK, Ishii T, Jaconi M, Jin Y, Kimber S, Kiselev S, Knowles BB, Kopper O, Kukharenko V, Kuliev A, Lagarkova MA, Laird PW, Lako M, Laslett AL, Lavon N, Lee DR, Lee JE, Li C, Lim LS, Ludwig TE, Ma Y, Maltby E, Mateizel I, Mayshar Y, Mileikovsky M, Minger SL, Miyazaki T, Moon SY, Moore H, Mummery C, Nagy A, Nakatsuji N, Narwani K, Oh SK, Oh SK, Olson C, Otonkoski T, Pan F, Park IH, Pells S, Pera MF, Pereira LV, Qi O, Raj GS, Reubinoff B, Robins A, Robson P, Rossant J, Salekdeh GH, Schulz TC, Sermon K, Sheik Mohamed J, Shen H, Sherrer E, Sidhu K, Sivarajah S, Skottman H, Spits C, Stacey GN, Strehl R, Strelchenko N, Suemori H, Sun B, Suuronen R, Takahashi K, Tuuri T, Venu P, Verlinsky Y, Ward-van Oostwaard D, Weisenberger DJ, Wu Y, Yamanaka S, Young L, Zhou Q. Screening ethnically diverse human embryonic stem cells identifies a chromosome 20 minimal amplicon conferring growth advantage. Nat Biotechnol. 2011;29:1132–44.
39. Iwashita T, Kruger GM, Pardal R, Kiel MJ, Morrison SJ. Hirschsprung disease is linked to defects in neural crest stem cell function. Science. 2003;301:972–6.
40. Kruger GM, Mosher JT, Bixby S, Joseph N, Iwashita T, Morrison SJ. Neural crest stem cells persist in the adult gut but undergo changes in self-renewal, neuronal subtype potential, and factor responsiveness. Neuron. 2002;35:657–69.
41. Kulkarni S, Zou B, Hanson J, Micci MA, Tiwari G, Becker L, Kaiser M, Xie XS, Pasricha PJ. Gut-derived factors promote neurogenesis of CNS-neural stem cells and nudge their differentiation to an enteric-like neuronal phenotype. Am J Physiol Gastrointest Liver Physiol. 2011;301:G644–55.
42. Lai FP, Lau ST, Wong JK, Gui H, Wang RX, Zhou T, Lai WH, Tse HF, Tam PK, Garcia-Barcelo MM, Ngan ES. Correction of Hirschsprung-associated mutations in human induced pluripotent stem cells via clustered regularly interspaced short palindromic repeats/Cas9, restores neural crest cell function. Gastroenterology. 2017;153(139–153):e138.
43. Li W, Huang L, Zeng J, Lin W, Li K, Sun J, Huang W, Chen J, Wang G, Ke Q, Duan J, Lai X, Chen R, Liu M, Liu Y, Wang T, Yang X, Chen Y, Xia H, Xiang AP. Characterization and transplantation of enteric

neural crest cells from human induced pluripotent stem cells. Mol Psychiatry. 2018;23:499–508.
44. Lindley RM, Hawcutt DB, Connell MG, Almond SL, Vannucchi MG, Faussone-Pellegrini MS, Edgar DH, Kenny SE. Human and mouse enteric nervous system neurosphere transplants regulate the function of aganglionic embryonic distal colon. Gastroenterology. 2008;135(205–216):e206.
45. Liu MT, Kuan YH, Wang J, Hen R, Gershon MD. 5-HT4 receptor-mediated neuroprotection and neurogenesis in the enteric nervous system of adult mice. J Neurosci. 2009;29:9683–99.
46. Liu W, Yue W, Wu R. Overexpression of Bcl-2 promotes survival and differentiation of neuroepithelial stem cells after transplantation into rat aganglionic colon. Stem Cell Res Ther. 2013;4:7.
47. Martucciello G, Brizzolara A, Favre A, Lombardi L, Bocciardi R, Sanguineti M, Pini Prato A, Jasonni V. Neural crest neuroblasts can colonise aganglionic and ganglionic gut in vivo. Eur J Pediatr Surg. 2007;17:34–40.
48. McCann CJ, Cooper JE, Natarajan D, Jevans B, Burnett LE, Burns AJ, Thapar N. Transplantation of enteric nervous system stem cells rescues nitric oxide synthase deficient mouse colon. Nat Commun. 2017;8:15937.
49. McKeown SJ, Mohsenipour M, Bergner AJ, Young HM, Stamp LA. Exposure to GDNF enhances the ability of enteric neural progenitors to generate an enteric nervous system. Stem Cell Reports. 2017;8:476–88.
50. Metzger M, Caldwell C, Barlow AJ, Burns AJ, Thapar N. Enteric nervous system stem cells derived from human gut mucosa for the treatment of aganglionic gut disorders. Gastroenterology. 2009;136(2214–2225):e2211–3.
51. Micci MA, Kahrig KM, Simmons RS, Sarna SK, Espejo-Navarro MR, Pasricha PJ. Neural stem cell transplantation in the stomach rescues gastric function in neuronal nitric oxide synthase-deficient mice. Gastroenterology. 2005a;129:1817–24.
52. Micci MA, Learish RD, Li H, Abraham BP, Pasricha PJ. Neural stem cells express RET, produce nitric oxide, and survive transplantation in the gastrointestinal tract. Gastroenterology. 2001;121:757–66.
53. Micci MA, Pattillo MT, Kahrig KM, Pasricha PJ. Caspase inhibition increases survival of neural stem cells in the gastrointestinal tract. Neurogastroenterol Motil. 2005b;17:557–64.
54. Mosher JT, Yeager KJ, Kruger GM, Joseph NM, Hutchin ME, Dlugosz AA, Morrison SJ. Intrinsic differences among spatially distinct neural crest stem cells in terms of migratory properties, fate determination, and ability to colonize the enteric nervous system. Dev Biol. 2007;303:1–15.
55. Natarajan D, Cooper J, Choudhury S, Delalande JM, McCann C, Howe SJ, Thapar N, Burns AJ. Lentiviral labeling of mouse and human enteric nervous system stem cells for regenerative medicine studies. Neurogastroenterol Motil. 2014;26:1513–8.
56. Natarajan D, Grigoriou M, Marcos-Gutierrez CV, Atkins C, Pachnis V. Multipotential progenitors of the mammalian enteric nervous system capable of colonising aganglionic bowel in organ culture. Development. 1999;126:157–68.
57. Nguyen HT, Geens M, Mertzanidou A, Jacobs K, Heirman C, Breckpot K, Spits C. Gain of 20q11.21 in human embryonic stem cells improves cell survival by increased expression of Bcl-xL. Mol Hum Reprod. 2014;20:168–77.
58. Olariu V, Harrison NJ, Coca D, Gokhale PJ, Baker D, Billings S, Kadirkamanathan V, Andrews PW. Modeling the evolution of culture-adapted human embryonic stem cells. Stem Cell Res. 2010;4:50–6.
59. Rollo BN, Zhang D, Stamp LA, Menheniott TR, Stathopoulos L, Denham M, Dottori M, King SK, Hutson JM, Newgreen DF. Enteric neural cells from hirschsprung disease patients form ganglia in autologous aneuronal colon. Cell Mol Gastroenterol Hepatol. 2016;2:92–109.
60. Sato Y, Heuckeroth RO. Retinoic acid regulates murine enteric nervous system precursor proliferation, enhances neuronal precursor differentiation, and reduces neurite growth in vitro. Dev Biol. 2008;320:185–98.
61. Schafer KH, Micci MA, Pasricha PJ. Neural stem cell transplantation in the enteric nervous system: roadmaps and roadblocks. Neurogastroenterol Motil. 2009;21:103–12.
62. Schlieve CR, Fowler KL, Thornton M, Huang S, Hajjali I, Hou X, Grubbs B, Spence JR, Grikscheit TC. Neural crest cell implantation restores enteric nervous system function and alters the gastrointestinal transcriptome in human tissue-engineered small intestine. Stem Cell Reports. 2017;9:883–96.
63. Stamp LA. Cell therapy for GI motility disorders: comparison of cell sources and proposed steps for treating Hirschsprung disease. Am J Physiol Gastrointest Liver Physiol. 2017;312:G348–54.
64. Stamp LA, Gwynne RM, Foong JPP, Lomax AE, Hao MM, Kaplan DI, Reid CA, Petrou S, Allen AM, Bornstein JC, Young HM. Optogenetic demonstration of functional innervation of mouse colon by neurons derived from transplanted neural cells. Gastroenterology. 2017;152:1407–18.
65. Stamp LA, Obermayr F, Pontell L, Young HM, Xie D, Croaker DH, Song ZM, Furness JB. Surgical intervention to rescue Hirschsprung disease in a rat model. J Neurogastroenterol Motil. 2015;21:552–9.
66. Trounson A, DeWitt ND. Pluripotent stem cells progressing to the clinic. Nat Rev Mol Cell Biol. 2016;17:194–200.
67. Tsai YH, Murakami N, Gariepy CE. Postnatal intestinal engraftment of prospectively selected enteric neural crest stem cells in a rat model of Hirschsprung disease. Neurogastroenterol Motil. 2011;23:362–9.
68. Uesaka T, Nagashimada M, Yonemura S, Enomoto H. Diminished Ret expression compromises neuronal

survival in the colon and causes intestinal aganglionosis in mice. J Clin Invest. 2008;118:1890–8.
69. Wester T, Granstrom AL. Hirschsprung disease-Bowel function beyond childhood. Semin Pediatr Surg. 2017;26:322–7.
70. Workman MJ, Mahe MM, Trisno S, Poling HM, Watson CL, Sundaram N, Chang CF, Schiesser J, Aubert P, Stanley EG, Elefanty AG, Miyaoka Y, Mandegar MA, Conklin BR, Neunlist M, Brugmann SA, Helmrath MA, Wells JM. Engineered human pluripotent-stem-cell-derived intestinal tissues with a functional enteric nervous system. Nat Med. 2017;23:49–59.
71. Zimmer J, Puri P. Knockout mouse models of Hirschsprung's disease. Pediatr Surg Int. 2015;31:787–94.

Pathophysiology of Hirschsprung's Disease

9

Anne Marie O'Donnell, Sandra Montedonico, and Prem Puri

Contents

A. M. O'Donnell · P. Puri (✉)
National Children's Research Centre, Our Lady's Children's Hospital, Crumlin, Dublin, Ireland
e-mail: prem.puri@ncrc.ie

S. Montedonico
National Children's Research Centre, Our Lady's Children's Hospital, Crumlin, Dublin, Ireland

Hospital Carlos Van Buren, Escuela de Medicina, Universidad de Valparaíso, Valparaíso, Chile

9.1 Introduction

The basic pathophysiologic feature in Hirschsprung's disease (HD) is a functional obstruction caused by a narrowed distal aganglionic colonic segment that prevents the propagation of peristaltic waves.

The digestive tract is unique among internal organs because it is exposed to a large variety of physicochemical stimuli from the external world in the form of ingested food. As a consequence, the intestine has developed a rich repertoire of coordinated movements of its muscular apparatus to ensure the appropriate mixing and propulsion of contents during digestion, absorption, and excretion. The normal motility of the gastrointestinal system is dependent on the interaction of a number of different tissues.

P. Puri (ed.), *Hirschsprung's Disease and Allied Disorders*,
https://doi.org/10.1007/978-3-030-15647-3_9

9.2 Organization of the Gut

9.2.1 The Gut Wall

The gut wall comprises two layers of smooth muscles. An outer thin layer of cells arranged along the length of the gut forms the longitudinal smooth muscle layer. A perpendicular, thicker layer of cells immediately inside the longitudinal muscle forms the circular smooth muscle layer. A well-developed, ganglionated nervous plexus is situated between both muscle layers, the myenteric plexus. On the luminal side of the circular muscle layer is the submucosa, which contains connective tissue, glands, small vessels, and a second ganglionated plexus, the submucous plexus. A thin muscle layer separates the submucosa from the mucosa. The mucosa is densely innervated by sensory nerve fibers from nerve cells in either of the plexuses. Enteroendocrine cells involved in the control of gut functions are common in the mucosal lining [1, 2].

9.2.2 "SIP" Syncytium

Gastrointestinal motility is controlled by four groups of cells, the enteric nervous system (ENS), smooth muscle cells (SMCs), interstitial cells of Cajal (ICCs), and platelet-derived growth factor receptor alpha-positive cells (PDGFRα^+ cells), commonly referred to as the "SIP" syncytium. SMCs are electrically coupled to ICC and PDGFRα^+ cells, forming an integrated unit [3]. SIP cells express a variety of receptors and ion channels, and conductance changes in any type of SIP cell affect the excitability and responses of the syncytium. SIP cells are known to provide pacemaker activity, propagation pathways for slow waves, transduction of inputs from motor neurons, and mechanosensitivity [3].

9.2.3 Smooth Muscle Cells

The smooth muscle cells are long thin cells with a large central nucleus. They are interconnected via gap junctions to operate as larger functional mechanical units. Electrical stimuli can spread between the cells through the gap junctions, causing parts of the muscle to act as one single unit [2]. The level of muscular activity depends on intrinsic, myogenic activity as well as on the neural apparatus. Electrical slow waves are cyclic changes in membrane potential that are responsible for rhythmic contractions of the muscles. The factors that trigger these slow waves are a network of pacemaker cells called interstitial cells of Cajal [2].

9.2.4 Interstitial Cells of Cajal

The interstitial cells of Cajal (ICCs) are mesenchymal cells, spindle shaped or with several processes that form networks that are widely distributed within the submucosal, intramuscular, and intermuscular layers of the gastrointestinal tract from the esophagus to the internal anal sphincter [4, 5]. Immunohistochemically, they can be localized by the expression of c-kit, a trans-cell membrane tyrosine-kinase receptor. ICCs act as pacemakers in the gut wall, by developing spontaneous slow waves, which spread to the smooth muscle cells. It has been demonstrated that ICCs also mediate enteric motor neurotransmission via synaptic-like contacts that exist between varicose nerve terminals and intramuscular ICC [5]. However, the integrative role of the ICC and the enteric nervous system in the control of gastrointestinal function is still unknown [6].

9.2.5 Platelet-Derived Growth Factor Receptor α-Positive Cells

PDGFRα^+ cells were, for many years, known as "fibroblast-like cells" or "ICC-like" cells, as they morphologically resembled ICCs, but were c-kit negative. PDGFRα^+ cells are found in close proximity to ICCs, enteric neurons, and SMCs. More recently, enhanced green fluorescent protein (eGFP) labeling of these cells, as well as commercial availability of antibodies directed against PDGFRα, has enabled specific and reliable identification of this cell type. PDGFRα^+ cells form discrete networks in the region of the myenteric plexus and within the circular and longitudinal muscle layer. PDGFRα^+

cells express the small-conductance Ca^{2+}-activated K^+ channel (SK3), which is an important mediator of purinergic neurotransmission in gastrointestinal smooth muscle [7].

9.2.6 Extrinsic Innervation

In addition to intrinsic myogenic activity and the involvement of ICC discussed above, the autonomic nervous system controls gut motility [8]. The autonomic nervous system controls several visceral functions that are not under conscious control. It can be divided into three main divisions: the cranial (parasympathetic) and the spinal (sympathetic and parasympathetic) systems, which relay extrinsic control, and the enteric nervous system, which is the intrinsic nervous system of the gut, and not only regulates the intestinal motility but also secretions, blood flow, and immune and endocrine functions [2]. The extrinsic innervation of the gut involves the vagus nerve and splanchnic nerves to the stomach and upper intestine and the pelvic nerves supplying the distal intestinal segments. Parasympathetic fibers running in the vagus nerve innervate the stomach; however, the majority of the fibers in the vagus are sensory fibers with their nerve cell bodies in the nodose ganglion. These fibers convey information from the stomach and other peripheral organs to the central nervous system. The splanchnic nerves are sympathetic, while the pelvic nerve contains both parasympathetic and sympathetic fibers. Sensory nerve fibers within the spinal nerves, running from the gut to the central nervous system, have their cell bodies located in the dorsal root ganglia.

9.2.7 Intrinsic Innervation: The Enteric Nervous System

The enteric nervous system (ENS) is the system of neurons and their supporting cells that are present within the wall of the gastrointestinal tract. It may act independently of extrinsic input, but both sympathetic and parasympathetic nerves can influence gut motility via enteric nerves [9]. The ENS is the largest division of the autonomic nervous system, and it contains about 100 million neurons, only comparable to the ones of the spinal cord [10, 11]. The neurons cell bodies are clustered together in ganglia. The ENS has two ganglionated plexuses, the myenteric and submucosal plexuses [12]. The myenteric plexus (Auerbach plexus) is positioned between the outer longitudinal and circular muscle layers throughout the digestive tract, from the esophagus to the anus. The submucous plexus is subdivided into separate plexuses: the inner submucous plexus (Meissner plexus) directly below the muscularis mucosae and the outer submucous plexus (Schabadasch or Henle plexus) directly adjacent to the circular muscle layer [11]. The submucosal plexus is absent from the esophagus and stomach, being only prominent in the intestines. This topography has functional relevance in that the myenteric plexus mainly regulates motor function, whereas the submucous plexus is mainly involved in control of blood flow, secretion, and absorption [11]. The density of neurons varies between myenteric and submucosal ganglia and between gut regions. Typically, myenteric ganglia are considerably larger than submucosal ganglia. The ENS neurons, although clustered into ganglia, do not form nuclei of morphologically similar neuron types as occur, for example, in the brain. Instead, each enteric ganglion contains many different neuron types, and neighboring ganglia will contain similar types of neurons although not always in identical proportions.

9.2.7.1 Classification of the Neurons of the ENS

Neurons of the ENS can be classified according to their morphological, neurochemical, or functional properties. These properties have been disclosed by different methods including light and electron microscopy, immunohistochemistry, electrophysiological analysis, intracellular dyes, and retrograde tracing of neuronal projections [13]. Seventeen different neuronal types, only 14 of which are functionally important, have been identified in the small intestine [12].

Morphology

According to their morphology, neurons are classified into Dogiel types I–VII and giant neurons. Most neurons are Dogiel types I–III [12]. Dogiel type I neurons have flat cell bodies with many short, lamellar dendrites and a single long axon, and they are implicated as enteric motor neurons. Dogiel type II neurons have relatively smooth cell bodies with short and long processes arising in a variety of configurations. The long processes may extend through interganglionic fiber tracts across several rows of ganglia. Shorter processes may project only within the home ganglion. Dogiel type III neurons are similar to the latest except that there are more processes and more of the processes are shorter in length [14].

Neurochemistry

Neurons usually express a combination of different neurotransmitters, a phenomenon known as *chemical coding* [15]. The chemical code depends on the type of neuron and the intestinal segment. The general mechanism of chemically mediated synaptic transmission is the same in the enteric nervous system as elsewhere in the body and seemingly as complex as in the central nervous system. More than 30 neurotransmitters have been identified in the ENS, which are usually colocalized according to their function, as shown in Table 9.1 [12]. Enteric neurotransmitters are either small molecules (norepinephrine, 5-HT), larger molecules (peptides), or gases (nitric oxide and carbon monoxide).

Table 9.1 Chemical coding of the enteric neurons

Function	Neurochemical coding
Sensory	Ach, Calb, CGRP, and SP
Ascending interneurons	Ach, Calret, ENK, and SP
Descending interneurons	5-HT, DYN, GRP, NO, somatostatin, and VIP
Short excitatory muscle motor neurons	Ach and SP
Long excitatory muscle motor neurons	Ach, Calret, and SP
Inhibitory muscle motor neurons	DYN, ENK, GRP, NO, and VIP
Secretomotor neurons	Ach, CCK, CGRP, DYN, NPY, somatostatin, and VIP

Ach acetylcholine, *NO* nitric oxide, *Calb* calbindin, *Calret* calretinin, *DYN* dynorphin, *GRP* gastrin-releasing peptide, *CGRP* calcitonin-generated peptide, *SP* substance P, *ENK* enkephalins, *5-HT* 5-hydroxytryptamine (serotonin), *NPY* neuropeptide Y, *VIP* vasoactive intestinal peptide

Functional Classification

Neurons are classified according to their function into sensory neurons, interneurons, and motor neurons.

Sensory Neurons

The sensory neurons are a dense network of extrinsic (vagal and spinal afferents with their cell bodies outside the gut wall) and intrinsic primary afferent neurons (IPANs, with their cell bodies within the gut wall) [16]. They communicate with each other and function together with enteroendocrine and immune cells. Whereas IPANs are essential for enteric nervous system control of digestion, extrinsic afferents notify the brain about processes that are relevant to energy and fluid homeostasis and the sensation of discomfort and pain [17]. Sensory neurons include mechano-, chemo-, and thermoreceptors. Mechanoreceptors are activated by distension and generate tonic muscle contractions, but if distension is maintained, they respond by generating peristaltic activity (Fig. 9.1). Besides direct activation of the IPANs, there are other specialized transducers, the enteroendocrine cells. These cells are strategically positioned in the mucosa to "taste" and sense luminal contents and release their mediators at the basolateral side to activate sensory nerve endings within the lamina propria, which synapse on excitatory or inhibitory motor neurons. While enteroendocrine cells are specialized for luminal nutrient sensing, subepithelial IPANs may also respond to luminal chemicals that freely diffuse across the epithelium [18]. There are regional and topographic differences in the distribution of enteroendocrine cells, with the highest frequency in the duodenum. The major transmitters are cholecystokinin (CCK), secretin, somatostatin, serotonin (5-hydroxytryptamine, 5-HT), and corticotropin-releasing factor. Cells containing 5-HT are present in all regions of the intestine and compose the single largest endocrine cell population.

Interneurons

Interneurons are usually Dogiel type II. At least one type of ascending and three types of descending interneurons have been described, most of them being the descending type. The ascending interneurons are mainly cholinergic, whereas the descending ones have a complex chemical cod-

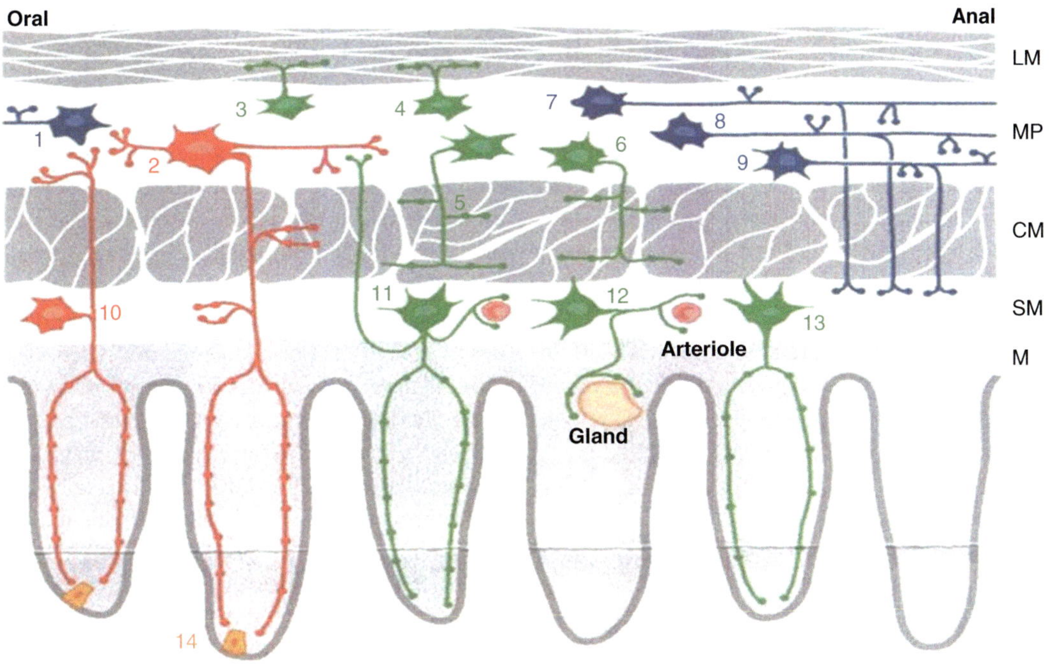

Fig. 9.1 The types of neurons in the small intestine. (1) Ascending interneuron, (2) myenteric intrinsic primary afferent neuron, (3) excitatory longitudinal muscle motor neuron, (4) inhibitory longitudinal muscle motor neuron, (5) excitatory circular muscle motor neuron, (6) inhibitory circular muscle motor neuron, (7) descending interneuron (local reflex), (8) descending interneuron (secretomotor reflex), (9) descending interneuron (migrating myoelectric complex), (10) submucosal intrinsic primary afferent neuron, (11) noncholinergic secretomotor/vasodilator neuron, (12) cholinergic secretomotor/vasodilator neuron, (13) cholinergic secretomotor (non-vasodilator) neuron, (14) enteroendocrine cell. LM longitudinal muscle, MP myenteric plexus, CM circular muscle, SM submucosal plexus, M mucosa

ing including acetylcholine, nitric oxide, vasoactive intestinal polypeptide, 5-HT, and somatostatin (Table 9.1 and Fig. 9.1).

Motor Neurons

Motor neurons are Dogiel type I. There are three types: muscle motor neurons, secretomotor neurons that are or are not vasodilators, and neurons innervating enteroendocrine cells. Muscle motor neurons innervate the longitudinal and circular muscles and the muscularis mucosae throughout the digestive tract. The muscle motor neurons are either excitatory or inhibitory and release transmitters that provoke muscle contraction or relaxation. For the excitatory neurons, transmission is predominantly muscarinic cholinergic and tachykinergic (substance P and neurokinin A). For the inhibitory neurons, the primary transmitter is nitric oxide [19] but also vasoactive intestine polypeptide, ATP, pituitary adenylate cyclase-activating polypeptide, and carbon monoxide (Table 9.1 and Fig. 9.1) [12].

9.3 Motility of the Gut

The different cell types mentioned in Sect. 9.2 must work in a coordinated manner in order to obtain an adequate intestinal motility. Two patterns of activity are recognized in the mammalian intestine, the activity of the interdigestive state and the fed pattern of activity [20].

9.3.1 Migrating Myoelectric Complex

In the interdigestive state, complexes of contractions traveling in an anal direction have been recorded. This is known as a migrating myoelectric complex (MMC), which passes along the intestine every 80–110 min in humans. The complex takes about 6–10 min to pass any point in the intestine, and as it passes, that region undergoes intense rhythmic contractions of the circular muscle [20]. These MMCs probably act as housekeepers, to transport waste products in the interdigestive stage, and they also control the bacterial flora, preventing overgrowth and returning bacteria to the large intestine [21]. The MMCs disappear soon after a meal is taken, to be replaced by the fed pattern of activity, the peristaltic movements. Both the interdigestive pattern and the fed pattern are generated through the ENS but are modified by the extrinsic nerves. The continuity of the ENS is necessary for the orderly progress of the MMC; if the intestine is interrupted surgically and then rejoined, the MMC does not always pass the lesion, and ectopic MMCs occur on the anal side [20].

9.3.2 Peristalsis

The fed pattern of activity both mixes and propels the contents. In one human study, about 45% of individual contractions did not propagate and about 35% propagated for less than 9 cm [22]. These non-propagating contractions correspond to the mixing activity. The propagated contractions are peristaltic waves, which consist of contraction of the circular muscle oral to a bolus in the lumen, the ascending excitatory reflex, and relaxation on the anal side, the descending inhibitory reflex. In addition, longitudinal muscle on the anal side may contract while the oral longitudinal muscle relaxes. Total extrinsic denervation of the bowel does not affect peristalsis [20]. All the neural elements for the peristaltic reflex are in the intestine; these are the intrinsic primary afferent neurons (IPANs), interneurons, and motor neurons. Passing the food may cause the release of 5-HT from an enteroendocrine cells in the mucosa stimulating sensory nerve endings from IPAN projecting from cells bodies in the myenteric or submucous plexus (Fig. 9.2 and Table 9.1). In addition, IPAN may be directly stimulated by distension of

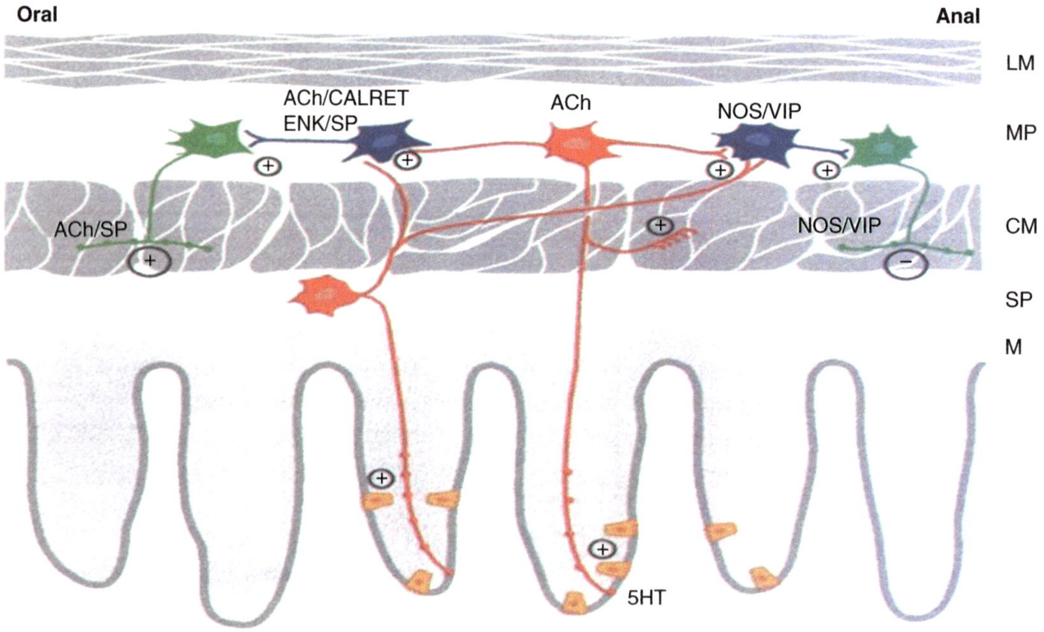

Fig. 9.2 A generalized picture of ascending and descending reflex pathways controlling intestinal peristalsis. Passage of food may cause release of 5-HT from enteroendocrine cells (yellow) in the mucosa stimulating sensory nerve endings from IPAN projecting from cells bodies in the myenteric or submucous plexus (red). In addition, IPAN may be directly stimulated by distension of the gut wall. The IPANs activate ascending (oral) and descending (anal) interneurons (blue). Orally projecting interneurons release acetylcholine, calretinin, enkephalins, and substance P that stimulate excitatory motor neurons innervating the circular muscle, which in turn release acetylcholine and substance P (green). Anally projecting interneurons contain nitric oxide and vasoactive intestinal peptide. These interneurons stimulate inhibitory motor neurons that release nitric oxide and vasoactive intestinal peptide among other neurotransmitters (green). Ach acetylcholine, NO nitric oxide, Calret calretinin, SP substance P, ENK enkephalins, 5-HT 5-hydroxytryptamine (serotonin), VIP vasoactive intestinal peptide, IPAN intrinsic primary afferent neuron, LM longitudinal muscle, MP myenteric plexus, CM circular muscle, SP submucous plexus, M mucosa

the gut wall. The IPANs activate ascending (oral) and descending (anal) interneurons. Orally projecting interneurons release acetylcholine calretinin, enkephalins, and substance P that stimulate excitatory motor neurons innervating the circular muscle, which in turn release acetylcholine and substance P. Anally projecting interneurons contain nitric oxide and vasoactive intestinal peptide. These interneurons stimulate inhibitory motor neurons that release nitric oxide and vasoactive intestinal peptide among other neurotransmitters (Fig. 9.2 and Table 9.1).

9.4 The Gut in Hirschsprung's Disease

The characteristic gross pathologic feature of Hirschsprung's disease (HD) is a narrowed distal colon with a funnel-shaped transition zone to a dilated and hypertrophied proximal colon. These features may vary with the duration of untreated disease. In the neonatal period, the intestine may appear normal; but as the child ages, the proximal intestine hypertrophies and becomes thicker and longer than normal. The taeniae disappear and the longitudinal muscle layer seems to completely surround the colon. In HD patients, there is a wide spectrum of clinical presentations, ranging from a nearly asymptomatic patient to an intestinal obstruction dating from the newborn period [23]. The absence of the enteric nervous system is the most remarkable finding in the narrow distal colon in HD. However, it has long been recognized that several other abnormalities have been described associated with HD that may contribute to its pathophysiology and may explain the clinical discrepancy among different patients.

9.4.1 Aganglionosis

The most striking finding in the distal intestine in HD is the absence of ganglion cells in the myenteric and submucous plexuses [24]. Aganglionosis typically extends to the rectosigmoid region in approximately 80% of cases. The aganglionosis is continuous and uninterrupted until the proximal transitional zone is reached. The length of this zone may vary and extend for several centimeters and is characterized by hypoganglionosis.

9.4.2 Cholinergic Hyperinnervation

In association with aganglionosis, there is a marked increase in cholinergic nerve fibers in the intermuscular zone and submucosa of the aganglionic segment. These fibers appear as thick nerve trunks and correspond to extrinsic preganglionic parasympathetic nerves [25, 26] The continuous acetylcholine release from the axons of these parasympathetic nerves results in an excessive accumulation of the enzyme acetylcholinesterase that is typically found in the lamina propria mucosae, muscularis mucosae, and circular muscle with histochemical staining techniques [24]. Both the thick nerve trunks and the increased acetylcholinesterase activity are most pronounced in the most distal aganglionic rectum and progressively diminish proximally as normal bowel is approached [27]. The proximal extent of increased cholinergic activity does not necessarily correspond to the extent of the aganglionosis, which usually extends more proximally to a variable degree. Pharmacologic investigations of the colon in HD have demonstrated higher acetylcholine release in the aganglionic segment at rest and after stimulation compared with the proximal ganglionic bowel [28]. Acetylcholinesterase concentration has also been found to be higher in the serum and erythrocytes from children suffering from HD [29]. Cholinergic nerve hyperplasia has been proposed as the cause of spasticity of the aganglionic segment since acetylcholine is the main excitatory neurotransmitter. However, in the chemical animal model of aganglionosis, after application of benzalkonium chloride or corrosive sublimate, the aganglionic bowel does not show hypertrophic nerve bundles, and the bowel still appears narrow and animals exhibit typical obstructive symptoms [30]. Therefore, the cholinergic hyperinnervation does not seem to be a prerequisite to the appearance of a narrow spastic segment.

9.4.3 Adrenergic Innervation

Fluorescent-histochemical studies for localization of adrenergic nerves have demonstrated that they are increased in number in the aganglionic colon of HD and have a chaotic distribution. They are also present in the circular and longitudinal muscle layers as well as in the mucosa, whereas they are almost never found in normal ganglionic colon [31]. However, the sensitivity of the aganglionic bowel to epinephrine is apparently not increased, despite the elevated number of adrenergic fibers [32]. Because adrenergic nerves normally act to relax the bowel, it is unlikely that adrenergic hyperactivity is responsible for increased tone in the aganglionic colon [33].

9.4.4 Nitrergic Innervation

Nitric oxide (NO) is considered to be one of the most important neurotransmitters involved in relaxation of the smooth muscle of the gut [34]. It is synthesized in a reaction catalyzed by nitric oxide synthase (NOS) and depends on L-arginine and molecular oxygen as co-substrates to form L-citrulline and NO. Nitric oxide binds to cytosolic guanylate cyclase and increases the production of 3′5′-cyclic guanosine monophosphate (cGMP) with subsequent relaxation of smooth muscle [35]. NOS has been shown to be colocalized with reduced nicotine adenine dinucleotide phosphate (NADPH) diaphorase, which has been demonstrated to have identical functions [36]. Several investigators have studied NOS distribution in the ganglionic and aganglionic bowel in patients with HD using nitric oxide synthase immunohistochemistry or NADPH diaphorase histochemistry [37–39]. In normal and ganglionic colon from patients with HD, there is a strong NADPH diaphorase staining of the submucous and myenteric plexuses and a large number of positive nerve fibers in the circular and longitudinal muscle as well as in the muscularis mucosae [40]. In the aganglionic segment of HD patients, there are no ganglia, and there is an absence or marked reduction of NADPH diaphorase-positive nerve fibers in both muscle layers and muscularis mucosae. The typical hypertrophied nerve trunks appear weakly stained [40]. Kusafuka and Puri [33] examined the expression of neural NOS mRNA in the aganglionic segment from seven patients who had HD and demonstrated that NOS mRNA expression was decreased at least 1/50 to 1/100 of the level expressed in ganglionic bowel. These findings indicate that there is impaired NO synthesis in the aganglionic bowel in HD, and this deficiency could prevent smooth muscle relaxation, thereby causing the lack of peristalsis in HD. In an interesting experiment, Bealer et al. [38] compared the effect of an exogenous source of NO, S-nitroso-N-acetylpenicillamine (SNAP), on the isometric tension of smooth muscle strips from aganglionic bowel and demonstrated a 70% reduction in resting tension. These results suggest that the defective distribution of nerves containing NOS may be involved in the pathogenesis of HD.

9.4.5 Interstitial Cells of Cajal

Abnormalities of ICC have been described in several disorders of human intestinal motility including HD. Vanderwinden et al. [41] using c-kit immunohistochemistry first described that ICCs were scarce, and its network appeared disrupted in aganglionic segments of HD, whereas the distribution of ICC in the ganglionic bowel of HD was similar to that observed in controls. Yamataka et al. [42, 43] found few c-kit-positive cells in the muscle layers in HD and a moderate number around the thick nerve bundles in the space between the two muscle layers in the aganglionic bowel. Horisawa et al. [44] reported no differences in c-kit immunopositive cells in aganglionic segments compared to the corresponding area of ganglionic bowel. Recently, Chen et al. [45] using confocal microscopy, flow cytometry, and transmission electron microscopy have shown that the content of ICC and its progenitors were significantly decreased in the narrow part of the HD colon. Rolle et al. [46, 47] using whole-mount and frozen sections stained with c-kit immunohistochemistry preparations showed an altered distribution of ICC in the entire resected bowel of HD patients and not only in the aganglionic segment. Moreover, gap junctions connecting ICC were immunolocalized by anti-Connexin 43 antibody and found to be absent from the aganglionic part of HD bowel and highly reduced from the transitional zone [48]. More recently, Coyle et al. have also demonstrated a reduction in the expression of Connexin 26 in the aganglionic bowel in HD compared with controls, as well as a moderate reduction in the ganglionic bowel in HD [49].

In recent years, it has come to light that the c-kit antibody, however, also labels mast cells in the circular smooth muscle, which calls into question its utility as a specific marker when evaluating ICC networks in the human colon. The Ca^{2+}-activated

Cl^- channel, anoctamin-1 (ANO1), has been demonstrated to be a highly specific marker of ICCs in the gastrointestinal tract [50]. ANO1 is preferential to c-kit in evaluating the ICC network in HD due to its specificity and functional importance. Coyle et al. reported ANO1 protein expression was reduced in both aganglionic and ganglionic HD colon relative to controls [51].

9.4.6 Platelet-Derived Growth Factor Receptor α-Positive Cells

Kurahashi et al. documented the first evidence of PDGFRα$^+$ cells in the human colon [7]. These cells are found to be distributed in a similar pattern to ICCs as well as morphologically resembling them. They have been found to play a role in inhibitory neurotransmission as they contain purinergic receptors and have been found to display gap junctions with SMCs [7]. O'Donnell et al. have reported a decreased expression of PDGFRα$^+$ cells in both aganglionic and ganglionic regions of HD colon, which suggests a role for this cell type in the pathophysiology of this condition [52].

9.4.7 Enteroendocrine Cells

Using the generic enteroendocrine cell immunohistochemical markers chromogranin A and synaptophysin, Soeda et al. [53] demonstrated that the number of enteroendocrine cells in the aganglionic colon in patients with HD was significantly increased compared with the number in the normal ganglionic segment. The increase in enteroendocrine cells in the mucosa of aganglionosis colon may well influence sustained contraction of the bowel wall mainly mediated by the release of 5-hydroxytryptamine.

9.4.8 Smooth Muscle

Since smooth muscle is the final effector for bowel motility, it is likely that it could also be abnormal in HD. The smooth muscle cell cytoskeleton consists of proteins whose primary function is to serve as a structural framework that surrounds and supports the contractile apparatus of actin and myosin filaments in the body of the smooth muscle cell. Nemeth et al. [35] studied the distribution of cytoskeleton in the smooth muscle of HD bowel by means of immunohistochemistry and found that dystrophin, vinculin, and desmin immunoreactivity were either absent or weak in the smooth muscle of aganglionic bowel, whereas it was moderate to strong in the smooth muscle of normal bowel and ganglionic bowel from patients with HD. Neural cell adhesion molecule (NCAM) is a cell surface glycoprotein involved in cell-cell adhesion during development that has been suggested to play an important role in the development and maintenance of the neuromuscular system [54]. NCAM is present in the innervation of normal infant bowel and, less densely, in some components of the enteric smooth muscle. Contradictory results have been published regarding the NCAM expression in the smooth muscle of aganglionic bowel. Kobayashi et al. [26] have described a lack of expression of NCAM in the muscularis propria of the aganglionic bowel compared with the ganglionic segment, whereas Romanska et al. [55] have found an increase in NCAM expression in muscle, particularly in the muscularis mucosae. Anyhow, both authors agree in that there is a strong expression of NCAM in the hypertrophic nerve trunks from the aganglionic segment.

9.4.9 Extracellular Matrix

Although extracellular matrix (EM) abnormalities have been described mainly related to the pathogenesis of HD, they could also have an influence on its pathophysiology. The lethal spotted mouse, an animal model which develops aganglionosis in its distal bowel, displays an abnormal distribution of EM components including laminin, collagen type IV, glycosaminoglycans, and proteoglycans in the smooth muscle layer [56]. Parikh et al. [57] have demonstrated that the laminin concentration in aganglionic bowel was twice as high as in the normoganglionic bowel of HD and three times higher than an age-matched control. Moreover, by means of immunohistochemistry, they found an uneven distribution of laminin and collagen type IV in the muscularis propria of aganglionic bowel, being more intensely expressed in the circular layer than in the longitudinal layer [58]. The same authors have described that EM components tenascin and fibronectin are more intensely expressed in aganglionic bowel from HD [59]. Moreover, Soret et al. [60] have recently described a HD animal model by upregulating the collagen 6α4 (col 6α4) gene. This upregulation increases total collagen VI protein levels that during development results in slower migration of neural crest cells.

9.4.10 Microbiome

In recent years, it has come to light that the microbiome has an enormous impact on intestinal physiology. Sustaining a balanced intestinal microbiota is key for maintaining intestinal health and preventing chronic inflammation. Rolig et al. [61] have demonstrated in an animal zebrafish model of HD that the enteric nervous system modulates gut microbiota to maintain intestinal health. The role of the microbiome in the pathophysiology of HD is still unclear. A recently published article showed that HD patients have an altered intestinal microbiome compared to healthy individuals characterized by a lack of richness and pathologic expansions of taxon, particularly Enterobacteria and Bacilli [62]. There is contradictory information regarding the role of probiotics in the prevention of HD-associated enterocolitis: El-Sawaf et al. [63] in a randomized controlled trial including 62 patients found no differences in the incidence of HD-associated enterocolitis in a 12-month period follow-up if given 3 months of probiotics postoperatively compared to placebo. On the other hand, Wang et al. [64], also in a randomized controlled trial including 60 patients, were able to demonstrate a significant reduction in the incidence and severity of enterocolitis in patients undertaking probiotics when they were followed up for 3 months after surgery. A recently published systematic review showed no significant reduction in the risk of HD-associated enterocolitis [65].

9.4.11 Alterations in the Proximal Ganglionic Segment

The goal of surgical treatment for HD is to enable the affected child to have regular spontaneous bowel motions without soiling. Advances in the management of HD afford most patients a satisfactory outcome following a properly performed pull-through operation. However, a substantial cohort of patients continues to have persistent bowel dysfunction despite adequate resection of the aganglionic bowel segment. The postoperative bowel dysfunction includes enterocolitis, constipation, and incontinence [66, 67]. Postoperative enterocolitis has been reported in 6%–20% of patients, and its incidence is unrelated to the timing of definitive surgery [68]. Constipation and soiling have been reported to occur in 11%–35% of patients after pull-through operations [66, 67]. While a proportion of these patients are found to have a treatable pathology such as strictures, residual aganglionosis, or transition zone, the majority have no identifiable cause for their ongoing bowel dysfunction. Persistent bowel problems in these patients after a properly performed pull-through operation have led to the increasing realization that within the pulled-through segment of bowel, the presence of normal ganglion cells is not sufficient as an indicator of satisfactory outcome.

Intestinal neuronal dysplasia (IND) is a malformation of the enteric nervous system characterized by the presence of giant ganglia in the submucous plexus, ectopic ganglion cells in the lamina propria of the mucosa, and an increased acetylcholinesterase activity in the lamina propria and around submucosal blood vessels [69]. In 1977, Puri et al. reported the first case of IND immediately proximal to a segment of aganglionic colon [70]. Since then, there have been several reports of the combined occurrence of these disorders. Some investigators have reported that 25–35% of patients with HD have associated IND [71, 72] and stressed that this could be the cause of persistent bowel symptoms after pull-through operation for HD [73–75]. Sandgren et al. [76] have studied in depth the proximal ganglionic bowel in the lethal spotted mice, a natural mutant model of rectosigmoid HD. They showed that the number of neurons was increased in the submucous plexus from the ileum and colon proximal to the aganglionosis, resembling human IND. They proposed that these findings might explain the persistence of dysmotility after operation for HD. Sandgren et al. also demonstrated that the expression of nitric oxide and vasoactive intestinal peptide was upregulated in the proximal ganglionic segment, whereas the expression of substance P was downregulated [76].

9.5 Gut Motility in Hirschsprung's Disease

In the 1940s, Swenson et al. recorded the peristaltic tracings of HD specimens. They found that the progressive contractions of the dilated proximal colon did not enter the more distal narrow segment [77]. These findings were the evidence of a physiological defect in the distal segment and led to the creation of a novel curative surgical procedure by resecting the rectosigmoid in these patients [78]. For many years, Kubota et al. studied the electrophysiological and pharmacological characteristics of the different bowel segments in surgically resected specimens of HD [79–81]. They found that while a single pulse stimulation is sufficient to induce a rapid membrane hyperpolarization followed by a spike generation in most cells in the dilated ganglionic bowel, in the transitional region, the amplitude of the hyperpolarization response decreases, and repetitive stimulation is necessary to induce a response. Even more so, in the narrow aganglionic segment, a repetitive stimulation evokes only a membrane depolarization in about 20% of the cells, and spike potential is generated only when the number of pulses is increased (Fig. 9.3). They showed that atropine completely abolishes the depolarization response in all segments and that a membrane hyperpolarization is insensitive to both cholinergic and adrenergic blockers and completely abolished by tetrodotoxin, demonstrating electrophysiologically, the presence of a non-adrenergic non-cholinergic inhibitory innervation. Then, by studying the regional changes in the amplitudes of the non-

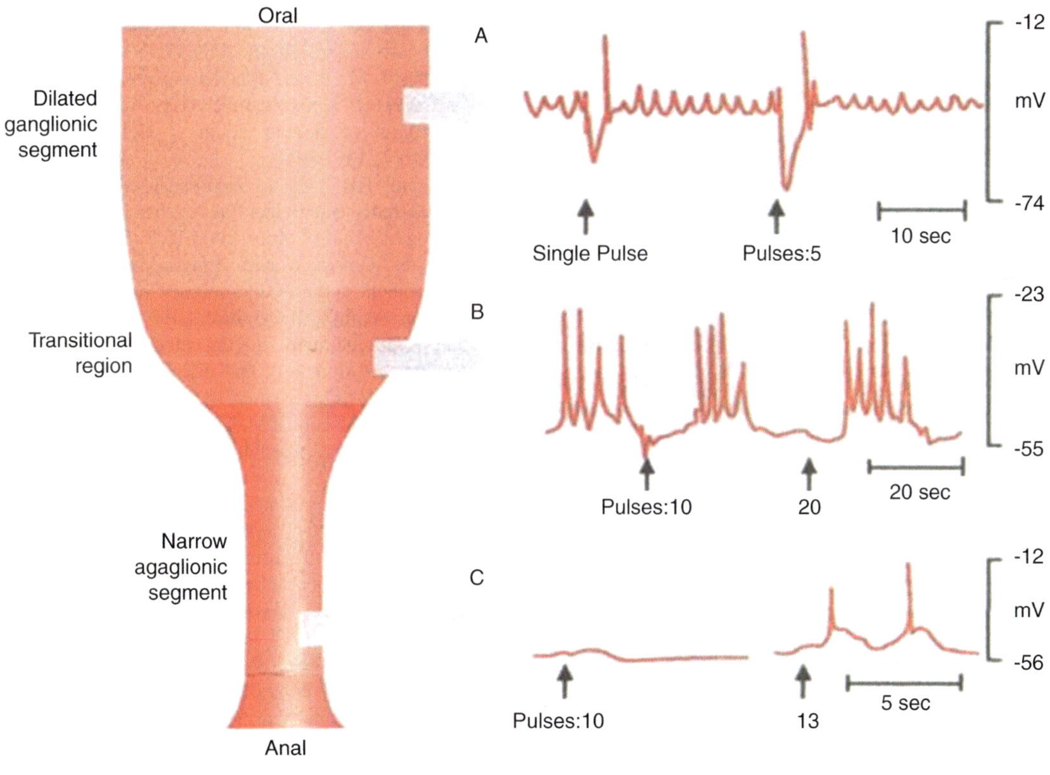

Fig. 9.3 Electrophysiological characteristics of the bowel in Hirschsprung's disease. In the dilated ganglionic bowel, a single pulse stimulation is sufficient to induce a rapid membrane hyperpolarization followed by a spike generation in most cells. In the transitional region, the amplitude of the hyperpolarization response decreases, and repetitive stimulation is necessary to induce a response. In the aganglionic segment, a repetitive stimulation evokes only a membrane depolarization in about 20% of the cells, and spike potential is generated only when the number of pulses is increased

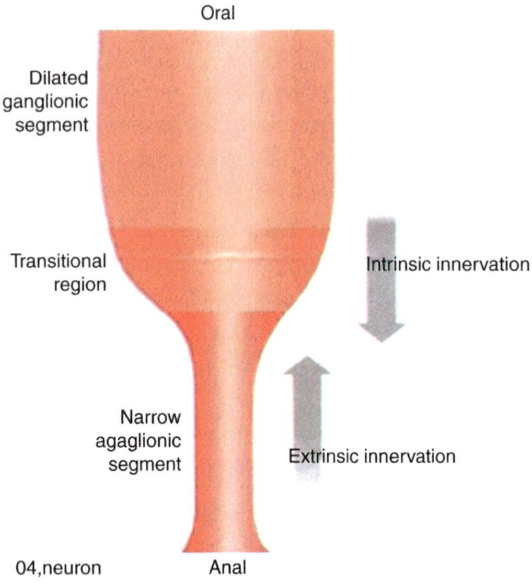

Fig. 9.4 Schematic view of the aganglionic bowel, which receives two nervous flows of different origins: the intrinsic inhibitory nervous flow from the ganglionic segment through the transitional region and the extrinsic excitatory nervous flow from the lower end of the aganglionic segment

adrenergic non-cholinergic inhibitory junction potentials, they concluded that the aganglionic segment receives two nervous flows of different origins: one is the intrinsic inhibitory nervous flow from the ganglionic segment through the transitional region and the other is the extrinsic excitatory nervous flow from the lower end of the aganglionic segment (Fig. 9.4). Since the transitional zone is the place where the stagnation of intestinal content takes place, they concluded that a decrease in the intrinsic inhibitory nervous flow might be the cause for the intestinal obstruction.

9.6 Final Remarks

Although the more striking histological feature in HD is the absence of ganglion cells, it is unlikely that this is the only cause of the increased intestinal wall tone provoking a functional intestinal obstruction. There are a number of other histopathological findings both in the aganglionic segment and in the proximal ganglionic segment in HD which may account for the frequent discrepancy encountered between the length of the non-functional bowel and the degree of obstruction and for the persistent obstructive symptoms after a pull-through operation.

References

1. Costa M, Brookes SJ, Hennig GW. Anatomy and physiology of the enteric nervous system. Gut. 2000;47 Suppl 4:iv15–9. discussion iv26
2. Olsson C, Holmgren S. The control of gut motility. Comp Biochem Physiol A Mol Integr Physiol. 2001;128(3):481–503.
3. Sanders K, Ward S, Koh S. Interstitial cells: regulators of smooth muscle function. Physiol Rev. 2014;94(3):859–907.
4. Takaki M. Gut pacemaker cells: the interstitial cells of Cajal (ICC). J Smooth Muscle Res. 2003;39(5):137–61.
5. Ward SM, Sanders KM, Hirst GD. Role of interstitial cells of Cajal in neural control of gastrointestinal smooth muscles. Neurogastroenterol Motil. 2004;16(Suppl 1):112–7.
6. Alberti E, et al. Motility patterns and distribution of interstitial cells of Cajal and nitrergic neurons in the proximal, mid- and distal-colon of the rat. Neurogastroenterol Motil. 2005;17(1):133–47.
7. Kurahashi M, et al. Platelet-derived growth factor receptor alpha-positive cells in the tunica muscularis of human colon. J Cell Mol Med. 2012;16(7):1397–404.
8. Berthoud HR, et al. Neuroanatomy of extrinsic afferents supplying the gastrointestinal tract. Neurogastroenterol Motil. 2004;16(Suppl 1):28–33.
9. Nagy N, Goldstein AM. Enteric nervous system development: a crest cell's journey from neural tube to colon. Semin Cell Dev Biol. 2017;66:94–106.
10. Ganz J. Gut feelings: studying enteric nervous system development, function, and disease in the zebrafish model system. Dev Dyn. 2018;247(2):268–78.
11. Schemann M, Neunlist M. The human enteric nervous system. Neurogastroenterol Motil. 2004;16(Suppl 1):55–9.
12. Furness JB. Types of neurons in the enteric nervous system. J Auton Nerv Syst. 2000;81(1–3):87–96.
13. Bornstein JC, Furness JB, Kunze WA. Electrophysiological characterization of myenteric neurons: how do classification schemes relate? J Auton Nerv Syst. 1994;48(1):1–15.
14. Brehmer A, Schrodl F, Neuhuber W. Morphological classifications of enteric neurons – 100 years after Dogiel. Anat Embryol. 1999;200(2):125–35.
15. Costa M, et al. Neurochemical classification of myenteric neurons in the guinea-pig ileum. Neuroscience. 1996;75(3):949–67.
16. Clerc N, Furness JB. Intrinsic primary afferent neurones of the digestive tract. Neurogastroenterol Motil. 2004;16(Suppl 1):24–7.

17. Holzer P. Sensory neurone responses to mucosal noxae in the upper gut: relevance to mucosal integrity and gastrointestinal pain. Neurogastroenterol Motil. 2002;14(5):459–75.
18. Dockray GJ. Luminal sensing in the gut: an overview. J Physiol Pharmacol. 2003;54(Suppl 4):9–17.
19. Matini P, et al. Nitric oxide producing neurons in the human colon: an immunohistochemical and histoenzymatical study. Neurosci Lett. 1995;193(1): 17–20.
20. Kunze WA, Furness JB. The enteric nervous system and regulation of intestinal motility. Annu Rev Physiol. 1999;61:117–42.
21. Vantrappen G, et al. The interdigestive motor complex of normal subjects and patients with bacterial overgrowth of the small intestine. J Clin Invest. 1977;59(6):1158–66.
22. Summers RW, Dusdieker NS. Patterns of spike burst spread and flow in the canine small intestine. Gastroenterology. 1981;81(4):742–50.
23. Heuckeroth RO. Hirschsprung disease - integrating basic science and clinical medicine to improve outcomes. Nat Rev Gastroenterol Hepatol. 2018;15(3):152–67.
24. Meier-Ruge W, Bruder E. Histopathological diagnosis and differential diagnosis in Hirschsprung's disease. In: Holschneider A, Puri P, editors. Hirschsprung's disease and allied disorders. Berlin, Heidelberg: Springer; 2008. p. 185–94.
25. Kakita Y, et al. Selective demonstration of mural nerves in ganglionic and aganglionic colon by immunohistochemistry for glucose transporter-1: prominent extrinsic nerve pattern staining in Hirschsprung disease. Arch Pathol Lab Med. 2000;124(9):1314–9.
26. Kobayashi H, O'Briain DS, Puri P. Nerve growth factor receptor immunostaining suggests an extrinsic origin for hypertrophic nerves in Hirschsprung's disease. Gut. 1994;35(11):1605–7.
27. Weinberg AG. Hirschsprung's disease – a pathologist's view. Perspect Pediatr Pathol. 1975;2:207–39.
28. Vizi ES, et al. Characteristics of cholinergic neuroeffector transmission of ganglionic and aganglionic colon in Hirschsprung's disease. Gut. 1990;31(9):1046–50.
29. Boston VE, Cywes S, Davies MR. Serum and erythrocyte acetylcholinesterase activity in Hirschsprung's disease. J Pediatr Surg. 1978;13(4):407–10.
30. Sato A, et al. Pathophysiology of aganglionic colon and anorectum: an experimental study on aganglionosis produced by a new method in the rat. J Pediatr Surg. 1978;13(4):399–435.
31. Nirasawa Y, et al. Hirschsprung's disease: catecholamine content, alpha-adrenoceptors, and the effect of electrical stimulation in aganglionic colon. J Pediatr Surg. 1986;21(2):136–42.
32. Hiramoto Y, Kiesewetter WB. The response of colonic muscle to drugs: an in vitro study of Hirschsprung's disease. J Pediatr Surg. 1974;9(1):13–20.
33. Kusafuka T, Puri P. Altered mRNA expression of the neuronal nitric oxide synthase gene in Hirschsprung's disease. J Pediatr Surg. 1997;32(7):1054–8.
34. Bult H, et al. Nitric oxide as an inhibitory non-adrenergic non-cholinergic neurotransmitter. Nature. 1990;345(6273):346–7.
35. Nemeth L, Rolle U, Puri P. Altered cytoskeleton in smooth muscle of aganglionic bowel. Arch Pathol Lab Med. 2002;126(6):692–6.
36. Hope BT, et al. Neuronal NADPH diaphorase is a nitric oxide synthase. Proc Natl Acad Sci U S A. 1991;88(7):2811–4.
37. Kobayashi H, O'Briain DS, Puri P. Lack of expression of NADPH-diaphorase and neural cell adhesion molecule (NCAM) in colonic muscle of patients with Hirschsprung's disease. J Pediatr Surg. 1994;29(2):301–4.
38. Bealer JF, et al. Effect of nitric oxide on the colonic smooth muscle of patients with Hirschsprung's disease. J Pediatr Surg. 1994;29(8):1025–9.
39. Larsson LT, et al. Lack of neuronal nitric oxide synthase in nerve fibers of aganglionic intestine: a clue to Hirschsprung's disease. J Pediatr Gastroenterol Nutr. 1995;20(1):49–53.
40. Rolle U, Nemeth L, Puri P. Nitrergic innervation of the normal gut and in motility disorders of childhood. J Pediatr Surg. 2002;37(4):551–67.
41. Vanderwinden JM, et al. Interstitial cells of Cajal in human colon and in Hirschsprung's disease. Gastroenterology. 1996;111(4):901–10.
42. Yamataka A, et al. A lack of intestinal pacemaker (c-kit) in aganglionic bowel of patients with Hirschsprung's disease. J Pediatr Surg. 1995;30(3):441–4.
43. Yamataka A, et al. Intestinal pacemaker C-KIT+ cells and synapses in allied Hirschsprung's disorders. J Pediatr Surg. 1997;32(7):1069–74.
44. Horisawa M, Watanabe Y, Torihashi S. Distribution of c-Kit immunopositive cells in normal human colon and in Hirschsprung's disease. J Pediatr Surg. 1998;33(8):1209–14.
45. Chen ZH, et al. Characterization of interstitial Cajal progenitors cells and their changes in Hirschsprung's disease. PLoS One. 2014;9(1):e86100.
46. Rolle U, et al. Altered distribution of interstitial cells of Cajal in Hirschsprung disease. Arch Pathol Lab Med. 2002;126(8):928–33.
47. Gfroerer S, Rolle U. Interstitial cells of Cajal in the normal human gut and in Hirschsprung disease. Pediatr Surg Int. 2013;29(9):889–97.
48. Nemeth L, Maddur S, Puri P. Immunolocalization of the gap junction protein Connexin43 in the interstitial cells of Cajal in the normal and Hirschsprung's disease bowel. J Pediatr Surg. 2000;35(6):823–8.
49. Coyle D, et al. Expression of connexin 26 and connexin 43 is reduced in Hirschsprung's disease. J Surg Res. 2016;206(1):242–51.
50. Gomez-Pinilla P, et al. Ano1 is a selective marker of interstitial cells of Cajal in the human and mouse gastrointestinal tract. Am J Physiol Gastrointest Liver Physiol. 2009;296(6):G1370–81.
51. Coyle D, et al. Use of anoctamin 1 (ANO1) to evaluate interstitial cells of Cajal in Hirschsprung's disease. Pediatr Surg Int. 2016;32(2):125–33.

52. O'Donnell AM, Coyle D, Puri P. Deficiency of platelet-derived growth factor receptor-alpha-positive cells in Hirschsprung's disease colon. World J Gastroenterol. 2016;22(12):3335–40.
53. Soeda J, O'Briain DS, Puri P. Mucosal neuroendocrine cell abnormalities in the colon of patients with Hirschsprung's disease. J Pediatr Surg. 1992;27(7):823–7.
54. Covault J, Sanes JR. Distribution of N-CAM in synaptic and extrasynaptic portions of developing and adult skeletal muscle. J Cell Biol. 1986;102(3):716–30.
55. Romanska HM, et al. Increased expression of muscular neural cell adhesion molecule in congenital aganglionosis. Gastroenterology. 1993;105(4):1104–9.
56. Tennyson VM, et al. Distribution of hyaluronic acid and chondroitin sulfate proteoglycans in the presumptive aganglionic terminal bowel of ls/ls fetal mice: an ultrastructural analysis. J Comp Neurol. 1990;291(3):345–62.
57. Parikh DH, et al. Abnormalities in the distribution of laminin and collagen type IV in Hirschsprung's disease. Gastroenterology. 1992;102(4 Pt 1):1236–41.
58. Parikh DH, et al. Quantitative and qualitative analysis of the extracellular matrix protein, laminin, in Hirschsprung's disease. J Pediatr Surg. 1992;27(8):991–5; discussion 995–6
59. Parikh DH, et al. The extracellular matrix components, tenascin and fibronectin, in Hirschsprung's disease: an immunohistochemical study. J Pediatr Surg. 1994;29(10):1302–6.
60. Soret R, et al. A collagen VI-dependent pathogenic mechanism for Hirschsprung's disease. J Clin Invest. 2015;125(12):4483–96.
61. Rolig AS, et al. The enteric nervous system promotes intestinal health by constraining microbiota composition. PLoS Biol. 2017;15(2):e2000689.
62. Neuvonen MI, et al. Intestinal microbiota in Hirschsprung disease. J Pediatr Gastroenterol Nutr. 2018;67(5):594–600.
63. El-Sawaf M, et al. Probiotic prophylaxis after pullthrough for Hirschsprung disease to reduce incidence of enterocolitis: a prospective, randomized, double-blind, placebo-controlled, multicenter trial. J Pediatr Surg. 2013;48(1):111–7.
64. Wang X, et al. Probiotics prevent Hirschsprung's disease-associated enterocolitis: a prospective multicenter randomized controlled trial. Int J Colorectal Dis. 2015;30(1):105–10.
65. Nakamura H, Lim T, Puri P. Probiotics for the prevention of Hirschsprung-associated enterocolitis: a systematic review and meta-analysis. Pediatr Surg Int. 2018;34(2):189–93.
66. Menezes M, Corbally M, Puri P. Long-term results of bowel function after treatment for Hirschsprung's disease: a 29-year review. Pediatr Surg Int. 2006;22(12):987–90.
67. Menezes M, et al. Long-term clinical outcome in patients with total colonic aganglionosis: a 31-year review. J Pediatr Surg. 2008;43(9):1696–9.
68. Mc Laughlin D, Friedmacher F, Puri P. Total colonic aganglionosis: a systematic review and meta-analysis of long-term clinical outcome. Pediatr Surg Int. 2012;28(8):773–9.
69. Puri P, Rolle U. Variant Hirschsprung's disease. Semin Pediatr Surg. 2004;13(4):293–9.
70. Puri P, et al. Neuronal colonic dysplasia: an unusual association of Hirschsprung's disease. J Pediatr Surg. 1977;12(5):681–5.
71. Fadda B, et al. Neuronal intestinal dysplasia. Critical 10-years' analysis of clinical and biopsy diagnosis. Z Kinderchir. 1983;38(5):305–11.
72. Scharli AF. Intestinal neuronal dysplasia. Cir Pediatr. 1992;5(2):64–5.
73. Kobayashi H, et al. Intestinal neuronal dysplasia is a possible cause of persistent bowel symptoms after pull-through operation for Hirschsprung's disease. J Pediatr Surg. 1995;30(2):253–7; discussion 257–9
74. Schmittenbecher PP, et al. Hirschsprung's disease and intestinal neuronal dysplasia – a frequent association with implications for the postoperative course. Pediatr Surg Int. 1999;15(8):553–8.
75. Banani SA, Forootan HR, Kumar PV. Intestinal neuronal dysplasia as a cause of surgical failure in Hirschsprung's disease: a new modality for surgical management. J Pediatr Surg. 1996;31(4):572–4.
76. Sandgren K, Larsson LT, Ekblad E. Widespread changes in neurotransmitter expression and number of enteric neurons and interstitial cells of Cajal in lethal spotted mice: an explanation for persisting dysmotility after operation for Hirschsprung's disease? Dig Dis Sci. 2002;47(5):1049–64.
77. Swenson O, Rheinlander H, Diamond I. Hirschsprung's disease: a new concept of the etiology. N Engl J Med. 1949;241:551–6.
78. Swenson O, Bill A. Resection of the rectum and rectosigmoid with preservation of the sphincter for benign spastic lesions producing megacolon. Surgery. 1948;24:212–20.
79. Kubota M, Ito Y, Ikeda K. Membrane properties and innervation of smooth muscle cells in Hirschsprung's disease. Am J Physiol. 1983;244(4): G406–15.
80. Kubota M, et al. Regional differences in the pattern of neurogenic responses in the aganglionic colon from congenitally aganglionic rats. J Pediatr Surg. 1989;24(9):911–9.
81. Kubota M, et al. Electrophysiological properties of the aganglionic segment in Hirschsprung's disease. Surgery. 2002;131(1 Suppl):S288–93.

Epidemiology and Clinical Characteristics of Hirschsprung's Disease

10

Prem Puri and Hiroki Nakamura

Contents

10.1 Introduction

Although Harald Hirschsprung first described this disease in 1888, the pathological features were not understood until the 1940s when Whitehouse and Kernohan demonstrated that the aganglionosis within the distal colon or rectum was the cause of the functional obstruction [56]. In 1948, Swenson and Bill reported rectosigmoidectomy with preservation of the sphincter as the optimal treatment for HSCR [51]. In recent years, the vast majority of cases of HSCR are diagnosed in the neonatal period, and many centers are now performing one-stage pull-through operations in the newborn period with minimal morbidity and encouraging results (Puri et al. 2018).

P. Puri (✉) · H. Nakamura
National Children's Research Centre, Our Lady's Children's Hospital, Crumlin, Dublin, Ireland
e-mail: prem.puri@ncrc.ie

10.2 Incidence

Several studies on the incidence of HSCR have been reported. The incidence of HSCR is estimated to be 1 in 5000 live births and ranges from 1 in 2000 to 1 in 12,000 live births (Table 10.1) [1, 6–8, 10, 18, 34, 39, 40, 49]. Recently, a large survey of HSCR cases from a population database in California found 2464 cases of HSCR among 9.3 million births during 1995–2013, with an incidence of 2.2 cases per 10,000 live births [3]. Incidence varied by race, with the highest rates seen among African Americans at 4.1 per 10,000 live births, Asian/Pacific children at 2.5 per 10,000 live births compared to 1.9 cases per 10,000 live births among white/Caucasian children. The incidence of HSCR in the UK and Ireland is reported to be 1.8 per 10,000 live births [9]. The incidence of HSCR is 1.91 per 10,000 live births in Sweden [25]. Recently, Taguchi et al. reported that the incidence of HSCR in Japan during 1978–2012 was 1.96 per 10,000 live births [54]. The incidence of HSCR in

P. Puri (ed.), *Hirschsprung's Disease and Allied Disorders*,
https://doi.org/10.1007/978-3-030-15647-3_10

Table 10.1 Incidence of Hirschsprung's disease

Author	Year	Incidence	Area
Althoff W	1962	1 in 12,000	Bremen
Bodian M et al.	1963	1 in 2000–10,000	Britain
Madsen C	1964	1 in 4700	Denmark
Passerge E	1967	1 in 5000	Cincinnati
Orr JD et al.	1983	1 in 4500	Southeast Scotland
Goldberg EL et al.	1984	1 in 5682	Baltimore
Ikeda K et al.	1984	1 in 4697	Japan
Spouge D et al.	1985	1 in 4417	British Columbia
Russell MB et al.	1994	1 in 7165	Denmark
Raja A. et al.	1997	1 in 3070	Oman
Torfs C et al.	1998	1 in 5405	California
Suita S et al.	2005	1 in 5343	Japan
Best KE et al.	2012	1 in 6135	North of England
Best KE et al.	2014	1 in 8840	Europe
Lof Granstrom A. et al.	2016	1 in 5236	Sweden
Chia ST et al.	2016	1 in 4545	Taiwan
Anderson JE et al.	2018	1 in 4545	California

Ontario, Canada, during 1991–2013 was 2.05 per 10,000 live births [32]. Recently, in a register-based study in Europe, a total 1374 cases of HSCR among 12,146,210 live births were reported, and the total prevalence was 1 in 8840 live births [7]. More recently, a nationwide survey from Taiwan found an incidence of HSCR of 1 in 4545 live births between 1998 and 2010 [10]. A European register-based study has revealed that there is no evidence of a significant increased risk of HSCR in cases born to women aged ≥35 years compared with those aged 25–29 [7]. A recent population-based case-control study found increased risk of obese females to have children with HSCR [25].

10.3 Extent of Aganglionosis

While the internal anal sphincter is the constant inferior limit, patients can be classified as classical segment HSCR when the aganglionic segment does not extend beyond the upper sigmoid, long-segment HSCR when aganglionosis extends to the splenic flexure or transverse colon, and total colonic aganglionosis when the aganglionic segment extends to the entire colon and a short segment of terminal ileum [38]. Table 10.2 shows the level of aganglionosis in different series with more than 100 patients studied [9, 22, 24, 33, 40, 42, 46, 47, 50, 52]. Total intestinal aganglionosis with absence of ganglion cells from the duodenum to the rectum is the rarest and most severe form of HSCR occurring in less than 1% of patients [30, 41, 44, 45].

10.4 Gender

It has been recognized that males are more commonly affected than females with a male-to-female ratio of 4:1 [6, 7, 18, 22, 24, 25, 33, 40, 42, 50, 54]. The male preponderance is less evident in long-segment HSCR, where the male-to-female ratio is 1:1–2:1 [24, 33, 42] and is even reversed in total colonic aganglionosis, where the male-to-female ratio is 0.8:1 [22]. The reason for these skewed ratios is unclear; no X-linked loci have been described in HSCR.

10.5 Birth Characteristics

A California population-based study comprising 2464 HSCR patients reported median gestational age of HSCR patients to be 39 weeks. This study found that a higher population of patients with HSCR were born preterm (<37 weeks) and a higher population of HSCR patients were low birth weight (<2500 g) compared to patients without HSCR. Duess et al. reported a prevalence rate of 6% of preterm infants born with HSCR [14]. Brandnock et al. reported that 12% of infants with HSCR were born prematurely [9].

10.6 Race

Epidemiological studies have suggested that there may be ethnic variations in the prevalence of HSCR. Recently, one of the largest

Table 10.2 Extent of aganglionosis

Author	Patients (*n*)	Rectosigmoid aganglionosis (%)	Long-segment aganglionosis (%)	Total colonic aganglionosis (%)
Swenson O et al.	498	72.5	23.7	3.8
Kleinhaus S et al.	998	74.0	17.0	9.0
Ikeda K et al.	1562	79.4	11.6	12.6
Orr JD et al.	103	81.6	18.4	–
Sherman JO et al.	874	74.6	22.0	3.5
Ryan ET et al.	179	88.8	3.9	7.3
Russell MB et al.	161	88.2	8.7	3.1
Singh SJ et al.	105	72.4	19.0	8.6
Suita S et al.	1103	77.6	13.0	9.4
Brandnock TJ et al.	270	73.3	22.2	3.0

population-based studies of the epidemiology of HSCR from California from 1995 to 2012 found that the incidence of HSCR varied by race [3]. The incidence was highest among African American (4.1/10,000 births) and Asians (2.5/10,000 births) compared to white/Caucasian and Hispanics (1.9/10,000 births). In another recent study, Chia et al. reported a total of 629 HSCR cases with an overall incidence of 2.2 in 10,000 live births in Taiwanese children [10]. Goldberg, in a previous epidemiological study, found the incidence of HSCR among nonwhite males to be 3.76 in 10,000 live births [18]. A survey of the Members of the Surgical Section of the AAP found that long-segment disease occurs significantly less frequently in nonwhites than in whites [24]. Sherman et al. later confirmed these findings [46]. Although the higher incidence of HSCR reported in the literature is 3.3 in 10,000 from a survey in Oman, this is unlikely to be due to racial differences but to a high consanguinity rate [39]. Recently, Taghavi et al. [53] reported a total of 246 patients with HSCR in New Zealand. The prevalence of HSCR was 2.6 in 10,000 live births for European, 1.5 in 10,000 among Maori, 5.5 in 10,000 among Pacific patients, 2.6 in 10,000 among Asian, and 1.8 in 10,000 among Middle Eastern. In New Zealand, the prevalence of HSCR was statistically significantly greater in Pacific People ($p < 0.0005$) [53]. The proportion of children with long-segment HSCR was also significantly greater in Pacific and Asian populations compared to others ($p = 0.04$) [53].

10.7 Heredity

HSCR is known to occur in families. The reported incidence of familial cases in rectosigmoid HSCR varies from 3.6% to 7.8% in different series [38]. A familial incidence of 15–21% has been reported in total colonic aganglionosis and 50% in the rare total intestinal aganglionosis [4]. Schiller et al. [43] reported 22 infants belonging to four families from Gaza, who had either documented or clinically suspected HSCR. Of these infants, 13 underwent laparotomy and multiple intestinal biopsies, 10 had total intestinal aganglionosis, 1 had total colonic aganglionosis, 1 had near total colonic aganglionosis, and only 1 had rectosigmoid HSCR. Engum et al. [16] reported 20 patients with HSCR in 12 kindreds. The level of aganglionosis was rectal or rectosigmoid in eight, left colon in two, transverse or right colon in two, and total colonic ganglionosis with variable small bowel involvement in eight. Recently, Moore and Zaahl [29] reported 45 patients with HSCR in 35 kindreds. Aganglionosis was significantly more frequent with total colonic aganglionosis in 40% familial cases. HSCR in twins is extremely rare. Henderson et al. [20] found HSCR in 24 of 36 twin subjects, of which 83% affected were males.

10.8 Syndromic Hirschsprung's Disease

HSCR occurs as an isolated trait in over 70% of patients. A chromosomal abnormality is associated with HSCR in 12% of patients, trisomy 21 being by far the most frequent (>90%). The clinical association between trisomy 21 (Down's syndrome) and HSCR is well-established, being of the order of 5%, and remains the most common congenital association with HSCR [27]. Other authors have reported the occurrence of Down's syndrome in 4.5–16% of all patients with HSCR [26, 28, 42]. Other chromosomal abnormalities that have been described in association with HSCR include interstitial deletion of distal 13q, partial deletion of 2p, reciprocal translation, and trisomy 18 mosaic. A number of unusual hereditary syndromes have been reported in patients with HSCR. These include Shah-Waardenburg syndrome, multiple endocrine neoplasia (MEN) type 2 syndrome, congenital central hypoventilation syndrome (Ondine's curse), Goldberg-Shprintzen syndrome, Kaufman-McKusick syndrome, Bardet-Biedl syndrome, Smith-Lemli-Opitz syndrome, cartilage-hair hypoplasia syndrome, and syndromes with HSCR and distal limbs anomalies (Table 10.3) [2, 17, 42]. In the European surveillance, Best et al. [7] reported, of the 1322 singleton cases, 15 (1.1%) occurred with genetic syndromes (including microdeletions) and 131 (9.9%) occurred with chromosomal anomalies. They have also reported that the most common genetic syndrome associated with a chromosomal anomaly was Down's syndrome [7].

Associated congenital anomalies have been reported in around 20% of HSCR patients [35] and include cardiac malformations, gastrointestinal malformations, kidney and urinary tract (CAKUT) malformations, craniofacial anomalies, cleft palate, and polydactyly. Associated congenital cardiac anomalies have been reported in 5–8% of patients with HSCR [13, 21, 55]. An associated urological anomaly has been reported in 4% of patients with HSCR [9, 21]. The association between HSCR and multiple endocrine neoplasia type 2a (MEN2A) has been reported rarely. Coyle et al. [12] found that while the overall incidence of HSCR co-occurring with MEN2A is low, both conditions occur with a relatively high frequency in families with a RET mutation at exon 10. In a literature search, they found that the co-occurrence of HSCR and MEN2A was recorded in 84 cases [12].

Table 10.3 Partial list of syndromes associated with Hirschsprung's disease

Syndrome	Features
Neurocristopathies	
Shah-Waardenburg	Pigmentary anomalies, deafness
Congenital central hypoventilation	Abnormal autonomic control of respiration
Multiple endocrine neoplasia 2A	Medullary thyroid carcinoma, pheochromocytoma, hyperplasia of the parathyroid
Non-neurocristopathies	
Goldberg-Shprintzen	Cleft palate, hypotonia, microcephaly, mental retardation
HSCR with limb anomalies	Polydactyly, brachydactyly, or nail hypoplasia with other assorted anomalies
BRESEK	Brain abnormalities, retardation, ectodermal dysplasia, skeletal malformations, Hirschsprung's disease, ear/eye anomalies, kidney dysplasia
Bardet-Biedl	Pigmentary retinopathy, obesity, hypogenitalism, mild mental retardation, postaxial polydactyly
Kaufman-McKusick	Hydrometrocolpos, postaxial polydactyly, congenital heart defect
Mowat-Wilson	Deviant facial features, defects of the central nervous system (agenesis of the corpus callosum), heart defects, and intestinal aganglionosis

10.9 Clinical Presentation

HSCR should be considered in any child who has a history of constipation dating back to the newborn period. The median age at which children are diagnosed with HSCR has progressively decreased over the past decades with greater awareness of the disease. Of all the cases of HSCR, 80–90% produce clinical symptoms and are diagnosed in the neonatal period. Delayed passage of meconium is the cardinal symptom in neonates with HSCR. Over 90% of affected patients fail to pass meconium in the first 24 hours of life. The usual presentation of HSCR in the neonatal period is with constipation, abdominal distention, and bile-stained vomiting. Recently, in a European surveillance, which collected 1039 isolated cases of HSCR between 1980 and 2009, Best et al. [7] reported that time of diagnosis was known in 803 (77.3%) isolated cases. A congenital anomaly was antenatally suspected in 11 (1.4%) isolated cases. HSCR was diagnosed at birth in 161 (20.0%) cases, in the first week in 354 (44.1%) cases, between 1 and 4 weeks in 116 (14.4%) cases, between 1 and 12 months in 95 (11.8%) cases, and after 12 months in 25 (3.1%) cases [7]. The remaining 41 cases were postnatally diagnosed but at an unknown time. The Australian Paediatric Surveillance Unit in a prospective survey from 1997 to 2000 has reported that the diagnosis of HSCR in the newborn period is made in 90.5% of patients [47]. The neonate with HSCR is usually a full-term baby [22, 23, 36, 42] and presents with a distended abdomen, with feeding intolerance with bilious aspirates or bilious vomiting, and classically, with delay in the passage of meconium (Fig. 10.1). In many cases a rectal examination or rectal irrigation causes passage of meconium and relief of acute intestinal obstruction.

Among normal full-term infants, 98% pass meconium in the first 24 hours of life and the remainder will pass their first stool by 48 hours [11, 37]. It has always been said that over 90% of HSCR infants fail to pass meconium in the first 24 hours of life [38]. However, several authors have found that more than 40% of HSCR newborns pass meconium in the first 24 hours of life [23, 47]. Thus, one should not be dissuaded from carrying out a rectal suction biopsy in the absence of a history of delayed passage of meconium. A prenatal history suggestive of intestinal obstruction is rare, except in children with total colonic aganglionosis [5]. Occasionally, a diagnosis of HSCR should be considered in the presence of unexplained perforation of the cecum or appendix, although this is a rare presentation [36, 48, 52]. Some children do not become obstructed in the neonatal period and present later in infancy or even adolescence or adulthood with severe constipation, chronic abdominal distension, and failure to thrive [38]. This is most common among breast-fed infants who may develop constipation around the time of weaning [38]. Rectal examination of patients with HSCR may show a tight anus [38]. The differential diagnosis for HSCR is shown in Table 10.4. After a careful history and physical examination, the diagnostic steps will include barium enema, anorectal manometry, and a rectal biopsy.

About one third of babies with HSCR present with diarrhea. Diarrhea in HSCR is always a symptom of enterocolitis, which is the commonest cause of morbidity and mortality. The

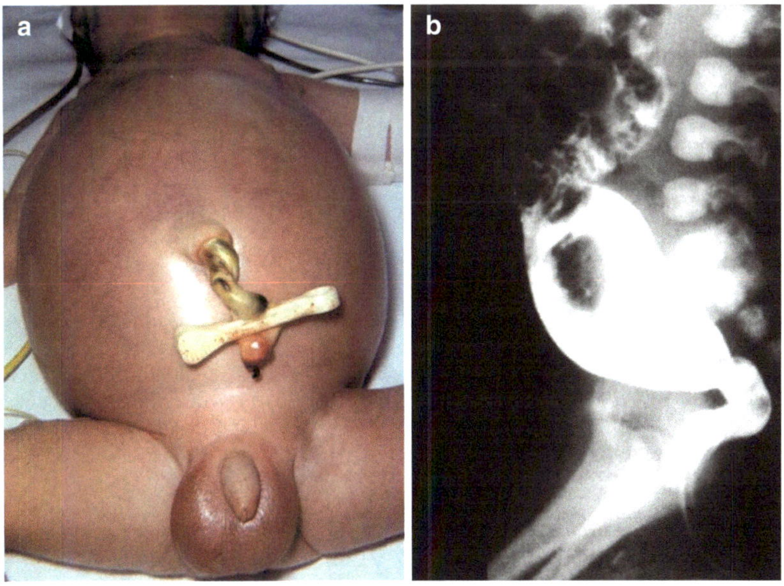

Fig. 10.1 (**a**) Newborn with Hirschsprung's disease. (**b**) Barium enema in the same infant showing clearly a transitional zone in rectosigmoid HSCR

Table 10.4 Differential diagnosis of Hirschsprung's disease

Neonatal bowel obstruction	Meconium ileus resulting from cystic fibrosis
	Ileal or colonic atresia
	Meconium plug syndrome
	Malrotation
	Congenital band
	Anorectal malformation
	Intestinal motility disorders/ pseudo-obstruction
	Necrotizing enterocolitis
	Medical causes: sepsis, electrolyte abnormalities, drugs, hypothyroidism, etc.
Chronic constipation	Functional megacolon
	Intestinal motility disorders/ pseudo-obstruction
	Medical causes: electrolyte abnormalities, drugs, hypothyroidism, etc.

classic symptoms of Hirschsprung-associated enterocolitis (HAEC) include abdominal distention, fever, and diarrhea. However, there is a broad clinical spectrum with which infants with HAEC may present, and other signs or symptoms may include vomiting, rectal bleeding, lethargy, loose stools, and obstipation [19]. The reported incidence of HAEC varies widely, ranging from 6% to 60% prior to definitive pull-through operation and from 25% to 37% postoperation [15, 19, 31]. While all patients with HSCR have a risk of HAEC, several features appear to be associated with an increased risk. These include Down's syndrome, long-segment aganglionosis, prior HAEC, and obstruction from any cause [19].

10.10 Conclusion

HSCR is a relatively common cause of functional bowel obstruction in the newborn. Several large population-based studies have shown evidence of a small increasing trend in HSCR and differences in prevalence by geographic distribution.

References

1. Althoff W. On the genetics of Hirschsprung's disease. Z Mensch Vererb Konstitutionsl. 1962;36:314–40.
2. Amiel J, Lyonnet S. Hirschsprung disease, associated syndromes, and genetics: a review. J Med Genet. 2001;38(11):729–39.
3. Anderson JE, Vanover MA, Saadai P, Stark RA, Stephenson JT, Hirose S. Epidemiology of Hirschsprung disease in California from 1995 to 2013. Pediatr Surg Int. 2018;34(12):1299–303.
4. Badner JA, Sieber WK, Garver KL, Chakravarti A. A genetic study of Hirschsprung disease. Am J Hum Genet. 1990;46(3):568–80.
5. Belin B, Corteville J, Langer J. How accurate is prenatal sonography for the diagnosis of imperforate anus and Hirschsprung's disease? Pediatr Surg Int. 1995;10:30–2.
6. Best KE, Glinianaia SV, Bythell M, Rankin J. Hirschsprung's disease in the North of England: prevalence, associated anomalies, and survival. Birth Defects Res A Clin Mol Teratol. 2012;94(6): 477–80.
7. Best KE, Addor MC, Arriola L, Balku E, Barisic I, Bianchi F, et al. Hirschsprung's disease prevalence in Europe: a register based study. Birth Defects Res A Clin Mol Teratol. 2014;100(9):695–702.
8. Bodian M, Carter C. A family study of Hirschsprung's disease. Ann Hum Genet. 1963;26:261–77.
9. Bradnock TJ, Knight M, Kenny S, Nair M, Walker GM. British association of paediatric surgeons congenital anomalies surveillance S. Hirschsprung's disease in the UK and Ireland: incidence and anomalies. Arch Dis Child. 2017;102(8):722–7.
10. Chia ST, Chen SC, Lu CL, Sheu SM, Kuo HC. Epidemiology of Hirschsprung's disease in Taiwanese children: a 13-year Nationwide Population-based Study. Pediatr Neonatol. 2016;57(3):201–6.
11. Clark DA. Times of first void and first stool in 500 newborns. Pediatrics. 1977;60(4):457–9.
12. Coyle D, Friedmacher F, Puri P. The association between Hirschsprung's disease and multiple endocrine neoplasia type 2a: a systematic review. Pediatr Surg Int. 2014;30(8):751–6.
13. Duess JW, Puri P. Syndromic Hirschsprung's disease and associated congenital heart disease: a systematic review. Pediatr Surg Int. 2015;31(8):781–5.
14. Duess JW, Hofmann AD, Puri P. Prevalence of Hirschsprung's disease in premature infants: a systematic review. Pediatr Surg Int. 2014;30(8): 791–5.
15. El-Sawaf M, Siddiqui S, Mahmoud M, Drongowski R, Teitelbaum DH. Probiotic prophylaxis after pullthrough for Hirschsprung disease to reduce incidence of enterocolitis: a prospective, randomized, double-blind, placebo-controlled, multicenter trial. J Pediatr Surg. 2013;48(1):111–7.

16. Engum SA, Petrites M, Rescorla FJ, Grosfeld JL, Morrison AM, Engles D. Familial Hirschsprung's disease: 20 cases in 12 kindreds. J Pediatr Surg. 1993;28(10):1286–90.
17. Gariepy CE. Genetic basis of Hirschsprung disease: implications in clinical practice. Mol Genet Metab. 2003;80(1–2):66–73.
18. Goldberg EL. An epidemiological study of Hirschsprung's disease. Int J Epidemiol. 1984;13(4): 479–85.
19. Gosain A, Frykman PK, Cowles RA, Horton J, Levitt M, Rothstein DH, et al. Guidelines for the diagnosis and management of Hirschsprung-associated enterocolitis. Pediatr Surg Int. 2017;33(5):517–21.
20. Henderson D, Zimmer J, Nakamura H, Puri P. Hirschsprung's disease in twins: a systematic review and meta-analysis. Pediatr Surg Int. 2017;33(8):855–9.
21. Hofmann AD, Duess JW, Puri P. Congenital anomalies of the kidney and urinary tract (CAKUT) associated with Hirschsprung's disease: a systematic review. Pediatr Surg Int. 2014;30(8):757–61.
22. Ikeda K, Goto S. Diagnosis and treatment of Hirschsprung's disease in Japan. An analysis of 1628 patients. Ann Surg. 1984;199(4):400–5.
23. Klein MD, Coran AG, Wesley JR, Drongowski RA. Hirschsprung's disease in the newborn. J Pediatr Surg. 1984;19(4):370–4.
24. Kleinhaus S, Boley SJ, Sheran M, Sieber WK. Hirschsprung's disease – a survey of the members of the Surgical Section of the American Academy of Pediatrics. J Pediatr Surg. 1979;14(5):588–97.
25. Lof Granstrom A, Svenningsson A, Hagel E, Oddsberg J, Nordenskjold A, Wester T. Maternal risk factors and perinatal characteristics for Hirschsprung disease. Pediatrics. 2016;138(1):e20154608.
26. Menezes M, Puri P. Long-term clinical outcome in patients with Hirschsprung's disease and associated Down's syndrome. J Pediatr Surg. 2005;40(5):810–2.
27. Moore SW. Advances in understanding the association between Down syndrome and Hirschsprung disease (DS-HSCR). Pediatr Surg Int. 2018;34:1127.
28. Moore SW, Zaahl MG. Intronic RET gene variants in Down syndrome-associated Hirschsprung disease in an African population. J Pediatr Surg. 2012;47(2):299–302.
29. Moore SW, Zaahl M. Clinical and genetic correlations of familial Hirschsprung's disease. J Pediatr Surg. 2015;50(2):285–8.
30. Nakamura H, Henderson D, Puri P. A meta-analysis of clinical outcome of intestinal transplantation in patients with total intestinal aganglionosis. Pediatr Surg Int. 2017;33(8):837–41.
31. Nakamura H, Lim T, Puri P. Probiotics for the prevention of Hirschsprung-associated enterocolitis: a systematic review and meta-analysis. Pediatr Surg Int. 2018;34(2):189–93.
32. Nasr A, Sullivan KJ, Chan EW, Wong CA, Benchimol EI. Validation of algorithms to determine incidence of Hirschsprung disease in Ontario, Canada: a population-based study using health administrative data. Clin Epidemiol. 2017;9:579–90.
33. Orr JD, Scobie WG. Presentation and incidence of Hirschsprung's disease. Br Med J (Clin Res Ed). 1983;287(6406):1671.
34. Passarge E. The genetics of Hirschsprung's disease. Evidence for heterogeneous etiology and a study of sixty-three families. N Engl J Med. 1967;276(3):138–43.
35. Pini Prato A, Rossi V, Mosconi M, Holm C, Lantieri F, Griseri P, et al. A prospective observational study of associated anomalies in Hirschsprung's disease. Orphanet J Rare Dis. 2013;8:184.
36. Polley TZ Jr, Coran AG, Wesley JR. A ten-year experience with ninety-two cases of Hirschsprung's disease. Including sixty-seven consecutive endorectal pull-through procedures. Ann Surg. 1985;202(3):349–55.
37. Puri P, Montedonico S. Hirschsprung's disease: clinical features. In: Holschneider AM, Puri P, editors. Hirschsprung's disease and allied disorders. 3rd ed. Berlin/Heidelberg: Springer; 2008. p. 107–13.
38. Puri P, Tomuschat C. Hirschsprung's disease. In: Puri P, editor. Newborn surgery. 4th ed. Florida: CRC Press; 2018. p. 667–83.
39. Rajab A, Freeman NV, Patton MA. Hirschsprung's disease in Oman. J Pediatr Surg. 1997;32(5):724–7.
40. Russell MB, Russell CA, Niebuhr E. An epidemiological study of Hirschsprung's disease and additional anomalies. Acta Paediatr. 1994;83(1):68–71.
41. Ruttenstock E, Puri P. A meta-analysis of clinical outcome in patients with total intestinal aganglionosis. Pediatr Surg Int. 2009;25(10):833–9.
42. Ryan ET, Ecker JL, Christakis NA, Folkman J. Hirschsprung's disease: associated abnormalities and demography. J Pediatr Surg. 1992;27(1): 76–81.
43. Schiller M, Levy P, Shawa RA, Abu-Dalu K, Gorenstein A, Katz S. Familial Hirschsprung's disease–a report of 22 affected siblings in four families. J Pediatr Surg. 1990;25(3):322–5.
44. Senyuz OF, Buyukunal C, Danismend N, Erdogan E, Ozbay G, Soylet Y. Extensive intestinal aganglionosis. J Pediatr Surg. 1989;24(5):453–6.
45. Sharif K, Beath SV, Kelly DA, McKiernan P, van Mourik I, Mirza D, et al. New perspective for the management of near-total or total intestinal aganglionosis in infants. J Pediatr Surg. 2003;38(1):25–8; discussion-8.
46. Sherman JO, Snyder ME, Weitzman JJ, Jona JZ, Gillis DA, O'Donnell B, et al. A 40-year multinational retrospective study of 880 Swenson procedures. J Pediatr Surg. 1989;24(8):833–8.
47. Singh SJ, Croaker GD, Manglick P, Wong CL, Athanasakos H, Elliott E, et al. Hirschsprung's disease: the Australian Paediatric Surveillance

Unit's experience. Pediatr Surg Int. 2003;19(4):247–50.
48. Soper RT, Opitz JM. Neonatal pneumoperitoneum and Hirschsprung's disease. Surgery. 1962;51:527–33.
49. Spouge D, Baird PA. Hirschsprung disease in a large birth cohort. Teratology. 1985;32(2):171–7.
50. Suita S, Taguchi T, Ieiri S, Nakatsuji T. Hirschsprung's disease in Japan: analysis of 3852 patients based on a nationwide survey in 30 years. J Pediatr Surg. 2005;40(1):197–201; discussion-2.
51. Swenson O, Bill AH Jr. Resection of rectum and rectosigmoid with preservation of the sphincter for benign spastic lesions producing megacolon; an experimental study. Surgery. 1948;24(2):212–20.
52. Swenson O, Sherman JO, Fisher JH. Diagnosis of congenital megacolon: an analysis of 501 patients. J Pediatr Surg. 1973;8(5):587–94.
53. Taghavi K, Goddard L, Evans SM, Hobson A, Beasley SW, Sankaran S, et al. Ethnic variations in the childhood prevalence of Hirschsprung disease in New Zealand. ANZ J Surg. 2018. https://doi.org/10.1111/ans.14857.
54. Taguchi T, Obata S, Ieiri S. Current status of Hirschsprung's disease: based on a nationwide survey of Japan. Pediatr Surg Int. 2017;33(4):497–504.
55. Tuo G, Pini Prato A, Derchi M, Mosconi M, Mattioli G, Marasini M. Hirschsprung's disease and associated congenital heart defects: a prospective observational study from a single institution. Front Pediatr. 2014;2:99.
56. Whitehouse FR, Kernohan JW. Myenteric plexus in congenital megacolon; study of 11 cases. Arch Intern Med (Chic). 1948;82(1):75–111.

Congenital Anomalies and Genetic Associations in Hirschsprung's Disease

11

Samuel William Moore

Contents

S. W. Moore (✉)
Division of Pediatric Surgery, Faculty of Medicine and Health Sciences, University of Stellenbosch, Stellenbosch, South Africa
e-mail: swm@sun.ac.za

11.1 Introduction

Hirschsprung's disease (HSCR) is a complex congenital disorder mostly of genetic origin, which, from a molecular perspective, appears to result from disruption of normal signalling during development of enteric nerve cells resulting in aganglionosis of the distal bowel. It is a frequent cause of neonatal intestinal obstruction and is not infrequently associated with congenital abnormalities (5–32%) and syndromic phenotypes [1, 2]. These have been linked to distinct genetic sites, indicating underlying genetic associations of the disease and probable gene-gene interaction in its pathogenesis. HSCR is a complex disease as is shown by the number of genes implicated in its pathogenesis (at least 11 genes and 5 gene loci have reportedly been associated with HSCR) [3]. In addition, these genetic variations account for more than 50% of the observed abnormalities associated with HSCR. These associations

P. Puri (ed.), *Hirschsprung's Disease and Allied Disorders*,
https://doi.org/10.1007/978-3-030-15647-3_11

are significant for at least two reasons: *Firstly*, the majority of associated anomalies may be attributed to abnormal genetic signalling and cross talk during development, yielding clues as to the genetic background of HSCR and its pathogenesis. *Secondly*, the associated anomalies influence the long-term prognosis of the patients. It therefore remains important to examine the roles of functionally related genes in HSCR and these associations to identify cell signalling pathways that interact to influence the final phenotypic expression. This is particularly true of deletions that encompass important gene areas.

A better understanding of the biological pathophysiologic signalling pathways, where genes and interactive mechanisms interact in the pathogenesis of HSCR, is necessary to understand related functional gastrointestinal (GIT) anomalies. In this endeavour, it is important to characterize phenotypic expression by exploring cell functionality and biology by researching clustered RNA sequences and microarray data to determine the interaction of involved genetically interlinked signalling systems and to assist understanding of the various phenotypic expressions of these fascinating conditions.

11.2 HSCR-Associated Conditions and Anomalies

Some of the syndromic phenotypes have been linked to distinct genetic sites, indicating underlying genetic associations of the disease and probable gene-gene interaction in its pathogenesis.

There are also a number of known associations between congenital anomalies and an increased risk of HSCR. These include Down syndrome (DS) [4], dominant sensorineural deafness [5], Waardenburg syndrome [4, 6], neurofibromatosis, neuroblastoma [4], phaeochromocytoma [4], the MEN Type IIB syndrome [7, 8] and other abnormalities [4].

11.2.1 Association of Trisomy 21 and Down Syndrome with Congenital Aganglionosis

The association between trisomy 21 and HSCR remains the most commonly encountered associated syndrome (Table 11.1).

Table 11.1 Congenital anomalies in HSCR

Author	Year	Country	No. of patients	Ass Anom%
Passarge [4]	1967	USA: Cincinnati	63	11.1
Kilcoyne [9]	1970	USA: Oakland, Cal	31	32.2
Ehrenpreiss [10]	1970	Norway	124	5
Spouge [11]	1985	Canada: Vancouver	178	29.7
Polley and Coran [12]	1986	USA: Ann Arbor	99	26
Ikeda and Goto [13]	1986	Japan	1628	11.1
Sieber [14]	1990	USA: Detroit	220	19
Lister & Rickham [15]	1990	UK: Liverpool	120	20.8
Swenson [16]	1990	USA: Chicago	172	26.1
Ryan [17]	1992	USA: Boston	321	22
Engum and Grosfeld [18]	1993	USA: Indianapolis	20	25
Klein [19]	1993	USA: Detroit	250	18
Moore [20]	1993	South Africa	370	16
Halevy [21]	1994	Israel	65	29.2
Sarioglu [22]	1997	Turkey: Ankara	302	27.4
Das [23]	2001	India	35	11.4
Holschneider and Ure [24]	2003	Germany: Cologne	203	35
Singh [25]	2003	Australia: Sydney	127	25.9
Pini [26]	2013	Italy: Genoa	106	57–5
Total			4434	24.9(av)

Apart from being the commonest congenital abnormality encountered in humans (occurring in approximately 1 out of every 800 live births worldwide), Down syndrome (trisomy 21) has a clear clinical association with aganglionosis of the colon (DS-HSCR). It occurs in approximately 5–7% of HSCR patients, and remains one of the consistent associations in most HSCR studies [4, 27, 28], appearing up to 50 times more frequently in association with HSCR than in the general population [29]. A review of 19 reported series is shown in Table 11.2, where the mean prevalence was 6.99%. This is higher than that usually quoted in the literature.

DS is characterized by clinically recognizable typical phenotypic features but also exhibits a fairly extensive phenotypic variability. The classical features include decreased muscle tone (floppy baby), skeletal defects (short stature, brachycephaly), neurological deficits (including learning difficulties and hearing deficits), congenital heart disease (especially cushion defects), and a number of other defects which lead to a variety of associated clinical problems.

Among the associated clinical problems are a variety of recognized associated congenital anomalies and malfunction of the gastrointestinal tract (GIT) which can be difficult for the individual patient. In addition to a number of associated structural anomalies, malfunction of the GIT is common affecting 77% of DS patients [38].

Many of these GIT problems relate to the abnormal function of the enteric nervous system (ENS) which represents the intricate intrinsic innervation of the GIT and is vital for normal GIT function at all stages of postnatal life.

The reasons for ENS involvement in trisomy 21 are, as yet, not completely clear. One potential reason is that central nervous system (CNS) developmental processes such as neural patterning, neuronal and axonal migration and synaptic development all appear to be affected in DS in general. Despite this, there has been little consensus as to the possible aetiologic and genetic factors influencing the association with HSCR and the ENS.

The various ways in which trisomy of chromosome influences the ENS is becoming clearer. The sum of these effects influences the outcome of surgery in DS-HSCR.

Table 11.2 Down syndrome associated with HSCR

Author	Year	Country	No. of patients	DS %
Bodian [30]	1963	London	220	1.47
Passarge [4]	1967	USA: Cincinnati	63	9.5
Kilcoyne [9]	1970	USA: Oakland, Cal	31	16.1
Goldberg [31]	1984	USA: Baltimore	33	9
Garver [32]	1985	USA: Pittsburgh	263	5.9
Spouge [11]	1985	Canada: Vancouver	178	2.8
Caniano [33]	1990	USA: Columbus; oh	80	2.8
Molander [34]	1990	Sweden: Stockholm	90	2.9
Ikeda [13]	1986	Japan	1628	15.5
Lister Lister	1990	UK: Liverpool	880	4.2
Swenson [16]	1990	USA: Chicago	172	3.2
Moore [35]	1991	South Africa	370	3.19
Ryan [17]	1992	USA: Boston	321	8.4
Russell [36]	1994	Denmark	224	2.24
Quinn [37]	1994	Eire: Dublin	135	12.59
Sarioglu [22]	1997	Turkey: Ankara	302	12.5
Das [23]	2001	India	35	5.71
Holschneider [24]	2003	Germany: Cologne	203	6
Singh [25]	2003	Australia	127	10.2
Pini [26]	2013	Italy: Genoa	106	7.54
Total			**5461**	**Mean 6.99**

Recent research has identified a number of levels at which ENS development is potentially affected in trisomy 21. These include a decreased central pool of available neuroblasts for migration into the ENS, abnormal neuroblast type, poor synaptic nerve function, and early germline gene-related influences on the migrating neuroblasts due to genetic mutations of a number of important developmental genes and possible somatic mutations resulting from alterations in the local tissue microenvironment.

There is evidence of both germline and somatic gene mutations suggesting causation of the association. Although the picture is complex, recent associations between specific *RET* proto-oncogene variations have been shown to be significant in HSCR in DS-HSCR patients as they probably interfere with vital RET functions in the development of the autonomic nervous system and ENS, increasing the risk of disturbed normal function. There is also the potential role of other susceptibility genes as well as potential other chromosome 21 gene actions and their influence on the microenvironment on the DS gastrointestinal tract.

These pathogenetic mechanisms include:

- A decreased pool of available neuroblasts for migration into the ENS. Histological studies have shown the DS brain to have both a decreased number and density of neurons in most brain regions in trisomy 21. There is little objective evidence of a decreased pool of ganglion cells in the ENS in DS patients. Reduction of oesophageal plexus ganglia neurons is documented in DS patients [39], where the mean number of neurons per ganglion of the deep submucous plexus in DS oesophagus was observed to be 69% of the control value and 75% in the Auerbach plexus. This may go some way to explain the oesophageal dysfunction, commonly encountered in DS.
- Abnormal neuronal cells in the DS nervous system

  Trisomy 21 affects the development processes of the enteric nervous system. Defective neural patterns with abnormal cellular morphology exist in DS with reductions in synaptic density and surface area along with a decreased number of postsynaptic spines. The existing spines appear abnormally long, thin or irregular in contour and appearance [40, 41].
- Effect of Trisomy 21 on nerve function

  It is becoming clear that the general process affecting the nervous system in DS appears to affect not only microanatomy of nerve cells but also nerve function. Significant differences in action potential and ionic current kinetics have been reported at the neuronal level in DS [42]. Animal experimental models have also shown alterations of intracellular Ca^{2+} signalling pathways in DS in response to a number of other neurotransmitters studied (i.e., glutamate, acetylcholine and GABA) [43].
- Early gene-related influences on the migrating neuroblasts

  Significant differences in action potential and ionic current kinetics have been reported at the neuronal level in DS [42]. Animal experimental models have also shown alterations of intracellular Ca^{2+} signalling pathways in DS in response to a number of other neurotransmitters studied (i.e., glutamate, acetylcholine and GABA) [43].
- Early gene influences on developing neuroblasts

  Variation in the RET proto-oncogene remains the most consistent genetic factor in HSCR pathogenesis, with allelic loss being found in over 80% of cases. However, thus far, no specifically identifiable *RET* mutations in the coding sequence in HSCR-DS have been identified. Results of DNA analysis in our series of DS-HSCR patients [44, 45] showed that, whereas RET variations could be identified in 94% of a DS-HSCR cohort, endothelin B receptor (EDNRB) gene variations occurred in 75%, with a preponderance of a variant in exon 4 (561C/T) in patients with co-existing Down syndrome. This 561C/T (rs 5349) variation has also subsequently been reported in other series [46].
- DSCAM and other special affected areas lie on chromosome 2

In DS-HSCR patients, *DSCAM,* which has been previously shown to map to the HSCR critical region [47] as well as in HSCR in a large Mennonite kindred [48], results in an increased HSCR risk [47].

Jannot et al. [49] have also advanced *DSCAM* as a predisposing locus to HSCR and DS-HSCR in a recent study of 26 DS-HSCR patients. Analysis of partial trisomy 21 phenotypes by Korbel et al. suggested that an extra copy of at least 1 of the 302 genes located in the 13 Mb interval from 33.5 to 46.25 Mb results in an increased HSCR risk [47].

The search for a significant DS Cam gene continues. It would appear to many that, based on available evidence, the flanking *COL6A1* gene is probably of greater importance in HSCR pathogenesis. A recent study [50] reported overexpression of the ATP50 gene from this area as a candidate region in DS HSCR.

- Potential epigenetic and other influences

  The addition of an extra chromosome in trisomy 21 has been shown to affect the methylation status of a number of CpG dinucleotide sites, thus resulting in a genome-wide transcriptional dysregulation. Trisomy 21 thus would appear to change DNA methylation in a variety of mechanisms [51].
- Alterations in the local tissue environment and potential somatic mutations are an important area of consideration in DS-HSCR.

  The local tissue environment (extracellular matrix) consists of a collection of collagen, non-collagenous glycoproteins and proteoglycans which surround the cells and tissues and regulates a number of vital cellular functions. It is well accepted that there are changes in extracellular matrix architecture of DS patients. This is as reflected in the umbilical cords of DS patients in which are found an abnormal amount of glycosaminoglycans and proteoglycans (particularly collagen 6 (ColVI)) [52].

It would therefore appear logical to surmise that a similar structural component to that occurring in the brain also exists in the ENS, leading to malfunction. This is not surprising as chromosome 21 contains the gene that codes for Type VI collagen. In trisomy 21, one subunit of this collagen is often overexpressed, resulting in connective tissue that has a more elastic composition.

A recent SNP association study suggested that excess of the DSCAM region may be important for HSCR pathogenesis in Down syndrome [49]. On the other hand, excess DSCAM has not been confirmed experimentally to cause HSCR-like disease in animal models.

11.3 Hirschsprung-Associated Enterocolitis (HAEC) and Trisomy 21

Despite a strong clinical suspicion, the rate of enterocolitis in children with DS HSCR has been shown not to differ from rates in children with HD alone [53]. However, clinical studies have shown a higher complication and mortality for this association, suggesting that, although possibly not more common, the impaired immune function of trisomy 21 patients carries a higher risk of severity.

Putting together all of the above factors, by which trisomy 21 influences the ENS function and development, it is not surprising that a large number of patients with DS-HSCR continue to have bowel dysfunction which persists after surgical pull-through for HSCR [54]. This suggests a wider ENS dysfunction than the aganglionosis, per se.

Although surgical correction can be achieved in DS-HSCR, patients may require ongoing help in the long term to facilitate acceptable bowel function. While some may achieve acceptable continence following surgical correction, patients with DS-HSCR are generally recognized as having a less confident prognosis [55].

Other strong associations such as dominant sensorineural deafness [5], Waardenburg syndrome [4, 6], neurofibromatosis, neuroblastoma [4], phaeochromocytoma [4], the MEN Type IIB syndrome [7, 8] and other abnormalities [4] will be discussed under their separate areas. These individual abnormalities are also of importance and will be dealt with under the relevant affected system of the body.

11.4 Prevalence of Individual Associated Anomalies

The incidence of particular HSCR-associated anomalies in reported series (4434 cases in 18 series) varied between 5% and 32% with a mean of 24.9% (Table 11.1). The spread of these associated anomalies is shown in the bar graph in Fig. 11.1.

11.4.1 Gastrointestinal Tract Anomalies (8.05%)

Other anomalies of the gastrointestinal system are some of the most frequent associations of HSCR. Signalling pathways and disruption of gene expression have currently been implicated in a number of gastrointestinal conditions, including HSCR, malrotation, anorectal anomalies, pyloric stenosis, Meckel's diverticulum, biliary atresia and pancreatic agenesis and heterotopia, among others.

It stands to reason that similar disrupted molecular pathways may underlie these congenitally acquired conditions.

11.4.1.1 Intestinal Malrotation

There appears to be a clinical association between HSCR and intestinal malrotation [56] with at least 28 infantile cases having been reported [57]. There is probably some measure of underreporting, but there are a number of reports [57–59]. There were also five additional cases in our reported series [20, 35] plus one recent unreported case as well as a further one of our own series (Fig. 11.2). This gives at least a total of 38 reported cases. Midgut volvulus has even been described in one of these malrotated HSCR patients [58].

In this connection, the association of malrotation with features of aganglionic colon has been reported in animal models [60] and more recently in humans and have been associated with Hedgehog signalling cascades.

The association of malrotation and imperforate anus is a further rare association with HSCR, which could possibly also be associated with the Hedgehog signalling pathway [61].

11.4.1.2 Anorectal Malformations (ARM)

It is generally accepted that the association between HSCR and ARM is an uncommon one [62]. We only encountered one out of 408 cases in our series [20, 35].

By way of contrast, anorectal malformations were identified in 2.5% of >1200 cases in another large collective series [63] and has been described in 9 cases from a single centre over

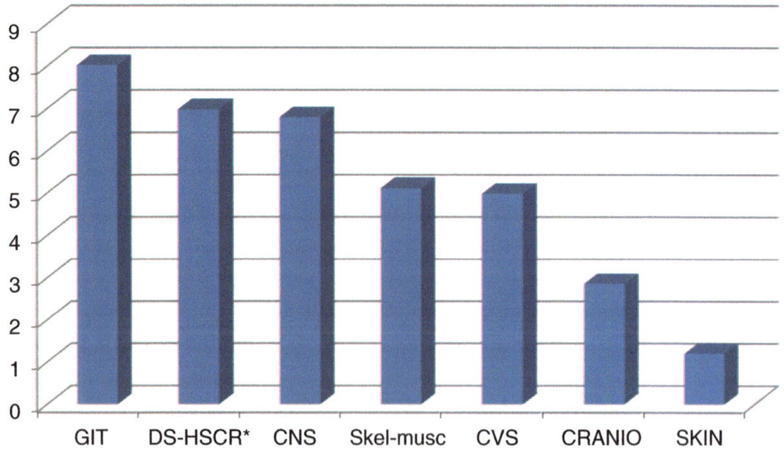

Fig. 11.1 Bar graph showing mean incidence of anomalies associated with HSCR based on analysis of 4434 reported cases in 19 complete series (Table 11.2)

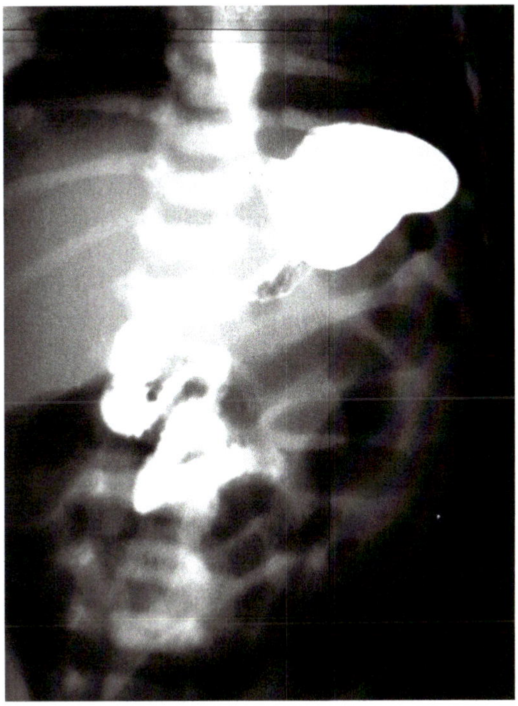

Fig. 11.2 Contrast enema showing malrotation with caecum on left and Hirschsprung's disease

a 10-year period [64]. It has furthermore been recorded in two siblings of consanguineous parents [65] as well as having a similar association with trisomy 21 [66].

Associations with ARM may lead to diagnostic delay of HSCR because of the initial diagnosis of the ARM and the fact that the defunctioning colostomy is proximal to the affected bowel. The association remains of interest due to common associations with major susceptibility genes [67].

11.4.1.3 Intestinal Atresia

Intestinal atresia is an infrequent association with HSCR occurring in at least 32 previously reported cases. Twenty-two of those reported were small bowel atresia in one report with a further eight cases involving the colon. A further 32 cases of small intestinal atresia and 26 colonic atresia have been reported. The association of these two conditions appears higher than the estimated population incidence of 1:2700 (0.04%) [13, 20, 35, 68, 69], and they occur mostly in association with long-segment HSCR [70] and in unfixed colon [69].

The most plausible explanation for the association between HSCR and intestinal atresia is the tendency of a malrotated, obstructed segment of bowel proximal to the aganglionic segment to undergo volvulus [71]. Much of the debate centres on the role of additional localized abnormalities (e.g. duplication cyst) resulting in intestinal volvulus and atresia and the role of HSCR per se [71].

11.4.2 CNS and Brain Anomalies (6.8%)

The incidence of CNS abnormalities and HSCR varies considerably from a mean of 8.3% in our overview of 6387 cases [44] but has been as high as 29% in one large series [22]. However, our calculation did not include those with Down syndrome, which would make a considerable difference to the prevalence. Giving associated neuronal migration brain disorders somewhere around a 23.5% prevalence if DS is included. The effect of trisomy 21 on the ENS is dealt with in another section. A number of reports include the co-segregation of HSCR with mental retardation and neurological impairment [72].

Various dysmorphic features exist within the CNS in HSCR patients, including the absence of the corpus callosum of the brain. Absence of the corpus callosum may occur as an isolated finding or in association with the Goldberg-Shprintzen [73] or Mowat-Wilson syndromes [74].

Anencephaly appears to be a common association with aganglionosis, and autopsies on 12 consecutive anencephalic newborns all showed some degree of aganglionosis [75].

Dandy-Walker abnormalities are possibly associated with chromosome 9 variations [76], a site associated with HSCR in previous reports [77].

The association between brain abnormalities and HSCR is not surprising as brain development is largely controlled by the same neural growth factors as the ENS. Other underlying reported defective signalling systems such as the L1 [78] and the ZFHX1B gene (renamed Zeb 2) [79] are also possible alternatives.

The L1 gene (L1CAM) associations with hydrocephalus and HSCR [80] appear to be more related to hydrocephalus [81]. This may be an important link because the X-linked gene, L1CAM, has been identified as the first modifier gene for members of the endothelin signalling pathway during development of the enteric nervous system.

Mutations in L1CAM may therefore modulate the severity of aganglionosis in some cases of HSCR [82]. On the other hand, the ZFHX1B (ZEB2) gene has also been associated with coloboma of the iris and chromosome 21-linked HSCR [83].

Meningomyelocoele appears to be a further relatively uncommon HSCR association [71, 84] but is significantly absent in a number of other large series [13, 85]. This may therefore be a chance occurrence. However, evidence of one further patient with spina bifida occulta in our series and two cousins of patients with HSCR known to have a meningomyelocoele [86] raises speculation as to the part played by the migration of nerve cells from the neural crest cells at the sacral level as a second source of neural precursor cells in the innervation of the hindgut.

11.4.2.1 Sensory Organs and HSCR

The linked embryology between the skin pigment cells and sensory organ embryology may partly explain the association of these congenital anomalies.

Progenitor melanoblasts migrate between mesodermal and ectodermal layers during embryogenesis to reach their final destinations in the skin epidermis, hair follicular bulbs, inner ear cochlea, choroids, ciliary body and iris. The eyes, therefore, in addition to the skin and hair, can exhibit pigmentary variation [87].

Omenn et al. [88] pointed out the association between HSCR and *Waardenburg syndrome*, which was then linked to the endothelin B receptor gene (EDNRB) [89].

Clinical syndromes associated with HSCR include Waardenburg syndrome and other dominant sensorineural deafness autosomal recessive syndromes, including the Shah-Waardenburg (WS4) syndromes [6].

Waardenburg syndrome is a group of genetic conditions characterized by deafness and pigmentary changes of the hair (white forelock), skin (hypopigmentation), and eyes (heterochromia). Distinctive hair pigmentation is a common sign, and a patch of white hair in front is typical (white forelock) or hair that becomes grey prematurely. The hearing loss is congenital (from birth).

Of the four recognized types of Waardenburg syndrome, Type IV (also known as Waardenburg-Shah syndrome) has signs and symptoms of both Waardenburg syndrome and HSCR (Fig. 11.3).

In addition to the RET proto-oncogene, EDNRB expression in spiral ganglion neurons (SGNs) in the inner ear is required for normal postnatal development of hearing in mice [90]. Significant variations of the endothelin receptor B (EDNRB) and its co-ligand SOX10 have been shown to result in a significantly increased risk of dominant sensorineural deafness in the HSCR patient. Homozygous mutations in both EDNRB alleles result in the full phenotype being expressed in this syndrome,

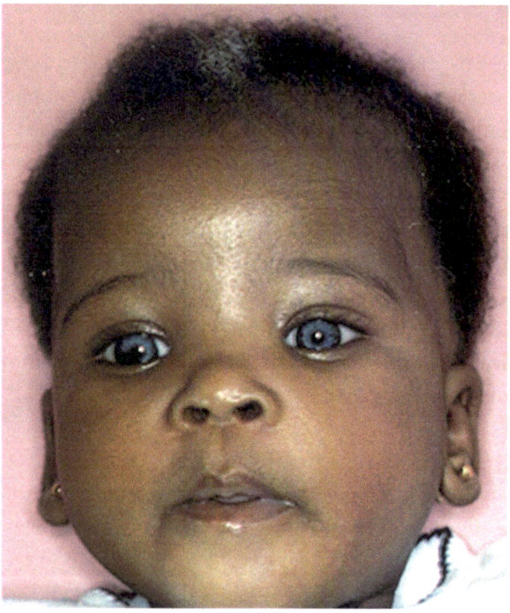

Fig. 11.3 Waardenburg syndrome and Hirschsprung's disease. Note heterochromia, white/grey forelock and hypopigmented patch on the chin. (Photograph per courtesy Prof P Beale)

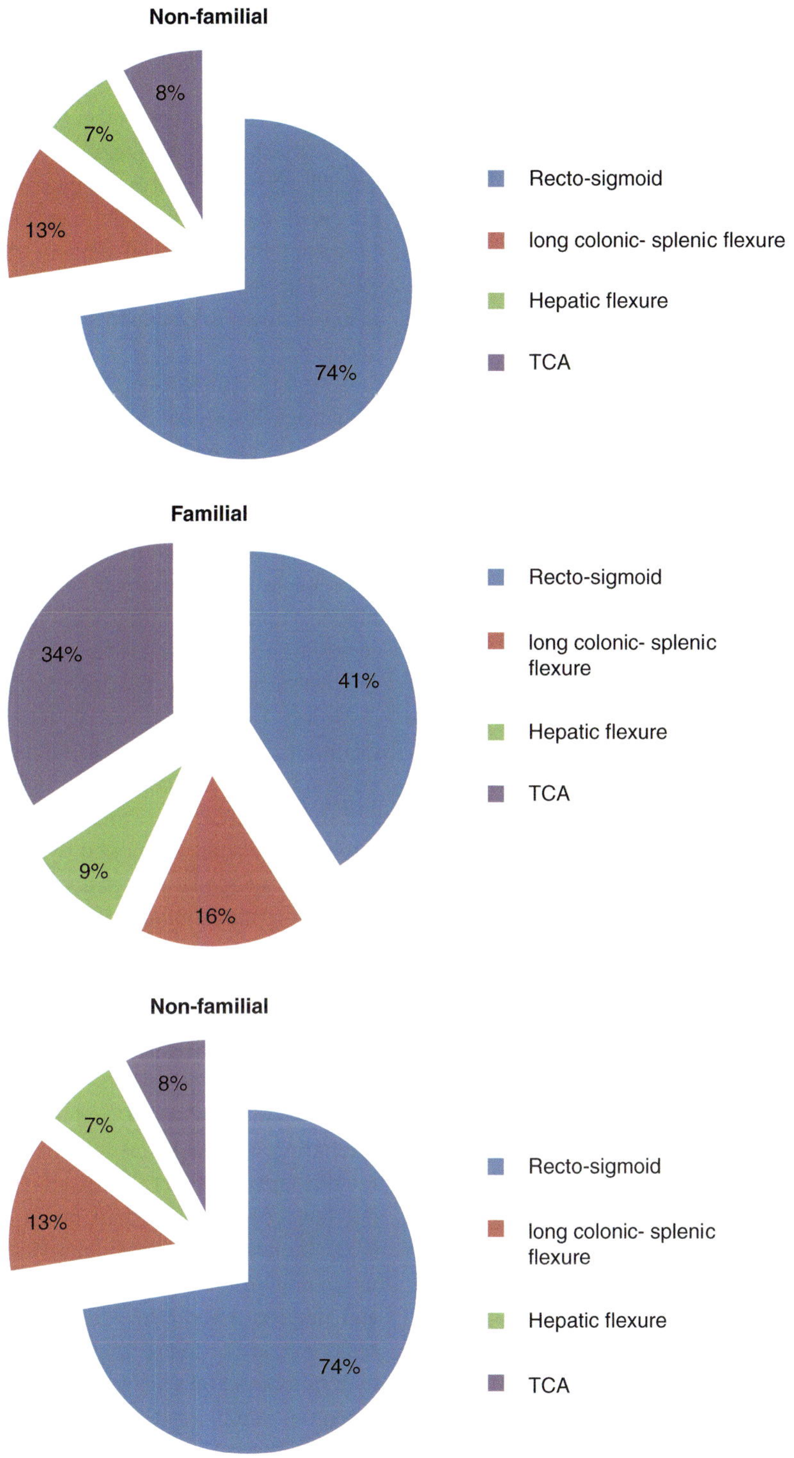

Fig. 11.3 (continued)

whereas heterozygous mutations may result in an isolated expression of HSCR (with or without minor pigmentary anomalies and/or sensorineural deafness) [91]. It has also been shown to play a role in Kallmann syndrome and the Yemenite deaf-blind hypopigmentation syndrome.

Y1062 is a vital autophosphorylation site on RET tyrosine kinase terminal residues that is essential for downstream signalling and normal development of the ENS and the kidney as well as other development. Study of this region has shown that interference with binding at the tyrosine 1062 (Y1062) phosphorylation of RET results in a syndromic form causing neurodegeneration of spiral ganglion neurons (SGNs) in mice resulting in non-syndromic age-related hearing loss [92].

SOX10 encodes a transcription factor expressed during the colonization of neural crest cells in the hindbrain [93]. Only *de novo* or *SOX10* mutations inherited in an autosomal dominant manner are reported in WS4 patients [94, 95]. Defects in *SOX10* have been reported in only a small number of individuals with HSCR and in none with isolated HSCR [96] (Fig. 11.4).

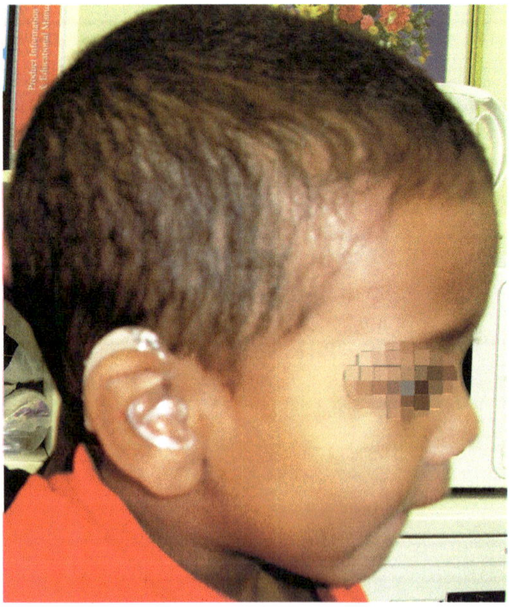

Fig. 11.4 Congenital sensorineural deafness and Hirschsprung's disease

11.4.3 Genitourinary Abnormalities (6.05%)

The reported incidence of genitourinary anomalies also shows considerable variation [1, 10, 20, 22, 35] and is of particular interest as they are much more commonly identified in the RET knockout mouse model than in clinical HSCR [97]. The RET ligands GDNF and GDNFα are also of known importance during its embryogenesis [98].

Certain HSCR-associated syndromes [e.g. McKusick-Kaufman syndrome [99]] include numerous genitourinary anomalies. Those described in association with HSCR include hypospadias as well as undescended testes, congenital kidney anomalies, ureteric duplications, hydronephrosis/hydroureter and disorders of bladder function [100]. Amiel and Lyonnet [1] reported a 4.4% renal agenesis (of particular interest because of RET gene involvement) plus a further 2–3% incidence of genital anomalies. Genitourinary anomalies can be divided between congenital (3%) and functional conditions (2.5–36%) [100]. A reported lack of Mullerian inhibiting substance reported by Cass et al. [101] would fit with the one patient with ambiguous genitalia reported in our series [35, 102].

11.4.4 Skeletal, Muscle and Limb Anomalies (5.12%)

Skeletal, muscle, limb and digital anomalies (including sacral agenesis and extremity defects) involve approximately 4.6% of HSCR patients but have been reported to be as high as 24% [22]. Skeletal and growth anomalies range from polydactyly/brachydactyly to limb anomalies and may be associated with renal anomalies or renal agenesis. There may also be associated hypertelorism and sensory organ defect of eye or ear and possible heart defects.

Muscular anomalies associated with HSCR include muscular dystrophy [103]. In addition, Fryns syndrome with diaphragmatic hernias [104] and distal limb anomalies [104] may be associated with HSCR. The Jeune asphyxiating thoracic dystrophy also affects the bone growth of the thoracic region.

Distal limb abnormalities are largely represented by polydactyly and limb hypoplasia but may also be associated with congenital deafness [105] or cardiac anomalies [106]. Polydactyly has been described as part of a syndrome of heart defects, laryngeal anomalies and HSCR [106] as well as other autosomal recessive syndromes in siblings [105]. HSCR has been associated with the Werner mesomelic dysplasia [107] which include digital and lower limb anomalies, short stature [108] and the BRESHEK syndrome [109]. The BRESHEK syndrome is a syndrome of brain abnormalities, retardation, ectodermal dysplasia, skeletal malformation, HSCR, ear or eye anomalies, kidney dysplasia and associated osteopetrosis. HSCR has also been reported in seven children with this syndrome resulting from consanguineous marriages [110].

Other rarely associated syndromes include *Fryns syndrome* (congenital diaphragmatic hernia) and *muscular dystrophies* (e.g. Fukuyama congenital muscular dystrophy).

11.4.5 Cardiac Abnormalities (4.99%)

A number of cardiovascular (CVS) anomalies were identified in the DS-HSCR patients in our series, as well as in non-Down-HSCR (4.8% DS vs. 0.3%) [20, 35].

Septal defects (ASD/VSD) [111] and conotruncal developmental defects [1] appear the most frequent lesions. This is understandable as the critical stage of cardiac development occurs at more or less the same time as the ENS and is dependent on neural crest cell proliferation, which then in turn links them to the neurocristopathies.

Neural crest cells originating from a specific hindbrain region have been shown to be essential for the normal development of the cardiac outflow tract and aorto-pulmonary septum, which is closely related to the cells which proliferate into the primitive gut to form the enteric ganglia [63].

In a 30-year nationwide survey of 216 DS-HSCR in Japan, the prevalence of cardiac anomalies had also increased in DS-HSCR patients over the last decade of the study.

In looking at the prevalence of cardiac lesions in DS-HSCR, it can be argued that the cause of the congenital cardiac defects lies outside of chromosome 21 because over half of all patients with DS have a normal heart. This suggests an interaction of modifier interaction with other dosage-sensitive genes to be the cause of the congenital heart disease [112]. Mutations in the CRELD1 gene which lies outside chromosome 21 have been associated with the aetiology of atrioventricular septal defects in DS patients [113].

Syndromes of polydactyly, HSCR and cardiac anomalies are not infrequently reported [106] as is the McKusick-Kaufman syndrome [99, 114] probably representing similar underlying genetic mechanisms.

11.4.6 Craniofacial Anomalies (2.86%)

Unusual facial appearances such as narrow palpebral fissures, broad nose base, cranial anomalies and developmental delay are encountered in association with HSCR and are of interest for a number of reasons. These include cleft palate (0.6–1.1%) as well as the Goldberg-Shprintzen [115], Pierre-Robin [18], Hanhart syndromes [micrognathia with craniofacial and distal limb anomalies] [12] as well as other craniofacial syndromes such as the Aarskog syndrome [faciogenital dysplasia linked to the FDG1 gene [116]] and Jeune asphyxiating frontonasal dysplasia [117]. In addition, some have characteristics of the DiGeorge syndrome [118].

Morphogenesis of the craniofacial region is known to be linked to neural crest development and involves common factors such as growth factor signalling [119, 120]. The SMAD binding protein 1 gene (SMADIP1, MIM 605802) at 2q22, previously linked to HSCR [121], has been recently identified as a disease-causing gene in a polytopic embryonic defect (MIM 235730) including midline anomalies, facial dysmorphic features and enteric nervous system malformation (HSCR) [122].

11.4.7 Ophthalmic Anomalies

Variable expression of reported HSCR-associated ophthalmological findings probably results from maldevelopment of neural crest cells from adjacent areas on the prosencephalon [63]. In our series, they occurred in 9 out of 408 patients studied (2.2%) and included micro/anophthalmos, congenital ptosis and coloboma [35], in keeping with other reports [83, 115, 123, 124]. Pini et al. found a high prevalence of visual disturbance and refractive errors in 43.4% (95% CI, 34.4–52.9%) [26].

Other reported HSCR-coloboma-associated clinical syndromes include the Goldberg-Shprintzen [HSCR, coloboma iris and microcephaly] [73, 125, 126], Rubinstein-Taybi (callosal agenesis, iris coloboma and megacolon) and 'cat's eye' syndromes [123].

Coloboma and the possibly related aniridia trait are often genetically linked to a 2p22 genetic variation [127] and the ZFHX1B gene [83] by autosomal dominant inheritance [128].The renal coloboma syndrome has also been associated with chromosome 2 [129] via Pax 2 [130].

The iris is pathologically involved in the Waardenburg-Shah association [6, 131] and chromosome 13 deletions [132, 133] as well as frame-shift and missense SOX10 mutations [134–136].

Abnormalities of the eye and autonomic nervous system are also frequent in the related congenital central hypoventilation syndrome (CCHS) especially when associated with HSCR [137]. Ophthalmic anomalies may also be included in those with auriculo-vertebral syndromes (e.g. Goldenhar syndrome) [138].

11.5 Skin and the Integumentary System

11.5.1 Pigmentary Skin Disorders

Pigmentary disturbances are anticipated in association with HSCR due to the established critical role of the endothelin system in HSCR, its association with the Waardenburg syndrome (WS4) [139] and its role in melanocyte development in EDNRB knockout mice [140].

Pigmentary disorders associated with HSCR include the neurocristopathy syndromes like the Shah-Waardenburg (WS4) and Yemenite deaf-blind hypopigmentation or BADS syndromes where pigmentary anomalies (white forelock, iris hypoplasia, patchy hypopigmentation) are associated with deafness, hearing loss and possible eye anomalies (microcornea, coloboma, nystagmus). The spectrum also includes patchy hypopigmentation of the skin (piebaldism) and possibly the retina of the eye.

It was Shah et al. [6] who described the white forelock, pigmentary disorder of irides, and long-segment Hirschsprung's disease. This possible variant of Waardenburg syndrome is now known as the Shah-Waardenburg syndrome. Hosada et al. showed in an animal model that targeted and natural (piebald-lethal) mutations of the endothelin-B receptor gene produce megacolon associated with spotted coat colour in mice [141].

Edery et al. then reported mutations of the endothelin-3 gene in Waardenburg-Hirschsprung's disease (Shah-Waardenburg syndrome) [131].

The Sox 10 gene was also shown to be connected and patients from four families with WS4 were shown to have mutations in SOX10, whereas no mutation could be detected in patients with HSCR alone. This points to an essential role of SOX10 in the development of two neural crest-derived human cell lineages [94]. Recent studies in transgene-insertion mutant mouse line (Hry) display incomplete aganglionosis, melanocyte loss and reduced Sox10 expression [142].

11.5.2 Other Associated Non-pigmentary Skin Conditions

Cartilage-hair hypoplasia is also rarely associated with HSCR and is a skeletal dysplasia, occurring in Finnish and Amish populations. It is characterized by short-limbed dwarfism, sparse hair, hypoplastic anaemia and a variety of immune defects and has an approximate 7–9% association with HSCR [143]. Inheritance is autosomal recessive, and the causative gene has been attributed to the endoribonuclease RNase MRP (*RMRP*) gene which is important in processing of nuclear ribosomal RNA and in mitochondrial DNA synthesis [144], which maps to chromosome 9p13 [145].

Other causes of hypopigmentation and white forelock are also encountered in the *ABCD* [146, 147] and *Yemenite deaf-blind hypopigmentation syndromes* which have now been shown to be associated with a SOX10 mutation [146]. Also included are Black locks albinism [148] and familial piebaldism [5]. Rarely, other skin conditions such as ichthyosis and the Clayton-Smith syndrome are associated with HSCR.

Familial ichthyosis [35, 149, 150] has been associated with HSCR, as has KID (keratitis, ichthyosis and deafness) syndrome [149]. Although the exact genetic links with ichthyoids are unknown, two recent publications identified Xp22.3 [151] and 2q35 [152], both of which are close to areas with known HSCR connections.

11.5.3 Central Hypoventilation and Related Syndromes

The *central hypoventilation* (Ondine's curse) *and related syndromes* (e.g. Haddad, congenital central hypoventilation syndromes) and autonomic nervous system disturbance (e.g., Riley-Day and hereditary sensory and autonomic neuropathy Type III (HSAN-III) syndromes) are rare life-threatening disorders of the autonomic nervous system. They affect the central and autonomic nervous system (which controls many of the automatic functions in the body such as temperature, heart rate, blood pressure, oxygen-level sensing and carbon dioxide levels in the blood). It is rare but is estimated to be 1000–1200 cases of CCHS worldwide affecting males and females equally.

By affecting breathing, it carries a significant mortality by causing the infant to hypoventilate (especially during sleep), resulting in a shortage of oxygen and a build-up of carbon dioxide in the blood. Current research has shown that the majority of affected children have mutations of the *PHOX2B* gene [153, 154]. The majority of these are called poly-alanine repeat expansion mutations or PARMs. Other affected children have unrelated *PHOX2B* mutations (non-poly-alanine repeat expansion mutations (NPARMs)), which also result in impaired function of the PHOX2B protein.

The connection to PHOX2B is not surprising as it is one of the known genes associated with HSCR. The PHOX2B gene on chromosome 4 encodes a protein known as neuroblastoma Phox (NBPhox). The PHOX2B gene is expressed exclusively in neurons mostly those controlling the viscera (cardiovascular, digestive and respiratory systems) and is required for their differentiation during development. As a result, there is a need for lifelong ventilatory support during sleep for many patients or all the time in others. There is currently no cure for CCHS.

The Haddad syndrome is a rare congenital disorder in which congenital central hypoventilation syndrome (CCHS), or Ondine syndrome, occurs concurrently with HSCR.

Other connections such as the *Riley-Day* and other syndromes affecting the autonomic nervous system are less obvious. Their link to HSCR is probably through modification of the RET proto-oncogene as it has been shown that PHOX2B and Sox10 act together with Nkx2.1 to modify RET signalling which may also contribute to HSCR susceptibility [155]. RET signalling has been shown to be essential for migration, axonal growth and axon guidance of developing sympathetic neurons [156].

Familial dysautonomia (FD; Riley-Day syndrome) is a hereditary sensory and autonomic neuropathy Type III (HSAN-III) which has been very rarely associated with HSCR [1]. The FD disorder of the autonomic nervous system affects the development and survival of sensory, sympathetic and some parasympathetic neurons in the autonomic and sensory nervous systems. It is largely confined to individuals of Ashkenazi Jewish descent and is characterized by two pathogenic variants of *ELP1* (*IKBKAP*) gene (c.2204+6T>C (formerly IVS20+6T>C)), which account for more than 99% of FD among the Ashkenazi Jews [157].

11.5.4 Mowat-Wilson Syndrome (MWS)

Clinically, MWS is a rare condition representing a spectrum of congenital dysmorphic features of the brain, head and face (microcephaly, corpus callosal agenesis, hypertelorism, prominent columella, pointed chin and uplifted earlobes) as well as GIT motility disturbances. The associations include HSCR (>50%) [158] and/or severe constipation [159]. In addition, genitourinary anomalies (especially hypospadias and renal tract anomalies), congenital heart defects, short stature and eye defects are not uncommon [74].

Since its initial description by Mowat et al. [158], MWS has been reported in countries mainly Europe, Australia and the USA. More recently, more than 179 cases from countries all over the world have been reported [160], with large series reported from countries like Japan [161], as well as a number of isolated cases from different countries. We reported the first confirmed cases of MWS in Africa with ZEB2 and an associated novel ZEB2 gene variation [162].

MWS has a genetic basis and has been reported to recur in families with an approximate 1% autosomal dominant recurrence risk [79]. Because the clinical diagnosis of MWS may prove difficult due to phenotypic variation and because of the progression of clinical features with time, molecular diagnosis of a ZEB2 mutation is required to confirm the diagnosis of MWS.

The association between MWS and HSCR is interesting as this association includes brain and facial development in addition to the congenital absence of ganglion cells in intermyenteric plexuses of the intestinal wall. HSCR is known to be a complex multigenic disorder resulting from the effects of genetic variations of at least 12 known susceptibility genes which affect a number of stages of the normal process of ENS development, including cell migration, differentiation and survival [163]. Although many of these genetic pathways influence the major susceptibility RET and EDNRB gene pathways, the mechanism of the ZEB2 gene in HSCR remains unclear.

11.5.5 HSCR Links to Cancer

There is a clear link between HSCR and a familial predisposition to certain tumours, including medullary carcinoma of the thyroid [164], phaeochromocytoma [4, 7, 165, 166] and other tumours related to the MEN2 phenotype and the RET proto-oncogene, which causes HSCR [7, 8], among others.

HSCR is also associated with a variety of tumours of neural crest origin which include neuroblastoma [4, 167], ganglioneuroma/ganglioneuroblastoma [168, 169] and retinoblastoma [170, 171]. It is fairly clear that these tumours result from oncogene upregulation and tumour suppressor gene inactivation. In addition, neurofibromatosis and other autonomic nervous system disturbances [172] may be related to neural tumours. The best known of these is the association with the MEN Type IIA and IIB syndromes [173]. In the autosomal dominant MEN 2A syndrome, HSCR is associated with medullary thyroid carcinoma due to the neoplastic transformation of C cells in the thyroid. It is also associated with parathyroid hyperplasia and adrenal medullary tumours (phaeochromocytoma). This association may be familial or sporadic in nature and is of particular importance as it is associated with a specific exon 10 genetic variation, the so-called 'Janus' gene [174, 175]. The medullary thyroid carcinoma is aggressive and may recur in families. The association exists because of the common factor of the *RET* gene being associated with these associations conditions [HSCR, MEN Type II and MTC]. This is an extremely interesting observation, as it involves both gain and loss of function of the same gene in the same patient. A single base-pair substitution in one of five cysteine radicals of *RET* results in dimerization of the receptor [176–178]. Our experience is of total colonic aganglionosis (TCA) in the index patient in all three families identified in our series [175]. It therefore appears that patients with long-segment HSCR carry the highest risk of developing MTC. They should have a detailed family history taken, and the presence of a long-segment HSCR should be an important selection criterion for gene testing in HSCR.

It is important to explore this concept further in families where HSCR and MTC co-exist, as it will yield possible RET gene associations and insights into possible molecular reasons for the phenotypic expression. It is generally accepted that aberrant RET protein synthesis, due to inactivating genetic variations, leads to HSCR. RET gene activation occurs in MEN2A.

The link between HSCR and MEN2B would appear to be more tenuous. MEN2B is related to a specific RET proto-oncogene mutation (*RET* (p.Met918Thr)) and is present in over 90% of patients; it produces diffuse ganglioneuromas of the alimentary canal, marfanoid skeletal features, medullary thyroid carcinoma (MTC) and pheochromocytoma. Although individuals with MEN2B may have a neonatal intestinal obstructive picture which may mimic HSCR, it results from the diffuse ganglioneuromatosis of the bowel [179].

11.5.6 Associations with Other Tumours

The major HSCR susceptibility genes [RET and EDNRB] do not appear to be involved in the familial neuroblastoma cases [180]. Familial neuroblastoma [181] and HSCR-NB associations [172, 182] have been reported with association of the PHOX2B gene, and together with the ALK gene (the majority), PHOX2B germline mutations account for 90% of hereditary neuroblastoma [183].

In addition to these known tumour associations, chromosome 10q LOH (including the RET site) has been described in early-stage chondrosarcomas [184] and T-cell lymphoma [185].

11.5.7 Other Less Common Associations with HSCR

Other less common associations with HSCR include syndromes related to cholesterol and fat metabolism such as the *Smith-Lemli-Opitz* [186–188].

Rarer associations with HSCR include Bardet-Biedl and Kaufman-McKusick syndromes that include genito-urinary, brain disorders and obesity.

The *Bardet-Biedl non-syndromic obesity* [BBS] [114, 189, 190] has a 2% overlap with HSCR [191]. The autosomal recessive association of progressive pigmentary retinopathy, obesity, postaxial polydactyly, hypogenitalism, renal abnormalities and variable intellectual disability are similar to many of the HSCR associations.

The connection between these conditions and HSCR is less clear.

A total of 19 genes have been identified for BBS, making the connection to HSCR less obvious. However, homozygosity for the common hypomorphic T allele plus a 11 bp deletion in the enhancer of RET, in association with missense mutations in the BBS genes, has been reported [192].

It would appear that epistasis between RET and *BBS* mutations may modulate enteric innervation and probably cause the association with syndromic *HSCR*.

The *McKusick-Kaufman syndrome occurs in 10% of BBS* [99] and has a 10% HSCR incidence [193]. McKusick-Kaufman syndrome has been linked to pathogenic variants of the *MKKS* gene [194].

The *Smith-Lemli-Opitz syndrome (SLOS)* can also probably be included here. The syndrome consists of microcephaly, congenital heart disease, growth and developmental delays, distinctive facial features, under-masculinization with hypospadias in males, and characteristically, syndactyly of toes two or three.

HSCR has been described in several individuals with this disorder, generally with more severe manifestations including HSCR [186, 195], although mild phenotypes of SLOS may be associated with HSCR [196]. Because the SLOS syndrome results from variations of the *DHCR7gene which e*ncodes the enzyme that catalyses cholesterol biosynthesis, it raises the potential link to cholesterol metabolism in HSCR.

Occasional reports of other associations with the Goldenhar, Lesch-Nyhan, Rubinstein-Taybi, Toriello-Carey and SEMDJL, associated syndromes and genetic variations have been identified.

As the search for environmental factors has yielded little in terms of meaningful results, it has become clear that HSCR is predominantly a genetic condition and there was a known target in the RET proto-oncogene.

11.6 Genetic Aspects of HSCR

11.6.1 Associated Genes and Genetic Associations

This huge list of associations with HSCR suggests genetic interaction/crosstalk that results in associated abnormal development of multiple systems during development. The pattern of conditions associated with HSCR has already been of great value in revealing many of the genetic associations of the disease and has been a major factor in identifying genes such as the EDNRB [48, 197] and SOX genes [142, 198] in the Waardenburg syndrome, the ZEB2 and ZFHX1B genes in the Mowat-Wilson syndrome [74, 199] and the SIP1 gene [200] and PHOX2B gene in congenital hypoventilation [153].

Other known HSCR associations such as Down syndrome [201], the Bardet-Biedl [189] and cholesterol-affecting syndromes [186], in addition to a number of other conditions, remain interesting areas of further research. Since genomic rearrangements in particularly sensitive areas of the RET proto-oncogene and/or associated genes may account for the HSCR phenotype in patients without other detectable RET variants, Serra et al. [202] set out to identify rearrangements in the coding sequence of RET as well as in three HSCR-associated genes (ZEB2, EDN3 and GDNF) in HSCR patients by using Multiplex Ligation-dependent Probe Amplification (MLPA). Their study did not identify any deletion or amplification in these four genes in all patients.

The roles of the major susceptibility genes on chromosome 10 (RET) and chromosome 13 (EDNRB) in the pathogenesis of HSCR are well established [203]. What is not always appreciated is that 9 of the 11 identified genes are related to these two major susceptibility gene signalling pathways: RET (RET; GDNF; GFRα; NTN) signalling cascade and EDNRB (EDN-3; ECE-1; PHOX2B and SOX10) signalling cascade.

11.6.2 Non-syndromic HSCR

Non-syndromic HSCR (in which HSCR occurs without other anomalies) has been associated with pathogenic variants in a number of genes [3, 204]. HSCR has been associated with high-penetrance mutations in at least 11 neuro-developmental genes, namely, RET, GDNF, NRTN, SOX10, EDNRB, EDN3, ECE1, ZFHX1B (ZEB2), PHOX2B, KIAA1279 and TCF4. The genes associated with non-syndromic HSCR fall into four major groups as follows:

- *RET* and its ligands *GDNF* and *NRTN*
- *EDNRB* and the related genes *EDN3* and *ECE1*
- The NRG signalling pathway (*NRG1* and *NRG3)*
- The *SEMA* signalling pathway (*SEMA3C and SEMA3D)*

There is a rare subgroup where RET coding sequence mutations with high penetrance have been reported. Forty-five percent of these cases are familial [49].

A recent population-based case group study which tested for associations between HSCR and common genetic variation [205] has confirmed the associations with RET,HOXB5 and PHOX2B variation but failed to demonstrate significant association with ASCL1, L1CAM and PROK1. The association with HOXB5 and PHOX2B is interesting as it supports the hypothesis that genes regulating enteric neuroblast proliferation, migration and differentiation may confer additional HSCR risk as modifiers. Although this study also showed a strong association between RET variants and HSCR (P 10(-3)-10(-31)), interethnic variation was observed in ethnic African-Americans which suggests interethnic variation in certain races or ethnic groups.

11.6.3 Chromosomal Anomalies in HSCR

A chromosome abnormality is present in approximately 12% of individuals with HSCR [1].

Although the main chromosomal anomaly associated with HSCR is trisomy 21, there are other reported chromosomal variations that are uncommonly HSCR associated.

These include chromosomal lesions associated with multiple congenital anomalies such as deletion of 20p [206], 18p monosomy and 18q trisomy [207] and XO/XX/XXX mosaicism [208].

It stands to reason that if a chromosomal deletion encompasses the area of a HSCR-associated gene, then it is probably significant.

The following have been reported:

- del13q22 (*EDNRB*) [209]
- del10q11.2 (*RET*) [210]
- del10q23.1 (*NRG3*) [211]
- del2q22 (*ZEB2*) [158, 212]
- del 4p12 (*PHOX2B*) [213]
- del 17q21/dup 17q21-q23 [3] has been described in individuals with HSCR, but the associated gene(s) are not identified as yet

There are at least two other chromosomal regions where genomic studies have re-emphasized an already suspected HSCR link. One of these is the association between HSCR and *2q37,* which arose because of a possible homology with the splotch mouse model [214]. Since the initial connections with this site, the SMAD interacting protein 1 gene (SIP-1) at 2q22-23 [121], partial duplication of chromosome 2 [212, 215] and the Mowat-Wilson syndrome with its ZEB2 mutations and deletions at 2q22-q24 [74, 215] have been associated with HSCR.

In addition, the *9q31* region has been identified in sibling pairs without significant RET variations [77]. This site has been previously associated with reports of tetrasomy of 9p [76] and the association with Riley-Day familial dysautonomia [216] whose IKBKAP gene has been linked to 9q31 [217]. The RMRP gene mutation in the cartilage-hair hypoplasia syndrome relates to a similar area [218].

HSCR is frequently associated with genetic anomalies, brain or systemic malformations (e.g. heart, orthopaedic, intestinal, urogenital and facial anomalies) and is also part of many syndromes. It also appears to be linked to chromosome 9 variations possibly explaining the HSCR connections [76, 77]. Dandy-Walker abnormalities have been reported associated with both HSCR [76] and Waardenburg-Shah syndrome [219].

Abnormalities of *chromosome 22 karyotype* have been reported to be associated with both malrotation and aganglionosis both in animal models [60] and in humans [220]. Associations related to this site include the cat's eye syndrome associated with trisomy 22pter-q11 [221] and the DiGeorge velocardiofacial syndrome at del22q11 [118], both of which have been associated with HSCR.

L1 gene (LiCAM) mutations have been associated with both hydrocephalus and HSCR [80]. Although there appears to be some association with L1 [222], it has recently been shown to not be causative in HSCR [205]. It may, however, act as a modifier gene for members of the endothelin signalling pathway during ENS development [223].

It is interesting to note that the majority of the reported chromosomal sites that lie outside of the major susceptibility genes have been identified in patients without major RET mutations, suggesting that these chromosomal sites may have a unique interaction resulting in HSCR [77].

11.6.4 A Multigenetic Aetiologic Hypothesis

It has become clear that HSCR is a very complex condition with multiple gene-gene interactions. A viable alternative to finding a specific modifier gene in trisomy 21 is that of a multigenetic aetiologic hypothesis [224]. Puffenberger et al. implicated the involvement of other susceptibility genes in HSCR pathogenesis quite early on [48].

Although gaps still remain in our knowledge, exploration of the genetic links with HSCR has helped to explain the phenotypic expression, and the condition is currently regarded as multigenetic and multi-factorial in origin. A hypothesis of a genetic interaction between mutations in RET and EDNRB as an underlying mechanism in ENS maldevelopment is supported by the observation of concurrent *EDNRB* variation with identified *RET* haplotypes [225]. This suggests that both genes may be promoting HSCR susceptibility. Other studies have also reported statistically significant joint transmission of RET and EDNRB alleles with interaction between RET and EDNRB pathways in HSCR-affected individuals [226].

References

1. Amiel J, Lyonnet S. Hirschsprung disease, associated syndromes, and genetics: a review. J Med Genet. 2001;38(11):729–39.
2. Moore SW. Chromosomal and related Mendelian syndromes associated with Hirschsprung's disease. Pediatr Surg Int. 2012;28(11):1045–58.
3. Amiel J, Sproat-Emison E, Garcia-Barcelo M, Lantieri F, Burzynski G, Borrego S, et al. Hirschsprung disease, associated syndromes and genetics: a review. J Med Genet. 2008;45(1):1–14.
4. Passarge E. The genetics of Hirschsprungs Disease. N Engl J Med. 1967;276:138–43.
5. Weinberg AG, Currarino G, Besserman M. Hirschsprungs disease and congenital deafness. Hum Genet. 1977;38:157–61.
6. Shah KN, Dalal SJ, Desai MP. White forelock, pigmentary disorder of irides and long segment Hirschsprung's disease: possible variant of Waardenburg syndrome. J Pediatr. 1981;99:432–5.
7. Bolande RP. The Neurocristopathies, a unifying concept of disease arising in neural crest maldevelopment. Hum Pathol. 1974;5:409–29.
8. Khan AH, Desjardin JG, Gregoire H, Seidman E. Gastrointestinal manifestations of the Sipple syndrome in children. J Pediatr Surg. 1987;22:719–23.
9. Kilcoyne RF, Taybi H. Conditions associated with congenital megacolon. Am J Roentgenol Radium Ther Nucl Med. 1970;108(3):615–20.
10. Ehrenpreiss TH. Hirschsprungs disease. Chicago: Year Book Medical Publishers; 1970.
11. Spouge D, Baird PA. Hirschsprungs Disease in a large birth cohort. Teratology. 1985;32:171–7.
12. Polley TZ, Coran AG. Hirschsprungs disease in the newborn. Pediatr Surg Int. 1986;1:80–3.
13. Ikeda K, Goto S. Additional anomalies in Hirschsprungs disease: an analysis based on a nationwide survey in Japan. Z Kinderchir. 1986;41:279–81.
14. Sieber W. Hirschsprungs disease. In: Welch KJ, Randolph JG, Ravitch M, editors. Paediatric surgery. 4th ed. Chicago: Year Book; 1986. p. 995–1020.
15. Lister J, Tam PK. Hirschsprungs disease. In: Lister J, Irving IM, editors. Neonatal surgery. 3rd ed. London: Butterworth; 1990. p. 523–46.
16. Swenson O, Raffensberger JG. Hirschsprungs disease. In: Raffensberger JG, editor. Swensons paediatric surgery. 5th ed. New York: Appleton and Lange; 1990. p. 555–78.
17. Ryan ET, Ecker JL, Christakis NA, Folkman J. Hirschsprung's disease: associated abnormalities and demography. J Pediatr Surg. 1992;27(1):76–81.
18. Engum SA, Petrites M, Rescorla FJ, Grosfeld JL, Morrison AM, Engles D. Familial Hirschsprung's disease: 20 cases in 12 kindreds. J Pediatr Surg. 1993;28(10):1286–90.
19. Klein MD, Philippart AI. Hirschsprung's disease: three decades' experience at a single institution. J Pediatr Surg. 1993;28(10):1291–3.
20. Moore SW. The study of the etiology of post-surgical obstruction in patients with Hirschsprungs disease. Doctoral Thesis, University of Cape Town; 1993. p. 1–373.
21. Halevy H, Mares A, Cohen Z, Finaly R, Freud E, Pilpel D. Hirschprung's disease in the Negev. Harefuah. 1994;127(5–6):148–54.
22. Sarioglu A, Tanyel FC, Buyukpamukcu N, Hicsonmez A. Hirschsprung-associated congenital anomalies. Eur J Pediatr Surg. 1997;7(6):331–7.
23. Das K, Alladi A, Kini U, Babu MK, D'Cruz AJ. Hirschsprung's disease, associated rare congenital anomalies. Indian J Pediatr. 2001;68(9):835–7.
24. Holschneider AM, Ure BM. Hirschsprung's disease. In: Ashcraft KW, Holcomb GW, Murphy J-P, editors. Pediatric surgery. 4th ed. Philadelphia: Elsevier Saunders; 2003. p. 453–68.
25. Singh SJ, Croaker GD, Manglick P, Wong CL, Athanasakos H, Elliott E, et al. Hirschsprung's disease: the Australian Paediatric Surveillance Unit's experience. Pediatr Surg Int. 2003;19(4):247–50.
26. Pini Prato A, Rossi V, Mosconi M, Holm C, Lantieri F, Griseri P, et al. A prospective observational study of associated anomalies in Hirschsprung's disease. Orphanet J Rare Dis. 2013;8:184.
27. Graivier L, Sieber WK. Hirschsprungs disease and mongolism. Surgery. 1966;60:458–61.
28. Badner JA, Sieber WK, Garver KL, Chakravarti A. A genetic study of Hirschsprung disease. Am J Hum Genet. 1990;46:568–80.
29. Bolk S, Pelet A, Hofstra RM, Angrist M, Salomon R, Croaker D, et al. A human model for multigenic inheritance: phenotypic expression in Hirschsprung disease requires both the RET gene and a new 9q31 locus. Proc Natl Acad Sci U S A. 2000;97([1]):268–73.
30. Bodian M, Carter CO. Family study of Hirschsprungs disease. Ann Hum Genet. 1963;26:261–71.
31. Goldberg EL. An epidemiological study of Hirschsprung's disease. Int J Epidemiol. 1984;13(4):479–85.

32. Garver K, Law J, Garver B. Hirschsprung disease: a genetic study. Clin Genet. 1985;28:503–8.
33. Caniano DA, Teitelbaum DH, Qualman SJ. Management of Hirschsprungs disease in children with Trisomy 21. Am J Surg. 1990;159:402–4.
34. Molander M-L. Hirschsprungs disease in mentally retarded patients: a bad prognostic combination. Pediatr Surg Int. 1990;5:339–40.
35. Moore SW, Rode H, Millar AJ, Albertyn R, Cywes S. Familial aspects of Hirschsprungs disease. Eur J Pediatr Surg. 1991;1:97–107.
36. Russell MB, Russell CA, Niebuhr E. An epidemiological study of Hirschsprung's disease and additional anomalies. Acta Paediatr. 1994;83(1):68–71.
37. Quinn FM, Surana R, Puri P. The influence of trisomy 21 on outcome in children with Hirschsprung's disease. J Pediatr Surg. 1994;29:781–3.
38. Spahis JK, Wilson GN. Down syndrome: perinatal complications and counseling experiences in 216 patients. Am J Med Genet. 1999;89(2):96–9.
39. Nakazato Y, Landing BH. Reduced number of neurons in esophageal plexus ganglia in Down syndrome: additional evidence for reduced cell number as a basic feature of the disorder. Pediatr Pathol. 1986;5(1):55–63.
40. Suetsugu M, Mehraein P. Spine distribution along the apical dendrites of the pyramidal neurons in Down's syndrome. A quantitative Golgi study. Acta Neuropathol. 1980;50(3):207–10.
41. Becker LE, Armstrong DL, Chan F. Dendritic atrophy in children with Down's syndrome. Ann Neurol. 1986;20(4):520–6.
42. Caviedes P, Caviedes R, Rapoport SI. Altered calcium currents in cultured sensory neurons of normal and trisomy 16 mouse fetuses, an animal model for human trisomy 21 (Down syndrome). Biol Res. 2006;39(3):471–81.
43. Saud K, Arriagada C, Cardenas AM, Shimahara T, Allen DD, Caviedes R, et al. Neuronal dysfunction in Down syndrome: contribution of neuronal models in cell culture. J Physiol Paris. 2006;99(2–3):201–10.
44. Moore SW. The contribution of associated congenital anomalies in understanding Hirschsprung's disease. Pediatr Surg Int. 2006;22(4):305–15.
45. Zaahl MG, du Plessis L, Warnich L, Kotze MJ, Moore SW. Significance of novel endothelin-B receptor gene polymorphisms in Hirschsprung's disease: predominance of a novel variant (561C/T) in patients with co-existing Down's syndrome. Mol Cell Probes. 2003;17(1):49–54.
46. Sanchez-Mejias A, Fernandez RM, Lopez-Alonso M, Antinolo G, Borrego S. New roles of EDNRB and EDN3 in the pathogenesis of Hirschsprung disease. Genet Med. 2010;12(1):39–43.
47. Korbel JO, Tirosh-Wagner T, Urban AE, Chen XN, Kasowski M, Dai L, et al. The genetic architecture of Down syndrome phenotypes revealed by high-resolution analysis of human segmental trisomies. Proc Natl Acad Sci U S A. 2009;106(29):12031–6.
48. Puffenberger E, Hosoda K, Washington SS, Nakao K, de Wit D, Yanagisawa M, et al. A missense mutation of the endothelin-B receptor gene in multigenic Hirschsprung's disease. Cell. 1994;79(7):1256–66.
49. Jannot AS, Pelet A, Henrion-Caude A, Chaoui A, Masse-Morel M, Arnold S, et al. Chromosome 21 scan in Down syndrome reveals DSCAM as a predisposing locus in Hirschsprung disease. PLoS One. 2013;8(5):e62519.
50. Cheng W. ATP50 on human chromosome 21 as a potential link between Hirschsprung disease and Down syndrome. Poster 15 5th international symposium on development of the enteric nervous system, Boston, 8–11 Apr 2018.
51. ves da Silva AF, Machado FB, Pavarino EC, Biselli-Perico JM, Zampieri BL, da Silva Francisco JR, et al. Trisomy 21 alters DNA methylation in parent-of-origin-dependent and -independent manners. PLoS One. 2016;11(4):e0154108.
52. Karousou E, Stachtea X, Moretto P, Viola M, Vigetti D, D'Angelo ML, et al. New insights into the pathobiology of Down syndrome – hyaluronan synthase-2 overexpression is regulated by collagen VI alpha2 chain. FEBS J. 2013;280(10):2418–30.
53. Kwendakwema N, Al-Dulaimi R, Presson A, Zobell S, Stephens A, et al. Enterocolitis and bowel function in children with Hirschsprung disease and trisomy 21. J Pediatr Surg. 2016;51(12):2001–4.
54. Friedmacher F, Puri P. Hirschsprung's disease associated with Down syndrome: a meta-analysis of incidence, functional outcomes and mortality. Pediatr Surg Int. 2013;29(9):937–46.
55. Catto-Smith AG, Trajanovska M, Taylor RG. Long-term continence in patients with Hirschsprung's disease and Down syndrome. J Gastroenterol Hepatol. 2006;21(4):748–53.
56. de Bruyn R, Hall CM, Spitz L. Hirschsprung's disease and malrotation of the mid-gut. An uncommon association. Br J Radiol. 1982;55(656):554–7.
57. Ko S, Fujii H, Yamamoto K, Sado S, Yamamoto M, Nakano H. Hirschsprung's disease associated with intestinal malrotation in an adult and a review of literature. Nippon Geka Gakkai Zasshi. 1991;92(4):469–72.
58. Jain SK, Singla SK, Sharma M, Pathania OP, Taneja SB. Hirschsprung's disease with intestinal malrotation and midgut volvulus: a rare association. Indian J Gastroenterol. 1989;8([3]):201.
59. Corsois L, Boman F, Sfeir R, Mention K, Michaud L, Poddevin F, et al. Extensive Hirschsprung's disease associated with intestinal malrotation. Arch Pediatr. 2004;11([10]):1205–8.
60. Ramalho-Santos M, Melton DA, McMahon AP. Hedgehog signals regulate multiple aspects of gastrointestinal development. Development. 2000;127(12):2763–72.
61. Arbell D, Gross E, Orkin B, Koplewitz BZ, Udassin R. Imperforate anus, malrotation, and Hirschsprung's disease: a rare and important association 2. J Pediatr Surg. 2006;41(7):1335–7.
62. Flageole H, Fecteau A, Laberge JM, Guttman FM. Hirschsprung's disease, imperforate anus, and Down's syndrome: a case report. J Pediatr Surg. 1996;31(6):759–60.

63. Meijers C, Mulder M. Anteroposterior differences within caudal hindbrain neural crest cell populations and the development of the enteric nervous system. Presented at the second international meeting: Hirschsprung disease and related neurocristopathies, Cleveland, Oct 1995.
64. Watanatittan S, Suwatanaviroj A, Limprutithum T, Rattanasuwan T. Association of Hirschsprung's disease and anorectal malformation. J Pediatr Surg. 1991;26(2):192–5.
65. Takada Y, Aoyama K, Goto T, Mori S. The association of imperforate anus and Hirschsprung's disease in siblings. J Pediatr Surg. 1985;20(3):271–3.
66. Clarke SA, Van der Avoirt A. Imperforate anus, Hirschsprung's disease, and trisomy 21: a rare combination. J Pediatr Surg. 1999;34(12):1874.
67. Moore SW, Zaahl M. Association of endothelin-receptor (*EDNRB*) gene variants with anorectal malformation patients in the diverse South African population. J Pediatr Surg. 2007;42(7):1266–70.
68. Romeo G, Ronchetto P, et al. Point mutations affecting the tyrosine kinase domain of the *RET proto-oncogene* in Hirschsprung's disease. Nature. 1994;367:378–80.
69. Fishman SJ, Islam S, Buonomo C, Nurko S. Nonfixation of an atretic colon predicts Hirschsprung's disease. J Pediatr Surg. 2001;36(1):202–4.
70. Gauderer MW, Rothstein FC, Izant RJ Jr. Ileal atresia with long-segment Hirschsprung's disease in a neonate. J Pediatr Surg. 1984;19(1):15–7.
71. Moore SW, Millar A, Rode H, Cywes S. Intestinal atresia and Hirschsprungs disease. Pediatr Surg Int. 1990;5(3):182–9.
72. Moore SW, Tshifularo N. Hirschsprung's disease in the neurologically challenged child 5. Int J Adolesc Med Health. 2011;23(3):223–7.
73. Shahar E, Shinawi M. Neurocristopathies presenting with neurologic abnormalities associated with Hirschsprung's disease. Pediatr Neurol. 2003;28(5):385–91.
74. Mowat DR, Wilson MJ, Goossens M. Mowat-Wilson syndrome. J Med Genet. 2003;40(5):305–10.
75. Mathew A. Anencephaly-associated aganglionosis. Am J Med Genet. 1998;80(5):518–20.
76. Melaragno MI, Brunoni D, Patricio FR, Corbani M, Mustacchi Z, dos Santos Rde C, et al. A patient with tetrasomy 9p, Dandy-Walker cyst and Hirschsprung disease. Ann Genet. 1992;35(2):79–84.
77. Bolk-Gabriel S, Salomon R, Pelet A, et al. Segregation at three loci explains familial and population risk in Hirschsprung disease. Nat Genet. 2002;31(1):89–93.
78. Okamoto N, Del Maestro R, Valero R, Monros E, Poo P, Kanemura Y, et al. Hydrocephalus and Hirschsprung's disease with a mutation of L1CAM. J Hum Genet. 2004;49([6]):334–7.
79. McGaughran J, Sinnott S, Moal FD, Wilson M, Mowat D, Sutton B, et al. Recurrence of Mowat-Wilson syndrome in siblings with the same proven mutation. Am J Med Genet A. 2005;137(3):302–4.
80. Okamoto N, Wada Y, Goto M. Hydrocephalus and Hirschsprung's disease in a patient with a mutation of L1CAM. J Med Genet. 1997;34(8):670–1.
81. Sztriha L, Frossard P, Hofstra RM, Verlind E, Nork M. Novel missense mutation in the L1 gene in a child with corpus callosum agenesis, retardation, adducted thumbs, spastic paraparesis, and hydrocephalus. J Child Neurol. 2000;15(4):239–43.
82. Wallace AS, Tan MX, Schachner M, Anderson RB. L1cam acts as a modifier gene for members of the endothelin signalling pathway during enteric nervous system development. Neurogastroenterol Motil. 2011;23(11):e510–22.
83. Gregory-Evans CY, Vieira H, Dalton R, Adams GG, Salt A, Gregory-Evans K. Ocular coloboma and high myopia with Hirschsprung disease associated with a novel ZFHX1B missense mutation and trisomy 21. Am J Med Genet A. 2004;131(1):86–90.
84. Merkler RG, Solish SB, Scherzer AL. Meningomyelocele and Hirschprung disease: theoretical and clinical significance. Pediatrics. 1985;76(2):299–300.
85. Sieber WK. Hirschsprungs disease. In: Welch KJ, Randolph JG, Ravitch MM, editors. Pediatric surgery. 4th ed. Chicago: Year Book; 1986. p. 995–1020.
86. Gordon H, Louw JH, Torrington M, Cywes S. A genetical study of Hirschsprungs disease. S Afr Med J. 1966;40:720–1.
87. Holbrook KA, Underwood RA, Vogel AM, Gown AM, Kimball H. The appearance, density and distribution of melanocytes in human embryonic and fetal skin revealed by the anti-melanoma monoclonal antibody, HMB-45. Anat Embryol. 1989;180(5):443–55.
88. Omenn GS, McKusick VA. The association of Waardenburgh syndrome and Hirschsprungs megacolon. Am J Med Genet. 1979;3:217–23.
89. Attie T, Pelet A, Edery P, et al. Diversity of *RET* proto-oncogene mutations in familial and sporadic Hirschsprung disease. Hum Mol Genet. 1995;4:1381–6.
90. Ohgami N, Tamura H, Ohgami K, Iida M, Yajima I, Kumasaka MY, et al. c-Ret-mediated hearing losses. nt. J Clin Exp Pathol. 2012;5(1):23–8.
91. Bondurand N, Fouquet V, Baral V, Lecerf L, Loundon N, Goossens M, et al. Alu-mediated deletion of SOX10 regulatory elements in Waardenburg syndrome type 4. Eur J Hum Genet. 2012;20(9):990–4.
92. Ohgami N, Ida-Eto M, Sakashita N, Sone M, Nakashima T, Tabuchi K, et al. Partial impairment of c-Ret at tyrosine 1062 accelerates age-related hearing loss in mice 9. Neurobiol Aging. 2012;33(3):626–34.
93. Bondurand N, Kobetz A, Pingault V, Lemort N, Encha-Razavi F, Couly G, et al. Expression of the SOX10 gene during human development 2. FEBS Lett. 1998;432(3):168–72.
94. Pingault V, Bondurand N, Kuhlbrodt K, Goerich DE, Prehu MO, Puliti A, et al. SOX10 mutations in patients with Waardenburg-Hirschsprung disease. Nat Genet. 1998;18([2]):171–3.

95. Southard-Smith EM, Angrist M, Ellison JS, Agarwala R, Baxevanis AD, Chakravarti A, et al. The Sox10(Dom) mouse: modeling the genetic variation of Waardenburg-Shah (WS4) syndrome. Genome Res. 1999;9([3]):215–25.
96. Sham MH, Lui VC, Fu M, Chen B, Tam PK. SOX10 is abnormally expressed in aganglionic bowel of Hirschsprung's disease infants. Gut. 2001;49(2):220–6.
97. Pingault V, Puliti A, Prehu M-O, Samadi A, Bondurand N, Goossens M. Human homology and candidate genes for the dominant megacolon locus, a mouse model of Hirschsprung disease. Genomics. 1997;39:86–9.
98. Sariola H, Saarma M. Novel functions and signalling pathways for GDNF. J Cell Sci. 2003;116(Pt 19):3855–62.
99. Hou JW. Bardet-Biedl syndrome initially presenting as McKusick-Kaufman syndrome. J Formos Med Assoc. 2004;103(8):629–32.
100. Kaiser G, Bettex M. Disorders and congenital malformations associated with Hirschsprungs disease. In: Holschneider AM, editor. Hirschsprung's disease. 1st ed. Stuttgart: Hipokrates-Verlag; 1982. p. 49–53.
101. Cass DT, Hutson J. Association of Hirschsprung's disease and Mullerian inhibiting substance deficiency. J Pediatr Surg. 1992;27(12):1596–9.
102. Brown RA, Cywes C. Disorders and congenital malformations associated with Hirschsprungs disease. In: Holschneider AM, Puri P, editors. Hirschsprungs disease. 3rd ed. Amsterdam: Harcourt; 2000. p. 137–45.
103. Mandel H, Brik R, Ludatscher R, Braun J, Berant M. Congenital muscular dystrophy with neurological abnormalities: association with Hirschsprung disease. Am J Med Genet. 1993;47(1):37–40.
104. Alkuraya FS, Lin AE, Irons MB, Kimonis VE. Fryns syndrome with Hirschsprung disease: support for possible neural crest involvement. Am J Med Genet A. 2005;132(2):226–30.
105. Santos H, Mateus J, Leal MJ. Hirschsprung disease associated with polydactyly, unilateral renal agenesis, hypertelorism, and congenital deafness: a new autosomal recessive syndrome. J Med Genet. 1988;25(3):204–5.
106. Huang T, Elias ER, Mulliken JB, Kirse DJ, Holmes LB. A new syndrome: heart defects, laryngeal anomalies, preaxial polydactyly, and colonic aganglionosis in sibs. Genet Med. 1999;1(3):104–8.
107. Goldenberg A, Milh M, de Lagausie P, Mesnage R, Benarif F, de Blois MC, et al. Werner mesomelic dysplasia with Hirschsprung disease. Am J Med Genet A. 2003;123([2]):186–9.
108. le Merrer M, Briard ML, Chauvet ML, Maroteaux P. Autosomal recessive metaphyseal chondrodysplasia and Hirschsprung's disease. Ann Pediatr (Paris). 1991;38(1):27–30.
109. Reish O, Gorlin RJ, Hordinsky M, Rest EB, Burke B, Berry SA. Brain anomalies, retardation of mentality and growth, ectodermal dysplasia, skeletal malformations, Hirschsprung disease, ear deformity and deafness, eye hypoplasia, cleft palate, cryptorchidism, and kidney dysplasia/hypoplasia (BRESEK/BRESHECK): new X-linked syndrome? Am J Med Genet. 1997;68(4):386–90.
110. Dudin AA, Rambaud-Cousson A. Syndrome of infantile osteopetrosis and Hirschsprung disease in seven children born to four consanguineous unions in two families. Am J Med Genet. 1993;47(7):1083–5.
111. Nowaczyk M, James AG, Superina R, Siegel-Bartelt J. Hirschsprung disease, postaxial polydactyly, and atrial septal defect. Am J Med Genet. 1997;68(1):74–5.
112. Li H, Cherry S, Klinedinst D, DeLeon V, Redig J, Reshey B, et al. Genetic modifiers predisposing to congenital heart disease in the sensitized Down syndrome population. Circ Cardiovasc Genet. 2012;5(3):301–8.
113. Maslen CL, Babcock D, Robinson SW, Bean LJ, Dooley KJ, Willour VL, et al. CRELD1 mutations contribute to the occurrence of cardiac atrioventricular septal defects in Down syndrome. Am J Med Genet A. 2006;140(22):2501–5.
114. Lorda-Sanchez I, Ayuso C, Ibanez A. Situs inversus and hirschsprung disease: two uncommon manifestations in Bardet-Biedl syndrome. Am J Med Genet. 2000;90(1):80–1.
115. Yomo A, Taira T, Kondo I. Goldberg-Shprintzen syndrome: Hirschsprung disease, hypotonia, and ptosis in sibs. Am J Med Genet. 1991;41(2):188–91.
116. Orrico A, Galli L, Cavaliere ML, Garavelli L, Fryns JP, Crushell E, et al. Phenotypic and molecular characterisation of the Aarskog-Scott syndrome: a survey of the clinical variability in light of FGD1 mutation analysis in 46 patients. Eur J Hum Genet. 2004;12(1):16–23.
117. Aurora P, Wallis CE. Jeune syndrome (asphyxiating thoracic dystrophy) associated with Hirschsprung disease. Clin Dysmorphol. 1999;8(4):259–63.
118. Kerstjens-Frederikse WS, Hofstra RM, van Essen AJ, Meijers JH, Buys CH. A Hirschsprung disease locus at 22q11? J Med Genet. 1999;36(3):221–4.
119. Young HM, Hearn CJ, Farlie PG, Canty AJ, Thomas PQ, Newgreen DF. GDNF is a chemoattractant for enteric neural cells. Dev Biol. 2001;229(2):503–16.
120. Farlie PG, McKeown SJ, Newgreen DF. The neural crest: basic biology and clinical relationships in the craniofacial and enteric nervous systems. Birth Defects Res C Embryo Today. 2004;72(2):173–89.
121. Wakamatsu N, Yamada Y, Yamada K, Ono T, Nomura N, Taniguchi H, et al. Mutations in SIP1, encoding Smad interacting protein-1, cause a form of Hirschsprung disease. Nat Genet. 2001;27(4):369–70.
122. Espinosa-Parrilla Y, Amiel J, Auge J, Encha-Razavi F, Munnich A, Lyonnet S, et al. Expression of the SMADIP1 gene during early human development. Mech Dev. 2002;114(1–2):187–91.

123. Guion-Almeida ML, Richieri-Costa A. Callosal agenesis, iris coloboma, and megacolon in a Brazilian boy with Rubinstein-Taybi syndrome. Am J Med Genet. 1992;43(6):929–31.
124. Ohnuma K, Imaizumi K, Masuno M, Nakamura M, Kuroki Y. Magnetic resonance imaging abnormalities of the brain in Goldberg-Shprintzen syndrome (Hirschsprung disease, microcephaly, and iris coloboma). Am J Med Genet. 1997;73(2):230–2.
125. Fryer AE. Goldberg-Shprintzen syndrome: report of a new family and review of the literature. Clin Dysmorphol. 1998;7(2):97–101.
126. Brooks AS, Breuning MH, Osinga J, vd Smagt JJ, Catsman CE, Buys CH, et al. A consanguineous family with Hirschsprung disease, microcephaly, and mental retardation (Goldberg-Shprintzen syndrome). J Med Genet. 1999;36([6]):485–9.
127. Webb GC, Keith CG, Campbell NT. Concurrent de novo interstitial deletion of band 2p22 and reciprocal translocation (3:7)(p21;q22). J Med Genet. 1988;25:125–7.
128. Lehman DM, Sponsel WE, Stratton RF, Mensah J, Macdonald JC, Johnson-Pais TL, et al. Genetic mapping of a novel X-linked recessive colobomatous microphthalmia. Am J Med Genet. 2001;101([2]):114–9.
129. Ferrell RE, Chakravarti A, Hittner HM, Riccardi VM. Autosomal dominant aniridia: probable linkage to acid phosphatase-1 locus on chromosome 2. Proc Natl Acad Sci U S A. 1980;77(3):1580–2.
130. Schimmenti LA, Manligas GS, Sieving PA. Optic nerve dysplasia and renal insufficiency in a family with a novel PAX2 mutation, Arg115X: further ophthalmologic delineation of the renal-coloboma syndrome. Ophthalmic Genet. 2003;24(4):191–202.
131. Edery P, Attie T, Amiel J, Pelet A, Eng C, Hofstra RM, et al. Mutation of the endothelin-3 gene in the Waardenburg-Hirschsprung disease (Shah-Waardenburg syndrome). Nat Genet. 1996;12(4):442–4.
132. Schocket LS, Beaverson KL, Rollins IS, Abramson DH. Bilateral Retinoblastoma, Microphthalmia, and Colobomas in the 13q Deletion Syndrome. Arch Ophthalmol. 2003;121:916–7.
133. Lansink PJ, Moll AC, Imhof SM, Schouten van Meeteren AY, Goverts ST. Variable expression of ophthalmological findings in the 13q deletion syndrome. Arch Ophthalmol. 2005;123(1):127–8.
134. Chan KK, Wong CK, Lui VC, Tam PK, Sham MH. Analysis of SOX10 mutations identified in Waardenburg-Hirschsprung patients: Differential effects on target gene regulation. J Cell Biochem. 2003;90(3):573–85.
135. Bondurand N, Kuhlbrodt K, Pingault V, Enderich J, Sajus M, Tommerup N, et al. A molecular analysis of the yemenite deaf-blind hypopigmentation syndrome: SOX10 dysfunction causes different neurocristopathies. Hum Mol Genet. 1999;8(9):1785–9.
136. Inoue K, Khajavi M, Ohyama T, Hirabayashi S, Wilson J, Reggin JD, et al. Molecular mechanism for distinct neurological phenotypes conveyed by allelic truncating mutations. Nat Genet. 2004;36(4):361–9.
137. Croaker GD, Shi E, Simpson E, Cartmill T, Cass DT. Congenital central hypoventilation syndrome and Hirschsprung's disease. Arch Dis Child. 1998;78(4):316–22.
138. Lankosz-Lauterbach J, Sanak M. Oculoauriculovertebral syndrome (Goldenhar syndrome) associated with Hirschsprung disease. Pediatr Pol. 1987;62(4):249–52.
139. Hofstra RM, Osinga J, Tan-Sindhunata G, Wu Y, Kamsteeg EJ, Stulp RP, et al. A homozygous mutation in the endothelin-3 gene associated with a combined Waardenburg type 2 and Hirschsprung phenotype (Shah-Waardenburg syndrome). Nat Genet. 1996;12(4):445–7.
140. Hou L, Pavan WJ, Shin MK, Arnheiter H. Cell-autonomous and cell non-autonomous signaling through endothelin receptor B during melanocyte development. Development. 2004;131([14]):3239–47.
141. Hosoda K, Hammer RE, Richardson JA, et al. Targeted and natural (piebald-lethal) mutations of endothelin-B receptor gene produce megacolon associated with spotted coat color in mice. Cell. 1994;79:1267–76.
142. Antonellis A, Bennett WR, Menheniott TR, Prasad AB, Lee-Lin SQ, Green ED, et al. Deletion of long-range sequences at Sox10 compromises developmental expression in a mouse model of Waardenburg-Shah (WS4) syndrome. Hum Mol Genet. 2006;15(2):259–71.
143. Makitie O, Heikkinen M, Kaitila I, Rintala R. Hirschsprung's disease in cartilage-hair hypoplasia has poor prognosis. J Pediatr Surg. 2002;37(11):1585–8.
144. Ridanpaa M, Jain P, McKusick VA, Francomano CA, Kaitila I. The major mutation in the RMRP gene causing CHH among the Amish is the same as that found in most Finnish cases. Am J Med Genet C Semin Med Genet. 2003;121(1):81–3.
145. Sulisalo T, Sistonen P, Hastbacka J, Wadelius C, Makitie O, de la Chapelle A, et al. Cartilage-hair hypoplasia gene assigned to chromosome 9 by linkage analysis. Nat Genet. 1993;3(4):338–41.
146. Gross A, Kunze J, Maier RF, Stoltenburg-Didinger G, Grimmer I, Obladen M. Autosomal-recessive neural crest syndrome with albinism, black lock, cell migration disorder of the neurocytes of the gut, and deafness: ABCD syndrome. Am J Med Genet. 1995;56(3):322–6.
147. Verheij JB, Kunze J, Osinga J, van Essen AJ, Hofstra R. ABCD Syndrome is caused by a homozygous mutation in the EDNRB Gene. Am J Med Genet. 2002;108(3):223–5.
148. Mahakrishnan A, Srinivasan MS. Piebaldness with Hirschsprung's disease. Arch Dermatol. 1980;116([10]):1102.

149. Mallory SB, Haynie LS, Williams ML, Hall W. Ichthyosis, deafness, and Hirschsprung's disease. Pediatr Dermatol. 1989;6(1):24–7.
150. Nadir E, Yerman S, Feldman M. A female neonate with Hirschsprung's disease and ichthyosis. Isr Med Assoc J. 2005;7([5]):342–3.
151. Lesca G, Sinilnikova O, Theuil G, Blanc J, Edery P, Till M. Xp22.3 microdeletion including VCX-A and VCX-B1 genes in an X-linked ichthyosis family: no difference in deletion size for patients with and without mental retardation. Clin Genet. 2005;67(4):367–8.
152. Kelsell DP, Norgett EE, Unsworth H, Teh MT, Cullup T, et al. Mutations in ABCA12 underlie the severe congenital skin disease harlequin ichthyosis. Am J Hum Genet. 2005;76(5):794–803.
153. Amiel J, Laudier B, Attie-Bitach T, Trang H, de Pontual L, Gener B, et al. Polyalanine expansion and frameshift mutations of the paired-like homeobox gene PHOX2B in congenital central hypoventilation syndrome. Nat Genet. 2003;33(4):459–61.
154. Ou-Yang MC, Yang SN, Hsu YM, Ou-Yang MH, Haung HC, Lee SY, et al. Concomitant existence of total bowel aganglionosis and congenital central hypoventilation syndrome in a neonate with PHOX2B gene mutation. J Pediatr Surg. 2007;42(2):e9–11.
155. Leon TY, Ngan ES, Poon HC, So MT, Lui VC, Tam PK, et al. Transcriptional regulation of RET by Nkx2-1, Phox2b, Sox10, and Pax3. J Pediatr Surg. 2009;44(10):1904–12.
156. Enomoto H, Crawford PA, Gorodinsky A, Heuckeroth RO, Johnson EM Jr, Milbrandt J. RET signaling is essential for migration, axonal growth and axon guidance of developing sympathetic neurons. Development. 2001;128(20):3963–74.
157. Dong J, Edelmann L, Bajwa AM, Kornreich R, Desnick RJ. Familial dysautonomia: detection of the IKBKAP IVS20(+6T --> C) and R696P mutations and frequencies among Ashkenazi Jews. Am J Med Genet. 2002;110(3):253–7.
158. Mowat DR, Croaker GD, Cass DT, Kerr BA, Chaitow J, Adès LC, Chia NL, Wilson MJ. Hirschsprung disease, microcephaly, mental retardation, and characteristic facial features: delineation of a new syndrome and identification of a locus at chromosome 2q22-q23. J Med Genet. 1998;35(8):617–23.
159. Garavelli L, Mainardi PC. Mowat-Wilson syndrome. Orphanet J Rare Dis. 2007;24(2):42.
160. Garavelli L, Zollino M, Mainardi PC, Gurrieri F, Rivieri F, Soli F, et al. Mowat-Wilson syndrome: facial phenotype changing with age: study of 19 Italian patients and review of the literature. Am J Med Genet A. 2009;149A(3):417–26.
161. Yamada Y, Nomura N, Yamada K, Matsuo M, Suzuki Y, Sameshima K, et al. The spectrum of ZEB2 mutations causing the Mowat-Wilson syndrome in Japanese populations. Am J Med Genet A. 2014;164A(8):1899–908.
162. Moore SW, Fieggen K, Honey E, Zaahl M. Novel Zeb2 gene variation in the Mowat Wilson syndrome (MWS). J Pediatr Surg. 2016;51(2):268–71.
163. Obermayr F, Hotta R, Enomoto H, Young HM. Development and developmental disorders of the enteric nervous system. Nat Rev Gastroenterol Hepatol. 2013;10:43–57.
164. Mulligan LM, Eng C, Healey CS, Ponder MA, Feldman GL, Li P, et al. A de novo mutation of the RET proto-oncogene in a patient with MEN 2A. Hum Mol Genet. 1994;3(6):1007–8. Related Articles, Links
165. Schocket E, Telok HA. Aganglionic megacolon, phaeochromocytoma, megaloureter and neurofibromatosis. Am J Dis Child. 1957;94:185–91.
166. Xing S, Furminger TL, Tong Q, Jhiang SM. Signal transduction pathways activated by RET oncoproteins in PC12 pheochromocytoma cells. J Biol Chem. 1998;273(9):4909–14.
167. Michna BA, McWilliams NB, Krummel TM, Hartenberg MA, Salzberg AM. Multifocal ganglioneuroblastoma coexistent with total colonic aganglionosis. J Pediatr Surg. 1988;23(1 Pt 2):57–9.
168. Hamel CJ, Severijnen RS, De Vaan GA. Neurocristopathy in mother (ganglioneuroblastoma) and daughter (aganglionosis): incidental or causal? Genet Couns. 1994;5(3):303–5.
169. Nemecek ER, Sawin RW, Park J. Treatment of neuroblastoma in patients with neurocristopathy syndromes. J Pediatr Hematol Oncol. 2003;25(2):159–62.
170. Weigel BJ, Pierpont ME, Young TL, Mutchler SB, Neglia JP. Retinoblastoma and Hirschsprung disease in a patient with interstitial deletion of chromosome 13. Am J Med Genet. 1998;77(4):285–8.
171. Sparkes RS, Sparkes MC, Kalina RE, Pagon RA, Salk DJ, Disteche CM. Separation of retinoblastoma and esterase D loci in a patient with sporadic retinoblastoma and del(13)(q14.1q22.3). Hum Genet. 1984;68:258–9.
172. Clausen N, Andersson P, Tommerup N. Familial occurrence of neuroblastoma, von Recklinghausen's neurofibromatosis, Hirschsprung's agangliosis and jaw-winking syndrome. Acta Paediatr Scand. 1989;78(5):736–41.
173. Decker RA, Peacock ML. Occurrence of MEN 2a in familial Hirschsprung's disease: a new indication for genetic testing of the RET proto-oncogene. J Pediatr Surg. 1998;33(2):207–14.
174. Arighi E, Popsueva A, Degl'Innocenti D, Borrello MG, Carniti C, Perala NM, et al. Biological effects of the dual phenotypic Janus mutation of ret cosegregating with both multiple endocrine neoplasia type 2 and Hirschsprung's disease. Mol Endocrinol. 2004;18(4):1004–17.
175. Moore SW, Zaahl M. Familial associations in Medullary thyroid carcinoma with Hirschsprungs disease: the role of the RET C620 "Janus" genetic variation. J Pediatr Surg. 2010;45:393–6.

176. Eng C, Clayton D, Schuffenecker I, Lenoir G, Cote G, Gagel RF, et al. The relationship between specific RET proto-oncogene mutations and disease phenotype in multiple endocrine neoplasia type 2. International RET mutation consortium analysis. JAMA. 1996;276([19]):1575–9.
177. Eng C, Mulligan LM. Mutations of the RET proto-oncogene in the multiple endocrine neoplasia type 2 syndromes, related sporadic tumours, and hirschsprung disease. Hum Mutat. 1997;9(2):97–109.
178. Sijmons RH, Hofstra RM, Wijburg FA, Links TP, Zwierstra RP, Vermey A, et al. Oncological implications of RET gene mutations in Hirschsprung's disease. Gut. 1998;43(4):542–7.
179. Smith VV, Eng C, Milla PJ. Intestinal ganglioneuromatosis and multiple endocrine neoplasia type 2B: implications for treatment. Gut. 1999;45(1):143–6.
180. Maris JM, Kyemba SM, Rebbeck TR, White PS, Sulman EP, Jensen SJ, et al. Molecular genetic analysis of familial neuroblastoma. Eur J Cancer. 1997;33(12):1923–8.
181. Trochet D, Bourdeaut F, Janoueix-Lerosey I, Deville A, de Pontual L, Schleiermacher G, et al. Germline mutations of the paired-like homeobox 2B (PHOX2B) gene in neuroblastoma. Am J Hum Genet. 2004;74(4):761–4.
182. Weese-Mayer DE, Berry-Kravis EM, Marazita ML. In pursuit (and discovery) of a genetic basis for congenital central hypoventilation syndrome. Respir Physiol Neurobiol. 2005;149(1–3):73–82.
183. Fisher JP, Tweddle DA. Neonatal neuroblastoma. Semin Fetal Neonatal Med. 2012;17(4):207–15.
184. Raskind WH, Conrad EU, Matsushita M. Frequent loss of heterozygosity for markers on chromosome arm 10q in chondrosarcomas. Genes Chromosomes Cancer. 1996;16(2):138–43.
185. Kondo H, Harigaya K, Kurosu K, Yumoto N, Mikata A. Peripheral T cell lymphoma (immunoblastic type, HTLV-1 negative) associated with aganglionosis of the intestine. Rinsho Ketsueki. 1994;35(5):495–500.
186. Cass D. Aganglionosis: associated anomalies. J Paediatr Child Health. 1990;26(6):351–4.
187. Patterson K, Toomey KE, Chandra RS. Hirschsprung disease in a 46,XY phenotypic infant girl with Smith-Lemli-Opitz syndrome. J Pediatr. 1983;103(3):425–7.
188. Rakheja D, Wilson GN, Rogers BB. Biochemical abnormality associated with Smith-Lemli-Opitz syndrome in an infant with features of Rutledge multiple congenital anomaly syndrome confirms that the latter is a variant of the former. Pediatr Dev Pathol. 2003;6(3):270–7.
189. Maeda T, Okazaki K, Tachibana M, Sakamoto Y, Sakaeda H, Yamamoto Y, et al. A case of Hirschsprung's disease associated with Laurence-Moon-Bardet-Biedl syndrome. Nihon Shokakibyo Gakkai Zasshi. 1984;81(3):912–6.
190. Islek I, Kucukoduk S, Erkan D, Bernay F, Kalayci AG, Gork S, et al. Bardet-Biedl syndrome: delayed diagnosis in a child with Hirschsprung disease. Clin Dysmorphol. 1996;5([3]):271–3.
191. Beales PL, Kopelman PG. Obesity genes. Clin Endocrinol (Oxf). 1996;45(4):373–8.
192. de Pontual L, Zaghloul NA, Thomas S, Davis EE, McGaughey DM, Dollfus H, et al. Epistasis between RET and BBS mutations modulates enteric innervation and causes syndromic Hirschsprung disease. Proc Natl Acad Sci U S A. 2009;18:13921–6.
193. Hurst JA, Markiewicz M, Kumar D, Brett EM. Unknown syndrome: Hirschsprung's disease, microcephaly, and iris coloboma: a new syndrome of defective neuronal migration. J Med Genet. 1988;25(7):494–7.
194. Stone DL, Slavotinek A, Bouffard GG, Banerjee-Basu S, Baxevanis AD, Barr M, et al. Mutation of a gene encoding a putative chaperonin causes McKusick-Kaufman syndrome. Nat Genet. 2000;25(1):79–82.
195. Curry CJ, Carey JC, Holland JS, Chopra D, Fineman R, Golabi M, et al. Smith-Lemli-Opitz syndrome-type II: multiple congenital anomalies with male pseudohermaphroditism and frequent early lethality. Am J Med Genet. 1987;26(1):45–57.
196. Mueller C, Patel S, Irons M, Antshel K, Salen G, Tint GS, et al. Normal cognition and behavior in a Smith-Lemli-Opitz syndrome patient who presented with Hirschsprung disease. Am J Med Genet A. 2003;123A(1):100–6.
197. McCallion AS, Chakravarti A. EDNRB/EDN3 and Hirschsprung disease type II. Pigment Cell Res. 2001;14(3):161–9.
198. Kelsh RN. Sorting out Sox10 functions in neural crest development 10. Bioessays. 2006;28(8):788–98.
199. Wilson M, Mowat D, Dastot-Le Moal F, Cacheux V, Kaariainen H, Cass D, et al. Further delineation of the phenotype associated with heterozygous mutations in ZFHX1B. Am J Med Genet A. 2003;119A(3):257–65.
200. Cacheux V, Dastot-Le Moal F, Kaariainen H, Bondurand N, Rintala R, Boissier B, Wilson M, Mowat D, Goossens M. Loss-of-function mutations in SIP1 Smad interacting protein 1 result in a syndromic Hirschsprung disease. Hum Mol Genet. 2001;10:1503–10.
201. Moore S, Johnson GA. Hirschsprung's disease: genetic and functional associations of Downs and Waardenburghs Syndromes. Semin Pediatr Surg. 1998;7(3):156–61.
202. Serra A, Gorgens H, Alhadad K, Ziegler A, Fitze G, Schackert HK. Analysis of RET, ZEB2, EDN3 and GDNF genomic rearrangements in 80 patients with Hirschsprung disease (using multiplex ligation-dependent probe amplification). Ann Hum Genet. 2009;73(2):147–51.
203. Borrego S, Ruiz A, Saez ME, Gimm O, Gao X, Lopez-Alonso M, et al. RET genotypes comprising

specific haplotypes of polymorphic variants predispose to isolated Hirschsprung disease. J Med Genet. 2000;37([8]):572–8.
204. Wartiovaara K, Salo M, Sariola H. Hirschsprung's disease genes and the development of the enteric nervous system. Ann Med. 1998;30(1):66–74.
205. Carter TC, Kay DM, Browne ML, Liu A, Romitti PA, Kuehn D, et al. Hirschsprung's disease and variants in genes that regulate enteric neural crest cell proliferation, migration and differentiation. J Hum Genet. 2012;57(8):485–93.
206. Venditti CP, Hunt P, Donnenfeld A, Zackai E, Spinner NB. Mosaic paternal uniparental (iso) disomy for chromosome 20 associated with multiple anomalies. Am J Med Genet A. 2004;124(3):274–9.
207. Prabhakara K, Wyandt HE, Huang XL, Prasad KS, Ramadevi AR. Recurrent proximal 18p monosomy and 18q trisomy in a family with a maternal pericentric inversion of chromosome 18. Ann Genet. 2004;47(3):297–303.
208. Hayward MD, Cameron AH. Triple mosaicism of the sex chromosomes in Turner syndrome and Hirschsprungs disease. Lancet. 1962;2:623.
209. Shanske A, Ferreira JC, Leonard JC, Fuller P, Marion RW. Hirschsprung disease in an infant with a contiguous gene syndrome of chromosome 13. Am J Med Genet. 2001;102(3):231–6.
210. Fewtrell MS, Tam PK, Thomson AH, Fitchett M, Currie J, Huson SM, et al. Hirschsprung's disease associated with a deletion of chromosome 10 (q11.2q21.2): a further link with the neurocristopathies? J Med Genet. 1994;31(4):325–7.
211. Tang CS, Cheng G, So MT, Yip B, Miao X, Wong E, et al. Genome-wide copy number analysis uncovers a new HSCR gene: NRG3. PLoS Genet. 2012; https://doi.org/10.1371/journal.pgen.1002687.
212. Lurie IW, Supovitz KR, Rosenblum-Vos LS, Wulfsberg EA. Phenotypic variability of del(2) (q22-q23): report of a case with a review of the literature. Genet Couns. 1994;5(1):11–4.
213. Benailly H, Lapierre J, Laudier B, Amiel J, Attie T, De Blois M, Vekemans M, Romana S. PMX2B, a new candidate gene for Hirschsprung's disease. Clin Genet. 2003;63(3):206–9.
214. Foy C, Newton V, Wellesley D, Harris R, Read AP. Assignment of the locus for Waardenburgh syndrome Type 1 to human chromosome 2q37 and possible homology to the splotch mouse. Am J Hum Genet. 1990;46:1017–23.
215. Mowat DR, Croaker GD, Cass DT, Kerr BA, Chaitow J, Ades LC, et al. Hirschsprung disease, microcephaly, mental retardation, and characteristic facial features: delineation of a new syndrome and identification of a locus at chromosome 2q22-q23. J Med Genet. 1998;35(8):617–23.
216. Azizi E, Berlowitz I, Vinograd I, Reif R, Mundel G. Congenital megacolon associated with familial dysautonomia. Eur J Pediatr. 1984;142(1):68–9.
217. Slaugenhaupt SA. Genetics of familial dysautonomia. Tissue-specific expression of a splicing mutation in the IKBKAP gene. Clin Auton Res. 2002;12(Suppl 1):I15–119.
218. Bonafe L, Schmitt K, Eich G, Giedion A, Superti-Furga A. RMRP gene sequence analysis confirms a cartilage-hair hypoplasia variant with only skeletal manifestations and reveals a high density of single-nucleotide polymorphisms. Clin Genet. 2002;61(2):146–51.
219. Yoder BJ, Prayson RA. Shah-Waardenburg syndrome and Dandy-Walker malformation: an autopsy report. Clin Neuropathol. 2002;21(5):236–40.
220. Hall T, Samuel M, Brain J. Mosaic trisomy 22 associated with total colonic aganglionosis and malrotation. J Pediatr Surg. 2009;44(1):e9–e11.
221. Mahboubi S, Templeton JM Jr. Association of Hirschsprung's disease and imperforate anus in a patient with "cat-eye" syndrome. A report of one case and review of the literature. Pediatr Radiol. 1984;14(6):441–2.
222. Hofstra RM, Elfferich P, Osinga J, Verlind E, Fransen E, Lopez Pison J, et al. Hirschsprung disease and L1CAM: is the disturbed sex ratio caused by L1CAM mutations? J Med Genet. 2002;39(3):E11.
223. Wallace DC. Mouse models for mitochondrial disease. Am J Med Genet. 2001;106(1):71–93.
224. Moore SW. Genetic impact on the treatment & management of Hirschsprung disease. J Pediatr Surg. 2017;52(2):218–22.
225. Burzynski GM, Nolte IM, Bronda A, Bos KK, Osinga J, Plaza Menacho I, et al. Identifying candidate Hirschsprung disease-associated RET variants. Am J Hum Genet. 2005;76(5):850–8.
226. Carrasquillo MM, McCallion AS, Puffenberger EG, Kaschuk CS, No N, Chakravarti A. Genome-wide association study as well as the study of mouse models help to identify the interaction between RET and EDNRB pathways in Hirschsprung disease. Nat Genet. 2002;32:237–44.

12 Association Between Hirschsprung's Disease and Multiple Endocrine Neoplasia

David Coyle and Prem Puri

Contents

D. Coyle
Temple Street Children's University Hospital, Dublin, Ireland

P. Puri (✉)
National Children's Research Centre, Our Lady's Children's Hospital, Crumlin, Dublin, Ireland
e-mail: prem.puri@ncrc.ie

Abbreviations

FMTC	familial medullary thyroid cancer
HSCR	Hirschsprung's disease
MEN	Multiple endocrine neoplasia
MTC	Medullary thyroid cancer
RET	Rearranged during transfection

12.1 Introduction

Hirschsprung's disease (HSCR) is frequently cited as an excellent example of a disease with a complex polygenic mechanism, with approximately 6–15% of cases being familial [1]. The association between multiple endocrine neoplasia type 2 (MEN 2) and gastrointestinal symptoms has long been recognised since the first descriptions of the subtypes of this hereditary cancer syndrome, MEN 2A and MEN 2B, in the mid-1900s [2, 3]. The first report highlighting the co-occurrence of HSCR in a large kindred with MEN 2 was published in 1982 [4]. In the intervening period, major advances in genetic diagnostic technology have greatly improved our knowledge about the association between these two neurocristopathies.

P. Puri (ed.), *Hirschsprung's Disease and Allied Disorders*,
https://doi.org/10.1007/978-3-030-15647-3_12

12.2 The *RET* Proto-oncogene

The *RET* (rearranged during transfection) proto-oncogene is the major susceptibility gene in HSCR and MEN 2. It encodes a tyrosine kinase receptor that is expressed during embryogenesis in neural crest-derived structures, such as the enteric nervous system, the para-follicular C-cells in the thyroid gland and the chromaffin cells of the adrenal gland [5]. It is located on chromosome 10 (10q11.22) and comprises at least 21 exons. RET is a cell surface protein which, when phosphorylated by the ligand glial cell line-derived neurotrophic factor (GDNF), exerts its physiological effects.

Its exact role during embryogenesis is unclear, but absent myenteric nerves throughout the GI tract have been demonstrated in *RET*-null mice [6]. It is thought that the pathogenesis of HSCR involves the presence of an inactivating mutation of the *RET* proto-oncogene, leading to abnormal processing of RET at the endoplasmic reticulum and reduced cell surface expression [7]. Defective *RET* signalling is also implicated in the development of congenital abnormalities of the kidney and urinary tract [8]. In addition, *RET* mutations have been demonstrated in a host of conditions in tissues derived from the neural crest, known collectively as neurocristopathies, which are discussed in further detail below.

12.3 Hirschsprung's Disease as a Neurocristopathy

The neural crest is a population of cells that arises at the junction of the neural and non-neural ectoderm in early embryonic development. These cells ultimately migrate to different parts of the embryo to give rise to a wide array of tissues and are grouped depending on which segment of the cephalocaudal axis they originate from—the cranial neural crest, the cardiac neural crest, the trunk neural crest and the sacral neural crest. The enteric neural crest cells that go on to form the enteric nervous system originate in the trunk and sacral neural crest [9].

The disease process that leads to the characteristic histological findings of aganglionosis and hypertrophic nerve trunks in HSCR is incompletely understood. However, the failure of enteric neural crest cells to migrate to their correct distal intestinal position, proliferate, differentiate or survive is thought to be the key inciting events in the pathogenesis of HSCR. The *RET* pathway plays a key role in all four of these events and is expressed on enteric neural crest cells [10].

Mutations in the *RET* pathway are associated with 10–15% of sporadic cases and more than 50% of familial cases of Hirschsprung's disease [10]. *RET* expression is modulated by numerous transcription factors such as PHOX2A and SOX10. Therefore, other neurocristopathies caused primarily by mutations of these transcription factors have HSCR as a characteristic disease association.

Congenital central hypoventilation syndrome, which is caused by a *PHOX2B* mutation, co-occurs with HSCR in up to 50% of cases [9]. Waardenburg syndrome is characterised by hearing loss and characteristic colour changes in the eyes, hair, and face. Those patients, whose Waardenburg syndrome is associated with a mutation of endothelin-3 or its receptor, endothelin receptor type B (EDNRB), have HSCR as part of their condition (type 4 Waardenburg syndrome/Shah-Waardenburg syndrome) [11]. Mowat-Wilson syndrome is a neurocristopathy association with a mutation of *ZEB2* gene, which is associated with intellectual and developmental delay and a characteristic facies, and, in approximately 45% of cases, HSCR [12]. While HSCR co-occurs with these neurocristopathies with high frequency, the co-occurrence of HSCR and MEN 2 is uncommon, but the study of this association has yielded interesting insights into the mechanism of both conditions.

12.4 Multiple Endocrine Neoplasia 2

Multiple Endocrine Neoplasia (MEN) is a collection of autosomal dominant conditions typified by the occurrence of neoplasms in two or more endocrine organs. Several different forms of MEN exist: MEN 1, MEN 2 and MEN 4. Patients with MEN 2 can be further sub-categorised as having MEN 2A, MEN 2B or familial medullary thyroid cancer (FMTC) [13, 14].

The key component of MEN 2 in all subtypes is the presence of medullary thyroid cancer (MTC). Other features of MEN 2A include the occurrence of pheochromocytoma and parathyroid adenoma or hyperplasia. Additionally, approximately 10% of patients with MEN 2A develop cutaneous lichen amyloidosis, a benign pruritic skin condition. In addition to MTC, MEN 2B is also characterised by marfanoid body habitus, enteric ganglioneuromatosis, mucosal neuromas and skeletal deformities. Those with MEN 2B appear to have a more aggressive phenotype of this condition, whereby the age of onset of MTC is much younger, often in early childhood [13, 14]. While those who have MEN 2B may experience chronic bowel symptoms related to intestinal ganglioneuromatosis, a small proportion of patients with MEN 2A will have HSCR in association with this.

12.5 Genetic Basis of the Association Between Multiple Endocrine Neoplasia Type 2 and Hirschsprung's Disease

The co-occurrence of HSCR and MEN 2A is a rare paradoxical phenomenon, as the former is caused by a loss-of-function mutation in *RET* while an activating mutation of *RET* is implicated in MEN 2A. One study wherein 36 families (426 individuals) at risk of hereditary MTC were screened for *RET* mutations found co-segregation of HSCR with MEN 2A in 6 families, with 15 individuals affected [15]. A small group of *RET* mutations on exon 10, corresponding to the cysteine-rich extracellular domain of RET, is associated with co-segregation of MEN2A and HSCR—C609, C611, C618 and, most commonly, C620, the so-called "Janus" mutations, named after the Roman god of doorways who could face in both directions [16]. One remarkable aspect of this HSCR–MEN 2A association is that the implicated *RET* mutation can vary in state from activated to suppressed across different generations of the same kindred and even in some cases across different time points in individual patients [17].

Mutations related to the C620 position on the *RET* gene, which corresponds with the transmembrane domain of the RET protein, have been most studied in this regard. This mutation has been reported to occur in up to 48.1% of individuals from kindreds where the HSCR–MEN 2A association is present. This series found that only 9% of individuals harbouring this mutation had neither HSCR or MEN 2A, while approximately one quarter of individuals harbouring a so-called "Janus" mutation had developed both conditions [16].

It has been proposed that the "dual personalities" of the *C620* mutation result from its promotion of cellular proliferation (the oncogenic gain-in-function capacity) coupled with cellular insensitivity to GDNF, which impairs the ability of enteric neural crest cells to migrate and branch and leads to apoptosis (the loss-of-function component) [18]. A mechanism for this disease relationship has been proposed based on the upregulation or downregulation of the *unfolded protein response*, a homeostatic stress response to the amount of an unfolded protein in the endoplasmic reticulum. Downregulation of this response as it relates to RET protein synthesis would push a cell, such as an enteric neural crest cell, toward apoptosis, leading to the characteristic findings in the enteric nervous system of the distal bowel in Hirschsprung's disease. Subsequent upregulation of this response leads to cellular changes that promote RET activation. RET is known to influence the activation of downstream pathways that are associated with tumour growth, such as insulin receptor substrate 2 signalling pathway. This may in turn promote carcinogenesis [7].

12.6 Abnormalities of the Enteric Nervous System in Multiple Endocrine Neoplasia Type 2B

MEN 2B is classically associated with a more aggressive phenotype of MTC. In addition, recognition of the typical morphological features associated with MEN 2B could enable earlier diagnosis and enhance survival from MTC. They appear marfanoid, with hypertrophied lips and thickened cornea, and may have joint laxity or kyphoscoliosis [14]. The major mutations identified in patients with MEN 2B are localised to exons 15 (*A883F*) and 16 (*M918 T*) of *RET* [19].

Essentially, all patients with MEN 2B develop gastrointestinal symptoms from infancy. They should be screened for HSCR. The underlying pathological mechanism for these symptoms is ganglioneuromatosis—the presence of multiple benign tumours of the nerve cells, which are demonstrable on biopsy—and the evolution of megacolon in the gastrointestinal tract. These tumours may cause obstructive symptoms which necessitate surgical intervention for resections and/or stoma formation. Approximately 1/3 of patients require operative intervention due to these symptoms [20]. Unlike HSCR, in which the abnormally innervated bowel can be removed with "curative" intent, surgical intervention for ganglioneuromatosis in MEN 2B should be carried out with the intent of palliating obstructive symptoms that cannot be controlled with non-operative treatment.

12.7 Clinical Aspects of Hirschsprung's Disease Co-occurring with Multiple Endocrine Neoplasia Type 2A

HSCR is the most common congenital gut motility disorder wherein approximately 80% of patients have rectosigmoid aganglionosis, with the remaining patients having long-segment disease, a quarter of whom have total colonic aganglionosis. It predominantly affects males, in whom it is 2–4 times more common than in females, although the male predilection is absent in those with long-segment disease and those with trisomy 21 [21].

In patients with Hirschsprung's disease associated with germ line *RET* mutations, the male/female ratio is similar to that of the general HSCR population. However, up to two thirds of such patients have long-segment aganglionosis, with total colonic aganglionosis affecting 40% [22]. Patients, in whom MEN 2A and HSCR co-segregate, have long-segment aganglionosis in approximately 30% of cases, with 17% having total colonic aganglionosis. These rates are considerably higher than in the general population. These findings are particularly referable to patients with *C620* and *C618 RET* mutations [16].

When C-cell hyperplasia or MTC are present in an individual with a so-called "Janus mutation", the median age at diagnosis of these conditions is approximately 21 years [16]. As the majority of cases of HSCR present in infancy, cases of MTC associated with a so-called Janus mutation will almost invariably be noted to arise in a patient with a pre-existing diagnosis of HSCR rather than vice versa. In one study from Finland, of 156 patients who were treated for HSCR over 36 years, 2 cases of MTC were noted in patients aged 35 and 37, the former of whom had familial HSCR. In addition, they identified four patients with *RET* mutations associated with the development of MTC, who at the time of follow-up had not gone on to develop any of the features of MEN 2A [23]. At present, there is no consensus as to whether it is beneficial to routinely offer testing for *RET* mutations to families of patients with HSCR.

12.8 Treatment of Multiple Endocrine Neoplasia Syndrome 2

Approximately 90% of patients with MEN 2 are classified as having either MEN 2A or FMTC. The most common tumours in patients with MEN 2A are medullary thyroid carcinomas, which occur in 90%, and pheochromocytomas, which occur in 50%. While the children with MEN 2A can start getting MTC from age 5 years, those with FMTC are more likely to have an onset of MTC in adulthood. Parathyroid hyperplasia and resultant hyperparathyroidism is a feature of MEN 2A only and occurs in a quarter of patients in midlife. MTC in children with MEN 2B has a much more aggressive phenotype and an earlier age of onset.

Approximately 40% of individuals with MEN 2B develop a pheochromocytoma [14].

In children with HSCR and a germ line *RET* mutation which pre-disposes them to MTC, a complete physical examination should be undertaken, with emphasis on the neck examination. An ultrasound scan of the thyroid should be performed and a serum calcitonin level measured. Of note, children under three have constitutively elevated levels of calcitonin, with boys having higher levels than girls [19].

In MEN 2A, *C634* mutations of the *RET* proto-oncogene represent a higher level of risk for development of MTC compared to the so-called "Janus" mutations. In such high-risk patients, a prophylactic total thyroidectomy has been recommended at or before 5 years of age contingent on serum calcitonin levels not already becoming elevated. In patients at moderate risk, which would include patients with MEN 2A co-segregating with HSCR, prophylactic thyroidectomy is recommended when the serum calcitonin starts to rise or at a point where parental preference is to discontinue clinical surveillance. Because of the aggressive nature of MTC associated with MEN 2B, prophylactic thyroidectomy is recommended in infancy, even in the first months of life with or without a level 4 lymph node dissection with autotransplantation of a parathyroid gland [19]. Patients with thyroid nodules, diagnosed with MTC, should undergo a total thyroidectomy with lymph node dissection. Those with metastatic MTC may also be managed with a combination of surgery, radiotherapy and a range of targeted therapies, such as tyrosine kinase inhibitors [24].

Pheochromocytoma is the first presenting tumour of MEN 2 in only approximately 10% of patients. They are generally benign and bilateral and typically occur in the fourth decade of life. Screening for pheochromocytoma typically begins at 11 years old for patients with the high-risk mutations of MEN 2B (*M918 T, A883F*) and in MEN 2A patients with *C634F* mutations. In patients with moderate-risk *RET* mutations, screening starts at 16 years old. Screening involves measurement of urinary and plasma metanephrines and normetanephrines and, in those with abnormal biochemistry, cross-sectional imaging of the adrenal gland with magnetic resonance imaging (MRI) or computed tomography (CT). Any patient planned to undergo intervention for MTC should be screened for a pheochromocytoma, as operative removal of the adrenal tumour should precede resection of the thyroid tumour [14, 19]. Resection of a pheochromocytoma can be performed as an open, laparoscopic or retroperitoneoscopic procedure and an adrenal-sparing procedure has even been described.

Screening for hyperparathyroidism begins in MEN 2 at the same time as screening for pheochromocytoma, with a serum ionised calcium, serum calcium corrected for albumin and serum parathyroid hormone levels. Surgical treatment with subtotal parathyroidectomy, total parathyroidectomy with auto-implantation or limited parathyroidectomy guided by intraoperative parathyroid level monitoring is offered as appropriate [19].

12.9 Conclusions and Future Directions

The co-occurrence of HSCR and MEN 2A is the result of an unusual *RET* mutation that can behave as both a "gain-of-function" (MEN 2) and a "loss-of-function" (HSCR) mutation, not just in the same kindred but in the same individual. Such mutations, located on exon 10 of chromosome 10, are associated with a moderate risk of developing MTC and are associated with a less aggressive phenotype than those mutations, which do not co-segregate with HSCR or the mutations found in individuals with MEN 2B. In the screening of patients with HSCR for *RET* mutations, the finding of a so-called "Janus" mutation—*C620, C618, C611* and *C609*—should prompt screening for MEN 2A in the individual patient, as well as associated family members. The corollary to this is that children born to parents with a family history of MEN 2A, who exhibit obstructive-type bowel symptoms, should be screened for HSCR. Children in whom MEN 2A co-segregates with HSCR are more likely to have long-segment or total colonic aganglionosis compared to the overall population with HSCR, with obvious ramifications for their long-term functional outcome. While the gastrointestinal symptoms exhibited by children with MEN 2B-associated ganglioneuromatosis and megacolon may be similar to those seen in HSCR, surgical intervention in this population should be reserved for those with mechanical obstruction. A more in-depth understanding of the mechanism of the "Janus mutation" seen in this disease association is required to shed light on the pathogenesis of Hirschsprung's disease but may also lead to insights that change our understanding of other illnesses with a genetic basis.

References

1. Godbole K. Many faces of Hirschsprung's disease. Indian Pediatr. 2004;41(11):1115–23.
2. Sipple JH. The association of pheochromocytoma with carcinoma of the thyroid gland. Am J Med. 1961;31:163–6.
3. Williams ED, Pollock DJ. Multiple mucosal neuromata with endocrine tumours: a syndrome allied to von Recklinghausen's disease. J Pathol Bacteriol. 1966;91(1):71–80. https://doi.org/10.1002/path.1700910109.
4. Verdy M, Weber AM, Roy CC, Morin CL, Cadotte M, Brochu P. Hirschsprung's disease in a family with multiple endocrine neoplasia type 2. J Pediatr Gastroenterol Nutr. 1982;1(4):603–7.
5. Eng C, Clayton D, Schuffenecker I, Lenoir G, Cote G, Gagel RF, Ploos Van Amstel HK, Lips CJM, Nishisho I, Takai SI, Marsh DJ, Robinson BG, Frank-Raue K, Raue F, Xue F, Noll WW, Romei C, Pacini F, Fink M, Niederle B, Zedenius J, Nordenskjold M, Komminoth P, Hendy GN, Gharib H, Thibodeau SN, Lacroix A, Frilling A, Ponder BAJ, Mulligan LM. The relationship between specific ret proto-oncogene mutations and disease phenotype in multiple endocrine neoplasia type 2: international RET mutation consortium analysis. J Am Med Assoc. 1996;276(19):1575–9.
6. Edery P, Eng C, Munnich A, Lyonnet S. RET in human development and oncogenesis. BioEssays. 1997;19(5):389–95. https://doi.org/10.1002/bies.950190506.
7. Moore SW, Zaahl M. The Hirschsprung's-multiple endocrine neoplasia connection. Clinics. 2012;67(Suppl):63–7.
8. Davis TK, Hoshi M, Jain S. To bud or not to bud: the RET perspective in CAKUT. Pediatr Nephrol. 2014;29(4):597–608. https://doi.org/10.1007/s00467-013-2606-5.
9. Vega-Lopez GA, Cerrizuela S, Tribulo C, Aybar MJ. Neurocristopathies: new insights 150 years after the neural crest discovery. Dev Biol. 2018; https://doi.org/10.1016/j.ydbio.2018.05.013.
10. Butler Tjaden NE, Trainor PA. The developmental etiology and pathogenesis of Hirschsprung disease. Transl Res. 2013;162(1):1–15. https://doi.org/10.1016/j.trsl.2013.03.001.
11. Read AP. Waardenburg syndrome. Adv Otorhinolaryngol. 2000;56:32–8.
12. Coyle D, Puri P. Hirschsprung's disease in children with Mowat-Wilson syndrome. Pediatr Surg Int. 2015;31(8):711–7. https://doi.org/10.1007/s00383-015-3732-x.
13. Peczkowska M, Januszewicz A. Multiple endocrine neoplasia type 2. Familial Cancer. 2005;4(1):25–36. https://doi.org/10.1007/s10689-005-0656-y.
14. Walls GV. Multiple endocrine neoplasia (MEN) syndromes. Semin Pediatr Surg. 2014;23(2):96–101. https://doi.org/10.1053/j.sempedsurg.2014.03.008.
15. Decker RA, Peacock ML. Occurrence of MEN 2a in familial Hirschsprung's disease: a new indication for genetic testing of the RET proto-oncogene. J Pediatr Surg. 1998;33(2):207–14.
16. Coyle D, Friedmacher F, Puri P. The association between Hirschsprung's disease and multiple endocrine neoplasia type 2a: a systematic review. Pediatr Surg Int. 2014;30(8):751–6. https://doi.org/10.1007/s00383-014-3538-2.
17. Moore SW, Zaahl M. Familial associations in medullary thyroid carcinoma with Hirschsprung disease: the role of the RET-C620 "Janus" genetic variation. J Pediatr Surg. 2010;45(2):393–6. https://doi.org/10.1016/j.jpedsurg.2009.10.080.
18. Arighi E, Popsueva A, Degl'innocenti D, Borrello MG, Carniti C, Perala NM, Pierotti MA, Sariola H. Biological effects of the dual phenotypic Janus mutation of ret cosegregating with both multiple endocrine neoplasia type 2 and hirschsprung's disease. Mol Endocrinol. 2004;18(4):1004–17.
19. Wells SA Jr, Asa SL, Dralle H, Elisei R, Evans DB, Gagel RF, Lee N, Machens A, Moley JF, Pacini F, Raue F, Frank-Raue K, Robinson B, Rosenthal MS, Santoro M, Schlumberger M, Shah M, Waguespack SG, American Thyroid Association Guidelines Task Force on Medullary Thyroid C. Revised American Thyroid Association guidelines for the management of medullary thyroid carcinoma. Thyroid. 2015;25(6):567–610. https://doi.org/10.1089/thy.2014.0335.
20. Cohen MS, Phay JE, Albinson C, DeBenedetti MK, Skinner MA, Lairmore TC, Doherty GM, Balfe DM, Wells SA Jr, Moley JF. Gastrointestinal manifestations of multiple endocrine neoplasia type 2. Ann Surg. 2002;235(5):648–54; discussion 654–645.
21. Kenny SE, Tam PK, Garcia-Barcelo M. Hirschsprung's disease. Semin Pediatr Surg. 2010;19(3):194–200. https://doi.org/10.1053/j.sempedsurg.2010.03.004.
22. Moore SW, Zaahl M. Clinical and genetic correlations of familial Hirschsprung's disease. J Pediatr Surg. 2015;50(2):285–8. https://doi.org/10.1016/j.jpedsurg.2014.11.016.

23. Virtanen VB, Pukkala E, Kivisaari R, Salo PP, Koivusalo A, Arola J, Miettinen PJ, Rintala RJ, Perola M, Pakarinen MP. Thyroid cancer and co-occurring RET mutations in Hirschsprung disease. Endocr Relat Cancer. 2013;20(4):595–602.
24. Wells SA Jr. Advances in the management of MEN2: from improved surgical and medical treatment to novel kinase inhibitors. Endocr Relat Cancer. 2018;25(2):T1–T13. https://doi.org/10.1530/ERC-17-0325.

Hirschsprung-Associated Enterocolitis

13

Laura V. Veras and Ankush Gosain

Contents

L. V. Veras
Division of Pediatric Surgery, Department of Surgery, University of Tennessee Health Science Center, Memphis, TN, USA
e-mail: lveras@uthsc.edu

A. Gosain (✉)
Division of Pediatric Surgery, Department of Surgery, University of Tennessee Health Science Center, Memphis, TN, USA

Children's Foundation Research Institute, Le Bonheur Children's Hospital, Memphis, TN, USA
e-mail: agosain@uthsc.edu

13.1 Introduction

Hirschsprung disease (HSCR, Online Mendelian Inheritance in Man #142623) is a common cause of neonatal bowel obstruction and was first described in 1886 by Harald Hirschsprung [42]. HSCR can lead to the feared complication of Hirschsprung-associated enterocolitis (HAEC), which is the condition that, in retrospect, Hirschsprung originally described. Broadly, HAEC is clinically characterized by abdominal distension, fever, and diarrhea, although there can be a variety of other associated symptoms, including colicky abdominal pain, lethargy, and the passage of bloodstained stools. At the time of his original description, Hirschsprung presented two children with constipation from birth who died after developing marked abdominal distension and loose stools; these would become the first reported cases of HAEC. Although the concept of HAEC was alluded to in the literature in 1950 by Burnard, Fisher and Swenson in 1956, and Dorman in 1957, it was not until 1962 that Bill and Chapman presented the first definitive description of the condition [11, 13, 22, 25].

HAEC can occur preoperatively or postoperatively and is the presenting symptom of HSCR in up to 25% of infants [26, 39, 63, 66]. The incidence of enterocolitis ranges from 20% to 60% [6, 24, 26, 30, 38]. HAEC can occur at any time from the neonatal period onwards into adulthood

P. Puri (ed.), *Hirschsprung's Disease and Allied Disorders*,
https://doi.org/10.1007/978-3-030-15647-3_13

and can be independent of the medical management or surgical procedure performed. Recurrent HAEC can occur even in the presence of a diverting colostomy and is termed "diversion enterocolitis" [49, 73].

Currently, the diagnosis of HAEC is predominantly based on clinical judgment. This has led to highly variable reports in the incidence rates of HAEC, ranging from 25% to 30% in recent series to as high as 60% in the past. Preoperative incidence is estimated at 6%–60%, and postoperative incidence ranges from 25% to 42% [23, 38, 77]. The overall mortality rate associated with HAEC ranges from 1% to 10%, with the majority of deaths occurring in newborns prior to definitive operation [63]. These newborn infants are at the highest risk of mortality among patients with HAEC. It is unclear whether these infants have higher mortality rates due to a delay in diagnosis, immature immune responses, or some other mechanism. Fortunately, the mortality rate appears to be declining over time, likely due to increasing recognition of this devastating complication. This includes earlier diagnosis of HSCR and HAEC and initiation of therapies such as rectal decompression, vigorous fluid resuscitation, and antibiotic therapy.

However, despite the improvement in mortality rates in HAEC, the morbidity has a profound impact on prolonged hospitalization with a mean of 13 days (ranging from 6 to 29 days). Teitelbaum et al. found that neonates with HAEC have a mortality rate of 5% and a morbidity rate of 30%, and their hospitalization is twice as long as neonates without HAEC [76]. The medical management of HSCR children with HAEC is 2.5 times costlier than of those without HAEC. Moreover, HSCR patients who develop HAEC have worse long-term bowel function than those who never develop HAEC, possibly secondary to inflammatory changes to the ENS [63].

In this chapter, we will review our current understanding of HAEC pathophysiology, risk factors, diagnosis, and treatment. We will additionally present areas of current research or controversy and topics for future investigation.

13.2 Pathophysiology

Despite multiple investigations and numerous theories, a complete understanding of the etiology of HAEC is still elusive. There are currently four prevailing theories regarding the etiology of HAEC: (1) dysmotility, (2) intestinal barrier function, (3) impaired mucosal immunity, and (4) abnormal microbiota.

13.2.1 Historical Considerations

Multiple small series or case reports have put forth etiologic considerations for HAEC.

In 1973, Ament and Bill presented the case of a 6-year-old boy with chronic enterocolitis following surgery for HSCR [3]. Clinical investigations revealed the presence of a sucrase-isomaltase deficiency, and the child recovered on a low sucrose diet. This led to the postulation that non-obstructed HAEC is caused by an inborn error of metabolism. It is important to note that this has not been replicated and that Ament and Bill acknowledged that the boy was an Eskimo and that 10% of Greenland Eskimos are sucrose-intolerant.

Berry and Frazer in 1968 suggested that HAEC is initiated by a sensitivity reaction similar to a Shwartzman reaction caused by intraluminal organisms invading the submucosa [9]. They injected endotoxin directly into the exteriorized rabbit bowel proximal to an obstruction and produced enterocolitis in six of nine animals.

A single case was reported by Lloyd-Still and Demers of HAEC with fulminant unresponsive diarrhea which revealed high PgE1 levels [47]. In response to cholestyramine, a 12-fold decrease in prostaglandin E (PgE) levels in the colostomy fluid was detected. It was postulated that increased PgE activity, enterotoxin, and bile acid malabsorption may be involved in HAEC.

In 1988 Wilson-Storey et al. postulated that defective white cell function may be a predisposing factor for HAEC [94]. White cell counts were analyzed in nine patients with HSCR, of whom five developed HAEC and ten age-matched controls. Their data showed statistically significant differences between the neutrophil count in those with HAEC, HSCR, and controls. This relative neutropenia worsened in three patients during and after an episode of HAEC. The authors also postulated that white cells in HAEC patients are "sluggish" in response to the inflammation.

While these series have not been confirmed in the basic science laboratory or larger clinical series, it is important to consider that there may be component contributions from these types of observations to the multifactorial process of HAEC.

13.2.2 Dysmotility

One of the earliest proposed causes for HAEC was impaired intestinal motility leading to functional obstruction with either subsequent bacterial stasis, overgrowth and translocation, or distension and ischemia [11, 74, 75]. Bill and Chapman argued that partial mechanical obstruction was involved in the pathogenesis of HAEC causing mechanical dilatation of the proximal bowel leading to fecal loading and stasis resulting in further dilatation and thus mucosal ischemia and bacterial invasion which was cured by colostomy [11]. This suggests that enterocolitis only occurs in dilated ganglionic proximal bowel. However, this theory does not explain the enterocolitis that occurs in distal colon with a defunctioning proximal stoma, the occurrence of enterocolitis in postoperative patients, or histological evidence of enterocolitis in aganglionic bowel [67, 72].

The ENS participates in host defense by modulation of secretory function and propulsion of luminal contents, thereby diluting and purging pathogens [71, 91]. The role of intestinal motility in the pathogenesis of inflammatory bowel disease is well described, with acute episodes of intestinal inflammation in Crohn's disease associated with decreased motility [10, 59]. It has been noted, in the $EdnrB^{NCC-/-}$ model, decreased neuronal density in the ganglionated bowel [96]. Further, there is a shift in neurotransmitter phenotypes, with overrepresentation of nitrergic (relaxation) neurons and underrepresentation of cholinergic (contractility) neurons. Similar findings have recently been published in the $EdnrB^{-/-}$ model and confirmed in human tissues, with a positive correlation between increased nitrergic neurons and postoperative enterocolitis [16].

13.2.3 Intestinal Barrier Dysfunction

The intestinal barrier plays a critical role in maintaining host health. Clinically the voluminous amount of mucus produced during HAEC is quite obvious and dramatic. Goblet cells produce mucus, which helps to maintain epithelial integrity by serving as a scaffold for bactericidal and bacteriostatic proteins. Abnormalities in mucin production, therefore, may contribute to the pathogenesis of HAEC.

In 1981, Akkary et al. studied rectal biopsies of HSCR patients and found a marked increase in the volume of mucin compared to control tissues [1]. Teitelbaum et al. hypothesized that HSCR involves an alteration in the composition of mucin in the colon, such that there is mucin retention and crypt dilation [76]. They proposed a histologic grading system which is unique to HSCR and cystic fibrosis. When they excluded patients with trisomy 21, whose histologic findings were often inconsistent with their clinical features, this grading system found that 100% of patients with HAEC had grade 3 or higher. Even though this system is not ideal for clinical use given the uneven distribution of histologic changes in resected specimens, it does demonstrate how the mucosa becomes susceptible to pathogens through local inflammatory responses.

A study of mucin turnover showed that HSCR patients who developed HAEC had turnover rates sevenfold lower than HSCR patients who did not develop HAEC [5]. Additionally, Hirschsprung's patients also have decreased MUC-2, the predominant mucin expressed in the human colon; MUC-2 is nondetectable in patients with HAEC [12, 51]. This may suggest an intrinsic problem that could allow for bacterial adherence and translocation. Finally, Thiagarajah et al. compared tissue from HSCR patients and the distal colon of *EdnrB*$^{-/-}$ mice and found increased goblet cell numbers when compared to controls [81]. They then used trans-epithelial resistance measurements to assess for functional differences and noted that trans-epithelial resistance and fecal dehydration were increased in the distal colon of *EdnrB*$^{-/-}$ mice. Additionally, they found increased mucus viscosity and therefore impaired particle diffusion in null mice.

Overall the evidence has not proven whether mucin alteration is due to the underlying aganglionic condition or a result of the enterocolitis. However, the balance of data supports the concept that the mucin variations are an expression of an altered mucosal barrier and the underlying aganglionic process itself [51]. Taken together, these findings suggest that alterations in mucus production and function may play a role in the development of HAEC.

13.2.4 Impaired Mucosal Immunity

Abnormal leukocyte function has been implicated in the development of HAEC.

Secretory IgA immunoglobulin provides a major immunological barrier in the gastrointestinal tract. IgA is the predominant immunoglobulin at all levels in the intestinal tract, both in the lumen and within the wall. Albanese et al. have shown that secreted IgA binds to bacteria and prevents bacterial translocation across an intact segment of viable intestinal tissue [2]. In the late 1980s, Wilson-Storey et al. conducted a series of studies which demonstrated that patients affected by HSCR have impaired transfer of secretory IgA across the GI mucosa [92, 94]. Specifically, they noted that although HSCR patients had increased IgA in their buccal mucosal tissue, there was a significant decrease of secretory IgA in the saliva. Similarly, the plasma cells in the lamina propria of the bowel were found to have significant increased levels of IgA, IgM, and IgG in HAEC bowel compared to non-HAEC bowel [44]. Those same HAEC patients were found to have decreased luminal IgA, suggesting decreased production or impaired transport into the lumen.

The most common genetic defects associated with HSCR are mutations of *rearranged during transfection* (*Ret*) and *endothelin receptor B* (*EdnrB*), which are both required for NCC migration and ENS formation [4]. Piebald mice, which have a naturally occurring *EdnrB* mutation, demonstrate congenital megacolon with absent distal ganglion cells and hence are an excellent model for HSCR [87]. A number of studies have established mucosal secretory function in HAEC in these animals [31, 32]. Two distinct patterns of mortality occur with the majority of mice (64%) characterized by becoming unwell acutely with evidence of acute enterocolitis at 3–4 weeks and then dying quickly or dying between 9 and 11 weeks due to ileus with massive abdominal distension and megacolon. Interestingly two different immunological responses were evident. Those with a more acute history had acute splenitis and a severe diffuse lymphocytic response in the intestinal submucosa and lamina propria with a significantly raised level of IgA in contrast to controls and the late death group. The late death group had increased plasma cell distribution within the deep layer of the lamina propria only. This increased level of plasma cell infiltration in the ganglionic segment of the colon in the early death group implies that the local antigenic stimulation is the principal pathological event. Interestingly, the finding of decreased luminal IgA has also been observed in *EdnrB*$^{NCC-/-}$ mice, in which *EdnrB* is deleted only in neural crest cells which form the ENS [34]. The *EdnrB*$^{NCC-/-}$ mouse develops colorectal aganglionosis and HAEC similar to human HSCR. A recent study showed not only that luminal IgA is reduced but that this finding is specific to the gut, with normal levels of bronchial and nasal IgA observed in these animals [34]. Overall it appears that IgA production by plasma cells is either normal or impaired and that transport into the lumen is further impaired [52].

Mucosal neuroendocrine (NE) cells mediate intestinal function through synthesis and storage of neuroendocrine neuropeptides and biogenic amines which act as chemical messengers [88]. Soeda et al. demonstrated that NE cells are increased in the aganglionic segment of bowel in

HSCR as opposed to the ganglionated bowel and normal controls [69]. They noted a marked reduction in NE cells in ganglionated bowel in HAEC compared to those without. These diminished NE cells may represent an impaired immune response or a deficiency which may facilitate the initialization of inflammation [70]. This impaired immune response theory is echoed in trisomy 21. The combination of HSCR and trisomy 21 is associated with a higher incidence of enterocolitis, with 50% of patients with trisomy 21 and HSCR developing HAEC in contrast to 29% among the normal population [4]. Infants with trisomy 21 have an intrinsic immune deficiency due to both decreased cytotoxic T lymphocytes and derangement in humoral function which may explain their increased risk of HAEC [56].

Histological evidence of enterocolitis consists of a number of features including crypt abscesses, leukocyte aggregates, ulceration, and Paneth cell metaplasia [31]. Paneth cells are normally present in the small bowel and secrete lysozymes which digest the bacterial wall membranes. Their presence in HAEC colon suggests an attempt at reinforcement of the mucosal immunity. ICAM-1 is a cell surface intercellular adhesion glycoprotein which is involved in leukocyte recruitment when inflammation occurs. Kobayashi et al. have demonstrated that ICAM-1 shows increased expression in the endothelium of both the ganglionated and aganglionic bowels in patients with HAEC [45]. This emphasizes the importance of endothelial cell activation in HAEC pathogenesis. Elhalaby et al. postulated that the occurrence of a single episode of HAEC can alter intrinsic intestinal immunity by causing a chronic change to the mucosa to an increased risk of further episodes [24]. This would help to explain the lower but real recurrence rate of HAEC following a "diversion" colostomy or a successful pull-through.

Splenic lymphopenia is also thought to contribute to an etiology of impaired immunity. This was first described in the *EdnrB*$^{-/-}$ mouse model by Cheng et al. [18]. These animals have abnormal splenic architecture and reduced total lymphocytes in the spleen. Specifically, they have a relative reduction in B as compared to T lymphocytes, as well as a negative correlation between splenic lymphocyte counts and intestinal inflammation on histologic analysis. This finding was confirmed in the *EdnrB*$^{NCC-/-}$ model, with the additional discovery of a decrease in marginal zone B lymphocytes, suggesting impaired B lymphocyte development or trafficking from the spleen to the Peyer's patches of the small intestine [34]. Another group attempted to understand the contribution of the *EdnrB* genotype to the clinical expression of HAEC by performing bone marrow transplants from *EdnrB* animals to *Rag2*$^{-/-}$ recipients and inducing bowel obstruction in wild-type animals [27]. They concluded that stress from obstruction resulted in similar lymphocyte alterations to those seen in HAEC models. However, they found that after surgical relief of obstruction, *EdnrB*$^{-/-}$ mice still carried a 40% risk of developing HAEC [97].

13.2.5 Abnormal Microbiota

Infectious etiologies have been linked to enterocolitis by a number of studies. *Clostridium difficile* was reported by Thomas et al. when high titers of the toxin were detected in four of six patients with HAEC [83]. They further detected the cytopathic toxin in 7 of 13 (54%), and *C. difficile* was isolated in 77% of children with HAEC [82]. In the control groups, *C. difficile* was isolated in 18% of those with HSCR and in 30% of children without. The authors postulated that the toxin was pathogenetic due to the incidence of toxin in the feces, the magnitude of the toxin levels, and the isolation rates for *C. difficile* which were significantly higher in HAEC patients than in those without HAEC or even HSCR. The possibility that HAEC could prevent the development of a "benign" colonic bacterial flora and aggressively treating *C. difficile* could improve this made this a very exciting theory. However, this has not been proven on subsequent investigations: 50% of all patients with HSCR have *C. difficile,* and there is no variation in incidence between before and after surgery [37]. Wilson-Storey et al. demonstrated a broad spectrum of organisms present in the stools with no significant difference in the *Clostridium* carriage rate between those with HAEC and those without HAEC or normal controls [93]. After an episode of enterocolitis, 70% of patients with HAEC have *C. difficile* present as opposed to 42% of those without HAEC. It is postulated that after the initiation of the enterocolitis episode, alteration in mucosal immunity allows *C. difficile* to flourish. Although it may not be causative, it may complicate the colitis. Pseudomembranous colitis with stools positive for *C. difficile* is rare and has been reported in four patients with a 50% mortality despite vancomycin therapy [8].

While several organisms have been found to be associated with HAEC (including *C. difficile*, *E. coli*, and rotavirus), none has been demonstrated to be causative. In the last 5 years, two mouse model studies have shed light on the relationship between host microbiome and development of HAEC.

Using the *EdnrB*$^{-/-}$ mouse model, Ward et al. demonstrated increasing microbiome diversity over 24 days, with a greater increase in HSCR mice versus wild type [86]. They identified clusters of microbiota in each group, showing that wild-type and HSCR mice had distinct microbiomes. Further, HSCR mice were found to have higher levels of *Bacteroidetes* and *Firmicutes* than controls. Similarly, Pierre et al. found evidence of comparable microbiomes between HSCR mice and controls early in the neonatal period, with divergence of the microbiota between HSCR and controls as the onset of HAEC approached [62]. HSCR mice expressed increased *Bacteroidetes* and *Clostridium* species, and *E. coli* was found only in HSCR mice. Both of these studies also showed decrease in *Lactobacillus* over time in HSCR mice. Another group used the *EdnrB*$^{-/-}$ model of HSCR/HAEC to demonstrate that survival could be extended to 36 days by changing to a liquid diet and the addition of oral antibiotics, further supporting a role for the microbiome in the development of HAEC [17].

Approaches to HAEC using genomics have also contributed to knowledge about alterations in the microbiome of HAEC patients. DeFilippo et al. used amplified ribosomal DNA restriction analysis to demonstrate distinct changes in the microbiota of a single child as he progressed from pre-enterocolitis through the acute episode and onto resolution [21]. Yan et al. used this technique in two patients with HAEC and two without and found different bacterial clustering in the patients with HAEC as compared to those without [95]. Recent studies are beginning to investigate a potential role for alterations in the fungal communities of the gut and their contribution to HAEC pathogenesis [29].

13.2.6 Summary

Impaired mucosal immunity, abnormal microbiota, intestinal barrier dysfunction, and dysmotility all appear to contribute to the pathogenesis of HAEC. ENS dysfunction can result in microbiome dysbiosis through impaired motility. When followed by impaired intestinal barrier function and an abnormal immune response, HAEC develops. This stepwise model is the target of current research endeavors by multiple groups (Fig. 13.1).

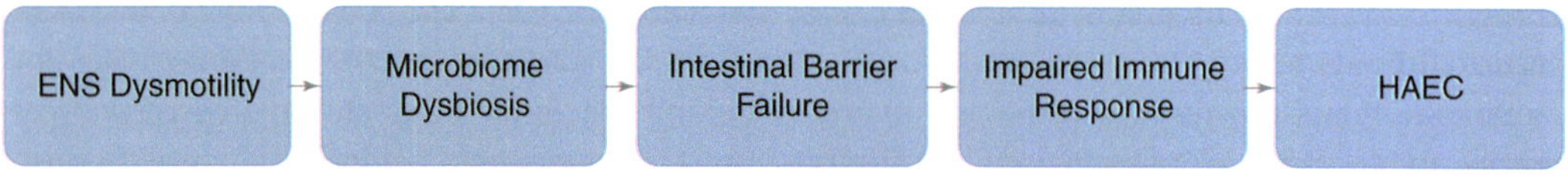

Fig. 13.1 Working model for Hirschsprung-associated enterocolitis pathogenesis. Enteric nervous system (ENS) dysfunction can result in microbiome dysbiosis through impaired motility. When followed by impaired intestinal barrier function and an abnormal immune response, HAEC may develop

13.3 Risk Factors

Many risk factors for HAEC have been identified. These factors include delay in the initial diagnosis of HSCR, gender, a family history of HSCR, and the presence of trisomy 21. Delays in the diagnosis of HSCR lead to a higher incidence of enterocolitis as the presenting condition [79]. In the neonatal period, the incidence of HAEC increases from 11% in the first week of life to 24% after.

The best-established risk factor for HAEC is trisomy 21 [14, 65, 79]. Patients with Down syndrome have been shown to have almost double the incidence of HAEC compared to other children with HSCR. The combination of HSCR and trisomy 21 is associated with a higher incidence of postoperative morbidity, prolonged hospitalization, and poor long-term bowel function. Infants with trisomy 21 have an intrinsic immune deficiency due to both decreased cytotoxic T lymphocytes and derangement in humoral function [56] which may explain their increased risk of HAEC. Of patients with trisomy 21, ~50% develop HAEC as opposed to 29% in the normal population [53, 65].

Other risk factors include family history of HSCR, male sex, delay in diagnosis of HSCR, and other genetic syndromes. There is growing evidence that genetic mutations may have a role in predisposition to HAEC: one study noted that 2/3 patients with HAEC had variants of integrin-β2, which is involved in cell surface-mediated signaling and has been associated with chronic colitis conditions [55]. Some have also postulated that the occurrence of a single episode of HAEC can alter intrinsic intestinal immunity leading to an increased risk of further episodes [24].

There has been conflicting evidence on whether or not the length of disease is related to recurrent HAEC, with longer disease involvement postulated to have a higher rate of recurrence [11, 24, 26, 43]. Studies have shown that HAEC is significantly more common in patients with aganglionic segments longer than the sigmoid [24, 43]. Neonates with total colonic aganglionosis may present with perforation of the ganglionic bowel. However, some studies on this condition have found no difference as regards length of the aganglionic bowel [11, 14, 26].

There is no evidence that the type of pull-through or presence of stoma after pull-through is related to the incidence of postoperative HAEC [64]. Swenson reported an HAEC incidence of 21% after pull-through in a 40-year follow-up [67]. However, Wildhaber et al. demonstrated no correlation between the incidence of HAEC and the type of pull-through performed [90]. Others have noted similar findings [64, 84, 89]. Additionally, no increase in HAEC has been found in the postoperative period after a primary pull-through without stoma formation [15].

After pull-through surgery, known risk factors for HAEC include anastomotic leak or stricture and postoperative intestinal obstruction secondary to adhesive disease. These increase the relative risk of HAEC by nearly threefold [36, 77]. Finally, although HAEC does occur with a diverting colostomy/enterostomy, its incidence appears substantially lower.

13.4 Diagnosis

The presentation of HAEC is highly variable in both symptoms and severity [35]. Due to the difficulty in making a definitive diagnosis and potential for morbidity or mortality with late diagnosis and treatment, most practitioners make a presumptive diagnosis and initiate therapy. Classic manifestations include abdominal distension, fever, and diarrhea. The broad spectrum of presentations is nonspecific, however, and likely contributes to the variable incidence of HAEC observed in the literature.

Mild cases may present with fever, mild distension, and diarrhea, mimicking viral gastroenteritis. More severe cases may include lethargy, rectal bleeding, and obstipation. In the neonate, the classical presentation consists of a history of constipation from birth associated with occasional loose foul-smelling stools and progressive abdominal distension [24, 30]. Among neonates with HSCR, 16%–33% present with diarrhea. The presence of diarrhea is pathognomonic of enterocolitis which occurs in 93% of patients with HAEC. Vomiting rarely occurs in HAEC. A markedly distended hyperresonant abdomen occurs in 32%–83%, vomiting in 9%–76%, pyrexia in 12%–54%, and less commonly rectal bleeding in 5%–9% of patients with HAEC.

Rectal examination, either by digit or soft catheter, is both diagnostic and therapeutic, resulting in a characteristically explosive foul smelly stool and gaseous decompression which once witnessed is never forgotten. Patients after a pull-through operation or those with a diverting stoma will present in the same fashion. The significant morbidity associated with HAEC occurs with the toxic megacolon which is characterized by bilious vomiting, fever, dehydration, marked abdominal distension, and signs of shock. Fortunately, bowel perforation is a rare complication occurring in only 2%–3% of patients [24].

Current diagnostic practice involves excluding other causes of colitis such as necrotizing enterocolitis in the infant and infectious colitis in older children. Stool studies and *Clostridium difficile* testing can be helpful to rule out the latter. Although in the majority of patients the diagnosis can be made easily on clinical evaluation, certain radiographic findings have been associated with HAEC in the context of a suspicious clinical history (Fig. 13.2). Simple anterior-posterior and lateral decubitus abdominal radiographs can show thickening of the bowel wall, mucosal irregularity ("sawtooth" appearance), dilated bowel loops, air-fluid levels, "cutoff" sign in the rectosigmoid colon, pneumatosis, pneumoperitoneum, and evidence of toxic megacolon (grossly dilated colonic loop) (Fig. 13.3). Contrast enema should be avoided during episodes of HAEC due to the risk of perforation.

A major barrier in the care of Hirschsprung patients has been the lack of a standardized method for diagnosing enterocolitis. In 2009, a large group of gastroenterologists and surgeons participated in a Delphi process to generate a diagnostic scoring system for HAEC [20, 60]. Using history, physical exam findings, laboratory findings, and imaging, they arrived at a 16-item list. Each item was assigned 1–2 points, with a summed score of 10 or greater being diagnostic of HAEC. Despite multidisciplinary expert input into the development of this definition, it was not designed for and has not been put into widespread clinical use. Recently, another collaborative reviewed the medical records of 116 children across 5 centers using the 16 Delphi criteria to create a more clinically useful scoring system [28]. The most common positive criteria included distended abdomen (31%), diarrhea with explosive stool (24%), diarrhea with foul-smelling stool (23%), and lethargy (19.8%). On multivariate analysis, diarrhea with explosive stool, decreased peripheral perfusion, lethargy, and dilated loops of bowel were independently associated with suspected HAEC episodes. Based on the calculated sensitivities and

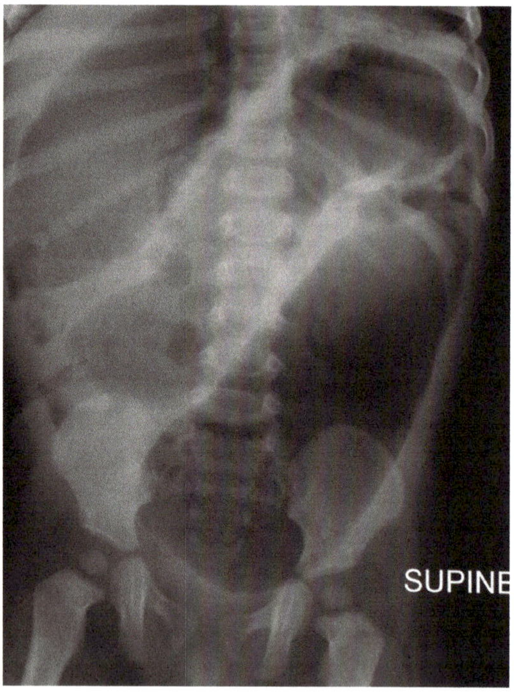

Fig. 13.2 Plain radiograph characteristics of Hirschsprung disease and Hirschsprung-associated enterocolitis. Abdominal radiograph demonstrating dilated bowel throughout, tapering to a blind end near the rectosigmoid junction. There is a paucity of colonic gas seen within the pelvis

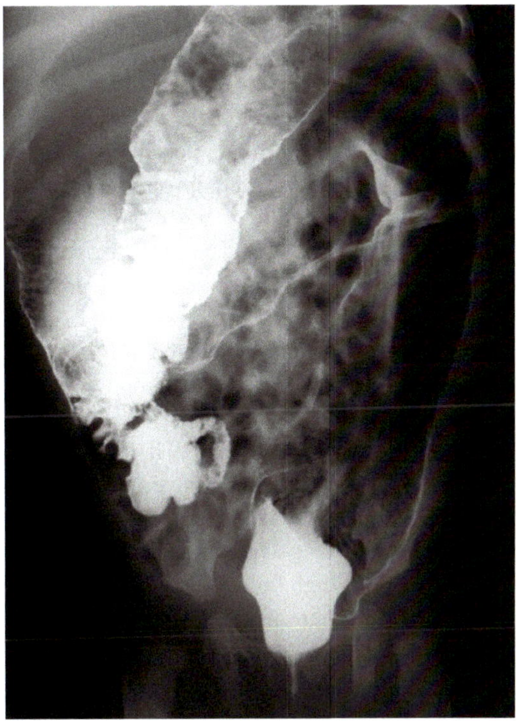

Fig. 13.3 Contrast enema characteristics of Hirschsprung disease and Hirschsprung-associated enterocolitis. Contrast enema demonstrating loss of the normal rectosigmoid ratio, where the sigmoid is expected to be larger in diameter than the rectum, in Hirschsprung disease. Also note colonic distension, speculation, edema, and mucosal nodularity ("sawtooth" appearance) of the distal rectum, indicative of active enterocolitis. Contrast enemas should be avoided during episodes of HAEC due to the risk of perforation

specificities for each score point, they demonstrated that a cutoff score of 4 points maximized the sensitivity (83.7%) and specificity (98.6%) in diagnosing HAEC. Using the same patient cohort, they then devised a new risk score based on these four criteria. However, this scoring system has not yet been prospectively verified.

The American Pediatric Surgery Association's (APSA) Hirschsprung Disease Interest Group also proposed a staging system for HAEC [35]. This system classifies HAEC into three stages based on many of the same history, physical exam, and radiologic features and is aimed toward aiding in both the diagnosis and management of HAEC (Table 13.1). However, it is hampered by the same primary weakness of the Delphi criteria – it relied on expert opinion in its development. There is an ongoing need to establish an evidence-based diagnosis and grading system for HAEC.

13.5 Treatment

There is currently no evidence-based, standard-of-care guideline or algorithm for the treatment of HAEC. Therapy is nonspecific and aimed at treating symptoms rather than a known etiology. Fluid resuscitation and correction of electrolyte abnormalities are critical in initial management.

Table 13.1 American Pediatric Surgical Association guideline for the diagnosis of Hirschsprung-associated enterocolitis

Grade	Description	Clinical history	Physical exam	Radiograph findings
1	Suspected HAEC	Anorexia Diarrhea	Mild abdominal distention	Normal Mild ileus gas pattern
2	Definite HAEC	History of past episode of HAEC Explosive diarrhea Fevers Lethargy	Fever Tachycardia Abdominal distention Abdominal tenderness Explosive gas/stool on DRE	Ileus gas pattern Air/fluid levels Dilated loops of bowel Rectosigmoid cutoff
3	Severe HAEC	Obstipation Obtunded	Decreased peripheral perfusion Hypotension Altered mentation Marked abdominal distention Peritonitis	Pneumatosis Pneumoperitoneum

Adapted from reference [35]
Guideline for the diagnosis and grading of HAEC from grade 1 (possible HAEC) to grade 3 (severe HAEC) based on clinical history, physical examination, and radiographic findings
HAEC Hirschsprung-associated enterocolitis, *DRE* digital rectal examination

Additional management strategies may include dietary changes, antibiotics, rectal irrigations, and intensive care unit admission.

13.5.1 Acute Illness

Treatment regimens should be tailored to the providers' clinical judgment of the severity of disease. The APSA HSCR interest group published guideline for the treatment of HAEC based on their diagnostic guidelines (Table 13.2) [35]. Three grades of disease severity are defined as suspected HAEC (grade 1), definite HAEC (grade 2), and severe HAEC (grade 3).

The APSA guidelines recommend that a patient with grade 1 HAEC may be safely treated as an outpatient with oral metronidazole and oral hydration. The optimal dosing, frequency, and duration of antibiotics for HAEC have not been determined. Rectal irrigations (washouts) can be considered in patients with abdominal distension or incomplete evacuation. Shim and Swenson recommended the use of a flatus or rectal tube to enable colonic decompression [68]. Rectal washouts are performed using a large-bore soft catheter with multiple side holes. The tube is well lubricated and advanced into the colon. In preoperative HAEC, the tube should be passed into the transition zone if technically possible. Repeated tube decompression and gentle rectal washouts with 10 mL/kg aliquots of warm or room-temperature normal saline make a significant clinical impact on these patients.

For grade 2 cases, inpatient or outpatient management is left to the provider's clinical judgment. Dietary restriction options include clear liquids or nothing by mouth. Broad-spectrum antibiotics and rectal irrigations/washouts are recommended.

Patients with severe cases of HAEC (grade 3) should be strongly considered for intensive care unit admission, bowel rest, broad-spectrum antibiotics, and rectal irrigations. These patients may require proximal diversion if there is failure to improve with nonoperative management. Clinical deterioration in the neonate, particularly those with long-segment disease, in which washouts have a high failure rate, may require an emergency decompression and diversion.

13.5.2 Recurrent HAEC

Treatment of recurrent HAEC begins with identifying the underlying cause. The workup for underlying etiology begins with assessing for causes of obstructive symptoms [46]. Anatomic etiologies can be identified with contrast enema, physical examination under anesthesia, and rectal biopsies to confirm the presence of ganglionated bowel. Anatomic abnormalities such as anastomotic stricture, transition zone pull-through, or

Table 13.2 American Pediatric Surgical Association guideline for the management of Hirschsprung-associated enterocolitis

Grade	Disposition	Diet	Antibiotics	Irrigations/ washouts	Surgery
1	Outpatient	Oral hydration	PO Metronidazole	Consider rectal irrigations	n/a
2	Outpatient, consider inpatient	Clear liquids or NPO IVF hydration	Metronidazole (PO or IV) Consider broad-spectrum coverage	Rectal irrigations	n/a
3	Inpatient	NPO IVF hydration	Metronidazole (IV) Broad-spectrum coverage	Rectal irrigations	Proximal diversion (ostomy) for failure to improve Surgical exploration for pneumoperitoneum

Adapted from reference [36]
Considerations for diet, antibiotics, rectal irrigations, and need for surgery are listed by grade
PO per os, *NPO* nothing per os, *ICU* intensive care unit, *IV* intravenous, *IVF* intravenous fluid

Duhamel spur should be treated surgically. Redo pull-through operations when appropriate appear to be as effective as primary procedures in terms of continence and stooling frequency and can decrease episodes of HAEC [78].

After excluding anatomic etiologies, non-relaxation of the internal anal sphincter should be considered. The use of botulinum injections for the treatment of postoperative HAEC has shown some promising results. In one study, 14 of 18 patients with persistent constipation, obstructive symptoms, or recurrent HAEC showed improvement in bowel function, and 5 of these had improvement that lasted longer than 6 months [54]. Multiple studies have shown a reduction in hospitalizations for HAEC following botulinum injections [61]. However, it is difficult to predict which patients will respond, and long-term outcomes have not been well studied.

Posterior myotomy/myectomy (POMM) can also be considered in children with recurrent episodes of HAEC 1–2 years after pull-through operation [19]. Although there has been some success in small trials, there have been mixed results regarding functional outcomes [40, 48, 64, 89]. An advantage to POMM is that redo pull-through can still be performed in the event that myectomy is not successful. Finally, end ileostomy or colostomy (diversion) can be considered as a last resort.

13.5.3 Prophylactic Measures

After pull-through surgery, some surgeons recommend routine anal dilations. Gao et al. reported an enterocolitis rate of 2/34 (6%) after using routine dilations for 3 months after surgery [33]. However, recent data questions these findings. A review by Temple et al. compared rates of stricture development and enterocolitis among children with HSCR and anorectal malformation undergoing either weekly calibration of the anastomosis by a surgeon or daily dilation by parents and observed no differences [80]. A separate review of HSCR patients had similar findings [7].

Concerns over the mortality rate due to fulminant enterocolitis in the postoperative period led Marty et al. to suggest routine postoperative rectal washout to decrease both the incidence and the severity of episodes of enterocolitis following definitive surgery [50]. They recommend a policy of rectal irrigation performed by the parents commencing 2 weeks following surgery twice daily for 3 months followed by once daily for 3 months. This policy reduced their incidence of HAEC from 36% (34 of 95 patients) to 10% (4 of 40 patients). A Spanish study of 37 children with HSCR treated between 1978 and 2005 found similar results [58].

Further research is needed to investigate what role probiotics might play in the prevention of HAEC. In one study, children undergoing surgery for HSCR were randomized to probiotic versus placebo postoperatively; this study did not show differences in HAEC rates between the two groups [23]. In contrast, another group similarly randomized patients and treated them for 4 weeks [85]. The probiotic group had reduced incidence and severity of HAEC over the following 3 months. A recent meta-analysis concluded that probiotics do not reduce the risk of HAEC [57].

13.6 Conclusion and Future Directions

HAEC remains a diagnostic and therapeutic challenge, despite recent advances in our understanding of the pathophysiology. Current research is focusing on a number of avenues including patient-specific microbiome analysis and targeted probiotic therapy and use of stem cell therapy to restore bowel function in HSCR [41]. Further studies on the underlying mechanisms of disease, accurate methods of diagnosis, and optimal treatment strategies will be needed in order to improve our ability to care for HSCR patients with HAEC.

References

1. Akkary S, Sahwy E, Kandil W, Hamdy MH. A histochemical study of the mucosubstances of the colon in cases of Hirschsprung's disease with and without enterocolitis. J Pediatr Surg. 1981;16(5):664–8.

2. Albanese CT, Smith SD, Watkins S, Kurkchubasche A, Simmons RL, Rowe MI. Effect of secretory IgA on transepithelial passage of bacteria across the intact ileum in vitro. J Am Coll Surg. 1994;179(6):679–88.
3. Ament ME, Bill AH. Persistent diarrhea due to sucrase-isomaltase deficiency in a postoperative child with Hirschsprung's disease. J Pediatr Surg. 1973;8(4):543–5.
4. Amiel J, Sproat-Emison E, Garcia-Barcelo M, Lantieri F, Burzynski G, Borrego S, Pelet A, Arnold S, Miao X, Griseri P, Brooks AS, Antinolo G, de Pontual L, Clement-Ziza M, Munnich A, Kashuk C, West K, Wong KK-Y, Lyonnet S, Chakravarti A, Tam PK-H, Ceccherini I, Hofstra RMW, Fernandez R, Hirschsprung Disease Consortium. Hirschsprung disease, associated syndromes and genetics: a review. J Med Genet. 2008;45(1):1–14.
5. Aslam A, Spicer RD, Corfield AP. Turnover of radioactive mucin precursors in the colon of patients with Hirschsprung's disease correlates with the development of enterocolitis. J Pediatr Surg. 1998;33(1):103–5.
6. Austin KM. The pathogenesis of Hirschsprung's disease-associated enterocolitis. Semin Pediatr Surg. 2012;21(4):319–27.
7. Aworanti O, Hung J, McDowell D, Martin I, Quinn F. Are routine dilatations necessary post pull-through surgery for Hirschsprung disease? Eur J Pediatr Surg. 2013;23(5):383–8.
8. Bagwell CE, Langham MR Jr, Mahaffey SM, Talbert JL, Shandling B. Pseudomembranous colitis following resection for Hirschsprung's disease. J Pediatr Surg. 1992;27(10):1261–4.
9. Berry CL, Fraser GC. The experimental production of colitis in the rabbit with particular reference to Hirschsprung's disease. J Pediatr Surg. 1968;3(1):36–42.
10. Bickelhaupt S, Pazahr S, Chuck N, Blume I, Froehlich JM, Cattin R, Raible S, Bouquet H, Bill U, Rogler G, Frei P, Boss A, Patak MA. Crohn's disease: small bowel motility impairment correlates with inflammatory-related markers C-reactive protein and calprotectin. Neurogastroenterol Motil. 2013;25(6):467–73.
11. Bill A, CHapman N. The enterocolitis of Hirschsprung's disease: its natural history and treatment. Am J Surg. 1962;103:70–4.
12. Buisine MP, Devisme L, Savidge TC, Gespach C, Gosselin B, Porchet N, Aubert JP. Mucin gene expression in human embryonic and fetal intestine. Gut. 1998;43(4):519–24.
13. Burnard ED. Hirschsprung's disease in infancy. Br Med J. 1950;1(4646):151–6.
14. Caniano DA, Teitelbaum DH, Qualman SJ. Management of Hirschsprung's disease in children with trisomy 21. Am J Surg. 1990;159(4):402–4.
15. Carcassonne M, Guys JM, Morrison-Lacombe G, Kreitmann B. Management of Hirschsprung's disease: curative surgery before 3 months of age. J Pediatr Surg. 1989;24(10):1032–4.
16. Cheng LS, Schwartz DM, Hotta R, Graham HK, Goldstein AM. Bowel dysfunction following pullthrough surgery is associated with an overabundance of nitrergic neurons in Hirschsprung disease. J Pediatr Surg. 2016;51(11):1834–8.
17. Cheng Z, Dhall D, Zhao L, Wang HL, Doherty TM, Bresee C, Frykman PK. Murine model of Hirschsprung-associated enterocolitis. I: phenotypic characterization with development of a histopathologic grading system. J Pediatr Surg. 2010;45(3):475–82.
18. Cheng Z, Wang X, Dhall D, Zhao L, Bresee C, Doherty TM, Frykman PK. Splenic lymphopenia in the endothelin receptor B-null mouse: implications for Hirschsprung associated enterocolitis. Pediatr Surg Int. 2011;27(2):145–50.
19. Coran AG, Teitelbaum DH. Recent advances in the management of Hirschsprung's disease. Am J Surg. 2000;180(5):382–7.
20. Dalkey N, Helmer O. An experimental application of the Delphi method to the use of experts. Manag Sci. 1963;9(3):458–67.
21. De Filippo C, Pini-Prato A, Mattioli G, Avanzini S, Rapuzzi G, Cavalieri D, Di Paola M, Stefanini I, Ceccherini I, Mavilio D, Lionetti P, Jasonni V. Genomics approach to the analysis of bacterial communities dynamics in Hirschsprung's disease-associated enterocolitis: a pilot study. Pediatr Surg Int. 2010;26(5):465–71.
22. Dorman GW. Hirschsprung's disease; a lethal problem in early infancy. AMA Arch Surg. 1957;75(6):906–13.
23. El-Sawaf M, Siddiqui S, Mahmoud M, Drongowski R, Teitelbaum DH. Probiotic prophylaxis after pullthrough for Hirschsprung disease to reduce incidence of enterocolitis: a prospective, randomized, double-blind, placebo-controlled, multicenter trial. J Pediatr Surg. 2013;48(1):111–7.
24. Elhalaby EA, Coran AG, Blane CE, Hirschl RB, Teitelbaum DH. Enterocolitis associated with Hirschsprung's disease: a clinical-radiological characterization based on 168 patients. J Pediatr Surg. 1995;30(1):76–83.
25. Fisher JH, Swenson O. Hirschsprung's disease during infancy. Surg Clin North Am. 1956:1511–5.
26. Foster P, Cowan G, Wrenn EL. Twenty-five years' experience with Hirschsprung's disease. J Pediatr Surg. 1990;25(5):531–4.
27. Frykman PK, Cheng Z, Wang X, Dhall D. Enterocolitis causes profound lymphoid depletion in endothelin receptor B- and endothelin 3-null mouse models of Hirschsprung-associated enterocolitis. Eur J Immunol. 2015a;45(3):807–17.
28. Frykman PK, Kim S, Wester T, Nordenskjöld A, Kawaguchi A, Hui TT, Teitelbaum DH, Granström AL, Rogatko A, HAEC Collaborative Research Group (HCRG). Critical evaluation of the Hirschsprung-associated enterocolitis (HAEC) score: a multicenter study of 116 children with Hirschsprung disease. J Pediatr Surg. 2018;53(4):708–17.
29. Frykman PK, Nordenskjold A, Kawaguchi A, Hui TT, Granstrom AL, Cheng Z, Tang J, Underhill DM, Iliev I, Funari VA, Wester T, H. C. R. Group. Characterization of bacterial and fungal microbiome

in children with Hirschsprung disease with and without a history of Enterocolitis: a multicenter study. PLoS One. 2015b;10(4):e0124172.
30. Frykman PK, Short SS. Hirschsprung-associated enterocolitis: prevention and therapy. Semin Pediatr Surg. 2012;21(4):328–35.
31. Fujimoto T. Natural history and pathophysiology of enterocolitis in the piebald lethal mouse model of Hirschsprung's disease. J Pediatr Surg. 1988a;23(3):237–42.
32. Fujimoto T, Reen DJ, Puri P. Inflammatory response in enterocolitis in the piebald lethal mouse model of Hirschsprung's disease. Pediatr Res. 1988;24(2):152–5.
33. Gao Y, Li G, Zhang X, Xu Q, Guo Z, Zheng B, Li P, Li G. Primary transanal rectosigmoidectomy for Hirschsprung's disease: preliminary results in the initial 33 cases. J Pediatr Surg. 2001;36(12):1816–9.
34. Gosain A, Barlow-Anacker AJ, Erickson CS, Pierre JF, Heneghan AF, Epstein ML, Kudsk KA. Impaired cellular immunity in the murine neural crest conditional deletion of Endothelin receptor-B model of Hirschsprung's disease. PLoS One. 2015;10(6):e0128822.
35. Gosain A, Frykman PK, Cowles RA, Horton J, Levitt M, Rothstein DH, Langer JC, Goldstein AM, American Pediatric Surgical Association Hirschsprung Disease Interest Group. Guidelines for the diagnosis and management of Hirschsprung-associated enterocolitis. Pediatr Surg Int. 2017;33(5):517–21.
36. Hackam DJ, Filler RM, Pearl RH. Enterocolitis after the surgical treatment of Hirschsprung's disease: risk factors and financial impact. J Pediatr Surg. 1998;33(6):830–3.
37. Hardy SP, Bayston R, Spitz L. Prolonged carriage of *Clostridium difficile* in Hirschsprung's disease. Arch Dis Child. 1993;69(2):221–4.
38. Haricharan RN, Seo J-M, Kelly DR, Mroczek-Musulman EC, Aprahamian CJ, Morgan TL, Georgeson KE, Harmon CM, Saito JM, Barnhart DC. Older age at diagnosis of Hirschsprung disease decreases risk of postoperative enterocolitis, but resection of additional ganglionated bowel does not. J Pediatr Surg. 2008;43(6):1115–23.
39. Harrison MW, Deitz DM, Campbell JR, Campbell TJ. Diagnosis and management of Hirschsprung's disease. A 25 year perspective. Am J Surg. 1986;152(1):49–56.
40. Heikkinen M, Rintala R, Luukkonen P. Long-term anal sphincter performance after surgery for Hirschsprung's disease. J Pediatr Surg. 1997;32(10):1443–6.
41. Heuckeroth RO. Hirschsprung disease – integrating basic science and clinical medicine to improve outcomes. Nat Rev Gastroenterol Hepatol. 2018;15(3):152–67.
42. Hirschsprung H. Stuhltragheit neugeborener infolge von dilatation and hypertrophies des colons. Jahrb Kinderheilkd. 1887;27:1–42.
43. Ikeda K, Goto S. Diagnosis and treatment of Hirschsprung's disease in Japan. An analysis of 1628 patients. Ann Surg. 1984;199(4):400–5.
44. Imamura A, Puri P, O'Briain DS, Reen DJ. Mucosal immune defence mechanisms in enterocolitis complicating Hirschsprung's disease. Gut. 1992;33(6):801–6.
45. Kobayashi H, Hirakawa H, Puri P. Overexpression of intercellular adhesion molecule-1 (ICAM-1) and MHC class II antigen on hypertrophic nerve trunks suggests an immunopathologic response in Hirschsprung's disease. J Pediatr Surg. 1995;30(12):1680–3.
46. Langer JC, Rollins MD, Levitt M, Gosain A, Torre L, Kapur RP, Cowles RA, Horton J, Rothstein DH, Goldstein AM. American Pediatric Surgical Association Hirschsprung Disease Interest Group. Guidelines for the management of postoperative obstructive symptoms in children with Hirschsprung disease. Pediatr Surg Int. 2017;33(5):523–6.
47. Lloyd-Still JD, Demers LM. Hirschsprung's enterocolitis, prostaglandins, and response to cholestyramine. J Pediatr Surg. 1978;13(4):417–8.
48. Marty TL, Matlak ME, Hendrickson M, Black RE, Johnson DG. Unexpected death from enterocolitis after surgery for Hirschsprung's disease. Pediatrics. 1995;96(1 Pt 1):118–21.
49. Marty TL, Seo T, Matlak ME, Sullivan JJ, Black RE, Johnson DG. Gastrointestinal function after surgical correction of Hirschsprung's disease: long-term follow-up in 135 patients. J Pediatr Surg. 1995;30(5):655–8.
50. Marty TL, Seo T, Sullivan JJ, Matlak ME, Black RE, Johnson DG. Rectal irrigations for the prevention of postoperative enterocolitis in Hirschsprung's disease. J Pediatr Surg. 1995;30(5):652–4.
51. Mattar AF, Coran AG, Teitelbaum DH. MUC-2 mucin production in Hirschsprung's disease: possible association with enterocolitis development. J Pediatr Surg. 2003;38(3):417–21; discussion 417-421
52. Medrano G, Cailleux F, Guan P, Kuruvilla K, Barlow-Anacker AJ, Gosain A. B-lymphocyte-intrinsic and -extrinsic defects in secretory immunoglobulin A production in the neural crest-conditional deletion of endothelin receptor B model of Hirschsprung-associated enterocolitis. FASEB J. 2019:fj201801913R. https://doi.org/10.1096/fj.201801913R.
53. Menezes M, Puri P. Long-term clinical outcome in patients with Hirschsprung's disease and associated Down's syndrome. J Pediatr Surg. 2005;40(5):810–2.
54. Minkes RK, Langer JC. A prospective study of botulinum toxin for internal anal sphincter hypertonicity in children with Hirschsprung's disease. J Pediatr Surg. 2000;35(12):1733–6.
55. Moore SW, Sidler D, Zaahl MG. The ITGB2 immunomodulatory gene (CD18), enterocolitis, and Hirschsprung's disease. J Pediatr Surg. 2008;43(8):1439–44.
56. Nair MP, Schwartz SA. Association of decreased T-cell-mediated natural cytotoxicity and interferon production in Down's syndrome. Clin Immunol Immunopathol. 1984;33(3):412–24.
57. Nakamura H, Lim T, Puri P. Probiotics for the prevention of Hirschsprung-associated enterocolitis: a sys-

tematic review and meta-analysis. Pediatr Surg Int. 2018;34(2):189–93.
58. Nunez R, Torres A, Agulla E, Moreno C, Marin D, Santamaria JI. Rectal irrigation and bowel decontamination for the prevention of postoperative enterocolitis in Hirschsprung's disease. Cir Pediatr. 2007;20(2):96–100.
59. Ohama T, Hori M, Fujisawa M, Kiyosue M, Hashimoto M, Ikenoue Y, Jinno Y, Miwa H, Matsumoto T, Murata T, Ozaki H. Downregulation of CPI-17 contributes to dysfunctional motility in chronic intestinal inflammation model mice and ulcerative colitis patients. J Gastroenterol. 2008;43(11):858–65.
60. Pastor AC, Osman F, Teitelbaum DH, Caty MG, Langer JC. Development of a standardized definition for Hirschsprung's-associated enterocolitis: a Delphi analysis. J Pediatr Surg. 2009;44(1):251–6.
61. Patrus B, Nasr A, Langer JC, Gerstle JT. Intrasphincteric botulinum toxin decreases the rate of hospitalization for postoperative obstructive symptoms in children with Hirschsprung disease. J Pediatr Surg. 2011;46(1):184–7.
62. Pierre JF, Barlow-Anacker AJ, Erickson CS, Heneghan AF, Leverson GE, Dowd SE, Epstein ML, Kudsk KA, Gosain A. Intestinal dysbiosis and bacterial enteroinvasion in a murine model of Hirschsprung's disease. J Pediatr Surg. 2014;49(8):1242–51.
63. Pini-Prato A, Rossi V, Avanzini S, Mattioli G, Disma N, Jasonni V. Hirschsprung's disease: what about mortality? Pediatr Surg Int. 2011;27(5):473–8.
64. Polley TZ, Coran AG, Wesley JR. A ten-year experience with ninety-two cases of Hirschsprung's disease. Including sixty-seven consecutive endorectal pull-through procedures. Ann Surg. 1985a;202(3):349–55.
65. Quinn FM, Surana R, Puri P. The influence of trisomy 21 on outcome in children with Hirschsprung's disease. J Pediatr Surg. 1994;29(6):781–3.
66. Rescorla FJ, Morrison AM, Engles D, West KW, Grosfeld JL. Hirschsprung's disease. Evaluation of mortality and long-term function in 260 cases. Arch Surg. 1992;127(8):934–41; discussion 941–932
67. Sherman JO, Snyder ME, Weitzman JJ, Jona JZ, Gillis DA, O'Donnell B, Carcassonne M, Swenson O. A 40-year multinational retrospective study of 880 Swenson procedures. J Pediatr Surg. 1989;24(8):833–8.
68. Shim WK, Swenson O. Treatmentof congenital megacolon in 50 infants. Pediatrics. 1966;38(2):185–93.
69. Soeda J, O'Briain DS, Puri P. Mucosal neuroendocrine cell abnormalities in the colon of patients with Hirschsprung's disease. J Pediatr Surg. 1992;27(7):823–7.
70. Soeda J, O'Briain DS, Puri P. Regional reduction in intestinal neuroendocrine cell populations in enterocolitis complicating Hirschsprung's disease. J Pediatr Surg. 1993;28(8):1063–8.
71. Spiller RC. Role of nerves in enteric infection. Gut. 2002;51(6):759–62.
72. Suita S, Taguchi T, Ieiri S, Nakatsuji T. Hirschsprung's disease in Japan: analysis of 3852 patients based on a nationwide survey in 30 years. J Pediatr Surg. 2005;40(1):197–201; discussion 201-192
73. Swenson O. Hirschsprung's disease—a complicated therapeutic problem: some thoughts and solutions based on data and personal experience over 56 years. J Pediatr Surg. 2004;39(10):1449–53.
74. Swenson O, Davidson FZ. Similarities of mechanical intestinal obstruction and aganglionic megacolon in the newborn infant: a review of 64 cases. N Engl J Med. 1960;262:64–7.
75. Swenson O, Fisher JH, Scott JE. Diarrhea following rectosigmoidectomy for Hirschsprung's disease. Surgery. 1960;48:419–21.
76. Teitelbaum DH, Caniano DA, Qualman SJ. The pathophysiology of Hirschsprung's-associated enterocolitis: importance of histologic correlates. J Pediatr Surg. 1989;24(12):1271–7.
77. Teitelbaum DH, Cilley RE, Sherman NJ, Bliss D, Uitvlugt ND, Renaud EJ, Kirstioglu I, Bengston T, Coran AG. A decade of experience with the primary pull-through for hirschsprung disease in the newborn period: a multicenter analysis of outcomes. Ann Surg. 2000;232(3):372–80.
78. Teitelbaum DH, Drongowski RA, Chamberlain JN, Coran AG. Long-term stooling patterns in infants undergoing primary endorectal pull-through for Hirschsprung's disease. J Pediatr Surg. 1997;32(7):1049–52; discussion 1052-1043
79. Teitelbaum DH, Qualman SJ, Caniano DA. Hirschsprung's disease. Identification of risk factors for enterocolitis. Ann Surg. 1988;207(3):240–4.
80. Temple SJ, Shawyer A, Langer JC. Is daily dilatation by parents necessary after surgery for Hirschsprung disease and anorectal malformations? J Pediatr Surg. 2012;47(1):209–12.
81. Thiagarajah JR, Yildiz H, Carlson T, Thomas AR, Steiger C, Pieretti A, Zukerberg LR, Carrier RL, Goldstein AM. Altered goblet cell differentiation and surface mucus properties in Hirschsprung disease. PLoS One. 2014;9(6):e99944.
82. Thomas DF, Fernie DS, Bayston R, Spitz L, Nixon HH. Enterocolitis in Hirschsprung's disease: a controlled study of the etiologic role of *Clostridium difficile*. J Pediatr Surg. 1986;21(1):22–5.
83. Thomas DF, Fernie DS, Malone M, Bayston R, Spitz L. Association between Clostridium difficile and enterocolitis in Hirschsprung's disease. Lancet. 1982;1(8263):78–9.
84. van Leeuwen K, Teitelbaum DH, Elhalaby EA, Coran AG. Long-term follow-up of redo pull-through procedures for Hirschsprung's disease: efficacy of the endorectal pull-through. J Pediatr Surg. 2000;35(6):829–33; discussion 833-824
85. Wang X, Li Z, Xu Z, Wang Z, Feng J. Probiotics prevent Hirschsprung's disease-associated enterocolitis: a prospective multicenter randomized controlled trial. Int J Color Dis. 2015;30(1):105–10.
86. Ward NL, Pieretti A, Dowd SE, Cox SB, Goldstein AM. Intestinal aganglionosis is associated with early and sustained disruption of the colonic microbiome. Neurogastroenterol Motil. 2012;24(9):874–e400.

87. Webster W. Aganglionic megacolon in piebald-lethal mice. Arch Pathol. 1974;97(2):111–7.
88. Wiedenmann B, Waldherr R, Buhr H, Hille A, Rosa P, Huttner WB. Identification of gastroenteropancreatic neuroendocrine cells in normal and neoplastic human tissue with antibodies against synaptophysin, chromogranin a, secretogranin I (chromogranin B), and secretogranin II. Gastroenterology. 1988;95(5):1364–74.
89. Wildhaber BE, Pakarinen M, Rintala RJ, Coran AG, Teitelbaum DH. Posterior myotomy/myectomy for persistent stooling problems in Hirschsprung's disease. J Pediatr Surg. 2004;39(6):920–6; discussion 920–926
90. Wildhaber BE, Teitelbaum DH, Coran AG. Total colonic Hirschsprung's disease: a 28-year experience. J Pediatr Surg. 2005;40(1):203–6; discussion 206-207
91. Wiles TJ, Jemielita M, Baker RP, Schlomann BH, Logan SL, Ganz J, Melancon E, Eisen JS, Guillemin K, Parthasarathy R. Host gut motility promotes competitive exclusion within a model intestinal microbiota. PLoS Biol. 2016;14(7):e1002517.
92. Wilson-Storey D, Scobie WG. Impaired gastrointestinal mucosal defense in Hirschsprung's disease: a clue to the pathogenesis of enterocolitis? J Pediatr Surg. 1989;24(5):462–4.
93. Wilson-Storey D, Scobie WG, McGenity KG. Microbiological studies of the enterocolitis of Hirschsprung's disease. Arch Dis Child. 1990;65(12):1338–9.
94. Wilson-Storey D, Scobie WG, Raeburn JA. Defective white blood cell function in Hirschsprung's disease: a possible predisposing factor to enterocolitis. J R Coll Surg Edinb. 1988;33(4):185–8.
95. Yan Z, Poroyko V, Gu S, Zhang Z, Pan L, Wang J, Bao N, Hong L. Characterization of the intestinal microbiome of Hirschsprung's disease with and without enterocolitis. Biochem Biophys Res Commun. 2014;445(2):269–74.
96. Zaitoun I, Erickson CS, Barlow AJ, Klein TR, Heneghan AF, Pierre JF, Epstein ML, Gosain A. Altered neuronal density and neurotransmitter expression in the ganglionated region of Ednrb null mice: implications for Hirschsprung's disease. Neurogastroenterol Motil. 2013;25(3):e233–44.
97. Zhao L, Dhall D, Cheng Z, Wang HL, Doherty TM, Bresee C, Frykman PK. Murine model of Hirschsprung-associated enterocolitis II: surgical correction of aganglionosis does not eliminate enterocolitis. J Pediatr Surg. 2010;45(1):206–11; discussion 211-202

Diagnosis of Hirschsprung Disease and Allied Disorders

14

Roisin Hayes and Jerry Kelleher

Contents

R. Hayes (✉) · J. Kelleher
Department of Radiology, Our Ladys Childrens Hospital, Crumlin, Dublin, Ireland
e-mail: roisin.hayes@olchc.ie

P. Puri (ed.), *Hirschsprung's Disease and Allied Disorders*,
https://doi.org/10.1007/978-3-030-15647-3_14

14.1 Radiological Diagnosis

Major advances have taken place in the histochemical diagnosis of Hirschsprung disease (HSCR) in recent years. While rectal biopsy is the gold standard, radiology still has an important role to play. The diagnosis of HSCR may be suggested on plain films, which may also demonstrate the serious complication of enterocolitis. Contrast enema is useful in confirming or excluding the diagnosis of HSCR, and in demonstrating the length of the distal aganglionic segment of bowel, which facilitates surgical planning.

14.2 Initial Radiographs

Most cases of HSCR present in the newborn period with delayed passage of meconium, abdominal distension and intolerance of feeds. Approximately 90% of patients fail to pass meconium in the first 24 hours of life. Supine and lateral decubitus plain films are performed routinely. The supine film will show gaseous distension of bowel loops with distribution of loops sometimes suggesting large bowel involvement. The level of obstruction may be indicated by the presence of undilated colon or rectum (Fig. 14.1a). The horizontal beam film may show multiple fluid levels in the distended bowel loops (Fig. 14.1b) and also

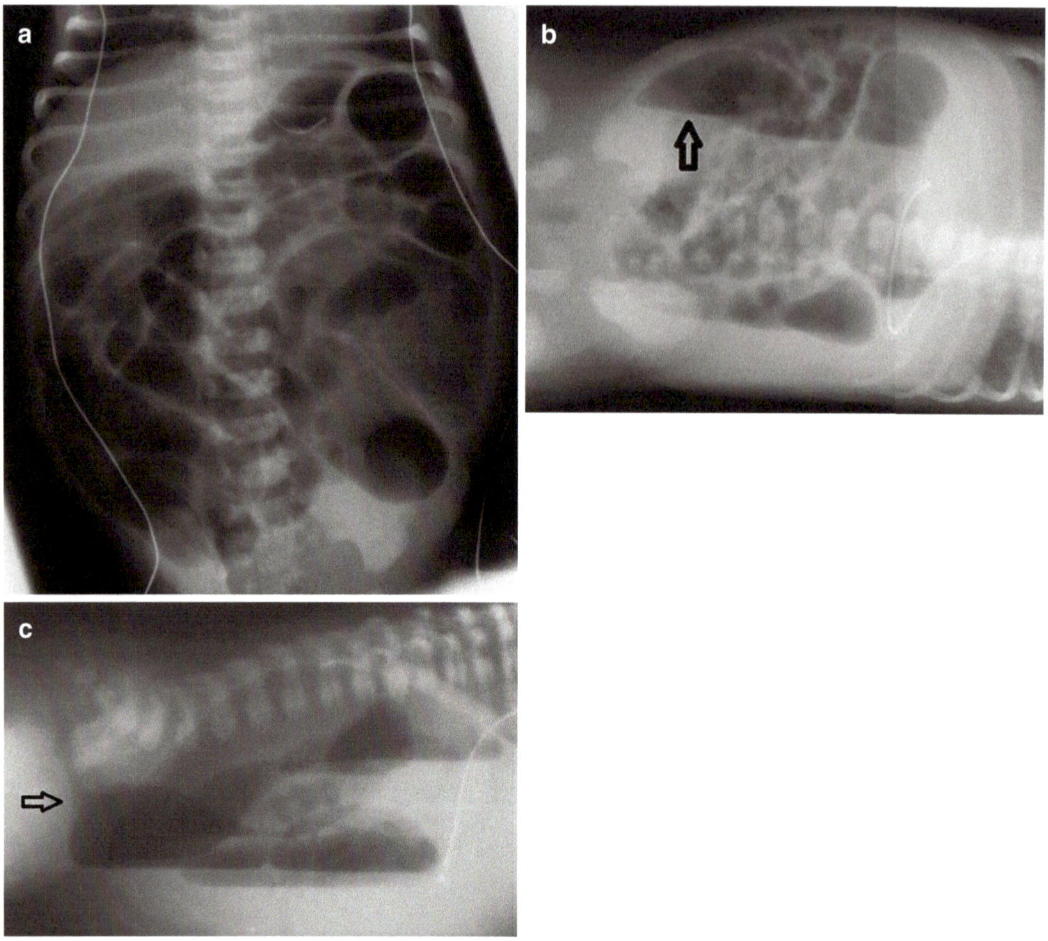

Fig. 14.1 (**a**–**c**) Abdominal imaging at 30 hours. (**a**) Supine. Marked gaseous distension of multiple bowel loops. Normal rectum. (**b**) Right-side up decubitus radiograph shows multiple air-fluid levels (open arrow). (**c**) Prone shoot-through shows transition zone at rectosigmoid junction (open arrow)

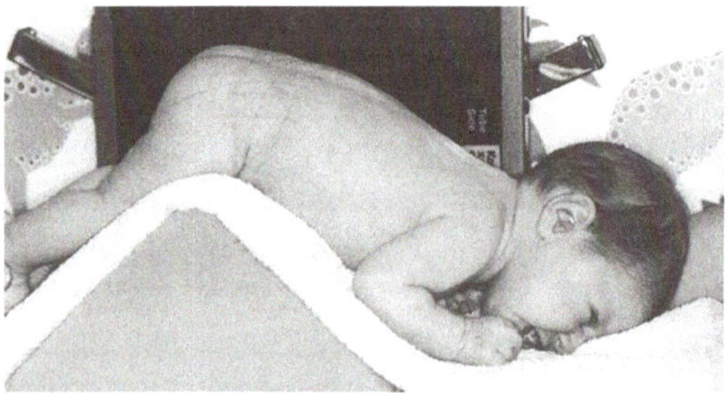

Fig. 14.2 Baby comfortably in position for prone lateral view with horizontal beam and buttocks elevated

serves to exclude perforation, which is a rare complication.

If the diagnosis is still uncertain, a prone, horizontal beam lateral view with buttocks elevated may be helpful (Fig. 14.2). The infant will be comfortable in this position for 10 minutes or longer, allowing gas to rise from the distended colon into the undilated rectum. A cone-shaped or funnel-like appearance of the transitional zone between the distended proximal bowel and the narrowed aganglionic distal segment may be shown (Fig. 14.1c).

14.3 Differential Diagnosis

Colonic atresia may give similar plain film findings to HSCR, but is readily excluded with a contrast enema, which will show complete mechanical obstruction. In cases of distal small bowel atresia, there is often marked dilatation of multiple loops of small bowel, with many abnormal air-fluid levels.

In meconium ileus, clear sharp air-fluid levels are usually not a feature on the lateral decubitus view. The bubbly appearance of gas trapped in the thick meconium has been found to be an unreliable indicator of meconium ileus [1]. HSCR can sometimes simulate meconium ileus on plain films, but the correct diagnosis is usually obvious on contrast enema.

Both meconium plug syndrome and neonatal small left colon syndrome probably represent part of a spectrum of similar functional disorders related to delayed "maturity" of the colon in the newborn [2]. Associated factors include prematurity, maternal diabetes, pre-eclampsia and maternal drug ingestion. In both of these conditions, the clinical presentation and plain film findings may suggest a diagnosis of HSCR. However, it is notable that in these conditions, the rectum is normally distensible, in contrast to true HSCR where the rectum remains abnormally narrow. The functional obstruction in both meconium plug syndrome and in the small left colon syndrome will usually resolve following contrast enema. However, if there is ongoing clinical concern, a rectal suction biopsy should be performed, as a minority of these infants will actually have HSCR.

14.4 Enema Technique

A carefully performed contrast enema is quite reliable in either confirming or excluding the diagnosis of HSCR [3] and, if positive, in identifying the transition zone. Rectal washouts are contraindicated, and even digital examination should be avoided or kept to a minimum prior to the contrast enema. Otherwise, the distended proximal bowel may be decompressed, with distortion of the transition zone leading to a false-negative diagnosis.

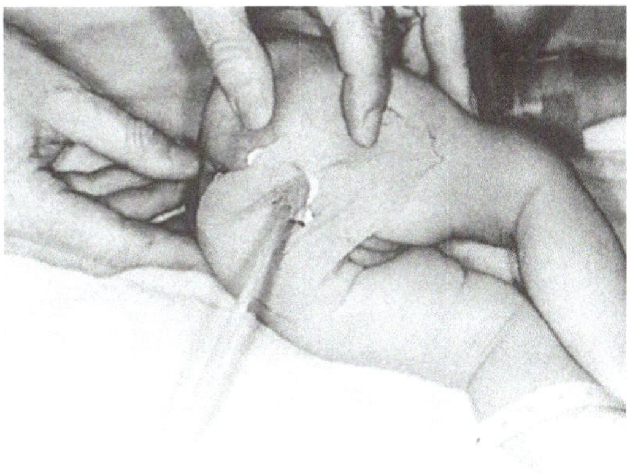

Fig. 14.3 Buttocks tightly strapped with adhesive tape. Tube is secured with a loop of tape

The fluoroscopy room should be warm. The baby should be well hydrated, with an intravenous line in place. A recent horizontal beam radiograph should be reviewed to exclude perforation.

A soft rubber catheter of appropriate size is inserted into the rectum and secured in position with firm strapping drawn tightly across the buttocks (Fig. 14.3). If a balloon catheter is used, the balloon should not be inflated due to the risk of perforation and of distortion of the transition zone by the distended balloon.

Regarding the choice of contrast medium, in the neonate with suspected intestinal obstruction of uncertain aetiology, we usually use an iso-osmolar, nonionic water-soluble contrast medium. In the event of a perforation, this is much safer than barium. In this group, there is no advantage to using barium. For older children, dilute barium can be used.

If HSCR has already been confirmed by rectal biopsy, we use contrast to identify the transition zone. In this case, we allow a period of

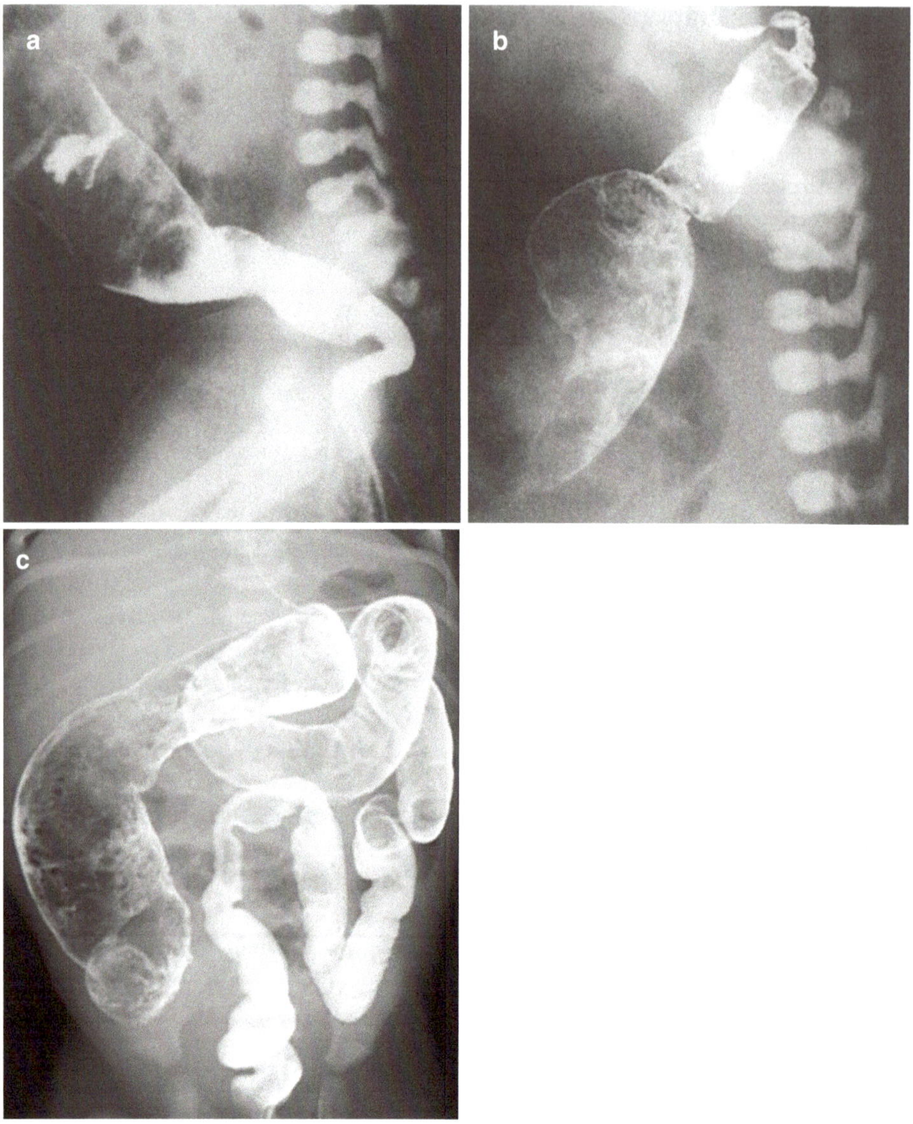

Fig. 14.4 (**a–c**) Contrast enemas in short- and long-segment Hirschsprung disease. (**a**) Distended sigmoid tapering to narrow rectum. (**b**) Transition zone more pronounced on delayed image. (**c**) Transition zone at splenic flexure

24–48 hours to elapse after suction biopsy before such an enema is performed.

Warmed contrast is injected slowly under fluoroscopic control using a 50-ml syringe with the baby in the lateral position. Slow injection of the contrast agent avoids over-distension and obliteration of a potential cone-shaped transition zone. This zone may be observed at the classical rectosigmoid level (Fig. 14.4a). Less frequently it will be seen at the splenic flexure (Fig. 14.4c).

Following identification of a transition zone, further contrast administration is usually not necessary.

14.5 Enema Findings

The rectosigmoid index (RSI) evaluates the ratio between the maximum diameter of the rectum on a lateral view and that of the sig-

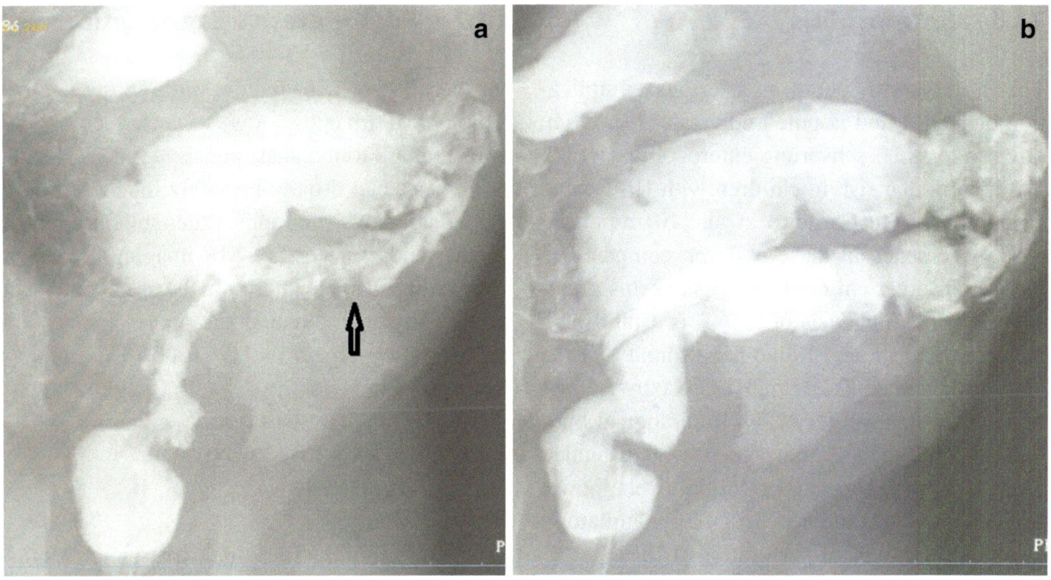

Fig. 14.5 (**a**) Irregular, sawtooth contractions in sigmoid colon (open arrow). (**b**) resolved after a few seconds

moid colon. In the absence of HSCR, it should be greater than 1. An abnormal RSI has been shown to be the most useful predictor of HSCR in neonates [3, 4]. The term "transition zone" refers to an abrupt transition from the narrow distal aganglionic segment to the normal or dilated proximal bowel. While it is a good predictor of HSCR in infants, it can be difficult to visualize in neonates. If the level of the transition zone is not clear initially, it may be accentuated on a delayed x-ray after 24 hours; this also facilitates assessment of the barium residue. Abnormal irregular, sawtooth colorectal contractions can be observed on fluoroscopy in infants with HSCR. These are usually very transient in nature (Fig. 14.5a, b) [5]; however, they are not seen frequently in neonates.

A modification of the contrast enema to incorporate the study of rectosphincteric reflex during balloon inflation of the rectum has been described by Nagasaki et al. [6]. Alternatively, cold contrast can be injected into the rectum [7, 8].

Total colonic aganglionosis is rare and often difficult to diagnose, as the colon may not be significantly narrowed. If reflux of contrast into a grossly dilated ileum is observed, the diagnosis should be strongly considered. However, the ileocaecal valve may be competent, preventing ileal filling (Fig. 14.6). In this situation, HSCR cannot be confidently differentiated from ileal atresia or meconium ileus, and a definitive diagnosis of total colonic HSCR may only be made histologically from frozen sections of surgical specimens.

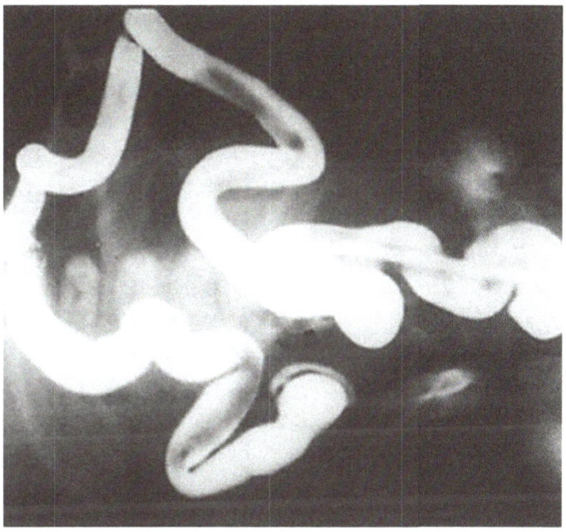

Fig. 14.6 Total colonic Hirschsprung's disease with generalized narrowing of the colon. Competent ileocaecal valve. Diagnosis made at surgery

If meconium ileus or meconium plug syndrome is diagnosed on contrast enema, dilute Gastrografin may be introduced to relieve the obstruction.

14.6 Enterocolitis

This is the most feared and serious complication of HSCR and is potentially fatal [9]. Often referred to as Hirschsprung enterocolitis (HEC), it is a particular risk in children with HSCR and trisomy 21, with Carneiro et al. [10] reporting a 50% incidence in these children compared to 29% in all other children. The risk seems greatest before the diagnosis of HSCR is established. However, Murthi and Raine have found that the highest incidence (22%) of HEC occurs following pull-through surgery [11]. Radiological findings in HEC include the presence of distended loops of bowel, abnormal air-fluid levels, bowel wall thickening, mucosal oedema, pneumatosis intestinalis or signs of perforation [12].

The presence of necrotizing enterocolitis (NEC) in a full-term infant should raise the possibility of HSCR, and a rectal biopsy should be performed at an appropriate time. A contrast enema should not be performed on a baby with suspected HEC (Fig. 14.7, films from an outside hospital).

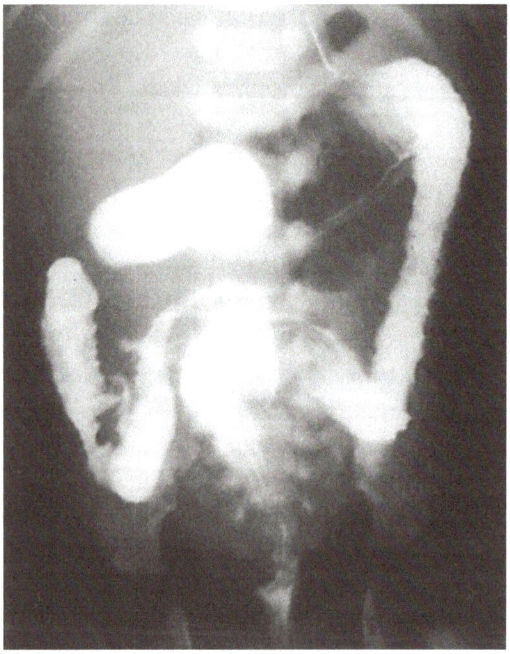

Fig. 14.7 Enterocolitis complicating Hirschsprung's disease. Mucosal oedema with fine ulceration throughout the distal colon

14.7 Postoperative Examinations

Most children will require little postoperative radiological imaging. Any suspected complications relating to the anastomosis, e.g. leak, fistula or abscess, can usually be safely diagnosed by a combination of sonography, water-soluble contrast enemas and, if necessary, MR imaging. Recently, there has been some interest in the use of endoanal sonography in evaluating the anal sphincters in children after surgery for HSCR [13–15].

14.8 Intestinal Neuronal Dysplasia

In most patients, intestinal neuronal dysplasia (IND) is clinically indistinguishable from HSCR at presentation [16, 17]. Our experience

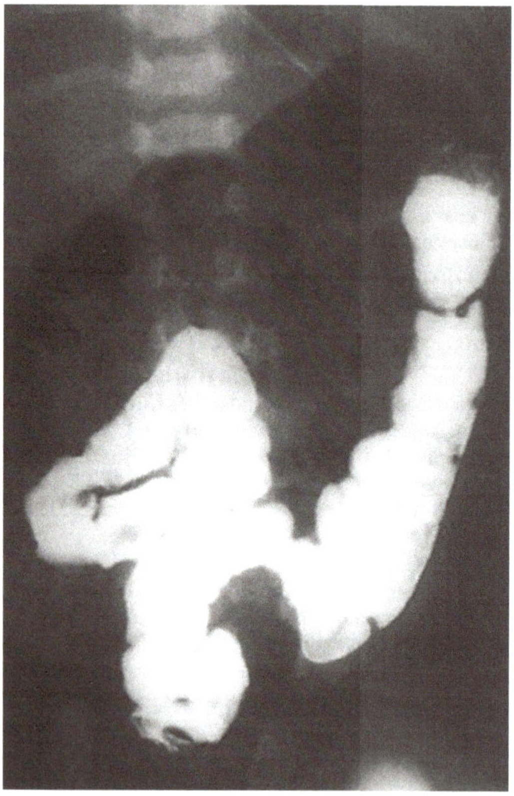

Fig. 14.8 Intestinal neuronal dysplasia. Delayed film at 24 hours shows significant residual contrast in colon. Rectal biopsy showed giant, ectopic ganglia and hyperganglionosis

of contrast enema in these patients suggests that the findings are often equivocal and could delay diagnosis (Fig. 14.8). It should be borne in mind that IND combined with HSCR occurs in 25–35% of patients with HSCR [18]. The diagnosis of IND is essentially histological and histochemical, but the paediatric radiologist should always keep this condition in mind when presented with a patient who does not easily satisfy the criteria for HSCR.

References

1. Carty H, Brereton RJ. The distended neonate. Clin Radiol. 1983;34:367–80.
2. LeQuesne G, et al. Functional immaturity of the large bowel in the newborn infant. Radiol Clin N Am. 1975;13:331.
3. Putnam L, John S, Greenfield S, Kellagher C, Austin M, Lally K, Tsao K. The utility of the contrast enema in neonates with suspected Hirschsprung disease. J Pediatr Surg. 2015;50:963–6.
4. Taxman T, Yulish B, Rothstein F. How useful is the barium enema in the diagnosis of infantile Hirschsprung's disease? Am J Dis Child. 1986;140:881–4.
5. Cremin BJ. Diagnosis of Hirschsprung's disease. In: Holschneider AM, editor. Hirschsprung's disease. Stuttgart: Hip- pokrates Verlag; 1982. p. 55–61.
6. Nagasaki A, Ikeda K, Hyashida Y. Radiological diagnosis of Hirschsprung's disease utilizing rectosphincteric reflex. Pediatr Radiol. 1984;14:384–7.
7. Vult von Steyern K, Wingren P, Wiklund M, Stenström P, Arnbjörnsson E. Visualisation of the rectoanal inhibitory reflex with a modified contrast enema in children with suspected Hirschsprung disease. Pediatr Radiol. 2013;43:950–7.
8. Orno A, Lovkvist H, Marsal K. Sonographic visualization of the rectoanal inhibitory reflex in children suspected of having Hirschsprung disease: a pilot study. J Ultrasound Med. 2008;27:1165–9.
9. Surana R, Quinn FMJ, Puri P. Evaluation of risk factors in the development of enterocolitis complicating Hirschsprung's disease. Pediatr Surg Int. 1994;9:234–6.
10. Carneiro PMR, Brereton RJ, Drake DP, et al. Enterocolitis in Hirschsprung's disease. Pediatr Surg Int. 1992;7:356–60.
11. Murthi GV, Raine PA. Preoperative enterocolitis is associated with poorer long-term bowel function after Soave-Boley endorectal pull-through for Hirschsprung's disease. J Pediatr Surg. 2003;38: 69–72.
12. Vieten D, Spicer R. Enterocolitis complicating Hirschsprung's disease. Semin Paediatr Surg. 2004;13:263–72.
13. Kuwahara M, Iwai N, Yanagihara J, Toliwa K, Fukata R. Endosonographic study of anal sphincters in patients after surgery for Hirschsprung's disease. J Pediatr Surg. 1999;34:450–3.
14. Jones NM, Smilgin-Humphreys M, Sullivan PB, Grant HW. Paediatric anal endosonography. Pediatr Surg Int. 2003;19:703–6.
15. Keshtgar AS, Ward HC, Clayden GS, de Sousa NM. Investigations for incontinence and constipation after surgery for Hirschsprung's disease in children. Pediatr Surg Int. 2003;19:4–8.
16. Fadda B, Pistor G, Meier-Ruge W. Symptoms, diagnosis and therapy of neuronal intestinal dysplasia masked by Hirschsprung's disease. Pediatr Surg Int. 1987;2:76–80.
17. Kobayashi H, Hirakawa H, Puri P. What are the diagnostic criteria for intestinal neuronal dysplasia? Pediatr Surg Int. 1995;10:459–64.
18. Ure BM, Holschneider AM, Schulten D, Meire-Ruge W. Clinical impact of intestinal neuronal malformations: a prospective study of 141 patients. Pediatr Surg Int. 1997;12:377–82.

Hirschsprung's Disease and Anorectal Manometry

15

Eleni Athanasakos and Stewart Cleeve

Contents

E. Athanasakos (✉) · S. Cleeve
Department of Paediatric Surgery, The Royal London Hospital, Barts Health, Whitechapel, London, UK
e-mail: Eleni.athanasakos@bartshealth.nhs.uk; StewartJames.Cleeve@bartshealth.nhs.uk

15.1 Normal Physiology of the Anorectum

Continence relies on a complex physiological interaction between motor and sensory function in the anorectum [1, 2]. An area of great growth in published work has been on sphincteric mechanisms. These consist of two muscular components: internal anal sphincter (IAS) and external anal sphincter (EAS) (Fig. 15.1). The IAS is responsible for about 85% of the total pressure of the anal canal at rest [3, 4]. The EAS is responsible for the increase in anal pressure when continence is challenged—such as when there is a rise in intrarectal/abdominal pressure [5, 6]. Dysfunction of the IAS results in decreased anorectal pressure, which is associated with passive faecal incontinence (FI): 'not [being] aware of defaecation' [7–10]. Dysfunction of the EAS leads to decreased squeeze anorectal pressures, which are associated with urge FI: 'the inability to hold on' [9, 11–13].

Continence is additionally maintained by the 'rectoanal inhibitory reflex' (RAIR), which refers to the relaxation of the caudal anus in response to rectal distension [14–16]. Gowers [17] was the first to describe the RAIR in 1877, and it was later confirmed by Denny-Brown and Robertson (1935) [18]. In a consensus statement on anorectal physiology (ARP), the RAIR has been described as 'the transient decrease in

P. Puri (ed.), *Hirschsprung's Disease and Allied Disorders*,
https://doi.org/10.1007/978-3-030-15647-3_15

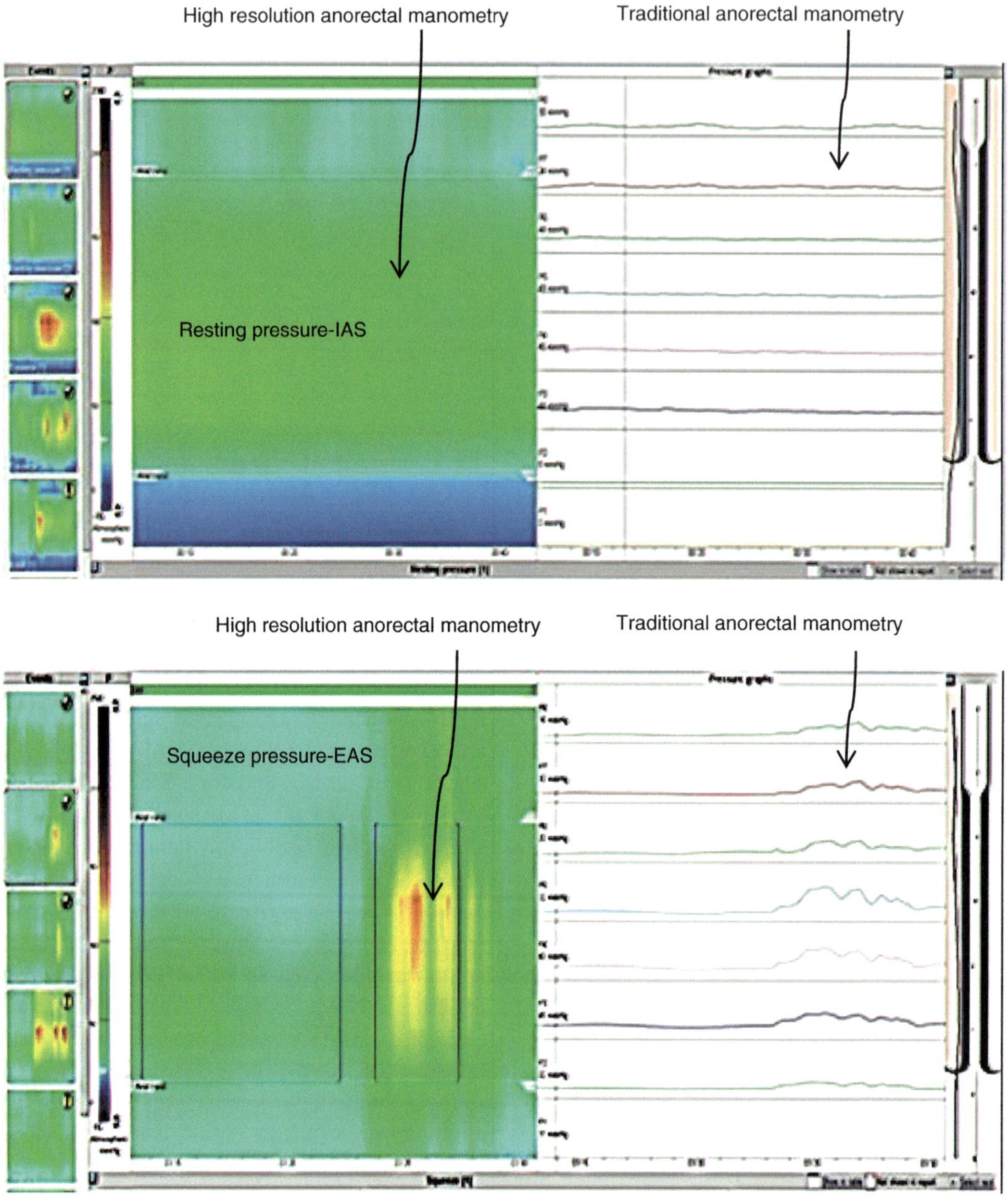

Fig. 15.1 Demonstration of the sphincteric mechanism (Source: Images are from the Children's Anorectal Physiology Service at the Royal London Hospital (MMS Ardmore Health)

resting anal pressure by ≥25% of basal pressure in response to rapid inflation of a rectal balloon with subsequent return to baseline' [19]. The RAIR is controlled by the sacral cord and myenteric neurons [20]. It has been suggested that the RAIR acts as a 'sampling reflex'—enabling the upper anal canal to discriminate between flatus and faeces [21, 22]. When the RAIR is absent, it is then that HSCR can be suspected, as will be discussed in further detail in this chapter.

Individuals may present with bowel symptoms—including FI—even if they have an anatomically intact and normal functioning sphincter complex. This highlights the importance of other pathophysiological mechanisms, such as rectal sensation [13, 23–30]. Studies have shown that stretch receptors located in the pelvic floor muscles, including the sphincteric complex, contribute to sensory discrimination [31]. Disruption of the afferent nerve pathway alters sensory perception, and this deficit has been associated with symptoms such as FI [24, 29]. The afferent pathway can be altered in multiple ways. An *elevated* sensory threshold will result in 'rectal *hypo*sensitivity'. Conversely, a *decreased* sensory threshold will result in 'rectal *hyper*sensitivity'.

Rectal hyposensitivity has been found in patients with functional constipation [32, 33]. Rectal hypersensitivity has been linked to autonomic neuropathy, congenital neurogenic anorectal malformation, spinal bifida, myelomeningocele, HSCR and functional and somatic alterations of the rectal reservoirs, such as megarectum and descending perineum syndrome [33]. Rectal hypersensitivity may underpin a heightened perception of rectal filling in FI [13, 34, 35], as well as the faecal urgency experienced by patients with 'urge' FI [9, 13, 34]. Disturbed sensory function has been reported in megarectum [24, 32, 36–38] and in children with idiopathic constipation [39].

15.2 ARP

ARP, also known as 'anorectal manometry', has been recognised for about 140 years. The first study of ARP was conducted by Gowers in 1877 [17]. Gowers demonstrated how to measure anal canal resting tone and RAIR. ARP provides an objective measurement of both motor and sensory functions—specifically pressures of the anal canal—for evaluation of the sphincteric mechanism in terms of contraction, relaxation and sensory rectal function [40, 41].

ARP has been considered the gold standard tool for [42] assessment of functional dysfunction in anal sphincter tone, [1] presence of the RAIR and [2] alteration of rectal sensory function. ARP is performed by placing a specifically designed catheter with a small balloon into the lower rectum and anal canal. The catheter is pressure-sensitive and is connected to a transducer, through which mechanical signals are converted into electronic signals that are recorded and displayed on a monitor.

Since Gower's initial work, there have been vast practical and technical advancements in the use of ARP, with high-resolution anorectal manometry (HRAM) becoming increasingly accepted worldwide [43–74]. Adult health services now perform HRAM to guide the management of bowel problems, such as constipation, FI, evacuation difficulties and dyssynergic defaecation. However, HRAM has yet to be fully recognised as a gold standard investigation in children. ARP for children is predominantly performed under sedation [48–55]—because the child is too young, insufficiently cooperative or being managed by clinicians who perceive ARP to be an invasive procedure [56, 57]. Traditional ARP in the awake child has been restricted to isolated research cases, or specific conditions such as HSCR [58–72]. Use of HRAM has been limited [73, 74].

Employment of ARP in both research and clinical practice remains hindered by a lack of uniformity among different institutions with regard to equipment, protocol and technique. Consequently, comparison of ARP data between centres is extremely limited, and it has been suggested in the literature that individual centre uses their own control values or, if using normative data from the literature, adopts a methodology similar to its author(s).

Despite variation among institutions, the use of ARP has revolutionised clinical practice in adult services. The authors hope that the service that is routinely available to adults will soon become routinely available to children.

15.3 ARP in Hirschsprung's Disease (HSCR)

15.3.1 Diagnostic Tests

ARP has been used in the diagnosis of HSCR, although there remain discrepancies concerning its accuracy and uncertainty, as to when it should be performed and whether it should be performed alongside other diagnostic tests. A 30-year retrospective study undertaken by [75] showed that the mean age at HSCR diagnosis could be decreased to 2.6 months through use of ARP, increased clinician awareness and early rectal suction biopsy.

HSCR must be distinguished in the neonate from other causes of intestinal obstruction. Later in development, HSCR must be further distinguished from idiopathic constipation or megacolon secondary to anal stenosis or stricture. HSCR predominately presents at birth and in males, with well-recognised signs of bilious vomiting, lack of passage of meconium or abdominal distension. Delayed passage of meconium can be an important early sign of HSCR [76, 77]. In rare cases, HSCR can be diagnosed later in life, in early childhood. According to the national institute for health and care excellence (NICE) guidelines (2004), constipation affects 5–30% of children in the United Kingdom [78]. In light of these figures, it is vital that idiopathic constipation is differentiated from HSCR in clinical practice.

Diagnostic tools used to diagnose HSCR include:

- *Barium enema* to locate the transition zone
- *Rectal suction biopsy* to confirm the absence of ganglion cells in the myenteric and subcutaneous plexi
- *Acetylcholinesterase (AChE) histochemistry* to show increased AChE activity
- *ARP* to establish the absence of the RAIR

A perfect investigation for the diagnosis of HSCR does not exist. The use of barium enema has been plagued with inaccuracies and technical difficulties, especially in the neonate. For example, the HSCR transition zone, which has been traditionally used as the hallmark for radiological diagnosis, has been shown to be falsely positive in 43% of infants [79]. There has been concern regarding the inadequacy of sampling at rectal biopsy, which had led to routine haemotoxylin and eosin (H&E) preparation which has shown imperfection with failure to reveal ganglion cells in 39% of patients without HSCR. AChE measurements were thought to improve the reliability of the rectal biopsy, but false-negative results have been demonstrated [80] in up to 29% in patients with HSCR. This error has been attributed to factors such as inhomogeneity, highly short-segment HSCR and incorrect sitting or sampling of rectal biopsy [81, 82]. Thus, only an increase in AChE activity contributes to the diagnosis of HSCR. The disease can be definitively excluded by the demonstration of ganglion cells histologically following conventional full-thickness rectal biopsy [83], but it depends on the adequacy of the sample.

In summary, an accurate diagnosis of HSCR is based on rectal biopsy [84, 85]—yet it is not necessarily needed to confirm the diagnosis of HSCR [86, 87]. The following section will discuss the diagnostic value and accuracy of ARP, with particular reference to the RAIR.

15.3.2 RAIR

The various reported applications of ARP in HSCR are listed in Table 15.1. As discussed previously, the diagnosis of HSCR on ARP is established by an absence of the reflex relaxation of the IAS (i.e. the RAIR) in response to rectal distention seen in the normal population (Fig. 15.2) [107, 108] (Fig. 15.3). The RAIR is induced by rapidly instilling air into a balloon in the rectum and studying the characteristics of the subsequent IAS relaxation. Air is withdrawn within 3–5 s of inflation [109]. The recommended maximum inflation volume for obtaining RAIR is 30 mL for infants, 60 mL for older children and more in patients with a megarectum [57].

Unfortunately, the accuracy of ARP has not been uniform, varying from 75% in neonates [110] to 90% [83] or close to 100% in children [110, 111]. One explanation for the variation in infant could be due to the technical difficulties in neonatal ARP due to the immaturity of the ganglion cells [110, 112, 113], particularly in premature and/or low birth weight babies [113, 114]. Yet other studies have been able to use ARP to diagnose HSCR in neonates with 90–92% accuracy [83, 88, 90, 115–117]. Low et al. [83] demonstrated that the accuracy of ARP was similar in neonates, infants and older children, and it was suggested that ARP should be done under sedation under the age of 4 years or older children

Table 15.1 Literature review of anorectal physiology in children

Author	Year	Sample	Healthy children	Traditional ARP	HRAM ARP	Diagnosis	Post-operative assessment
Boston et al. [88]	1976	63 HSCR neonates		√		√	
Zaslavsky et al. [63]	2003	35 HSCR children		√		√	√
Martins et al. [89]	2009	42 HSCR children		√			
Noviello et al. [68]	2010	185 suspected HSCR		√		√	
Low et al. [83]	1989	50 constipated children		√		√	
Boston et al. [90]	1977	101 HSCR neonates		√		√	
Demirbag et al. [64]	2012	18 HSCR children		√			√
Lanfranchi et al. [91]	1984	34 suspected HSCR		√		√	
Nagasaki et al. [92]	1980	30 healthy children 22 HSCR children	√	√			√
Iwai et al. [93]	1979	9 HSCR children 10 idiopathic constipation		√		√	
Bigelli et al. [94]	2005	20 constipation children		√			
Ambartsumyan et al. [73]	2012	30 constipation children			√		
de Lorijn et al. [77]	2003	16 healthy neonates	√	√		√	
Nagasaki et al. [95]	1989	48 HSCR children 61 healthy children	√	√		√	
Keshtgar et al. [60]	2003	16 HSCR children		√			√
Kumar et al. [96]	2009	90 healthy children	√	√			
Fathy et al. [70]	2013	150 constipated children 50 healthy children	√	√			
van Ginkel et al. [97]	2001	212 constipated children		√			
Morikawa et al. [98]	1989	82 HSCR children		√			√
Chiarioni et al. [52]	2005	15 constipated children 12 healthy children	√	√			
Yokoyama et al. [99]	1989	268 constipated children 95 HSCR children		√		√	
Benninga et al. [100]	2001	22 healthy neonates	√	√			
Hsu et al. [101]	1999	35 HSCR children		√			√
Bjornland et al. [102]	1998	48 HSCR children		√			√
Tang et al. [74]	2014	180. asymptomatic newborns, 181. 16 newborns suspicious of HSCR			√	√	
Iwai et al. [103]	1988	79 constipated children		√		√	
Jarvi et al. [52]	2009	81 suspected HSCR 33 HSCR children 48 healthy children	√	√		√	
Stensrud et al. [104]	2015	52 HSCR children		√			√
Banasiuk et al. [105]	2016	14 HSCR children			√		√

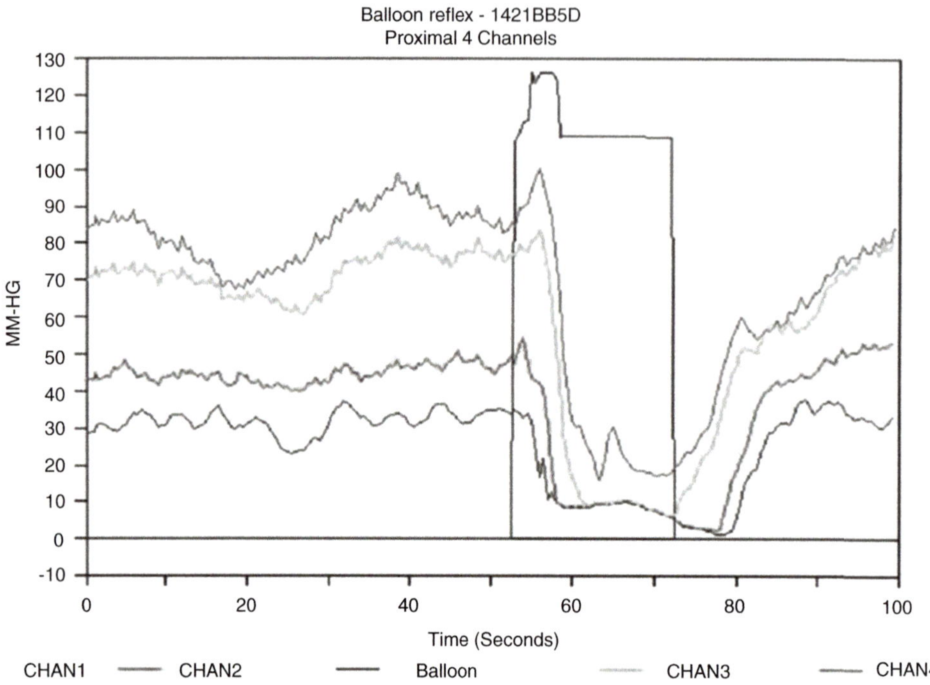

Fig. 15.2 Presence of RAIR [106]. (Source: Images are from the Children's Anorectal Physiology Service at the Royal London Hospital (MMS Ardmore Health)

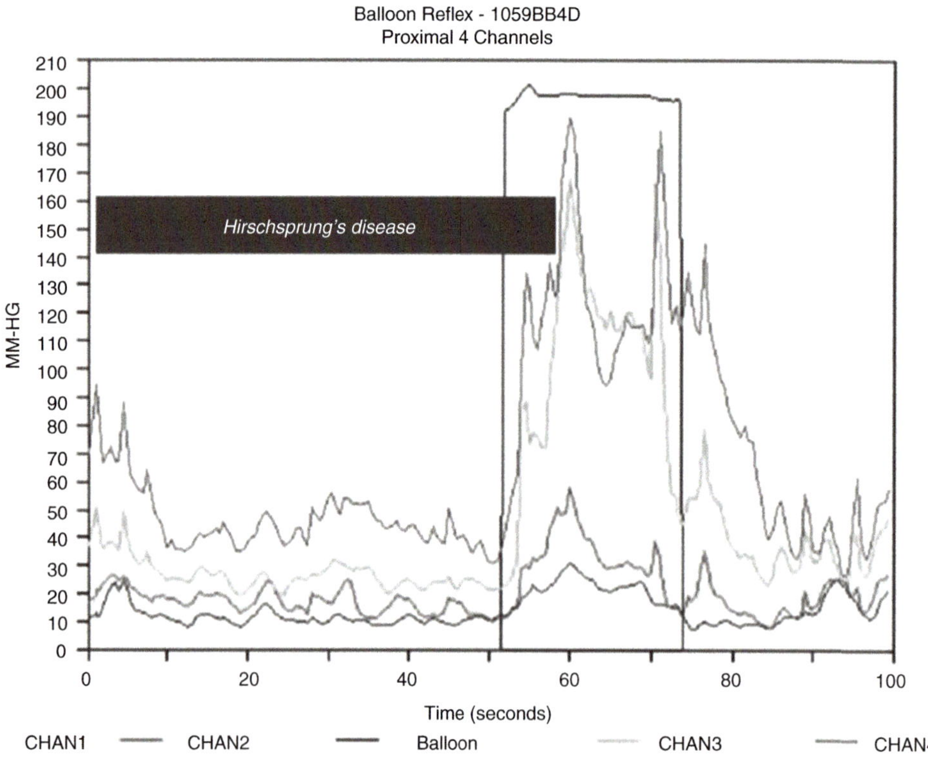

Fig. 15.3 Absence of RAIR in Hirschsprung's disease. (Source: Images are from the Children's Anorectal Physiology Service at the Royal London Hospital (MMS Ardmore Health)

who are uncooperative. Sedation does not appear to have any effect on the RAIR [95, 111, 118, 119]. Nagasaki et al. [95] suggested that indistinct reflexes often occur in neonates, possibly due to the weak constriction of the anal canal, and that using prostaglandin F2 alpha, electrical stimulation or cold water could improve the reliability of conventional ARP.

Variability in the accuracy of conventional ARP might also be attributed to other sources of variation, such as the volume of air required to elicit the RAIR [83, 111]. The literature is divided on the resting anal pressure in HSCR. Slightly higher resting pressures have been observed in patients with HSCR, yet these values do not differ markedly to individuals with a normal RAIR [115] and pronounced IAS contraction [93]. Indeed, some studies have found a lower anal resting pressure in patients with HSCR [91] and others no difference in anal resting pressures [95].

Further technical factors known to influence ARP results are incorrect positioning of the catheter, air leak in the circuit and performance of the test during faecal impaction. The pressure exerted by a solid mass of faeces can give false readings of inflation volume and increase the time needed to elicit the RAIR. Steyern et al. [93] used ARP in a group of 95 patients without signs of HSCR and reported the RAIR to be inconclusive or absent in 16 patients. The authors ventured several explanations for this finding, including difficulty in inducing the RAIR due to severe constipation, colitis and motility disorders and limitations in their broader methodology, which involved modified contrast enema supplemented with injections of cold agent in the rectum.

Reflecting on the literature, it appears that in patients with a neonatal onset of constipation and related symptoms, a rectal suction biopsy is the superior diagnostic tool. As discussed earlier in this chapter, it is vital for neonatal surgeons to detect HSCR. However, in the context of the high incidence of constipation in children, the balance of probability and specificity of symptoms shift massively in childhood [78]. Clearly it would be preferable to avoid exposing constipated children who do not have HSCR, the vast majority, to rectal biopsy. It is clear that ARP is a non-invasive screen test for the diagnosis of HSCR, especially when sedation is not necessary. Ultimately, as HSCR is a histological diagnosis, rectal biopsy is necessarily the clinician's final arbiter in the diagnostic process.

It is important to adjust for the presence of a megarectum in estimating the likelihood of HSCR in a constipated patient. In patients with a megarectum, regardless of the cause of the rectal distention, the RAIR is not always seen. The larger rectum, understandably, requires larger volumes to trigger the sphincter response [108, 120]. The recommended volumes for eliciting this response are 50–80 cc in a megarectum patient [106].

While the RAIR is normally reported as 'present' or 'absent', it may be of some use to describe the various characteristics of the RAIR, such as its latency, duration and amplitude at both the proximal and distal ends of the sphincter [106, 121, 122]. The amplitude and duration of the RAIR is influenced by the frequency and volume of rectal distention: with increasing rectal volumes, the RAIR residual pressure will decrease, and its duration will increase [123, 124]. Limited publications feature an analysis of these different phases of the RAIR. Zbar et al. [120] separated the RAIR into different sphincter segments in normal controls, constipated patients and patients with FI. They revealed significant linear trends for most parameters at each sphincter level. Recovery time and area under the inhibitory curve differed between the sphincter levels and patient groups, with the most rapid recovery occurring in the distal sphincter of incontinent patients ($P < 0.001$).

15.3.3 Contemporary Use of Anorectal Physiology in Infants and Children Older Than Six Months

Clinicians are referred patients with constipation, painful or difficult defaecation and withholding. Eighty-five percent of patients with HSCR will have been diagnosed before 6 months of age. Therefore, the pretest probability of a patient older than 6 months having HSCR is approximately 1 in 20,000, or 0.005%. [Assuming [42] incidence of HSCR is 1 in 3000 and [1] 85% of children with HSCR are diagnosed in the first

6 months of life.] The incidence of constipation in children is 5–30% (NICE) [78]. Using this data, a child's constipation is 1000 times more likely to be idiopathic in origin than attributable to HSCR.

We acknowledge that a degree of filtering by referring general practitioners, paediatricians, and paediatric gastroenterologists will occur. It is indisputable that the prevalence of idiopathic constipation is much greater than HSCR in infants over 6 months. ARP may be the investigation of choice for severe idiopathic constipation. The authors suggest that ARP may assist in screening which patients ultimately will need a rectal biopsy, thus increasing the pretest probability of the procedure in children older than 6 months and decreasing the number of normal rectal biopsies performed. The authors acknowledge that rectal biopsy is useful in diagnosing rare forms of dysganglionosis (e.g. hypoganglionosis, hyperganglionsis, intestinal neuronal dysplasia, immature ganglion cells, ganglioneuromata associated with neurofibromatosis and multiple endocrine neoplasia type 2B (MEN 2B)).

15.3.4 A Post-Surgical Role for ARP in HSCR

Studies of patients with HSCR have investigated changes in ARP following surgery.

Research has demonstrated that a RAIR can develop in children after a pull-through operation for HSCR [92, 98, 125, 126]—particularly following transanal procedures [127]. Morikawa et al. [98] demonstrated the presence of a RAIR in 39% of patients with HSCR after the Soave-Denda technique. A relationship has been identified in patients with HSCR between specific operative techniques and post-surgical changes in resting pressure [128]. Resting pressures have been found to be lower than normal in patients who undergo the Duhamel technique. Lower resting pressures can be explained by the IAS myotomy performed during the pull-through procedure when the septum between the rectum and the ganglionic segment is resected and partly by the anal dilation performed during the procedure [102].

Other authors contend that the majority of patients with HSCR continue to have an abnormal RAIR and a non-relaxing IAS after surgery [63, 102, 116, 128–132]. Zaslavsky et al. [63] studied 35 patients after corrective surgery for HSCR, and of the 16 who received ARP, all had persistent absence of RAIR, regardless of surgical technique. In fact, there was no difference found in anal resting pressure between patients with or without sphincterotomy. Thus, Zaslavsky et al. concluded that propulsive waves were not a prognostic indicator for achieving bowel control. Questions have been raised regarding the necessity of performing post-surgical ARP in HSCR, as normal findings are returned in many patients [63, 89, 127, 133] who have persistent symptoms of FI [64, 102, 104, 134, 135]. Stensrud et al. [104] reported no association between IAS defects in HSCR and low resting pressures on ARP after endorectal pull-through surgical approach, contrary to the findings of a comparable study, where IAS disruption was shown to correlate with low resting pressure after a Duhamel procedure [102].

Studies that have shown association between anal resting pressure and FI after different types of surgical procedures for HSCR have frequently used sedation when performing ARP. [60, 130]. Several studies have demonstrated the usefulness of ARP as an indicator of bowel function (particularly FI) after surgery for HSCR [60, 101, 114, 125, 128, 136–139]. Persistent symptoms in HSCR have been attributed to abnormalities of the enteric plexus, which may be associated with a diverse range of pathologies, including impaired colonic propulsive forces (or anorectal dyssynergia), [60, 64] anal stenosis, an enlarged Duhamel pouch, residual aganglionic segment or intestinal neuronal dysplasia [1, 128, 138, 140].

15.4 HRAM and Hirschsprung's Disease

HRAM is a novel technique for assessing motor and sensory function in the anorectum, with several potential advantages over traditional ARP. The primary advantage of HRAM is that HRAM allows computerised data acquisition and display-utilised colour-coded amplitude depiction, enabling enhanced visual and analytic assessment of the sphincter complex [141]. HRAM provides a better understanding of pressure profiles and synchronised events over time than can be derived from the traditional line traces seen on ARP [142, 143]. Moreover, HRAM can use either solid or water-perfused systems and two-dimensional or three-dimensional—albeit with limited guidance from the literature as to which is superior, due to limited studies. There has been a preference for solid-state catheters in HRAM. It has been suggested that traditional ARP method were cumbersome and required the placement of the recording sensors precisely within the anal sphincter for accurate diagnosis, as catheter movement with anorectal manoeuvres could confound the values.

Studies have demonstrated the efficacy of using HRAM to diagnose HSCR [74]. A few authors maintain that the RAIR cannot be elicited in newborns less than 1-week-old on account of their immature anorectum [77, 100], yet numerous studies [97, 144] have demonstrated that this can be done using HRAM with high sensitivity (89%) and specificity (83%). However, we face the same dilemma as we did with traditional ARP: there is variation in technique between centres, and an absence of robust normative data within paediatrics.

At the Royal London Hospital, Barts Health NHS (London, UK), the Children's Anorectal Physiology Service (CAPS) was established in August 2016. The service uses a combination of HRAM (2D) water-perfused ARP and complementary investigations including endoanal ultrasound, colonic transit study and proctogram. The service has seen 135 children suffering from chronic constipation with or without FI, HSCR or anorectal malformations, for both diagnostic and management purposes. Most investigations are performed when children are awake (90%) with a small number done under sedation (ketamine). All patients are discussed at a multidisciplinary team meeting with input from up to seven specialists: paediatric surgeon, paediatric gastroenterologist, clinical nurse specialist, health play specialist, clinical psychologist, paediatric radiologist and paediatric clinical scientist. Investigations are used to direct management, taking into consideration information from validated bowel assessment, psychological evaluation and medical history. The service believes in using both scientific diagnostic evidence and multi-professional input to manage these patients. The RAIR is measured in all patients using a 2D HRAM water-perfused machine (Figs. 15.4 and 15.5). Out of 135 patients seen at CAPS, 10 (7%) had HSCR, and ARP was performed in each to assess sphincteric

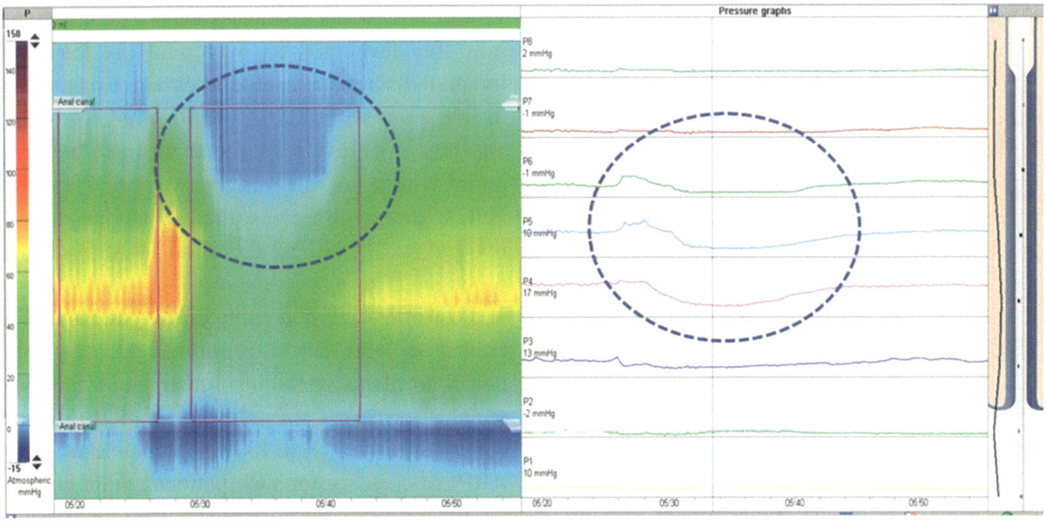

Fig. 15.4 Presence of RAIR in a symptomatic patient. (Source: Images are from the Children's Anorectal Physiology Service at the Royal London Hospital (MMS Ardmore Health)

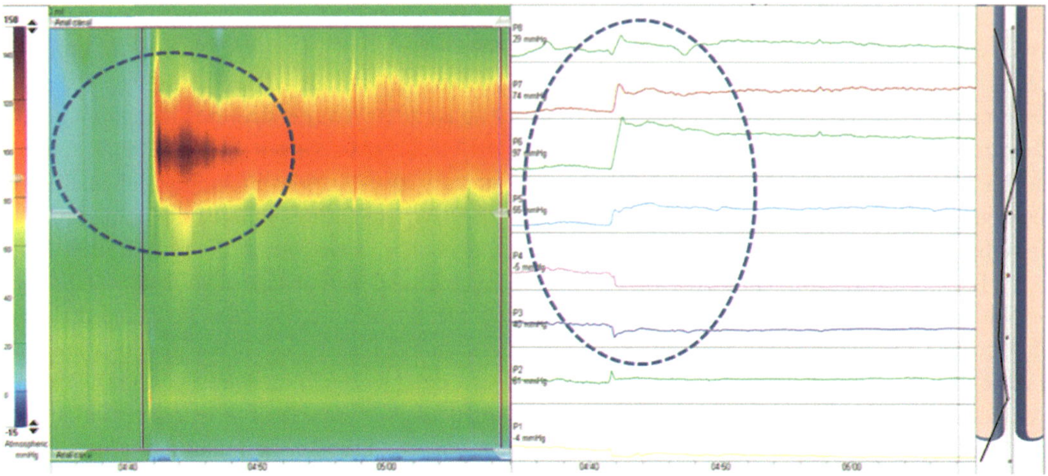

Fig. 15.5 Absence of RAIR in Hirschsprung's disease patient. (Source: Images are from the Children's Anorectal Physiology Service at the Royal London Hospital (MMS Ardmore Health)

pressures (IAS/EAS), RAIR, enhanced squeeze, cough reflex, defaecatory function ('push') and rectal sensation (unpublished work). RAIR was absent in all known patients with HSCR.

Banasiuk et al. [105] have argued that 3D HRAM is the most precise method for assessment of anal sphincter function and may help to direct surgical procedures. It was suggested from Banasiuk et al. that using 3D HRAM gives the opportunity to assess the anal sphincter both longitudinally and circumferentially; however, there is limited understanding of how such measurements are practical in understanding further the pathophysiological role and characteristics in patients with bowel dysfunction and HSCR.

The main limitation with using HRAM in children is the lack of normative data available in the professional literature—unlike in adults, for whom we have normal values to compare patients to, despite wide variation in technique, protocol and manometric equipment [43, 44].

15.5 Concluding Remarks

This chapter has discussed ARP as one of multiple ways to investigate HSCR. There has been considerable debate as to which diagnostic tool is the most appropriate and accurate, as is often the case when the perfect investigation does not exist. Rectal suction biopsy and ARP are generally considered to be the most accurate tests [52, 145].

ARP has been demonstrated in the literature to be a reliable, cost-effective and non-invasive scientific tool for the diagnosis of HSCR [68, 91, 95, 99, 103, 116]. Nevertheless, it is clear that rectal biopsy is the investigation of choice in neonates. It has been proposed that in children under the age of 1 year, HSCR is very unlikely in the presence of a RAIR. Based on the specificity and positive predictive value of ARP for the diagnosis of HSCR, it remains inferior to other diagnostic tools (i.e. rectal suction biopsy) and should not be used solely [52, 84]. Guidelines must be developed to overcome the variability and discrepancies found when using ARP in patients with HSCR—both diagnostically and post-operatively. While there may be clear understanding of the various ways to diagnose HSCR among clinicians, there exists no definitive pathway for the integration of ARP in this process.

Post-operatively, a number of patients with HSCR will present with short- and long-term bowel problems, including constipation, FI, anorectal dyssynergia and intestinal motility disturbances [125, 128, 136, 137]. It is unclear whether ARP is necessary for such patients: their sphincter function can be normal, as made evident in recent research. Significant discussion has been devoted in this chapter to the presence or absence of the RAIR post-operatively in patients with HSCR, yet understanding about the other parameters of the RAIR remains rudimentary—limiting the extent to which it may be used to predict functional outcome.

It is clear that there are obstacles which need to be confronted to gain uniformity in the use of ARP, for HSCR or other bowel conditions. In adults [40, 43, 146, 147], there is no standardisation in ARP for either protocol or equipment—this is also the case within paediatrics. Furthermore, there is a lack of normative data for scientific comparison of findings within paediatrics, as every institution performs the investigation on children differently (whether it be awake or under sedation), and there remains variation in ARP protocol and catheter use (solid/liquid, 2D/3D), making it impossible for scientific comparisons. It is important to keep in mind that, when comparing results, ARP should be performed with identical techniques in the same institution.

ARP is a useful tool for identifying the pathophysiology of a patient's anorectal dysfunction, which may be complex and multifactorial. Specifically, in the age of HRAM, we have the ability to assess the coordination of pelvic floor mechanisms, observing for dysfunction both when the patient is asked to squeeze and when they are asked to 'push' as a demonstration of their muscle activity during defaecation. Information gained from these observations can be used to direct biofeedback management. In conclusion, ARP does improve understanding of the pathophysiological mechanisms involved in HSCR. The primary ambition should be the establishment of an internationally agreed paediatric standardised protocol using uniform equipment. Future research will then be universally comparable and can proceed to improvements in investigation and, most importantly, outcomes for children and adults with HSCR.

References

1. Rao SS, Mudipalli RS, Stessman M, Zimmerman B. Investigation of the utility of colorectal function tests and Rome II criteria in dyssynergic defecation (Anismus). Neurogastroenterol Motil. 2004;16:589–96.
2. Rao SS, Azpiroz F, Diamant N, Enck P, Tougas G, Wald A. Minimum standards of anorectal manometry. J Neurogastroenterol Motil. 2002;14:553–9.
3. Cooper ZR, Rose S. Fecal incontinence: a clinical approach. Mt Sinai J Med. 2000;67:96–105.
4. Fernández-Fraga X, Azpiroz F, Malagelada JR. Significance of pelvic floor muscles in anal incontinence. Gastroenterol. 2002;123:1441–50.
5. Chatoor DR, Taylor SJ, Cohen CR, Emmanuel AV. Faecal incontinence. Br J Surg. 2007;94:134–44.
6. Cheetham MJ, Malouf AJ, Kamm MA. Fecal incontinence. Gastroenerol Clin North Am. 2001;30:115–30.
7. Salvioli B, Bharucha AE, Rath-Harvey D, Pemberton JH, Phillips SF. Rectal compliance, capacity, and rectoanal sensation in fecal incontinence. Am J Gastroenterol. 2001;96:2158–68.
8. Read NW, Bartolo DC, Read MG. Differences in anal function in patients with incontinence to solids and in patients with incontinence to liquids. Br J Surg. 1984;71:39–42.
9. Engel AF, Kamm MA, Bartram CI, Nicholls RJ. Relationship of symptoms in faecal incontinence to specific sphincter abnormalities. Int J Colorectal Dis. 1995;10:152–5.
10. Vaizey CJ, Kamm MA, Bartram CI. Primary degeneration of the internal anal sphincter as a cause of passive faecal incontinence. Lancet. 1997;349:612–5.
11. Deutekom M, Dobben AC, Terra MP, Engel AF, Stoker J, Bossuyt PM, Boeckxstaens GE. Clinical presentation of fecal incontinence and anorectal function: what is the relationship? Am J Gastroenterol. 2007;102:351–61.
12. Gee AS, Durdey P. Urge incontinence of faeces is a marker of severe external anal sphincter dysfunction. Br J Surg. 1995;82:1179–82.
13. Chan CL, Lunniss PJ, Wang D, Williams NS, Scott SM. Rectal sensorimotor dysfunction in patients with urge faecal incontinence: evidence from prolonged manometric studies. Gut. 2005a;54:1263–72.
14. Shafik A, El-Sibai AI. Parasympathetic reflex: role in defecation mechanisms. World J Surg. 2002;26:737–40.
15. O'Riordain MG, Molloy RG, Gillen P, Horgan A, Kirwan WO. Rectoanal inhibitory reflex following low stapled anterior resection of the rectum. Dis Colon Rectum. 1992;35:874–8.
16. Netinho JG, Ayrizono M, Coy R, Fagundes JJ, Goes RN. Amplitude and recovery velocity of relaxation induce by rectoanal inhibitory reflex and its importance for obstructive evacuation. Arch Gastroenterol. 2005;42:19–23.
17. Gowers WR. The autonomic action of the sphincter ani. Proc R Soc Med. 1877;26:77–84.
18. Denny-Brown D, Robertson EG. An investigation of the nervous control of defecation. Brain. 1935;58:256–310.
19. Lowry AC, Simmang CL, Boulos P. Consensus statement of definitions for anorectal physiology and rectal cancer. Col Dis. 2001;3:272–5.
20. Kaur G, Gardiner A, Duthie GS. Rectoanal reflex parameters in incontinence and constipation. Dis Colon Rectum. 2002;45:928–33.

21. Duthie HL, Bennett RC. The relation of sensation in the anal canal to the function and anal sphincter: a possible factor in anal continence. Gut. 1963;4:179–82.
22. Miller R, Bartolo DCC, Cervero F, Mortensen NJM. Anorectal sampling: a comparison of normal and incontinent patients. British Journal of Surgery. 1988;75:44–7.
23. Athanasakos EP, Ward HC, Williams NS, Scott SM. Importance of extrasphincteric mechanisms in the pathophysiology of faecal incontinence in adults with a history of anorectal anomaly. Br J Surg. 2008;9:1394–400.
24. Vasudevan SP, Scott SM, Gladman MA, Lunniss PJ. Rectal hyposensitivity: evaluation of anal sensation in female patients with refractory constipation with and without faecal incontinence. Neurogastroenterol Motil. 2007;19:660–7.
25. Bharacha AE. Pelvic floor: anatomy and function. Neurogastroenterol and Motility. 2006;18:507–19.
26. Roe AM, Bartolo DC, Mortensen NJ. New method for assessment of anal sensation in various anorectal disorders. Brit J Surg. 1986;73:310–2.
27. Burgell R, Scott M. Rectal hyposensitivity. J Neurogastroenterol Motil. 2012;18:373–84.
28. Scott SM, Berg VD, Benninga MA. Rectal sensorimotor dysfunction in constipation. Best Pract Res Clin Gastroenterol. 2011;25:103–18.
29. Gladman MA, Aziz Q, Scott SM, Williams NS, Lunniss PJ. Rectal hyposensitivity: pathophysiological mechanisms. Neurogastroenterol Motil. 2009;21:508–e5.
30. Gladman MA, Scott SM, Chan CL, Williams NS, Lunniss PJ. Rectal hyposensitivity: prevalence and clinical impact in patients with intractable constipation and fecal incontinence. Dis Colon Rectum. 2003;46(2):238–46.
31. Ramussen OO, Petersen IK, Christiansen J. Anorectal function following low anterior resection. Colorectal Dis. 2003;5:258–61.
32. Gladman MA, Dvorkin LS, Lunniss PJ, Williams NS, Scott SM. Rectal hyposensitivity: a disorder of the rectal wall or the afferent pathway? An assessment using the barostat. Am J Gastroenterol. 2005;100:106–14.
33. Hancke E, Schürholz M. Impaired rectal sensation in idiopathic faecal incontinence. Int J Colorectal Dis. 1987;2:146–8.
34. Chan CL, Scott SM, Williams NS, Lunniss PJ. Rectal hypersensitivity worsens stool frequency, urgency, and lifestyle in patients with urge fecal incontinence. Dis Colon Rectum. 2005b;48:134–40.
35. Azpiroz F, Bouin M, Camilleri M, Mayer EA, Poitras P, Serra R, Spllier C. Mechanisms of hypersensitivity in IBS and functional disorders. Neurogastroenterol and Motility, Supplement. 2007;1:62–88.
36. Tuteja AK, Rao SS. Review article: recent trends in diagnosis and treatment of faecal incontinence. Aliment Pharmacol Ther. 2004;19(8):829–40.
37. Lubowski DZ, Nicholls RJ. Faecal incontinence associated with reduced pelvic sensation. Br J Surg. 1988;75:1086–8.
38. Rogers J, Henry MM, Misiewicz JJ. Combined sensory and motor deficit in primary neuropathic faecal incontinence. Gut. 1988;29:5–9.
39. van der Plas RN, Benninga MA, Staalman CR, Akkermans LM, Redekop WK, Taminiau JA, Buller HA. Megarectum in constipation. Arch Dis Child. 2000;83:52–8.
40. Azpiroz F, Enck P, Whitehead WE. Anorectal functional testing: review of collective experience. Am J Gastroenerol. 2002;97:232–40.
41. Rao SS, Patel RS. How useful are manometric tests of anorectal function in the management of defecation disorders? Am J Gastroenterol. 1997;92:469–75.
42. Potts WJ. The surgeon and the child. Philadelphia: WB Saunders Company; 1959.
43. Carrington EV, Brokjaer A, Craven H, Zarate N, Horrocks EJ, Palit S, Jackson W, Duthie GS, Knowles CH, Lunniss PJ, Scott SM. Traditional measures of normal anal sphincter function using high-resolution anorectal manometry (HRAM) in 115 healthy volunteers. Neurogastrol Motil. 2014;26:625–35.
44. Carrington EV, Heinrich H, Knowles CH, Rao SS, Fox M, Scott SM. International Anorectal Physiology Working Party Group (IAPWG). Methods of anorectal manometry vary widely in clinical practice: results from an international survey. Neurogastroenterol Motil. 2017;29:e13016.
45. Dinning PG, Carrington EV, Scott SM. The use of colonic and anorectal high-resolution manometry and its place in clinical work and in research. Neurogastroenterol Motil. 2015;27:1693–708.
46. Sharma A, Rao S. Constipation: pathophysiology and current therapeutic approaches. Handb Exp Pharmacol. 2017;239:59–74.
47. Prichard DO, Lee T, Parthasarathy G, Fletcher JG, Zinsmeister AR, Bharucha AE. High-resolution anorectal manometry for identifying defecatory disorders and rectal structural abnormalities in women. Clin Gastroenterol Hepatol. 2016;15:412–20.
48. Keshtgar AS, Athanasakos E, Clayden GS, Ward HC. Evaluation of outcome of anorectal anomaly in childhood: the role of anorectal manometry and endosonography. Pediatr Surg Int. 2008;24:885–92.
49. Keshtgar AS, Ward HC, Clayden GS. Pathophysiology of chronic childhood constipation: functional and morphological evaluation by anorectal manometry and endosonography and colonic transit study. J Pediatr Surg. 2012;48:806–12.
50. Tran K, Kuo B, Zibaitis A, Bhattacharya S, Cote C, Belkind-Gerson J. Effect of propofol on anal sphincter pressure during anorectal manometry. J Pediatr Gastroenterol Nutr. 2014;58:495–7.
51. Sangkhathat S, Patrapinyokul S, Osatakul N. Crucial role of rectoanal inhibitory reflex in emptying function after anoplasty in infants with anorectal malformations. Asian J Surg. 2004;27:125–9.
52. Jarvi K, Koivusalo A, Rintala RJ, Pakarinen MP. Anorectal manometry with reference to operative rectal biopsy for the diagnosis/exclusion of Hirschsprungs disease in children under 1 year of age. Int J Colorectal Dis. 2009;24:451–4.

53. Ruttenstock EM, Zani A, Huber-Zeyringer A, Höllwarth ME. Pre- and postoperative rectal manometric assessment of patients with anorectal malformations: should we preserve the fistula? Dis Colon Rectum. 2013;56:499–504.
54. Raghunath N, Glassman MS, Halata MS, Berezin SH, Stewart JM, Medow MS. Anorectal motility abnormalities in children with encopresis and chronic constipation. J Pediatr. 2010;158:293–6.
55. Kubota M, Okuyama N, Hirayama Y, Kobayashi K, Satoh K. Effect of sacral magnetic stimulation on the anorectal manometric activity: a new modality for examining sacro-rectoanal interaction. Pediatr Surg Int. 2007;23:741–5.
56. Rodriguez L, Sood M, Di Lorenzo C, Saps M. An ANMS-NASPGHAN consensus document on anorectal and colonic manometry in children. Neurogastroetnerol Motil. 2016;29:1–8.
57. Di Lorenzo C, Hillemeier C, Hyman P, Loening-Baucke V, Nurko S, Rosenberg A, Taminiau J. Manometry studies in children: minimum standards for procedures. Neurogastroenterol Motil. 2002;14:411–20.
58. Marques GM, Martins JL, Nobre VD. Comparison between perfusion and balloon techniques for performing anorectal manometry in children with intestinal constipation. Acta Cir Bras. 2008;23:405–11.
59. Li ZH, Dong M, Wang ZF. Functional constipation in children: investigation and management of anorectal motility. World J Pediatr. 2008;4:45–8.
60. Keshtgar AS, Ward HC, Clayden GS, de Sousa NM. Investigations for incontinence and constipation after surgery for Hirschsprung's disease in children. Pediatr Surg Int. 2003;19:4–8.
61. Arnoldi R, Macchini F, Gentilino V, Farris G, Morandi A, Brisighelli G, Leva E. Anorectal malformations with good prognosis: variables affecting the functional outcome. J Pediatr Surg. 2014;49: 1232–6.
62. Chiarioni G, de Roberto G, Mazzocchi A, Morelli A, Bassotti G. Manometric assessment of idiopathic megarectum in constipated children. World J Gastroenterol. 2005;14:6027–30.
63. Zaslavsky C, Loening-Baucke V. Anorectal manometric evaluation of children and adolescents post surgery for Hirschsprung's disease. J Pediatr Surg. 2003;38:191–5.
64. Demirbag S, Tiryaki T, Purtuloglu T. Importance of anorectal manometry after definitive surgery for Hirschsprung's disease in children. Afr J Paediatr Surg. 2013;10:1–4.
65. Morera C, Nurko S. Rectal manometry in patients with isolated sacral agenesis. J Pediatr Gastroenterol Nutr. 2003;37:47–52.
66. Velde SV, Pratte L, Verhelst H, Meersschaut V, Herregods N, Van Winckel M, Van Biervliet S. Colon transit time and anorectal manometry in children and young adults with spina bifida. Int J Colorectal Dis. 2013;28:1547–53.
67. Noviello C, Cobellis G, Papparella A, Amici G, Martino A. Role of anorectal manometry in children with severe constipation. Colorectal Dis. 2009;11:480–4.
68. Noviello C, Cobellis G, Romano M, Amici G, Martino A. Diagnosis of Hirschsprungs disease: an age related approach in children below or above one year. Colorectal Dis. 2010;12:1044–8.
69. Caldaro T, Romeo E, De Angelis P, Gambitta RA, Rea F, Torroni F, Foschia F, di Abriola GF, Dall'Oglio L. Three-dimensional endoanal ultrasound and anorectal manometry in children with anorectal malformations: new discoveries. J Pediat Surg. 2012;47:956–63.
70. Fathy A, Megahed A, Barakat T, Abdalla AF. Anorectal functional abnormalities in Egyptian children with chronic functional constipation. Arab J Gastroenterol. 2013;14:6–9.
71. Kyrklund K, Pakarinen MP, Rintala RJ. Manometric findings in relation to functional outcomes in different types of anorectal malformations. J Pediatr Surg. 2016;52:563–8.
72. Benninga MA, Voskuijl WP, Akkerhuis GW, Taminiau JA, Büller HA. Colonic transit times and behaviour profiles in children with defecation disorders. Arch Dis Child. 2004;89:13–6.
73. Ambartsumyan L, Rodriguez L, Morera C, Nurko S. Longitudinal and radial characteristics of intra-anal pressures in children using 3D high-definition anorectal manometry: new observations. Am J Gastroenterol. 2013;108:1918–28.
74. Tang YF, Chen JG, An HJ, Jin P, Yang L, Dai ZF, Huang LM, Yu JW, Yang XY, Fan RY, Li SJ, Han Y, Wang JH, Gyawali CP, Sheng JQ. High-resolution anorectal manometry in newborns: normative values and diagnostic utility in Hirschsprung disease. Neurogastroenterol Motil. 2014;26:1565–72.
75. Klein MD, Phillippart AI. Hirschsprung's disease: Three decades' experience at a single institution. J Pediatr Surg. 1993;28:1291–3.
76. Lewis NA, Levitt MA, Zallen GS, Zafar MS, Iacono KL, Rossman JE, Caty MG, Glick PL. Diagnosing Hirschsprung's disease: increasing the odds of a positive rectal biopsy result. J Pediat Surg. 2003;38:412–6.
77. de Lorijn F, Omari TI, Kok JH, Taminiau JA, Benninga MA. Maturation of the rectoanal inhibitory reflex in very premature infants. J Pediatr. 2003;143:630–3.
78. NICE Guidelines: insert website. https://cks.nice.org.uk/constipation-in-children#!topicSummary
79. Taxman TL, Yulish BS, Rothstein FC. How useful is the barium enema in the diagnosis of infantile Hirschsprungs disease. Am J Dis Child. 1986;140:881–4.
80. Hamoudi AB, Reiner CB, Boles ET Jr, HJ MC, Kerzner B. Acetylthiocholinesterase staining activity of rectal mucosa. Its use in the diagnosis of Hirschsprung's disease. Arch Pathol Lab Med. 1982;106:670–2.
81. Bonham JR, Dale G, Scott DJ, Wagget J. A 7-year study of the diagnostic value of rectal mucosal acetylcholinesterase measurement in Hirschsprung's disease. J Pediatr Surg. 1987;22:150–2.

82. Wells FE, Addison GM. Acetylcholinesterase activity in rectal biopsies: an assessment of its diagnostic value in Hirschsprung's disease. J Pediatr Gastroenterol Nutr. 1986;5:912–9.
83. Low PS, Quak SH, Prabhakaran VT, Gilbert J, Chiang GS, Aiyathurai E. Accuracy of anorectal manometry in the diagnosis of Hirschsprungs disease. J Pediatr Gastroenterol Nutri. 1989;9:342–6.
84. Pini-prato A, Avanzini S, Gentilino V, Martuciello G, Mattioli G, Coccia C. Rectal suction biopsy in the workup of childhood constipation: indication and diagnostic value. Pediatr Surg Int. 2007;23:117–22.
85. Martucciello G, Pini Prato A, Puri P, Holschneider AM, Meier-Ruge W, Jasonni V, Tovar JA, Groseld JL. Controversies concerning diagnostic guidelines for anomalies of the enteric nervous system: a report from the fourth International Symposium on Hirschsprungs disease and related neurocristopathies. J Pediatr Surg. 2005;40:1527–31.
86. de Lorijn F, Kremer LC, Reitsma JB, Benninga MA. Diagnostic tests in Hirschsprung disease: a systematic review. J Pediatr Gastroenterol Nutr. 2006;42:496–505.
87. Emir H, Akman M, Sarimurat N, Kilic N, Erdogan E, Sovlet Y. Anorectal manometry during the neonatal period: its specificity in the diagnosis of Hirschsprungs disease. Eur J of Pediatr Surg. 1999;9:101–3.
88. Boston VE, Scott JES. Anorectal manometry as a diagnostic method in the neonatal period. J of Pediat Surg. 1976;11:9–16.
89. Martins EC, Peterlini FL, Fagundes DJ, Martins JL. Clinical, manometric and profilometric evaluation after surgery for Hirschsprung's disease: comparison between the modified Duhamel and the transanal rectosigmoidectomy techniques. Acta Cir Bras. 2009;24:416–22.
90. Boston VE, Cywes S, Davies MR. Qualitative and quantitative evaluation of internal anal sphincter function in the newborn. Gut. 1977;18:1036–44.
91. Lanfranchi GA, Bazzocchi G, Federici S, Brignola C, Campieri M, Rossi F, Domini R, Labo G. Anorectal manometry in the diagnosis of Hirschsprung's disease-comparison with clinical and radiological criteria. Am J Gastroenterol. 1984;79:270–5.
92. Nagasaki A, Ikeda K, Suita S. Postoperative sequential anorectal manometric study of children with Hirschsprung's disease. J Pediatr Surg. 1980;15:615–9.
93. Iwai N, Ogita S, Kida M, Nishioka B, Fujita Y, Majima S. A manometric assessment of anorectal pressures and its significance in the diagnosis of Hirschsprung's disease and idiopathic megacolon. Jpn J Surg. 1979;9:234–40.
94. Bigelli R, Fernandes M, Vicente Y, Dantas R, Galvao L, Campos A. Anorectal manometry in children with chronic functional constipation. Arq Gastroenterol. 2005;42:178–81.
95. Nagasaki A, Sumitomo K, Shono T, Ikeda K. Diagnosis of Hirschsprung's disease by anorectal manometry. Prog Pediatr Surg. 1989;24:40–8.
96. Kumar S, Ramadan S, Gupta V, Helmy S, Atta I, Alkholy A. Manometric tests of anorectal function in 90 healthy children: a clinical study from Kuwait. J Pediatr Surg. 2009;44:1786–90.
97. Van Ginkel RV, Voskuijl WP, Benninga MA, Taminiau JAJ, Boeckxstaens GE. Alterations in rectal sensitivity and motility in childhood irritable bowel syndrome. Gastroenterol. 2001;120:31–8.
98. Morikawaw Y, Matsufugi H, Hirobe S, Yokoyama J, Katsumata K. Motility of the anorectal after the Soave-Denda operation. Prog Pediatr Surg. 1989;24:67–76.
99. Yokoyama J, Kuroda T, Matsufugi H, Hirobe S, Hara S, Katsumata K. Problems in diagnosis of Hirschsprungs disease by anorectal manometry. Prog Pediatr Surg. 1989;24:49–58.
100. Benninga MA, Omari TI, Haslam RR, Barnett CP, Dent J, Davidson GP. Characterization of anorectal pressure and the anorectal inhibitory reflex in healthy preterm and term infants. J Pediatr. 2001;139:233–7.
101. Wm H, Chen CC. Clinical and manometric evaluation of postoperative fecal soiling in patients with Hirschsprungs disease. Journal of Formos Medical Association. 1999;98:410–4.
102. Bjornland K, Diseth TH, Emblem R. Long-term functional, manometric, and endosonographic evaluation of patients operated upon with the Duhamel technique. Pediat Surg Int. 1998;13:24–8.
103. Iwai N, Yanagihara J, Tokiwa K, Deguchi E, Perdzynski W, Takahashi T. Reliability of anorectal manometry in the diagnosis of Hirschsprung's disease. Z Kinder. 1988;43:405–7.
104. Stensrud KJ, Emblem R, Bjørnland K. Anal endosonography and bowel function in patients undergoing different types of endorectal pull-through procedures for Hirschsprung disease. J Pediatr Surg. 2015;50:1341–6.
105. Banasiuk M, Banaszkiewic A, Piotrowski D, Albrecht P, Kaminski A, Radzikowski A. 3D high-definition manometry in evaluation of children after surgery for Hirschsprung's disease: a pilot study. Adv Med Sci. 2016;61:18–22.
106. Roberts PL. Rectoanal inhibition. In: Wexner SD, Zbar AP, Pescatori M, editors. Complex anorectal disorders: investigation and management, Chapter 2.2. London: Springer; 2005. p. 41–4.
107. Loening-Baucke V. Anorectal manometry: experience with strain gauge pressure transducers for the diagnosis of Hirschsprung's disease. J Pediatr Surg. 1983;18:595–600.
108. Loening-Baucke V, Pringle KC, Ekwo EE. Anorectal manometry for the exclusion of Hirschsprung's disease in neonates. J Pediatr Gastroenterol Nutr. 1985;4:596–603.
109. Hong J. Clinical applications of gastrointestinal manometry in children. Pediatr Gastroenterol Hep Nutri. 2014;17:23–30.
110. Meunier PD, Gallavardin D. Anorectal manometry: the state of the art. Dig Dis. 1993;11:252–64.

111. Rosenberg AJ, Velda R. A simplified technique for paediatric anorectal manometry. Pediatr. 1983;71:240–5.
112. Ito Y, Donahoe PK, Hendron WH. Maturation of the rectoanal response in premature and perinatal infants. J Pediat Surg. 1977;12:477–82.
113. Howard ER, Nixon HH. Internal anal sphincter: observation on development and mechanisms of inhibiting resources in premature infants and children with Hirschsprungs disease. Arch Dis Child. 1968;43:539–78.
114. Holschneider AM, Kellner E, Streibl P, Sippell WG. The development of anorectal continence and the significance in the diagnosis of Hirschsprung's disease. J Pediat Surg. 1976;11:151–6.
115. Aaronson I, Nixon HH. A clinical evaluation of anorectal pressure studies in the diagnosis of Hirschsprungs disease. Gut. 1972;13:138–46.
116. Suzuki H, White JJ, El Shafie M, Shaker IJ, Haller JA, Schnaufer L. Nonoperative diagnosis of Hirschsprung's disease in the neonates. Pediatr. 1973;51:188–91.
117. Verder H, Krasilnikoff PA, Scheibel E. Anal Tonometry in the neonatal period in mature and premature children. Acta Paediatrica Scandinavica. 1975;64:592–6.
118. Ustach TJ, Tobon F, Schuster MM. Simplified method for diagnosis of Hirschsprungs disease. Arch Dis Child. 1969;44:694–7.
119. Constantinides CG, Nixon HH. Anorectal manometry under anaesthesia in the investigation of children with chronic constipation. Dis Colon Rectum. 1982;25:125–30.
120. Zbar A, Aslam M, Gold DM, Gatzen C, Gosling A, Kmiot WA. Parameters of the rectoanal inhibitory reflex in patients with idiopathic fecal incontinence and chronic constipation. Dis Colon Rectum. 1998;41:200–8.
121. Sangwan YP, Coller JA, Barrett RC, Murray JJ, Roberts PL, Schoetz DJ Jr. Distal rectoanal excitatory reflex: a reliable index of pudendal neuropathy. Dis Colon Rectum. 1995;38:916–20.
122. Sangway UP, Coller JA, Schoetz DJ Jr, Murray JJ, Roberts PL. Latency measurement of rectoanal reflexes. Dis Colon Rectum. 1995;38:1281–5.
123. Sun WM, Read NW, Prior A, Daly JA, Cheah SK, Grundy D. Sensory and motor responses to rectal distention vary according to rate and pattern of balloon inflation. Gastroenterol. 1990;99:1008–15.
124. Monteiro FJ, Regadas FS, Muirad-Regadas SM, Rodrigues LV, Leal VM. Comparative evaluation of the effect of sustained inflation and rapid inflation/deflation of the intrarectal balloon upon rectoanal inhibitory reflex parameters in asymptomatic subjects. Tech Coloproc. 2007;11:323–6.
125. Heij HA, de Vries X, Bremer I. Long-term anorectal function after Duhamel operation for Hirschsprung's disease. J Pediatr Surg. 1995;30:430–2.
126. Suzuki H, Tsukamoto Y, Amano S, Sakarai A. Motility of the anorectum after 'rectoplasty with posterior triangular colonic flap' in Hirschsprung's disease. Jpn J Surg. 1984;14:335–8.
127. Van Leeuwen K, Geiger JD, Barnett JL, Coran AG, Teitelbaum DH. Stooling and manometric findings after primary pull-throughs in Hirschsprung's disease: perineal versus abdominal approaches. J Pediatr Surg. 2002;37:1321–5.
128. Mishalany HG, Wooley MM. Postoperative functional and manometric evaluation of patients with Hirschsprung's disease. J Pediatr Surg. 1987;22:443–6.
129. Banani SA, Forootan H. Role of anorectal myectomy after failed endorectal pull-through in Hirschsprung's disease. J of Pediatr Surg. 1994;29:1307–90.
130. Heikkinen M, Rintala R, Luukkonen P. Long-term anal sphincter performance after surgery for Hirschsprung's disease. J Pediatr Surg. 1997;32:1443–6.
131. Iwai N, Yanagihara T, Tsuto T. Clinical and manometric assessment of anorectal function after Martin's operation. Z Kinder. 1987;42:235–7.
132. Frenckner B, Lindstrom O. Ano-rectal function assessed by manometric and electromyography after endoanal pull-through for Hirschsprungs disease. Z Kinderchir. 1983;38:101–4.
133. Raizada V, Bhargava V, Karsten A, Mittal RK. Functional morphology of anal sphincter complex unveiled by high definition anal manometry and three dimensional ultrasound imaging. Neurogastroenterol Motil. 2011;23:1013–9.
134. Kaur A, Garza JM, Connor FL, Cocjin JT, Flores AF, Hyman PE, Di Lorenzo C. Colonic hyperactivity results in frequent fecal soiling in a subset of children after surgery for Hirschsprung disease. J Pediatr Gastroenterol Nutr. 2011;52:433–6.
135. Langer JC. Persistent obstructive symptoms after surgery for Hirschsprung's disease: development of a diagnostic and therapeutic algorithm. J Pediatr Surg. 2004;39:1458–62.
136. Marty TL, Seo T, Matlak ME, Sullivan JJ, Black RE, Johnson DG. Gastrointestinal function after surgical correction for Hirschsprung's disease: Long term follow up in 135 patients. J Pediatr Surg. 1995;30:655–8.
137. Moore SW, Millar AJ, Cywes S. Long term clinical manometric and histologic evaluation of obstructive symptoms in the postoperative Hirschsprung's patient. J Pediatr Surg. 1994;29:106–11.
138. Kobayashi H, Hirakawa H, Surana R, O'Brien DS, Puri P. Intestinal neuronal dysplasia is a possible cause of persistent bowel symptoms after pull through operation for Hirschsprung's disease. J Pediat Surg. 1995;30:253–7.
139. Catto-Smith AG, Coffey CMM, Nolan TM, Hutson JM. Fecal incontinence after surgical treatment of Hirschsprung disease. J Pediatr. 1995;127:954–7.
140. Bandre E, Kabore RA, Ouedraogo I, Sore O, Tapsoba T, Bambara C. Hirschsprung's disease: management problem in a developing country. Afri J of Paediat Surg. 2010;7:166–8.
141. Noelting J, Sk R, Bharucha AE, Harvey DM, Ravi K, Zinsmeister AR. Normal values for high-resolu-

tion anorectal manometry in healthy women: effects of age and significance of rectoanal gradient. Am J Gastroenterol. 2012;107:1530–6.
142. Clouse RE, Staiano A, Alrakawi A, Haroian L. Application of topographical methods to clinical oesophageal manometry. Am J Gastroterol. 2000;95:2720–30.
143. Sk G, Pandolfino JE, Zhang Q, Jarosz A, Shah N, Kahrilas PJ. Quantifying oesophageal peristalsis with high-resolution manometry: a study of 75 asymptomatic volunteers. Am J Physiol Gastrointest Liver Physiol. 2009;290:G988–97.
144. Wu JF, Lu CH, Yang CH, Tsai IJ. Diagnostic role of anal sphincter relaxation integral in high-resolution anorectal manometry for Hirschsprung disease in infants. J Pediatr. 2018;194:136–141.e2. https://doi.org/10.1016/j.jpeds.2017.10.017. Epub 2017 Dec 6.
145. De Lorijn F, Reitsma JB, Voskuijl WP, Aronson DC, Ten Kate FJ, Smets AM, Taminiau JA, Benninga MA. Diagnosis of Hirschsprung's disease: a prospective, comparative accuracy study of common tests. J Pediatr. 2005;146:787–92.
146. Barnett JL, Hasler WL, Camilleri M. American Gastroenterological Association medical position statement on anorectal testing techniques. American Gastroenterological Association. Gastroenterol. 1999;116:732–60.
147. Keighley MR, Henry MM, Bartolo DC, Mortensen NJ. Anorectal physiology measurement: report of working party. Br J Surg. 1989;76:356–7.

Rectal Biopsy for the Diagnosis of Hirschsprung's Disease

16

Florian Friedmacher and Prem Puri

Contents

16.1 Introduction

To meet the diagnostic criteria for Hirschsprung's disease (HSCR), the histological evaluation of adequate rectal wall biopsies showing a combination of aganglionosis and hypertrophic nerve trunks is necessary [1, 2]. Therefore, the diagnosis of HSCR can be difficult, as it relies on histological confirmation of complete absence of enteric ganglion cells in the myenteric and submucosal plexuses of the distal rectum, which extends proximally for varying distances. It also requires an experienced histopathologist, who is familiar with the various staining methods used in the diagnostic work-up of HSCR including hematoxylin and eosin staining, acetylcholinesterase, and calretinin immunohistochemistry, in order to avoid false-positive or false-negative results [3–5].

Sampling of the necessary mucosal and submucosal tissue was revolutionized in 1965, when Dobbins and Bill first described the technique for rectal suction biopsy (RSB) [6], a relatively simple and less traumatic procedure to exclude the diagnosis of HSCR. This approach was further refined by Helen R. Noblett in 1969 with the introduction of a specific RSB tube particularly for the use in neonates and young infants [7]. Today, RSB has mostly superseded the former techniques of open rectal biopsy and punch biopsy with a sigmoidoscope or speculum [8, 9] and is widely considered to be the gold standard in the diagnostic work-up of patients with suspected HSCR [10].

16.1.1 Rectal Suction Biopsy

Although RSB is a rather simple surgical procedure that can be taught with relative ease to trainees, it needs to be carried out with meticulous attention to detail in order to obtain a suitable diagnostic specimen. In fact, some histopathologists remain reluctant to confirm the presence or absence of enteric ganglion cells

F. Friedmacher
Department of Pediatric Surgery, The Royal London Hospital, Whitechapel, London, UK

National Children's Research Centre, Our Lady's Children's Hospital, Crumlin, Dublin, Ireland

P. Puri (✉)
National Children's Research Centre, Our Lady's Children's Hospital, Crumlin, Dublin, Ireland

Conway Institute of Biomolecular and Biomedical Research, School of Medicine & Medical Science, University College Dublin, Dublin, Ireland
e-mail: prem.puri@ncrc.ie

P. Puri (ed.), *Hirschsprung's Disease and Allied Disorders*,
https://doi.org/10.1007/978-3-030-15647-3_16

merely on the basis of RSBs [11], as it necessitates a thick specimen with enough submucosal tissue to be considered as adequate [12]. Consequently, insufficient tissue samples are not uncommon and often result in a diagnostic delay with need for repeat RSB or full-thickness rectal biopsy, causing considerable parental anxiety, prolonged hospital stay, and increased costs [13]. It has recently been reported that RSB identifies HSCR in patients <39 days of age with a sensitivity of only 50%, thus frequently leading to inconclusive results [14]. In addition, RSB has been found to provide often inconsistent results in older infants and children, probably because their submucosal tissue is more fibrous [15], raising concern of a decreased diagnostic yield. However, with an adequacy of 90.5% for patients older than 5 years of age in their series, Brady et al. [16] have proven that RSB is also effective in evaluating older children with suspected HSCR.

16.1.1.1 Preoperative Considerations

Before undertaking an RSB, a thorough history, physical examination, and contrast enema or anorectal manometry should be performed to reliably identify patients unlikely to have HSCR, thus sparing them from an unnecessary RSB [17]. In fact, some authors suggest performing RSB only in newborn infants with neonatal onset of symptoms [17, 18], whereas others also advocate this in patients who present symptoms later in life [19, 20]. An RSB may be accomplished on the ward or in an outpatient setting without general anesthesia. It is normally a painless procedure provided the specimen is taken at least 2.0 cm above the anal verge in neonates and 3.5 cm in older children. In general, it is recommended to give prophylactic antibiotics beforehand. In neonates, it is important to ensure that vitamin K has been given.

16.1.1.2 Instrumentation

Although various types of RSB devices exist, the most common ones currently in use are the rbi2 (Aus systems, Allenby Gardens, Australia) (Fig. 16.1) and Solo-RBT (SAMO Biomedica, Bologna, Italy) [21]. These instruments are either made up of a single-use capsule or hollow tube system with depth measuring indicators, which houses a 3-mm-diameter side hole 1 cm away from the blunt-ended tip and a concealed, ultrasharp blade for a clean, precise cut.

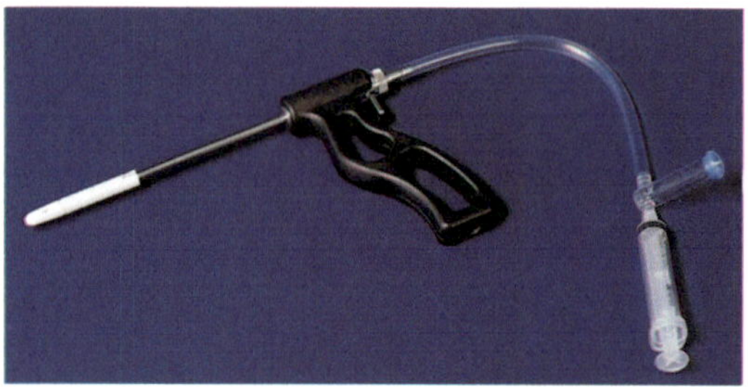

Fig. 16.1 rbi2 (Aus systems, Allenby Gardens, Australia) – an RSB system consisting of a sterile, single-use capsule, a sterilizable handpiece, and a negative pressure manometer with connected 10 mL syringe

16.1.1.3 Patient Positioning

Neonates and young infants are usually held in the lithotomy position, whereas the left lateral position with bent knees is more comfortable for older children.

16.1.1.4 Operative Technique

The lubricated RSB instrument is inserted into the anus and the side hole positioned approximately 2–3 cm from the anal verge. This is the minimum distance as the distal 1–2 cm of rectum is normally hypoganglionic, and thus sampling from this area may lead to a false impression of aganglionosis causing diagnostic confusion [22, 23]. In order to reduce the risk of perforation into the rectovesical or rectovaginal pouch, biopsy specimens should always be taken from the posterior or lateral rectal wall. It is advised to gently approximate the instrument tip in neutral position to the rectal wall and not to push or force as this may stretch and tighten the mucosa, making it more difficult to withdraw sufficient tissue into the side hole. It is not enough to insert the instrument into the rectum only. The most important point for a successful RSB is an adequate suction level. Irrespective of whether a conventional syringe (3–20 mL air) or wall/machine suction is used (−150 to −300 cm H_2O) [24], it requires the appropriate technique of maintaining adequate suction and usage of a sharp, clean-cutting blade [25]. Results from an international survey among 87 pediatric surgeons have shown that less than 30% of respondents use a defined negative suction pressure or manometer device for obtaining an RSB [21], which can have a huge impact on the specimen size and patient safety. A manometric suction control guarantees not only the grasping of sufficient submucosal tissue but also minimizes the risk of perforation. For accuracy and safety, some authors further recommend that RSB should be performed under direct vision after anal dilatation with the patient under general anesthesia [26, 27]. After 2–3 seconds of continuous suction, the trigger is fired and the blade cuts the specimen. As a general rule, a successful biopsy will be achieved when the side hole is fully covered by mucosa. The suction is then released to neutral pressure before withdrawing the instrument from the patient for specimen retrieval. This usually measures approximately 3 × 1 mm, and the critical submucosa can be recognized as a definite whitish layer. The International Working Group of the 2009 World Congress of Gastroenterology advocates that the diagnosis of HSCR requires a biopsy specimen of at least 3 mm diameter and a minimum of one-third of the sample should include submucosa to be considered adequate [12]. Interestingly, a recent study from the USA has demonstrated that tissue specimens obtained by RSB are significantly smaller than those obtained by full-thickness biopsy, especially in older children [28]. However, the authors also found that RSB and open rectal biopsy appear equivalent in their ability to provide sufficient submucosa [28].

Although there is no consensus, it is recommended to repeat the procedure at 3.5 cm and 4 cm above the anal verge with two and four specimens obtained.

16.1.1.5 Specimen Processing

The method of processing RSBs must be clarified with the histopathologist before the procedure, as dictated by specific laboratory requirements. All specimens must be marked with the exact level of biopsy. Usually, two formalin-fixed and paraffin-embedded samples are needed for routine hematoxylin and eosin staining with an additional specimen on saline wet gauze for acetylcholinesterase (AChE) immunohistochemistry of frozen sections (Fig. 16.2). When properly oriented and cut adequately, 50–75 sections should be generally sufficient to exclude the presence of submucosal ganglion cells [11, 15]. However, numerous other staining methods are currently in use to facilitate the diagnosis of HSCR, including calretinin, neural cell adhesion molecule, neuron-specific enolase, nicotinamide adenine dinucleotide phosphate diaphorase, lactate and succinic dehydrogenase, peripherin, protein gene product 9.5, and S-100 protein [21, 29].

16.1.1.6 Postoperative Care

Any rectal manipulation should be avoided for the first 24 hours after RSB.

16.1.1.7 Complications

There have been a few reports of serious and potentially life-threatening adverse events associated with RSB [25, 30–34], but the overall number of complications in clinical practice appears to be very small. Immediately after the procedure, the patient may experience slight transient rectal bleeding, which usually settles spontaneously. Although rare, persistent rectal bleeding requiring blood transfusion [25, 30], bowel perforation [31], and pelvic sepsis [31–33] has been reported, which in turn adds a further risk to the patient. Rectal perforations seem to be more probable in neonates and young infants due to the varying thickness of the circular muscle layer in this age group compared with older patients. Very rare, but devastating, adverse events have been described in the literature, including injury to the common iliac artery [34], peripheral limb gangrene [33], and death [31]. A recent systematic review has indicated that the likelihood of RSB-related complications appears to be higher in newborns and young infants compared to older children [35]. In contrast, Keyzer-Dekker et al. [36] found that RSB can also be reliably and safely performed in preterm infants, which implies there is no reason to postpone an RSB in these patients.

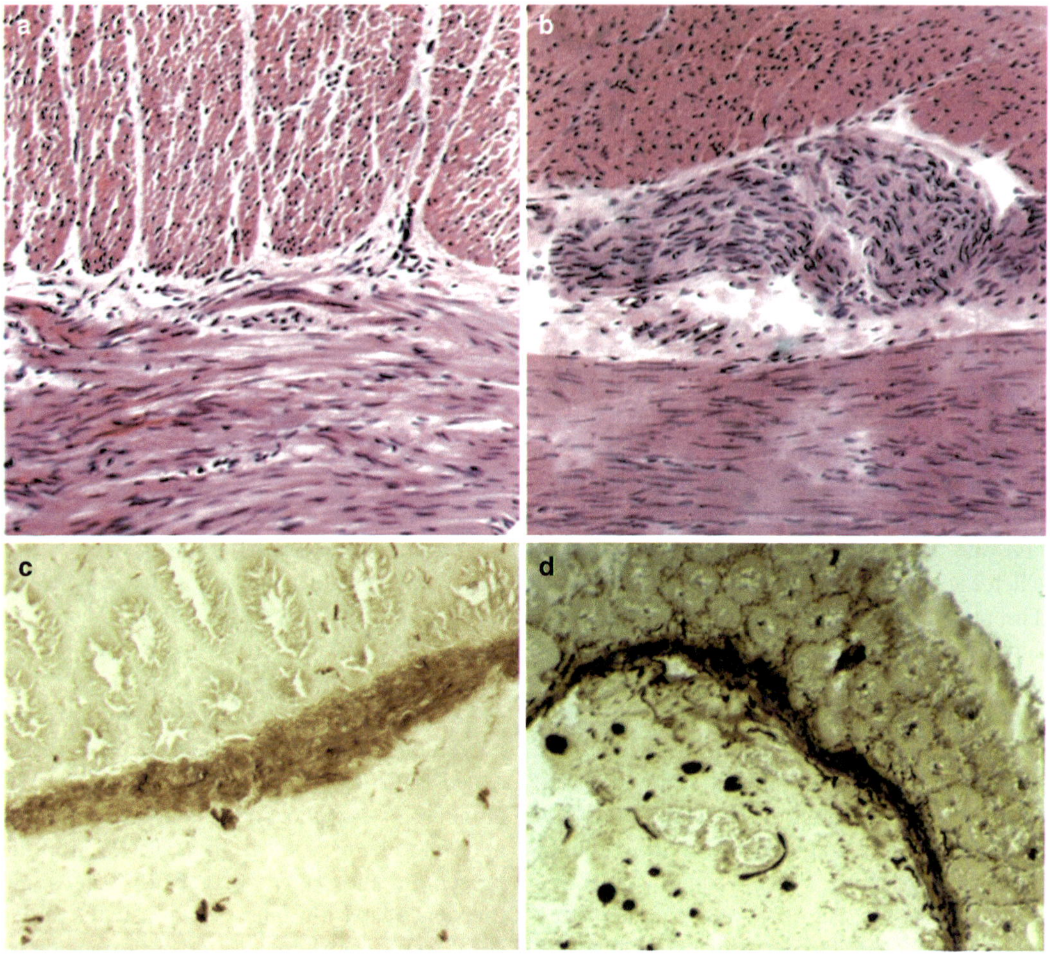

Fig. 16.2 Rectal biopsies showing presence of ganglionic cells in the myenteric and submucosal plexuses of normal bowel (**a**) and absence with replacement by hypertrophied nerve trunks in a patient with HSCR (**b**). Normal rectal biopsy showing minimal AChE staining in mucosa, lamina propria, and muscularis mucosae (**c**), whereas a marked increase in AChE-positive nerve fibers is found in the lamina propria and muscularis mucosae of a patient with HSCR (**d**)

Clearly, great care should always be taken, particularly when the procedure is performed in children younger than 1 year of age [37].

16.1.2 Open Rectal Biopsy

In circumstances where the specimen obtained with the RSB instrument is insufficient or the child is older, an open full-thickness rectal biopsy under general anesthesia is generally required. The same preoperative considerations as for RSB apply also for open rectal biopsy.

16.1.2.1 Patient Positioning

Infants are usually held in the lithotomy position, whereas older children will need to be placed in stirrups.

16.1.2.2 Operative Technique

The anal opening is digitally dilated and held open with a self-retaining retractor or alternatively by an assistant holding either a speculum or two small Langenbeck retractors. A strong polyglycol stay suture is placed on the midline of the posterior rectal wall at least 2 cm above the pectinate line. Applying traction on this suture, the surgeon then places a further stay suture approximately 2 cm higher, which is tied, and the needle is left intact as this will be used to repair the defect once the specimen has been taken [38]. A specimen comprising sufficient submucosal tissue or full-thickness is then obtained between the stay sutures using sharp-pointed scissors. Adequate hemostasis is normally achieved by suturing the defect with a running locking suture in one or two layers from above. Alternately, bipolar diathermy may be used.

16.1.2.3 Postoperative Care

The same postoperative care as for RSB should also apply for patients undergoing open rectal biopsy.

16.1.2.4 Complications

Complications mainly consist of rectal bleeding and postoperative infection.

References

1. Kapur RP. Hirschsprung disease and other enteric dysganglionoses. Crit Rev Clin Lab Sci. 1999;36:225–73.
2. Monforte-Muñoz H, Gonzalez-Gomez I, Rowland JM, Landing BH. Increased submucosal nerve trunk caliber in aganglionosis: a "positive" and objective finding in suction biopsies and segmental resections in Hirschsprung's disease. Arch Pathol Lab Med. 1998;122:721–5.
3. Martucciello G. Hirschsprung's disease, one of the most difficult diagnoses in pediatric surgery: a review of the problems from clinical practice to the bench. Eur J Pediatr Surg. 2008;18:140–9.
4. Barshack I, Fridman E, Goldberg I, Chowers J, Kopolovic J. The loss of calretinin expression indicates aganglionosis in Hirschsprung's disease. J Clin Pathol. 2004;57:712–6.
5. Meier-Ruge W, Lutterbeck PM, Herzog B, Morger R, Moser R, Schärli A. Acetylcholinesterase activity in suction biopsies of the rectum in the diagnosis of Hirschsprung's disease. J Pediatr Surg. 1972;7:11–7.
6. Dobbins WO 3rd, Bill AH Jr. Diagnosis of Hirschsprung's disease excluded by rectal suction biopsy. N Engl J Med. 1965;272:990–3.
7. Noblett HR. A rectal suction biopsy tube for use in the diagnosis of Hirschsprung's disease. J Pediatr Surg. 1969;4:406–9.
8. Kurer MH, Lawson JO, Pambakian H. Suction biopsy in Hirschsprung's disease. Arch Dis Child. 1986;61:83–4.
9. Yunis EJ, Dibbins AW, Sherman FE. Rectal suction biopsy in the diagnosis of Hirschsprung disease in infants. Arch Pathol Lab Med. 1976;100:329–33.
10. Martucciello G, Pini Prato A, Puri P, Holschneider AM, Meier-Ruge W, Jasonni V, et al. Controversies concerning diagnostic guidelines for anomalies of the enteric nervous system: a report from the fourth International Symposium on Hirschsprung's disease and related neurocristopathies. J Pediatr Surg. 2005;40:1527–31.
11. Qualman SJ, Jaffe R, Bove KE, Monforte-Muñoz H. Diagnosis of Hirschsprung disease using the rectal biopsy: multi-institutional survey. Pediatr Dev Pathol. 1999;2:588–96.
12. Knowles CH, De Giorgio R, Kapur RP, Bruder E, Farrugia G, Geboes K, et al. The London classification of gastrointestinal neuromuscular pathology: report on behalf of the Gastro 2009 International Working Group. Gut. 2010;59:882–7.
13. Hall NJ, Kufeji D, Keshtgar A. Out with the old and in with the new: a comparison of rectal suction biopsies with traditional and modern biopsy forceps. J Pediatr Surg. 2009;44:395–8.
14. Meinds RJ, Kuiper GA, Parry K, Timmer A, Groen H, Heineman E, et al. Infant's age influences the accuracy of rectal suction biopsies for diagnosing of Hirschsprung's disease. Clin Gastroenterol Hepatol. 2015;13:1801–7.
15. Kapur RR. Practical pathology and genetics of Hirschsprung's disease. Semin Pediatr Surg. 2009;18:212–23.
16. Brady AC, Saito JM, Lukas K, Guthrie T, Utterson EC, White FV, et al. Suction rectal biopsy yields adequate tissue in children. J Pediatr Surg. 2016;51:966–9.
17. Lewis NA, Levitt MC, Zallen GS, Zafar MS, Iacono KL, Rossman JE, et al. Diagnosing Hirschsprung's disease: increasing the odds of a positive rectal biopsy result. J Pediatr Surg. 2003;38:412–6.
18. Ghosh A, Griffiths DM. Rectal biopsy in the investigation of constipation. Arch Dis Child. 1998;79:266–8.
19. Simpson BB, Ryan DP, Schnitzer JJ, Flores A, Doody DP. Surgical evaluation and management of refractory constipation in older children. J Pediatr Surg. 1996;31:1040–2.
20. Wheatley MJ, Wesley JR, Coran AG, Polley TZ Jr. Hirschsprung's disease in adolescents and adults. Dis Colon Rectum. 1990;33:622–9.
21. Friedmacher F, Puri P. Current practice patterns of rectal suction biopsy in the diagnostic work-up of Hirschsprung's disease: results from an international survey. Pediatr Surg Int. 2016;32:717–22.
22. Aldridge RT, Campbell PE. Ganglion cell distribution in the normal rectum and anal canal. A basis for the diagnosis of Hirschsprung's disease by anorectal biopsy. J Pediatr Surg. 1968;3:475–90.
23. Venugopal S, Mancer K, Shandling B. The validity of rectal biopsy in relation to morphology and distribution of ganglion cells. J Pediatr Surg. 1981;16:433–7.
24. Ali AE, Morecroft JA, Bowen JC, Bruce J, Morabito A. Wall or machine suction rectal biopsy for Hirschsprung's disease: a simple modified technique

can improve the adequacy of biopsy. Pediatr Surg Int. 2006;22:681–2.
25. Pini-Prato A, Carlini C, Pesce F, Jasonni V, Seymandi P. Massive bleeding after rectal suction biopsy: uncommon and unexpected delayed onset. World J Pediatr. 2011;7:83–5.
26. Kobayashi H, Li Z, Yamataka A, Lane GJ, Miyano T. Rectal biopsy: what is the optimal procedure? Pediatr Surg Int. 2002;18:753–6.
27. Croffie JM, Davis MM, Faught PR, Corkins MR, Gupta SK, Pfefferkorn MD, et al. At what age is a suction rectal biopsy less likely to provide adequate tissue for identification of ganglion cells? J Pediatr Gastroenterol Nutr. 2007;44:198–202.
28. Muise ED, Hardee S, Morotti RA, Cowles RA. A comparison of suction and full-thickness rectal biopsy in children. J Surg Res. 2016;201:149–55.
29. Zani A, Eaton S, Morini F, Puri P, Rintala R, Heurn EV, et al. European Paediatric Surgeons' Association survey on the management of Hirschsprung disease. Eur J Pediatr Surg. 2017;27:96–101.
30. Dahshan A. Serious rectal bleeding complicating suction rectal biopsy in a child. W V Med J. 2014;110:34–5.
31. Rees BI, Azmy A, Nigam M, Lake BD. Complications of rectal suction biopsy. J Pediatr Surg. 1983;18:273–5.
32. Alizai NK, Batcup G, Dixon MF, Stringer MD. Rectal biopsy for Hirschsprung's disease: what is the optimum method? Pediatr Surg Int. 1998;13:121–4.
33. Jani BR, Brereton RJ, Dillon MJ. Peripheral limb gangrene following rectal biopsy. Treatment with prostacyclin and exchange transfusion. Clin Pediatr (Phila). 1989;28:585–8.
34. de Brito IA, Maksoud JG. Evolution with age of the acetylcholinesterase activity in rectal suction biopsy in Hirschsprung's disease. J Pediatr Surg. 1987;22:425–30.
35. Friedmacher F, Puri P. Rectal suction biopsy for the diagnosis of Hirschsprung's disease: a systematic review of diagnostic accuracy and complications. Pediatr Surg Int. 2015;31:821–30.
36. Keyzer-Dekker CM, Sloots CE, Schokker-van Linschoten IK, Biermann K, Meeussen C, Doukas M. Effectiveness of rectal suction biopsy in diagnosing Hirschsprung disease. Eur J Pediatr Surg. 2016;26:100–5.
37. Pini-Prato A, Martucciello G, Jasonni V. Rectal suction biopsy in the diagnosis of intestinal dysganglionoses: 5-year experience with Solo-RBT in 389 patients. J Pediatr Surg. 2006;41:1043–8.
38. Zani A, Davenport M. Rectal biopsies. In: Spitz L, Coran AG, editors. Operative pediatric surgery. 7th ed. Boca Raton/London/New York: CRC Press/Taylor & Francis Group; 2013. p. 544–8.

Anatomic Pathology of Hirschsprung Disease

17

Raj P. Kapur

Contents

R. P. Kapur (✉)
Department of Pathology, Seattle Children's Hospital and University of Washington, Seattle, WA, USA
e-mail: raj.kapur@seattlechildrens.org

17.1 Introduction

The pathology of Hirschsprung disease (HSCR) includes primary malformations of the enteric nervous system and secondary consequences in the bowel that result from the physiological effects of aganglionosis. Some of these alterations are pathophysiologically significant and likely contribute to the obstructive symptoms that characterize these patients. The clinical relevance and appropriate management of other alterations are either controversial or non-specific findings that may or may not have physiologic relevance. The first part of this chapter is an overview of primary and secondary pathological features of HSCR. This is followed by a practical discussion of HSCR-related surgical pathology in the contexts of diagnosis, operative management, and postoperative complications.

17.2 Primary Malformations

17.2.1 Aganglionosis

Congenital aganglionosis of the distal rectum and a variable length of contiguous proximal bowel is the most obvious and diagnostically important malformative aspect of HSCR. In approximately 80% of patients, aganglionosis is restricted to the rectosigmoid colon, a condition termed short-segment HSCR (ssHSCR) [82]. Longer agan-

P. Puri (ed.), *Hirschsprung's Disease and Allied Disorders*,
https://doi.org/10.1007/978-3-030-15647-3_17

glionic segments are subdivided by the proximal extent of the aganglionic segment into colonic (left colon), long-segment (transverse or right colon), total colonic (ileum), small intestinal (jejunum), or pan-intestinal (gastric) variants. In some contexts, it is useful to segregate aganglionosis limited to 2–3 cm of the distal-most rectum as very short-segment HSCR (vssHSCR) because these patients often pose unique diagnostic challenges for the clinician and pathologist [29, 53]. The use of the term "ultrashort-segment HSCR" is discouraged because it has been used ambiguously in the past to refer to either patients with vssHSCR or non-HSCR patients with HSCR-like abnormal anorectal manometry findings [62].

The aganglionic segment is devoid of myenteric and submucosal ganglion cells, but in other respects, the mucosal, submucosal, and muscular tunics are relatively intact with age-appropriate differentiation of epithelium, vasculature, and smooth muscle cells. In the absence of intrinsic ganglion cells, extrinsic innervation persists but is abnormal. Specifically, nerves derived primarily from cholinergic autonomic neurons ramify through the full-thickness of the bowel wall, including the mucosa [23, 52, 66]. A major source of these nerves is pelvic autonomic ganglion cells [66], with additional contributions from spinal sensory ganglia and paravertebral sympathetic ganglia (Fig. 17.1). These extrinsic nerves tend to course through the muscularis interna perpendicular to the surface of the bowel toward the mucosa [50]. In addition, downstream projections from the ganglionic segment are also present, but these are likely short, innervate 1–2 cm distal to the aganglionic/ganglionic interface, and, within the muscularis interna, run parallel to the bowel surface. Included in these intrinsic downstream projections are calretinin-immunoreactive mucosal nerves and inhibitory motor neurons in the muscularis propria, which express neuronal nitric oxide synthase (nNOS) (Fig. 17.2).

Apart from the proximal aganglionic segment, where projections from upstream neurons are found, immunohistochemical markers selective for intrinsic neurons are absent. These include antigens localized to the cell soma of most or all neurons (e.g., Hu C/D, Phox2B) [9], as well as antigens expressed in the cell soma and/or neuronal processes of selected subsets of neurons (e.g., calretinin, nNOS, bcl2) [6, 50, 71]. nNOS is expressed in a subset of neurites in extrinsic nerves in the distal aganglionic segment, but the intramuscular extension of these nerves is very sparse in comparison with that of the euganglionic bowel (Fig. 17.2). Immunohistochemical assessment of calretinin-immunoreactive mucosal innervation is particularly useful diagnosti-

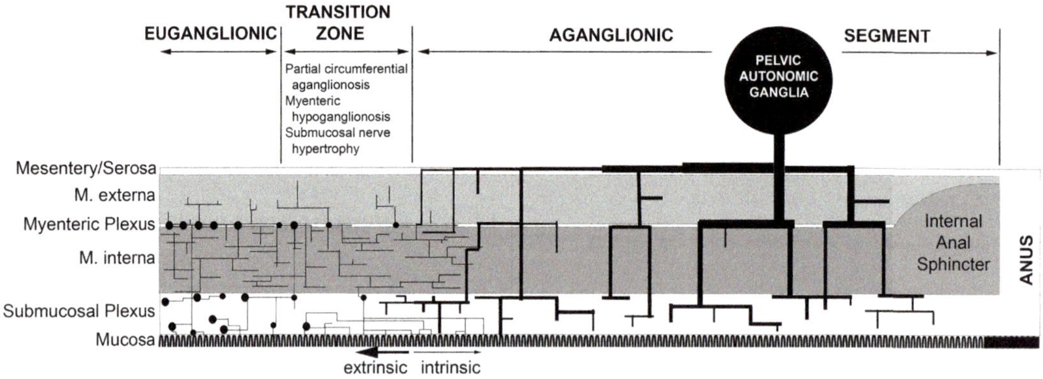

Fig. 17.1 Diagrammatic representation of some features of the extrinsic and intrinsic innervation in HSCR. Intrinsic innervation is absent in the aganglionic segment and hypoplastic (reduced density of ganglion cells) in the transition zone but appears histologically normal further rostrally in the euganglionic bowel. At the distal end of the transition zone, nerves (e.g., nNOS- and calretin-immunoreactive) project from ganglionic bowel into the proximal 1–2 cm of the aganglionic segment. Extrinsic innervation includes nerves from pelvic autonomic ganglia, in addition to projections from sympathetic ganglia and sensory ganglia. The former predominantly cholinergic nerves enter the bowel in the distal rectum and project rostrally along and into the left colon. In the aganglionic segment and distal transition zone, extrinsic cholinergic nerves are abnormally large and numerous and ramify through the entire thickness of the bowel wall

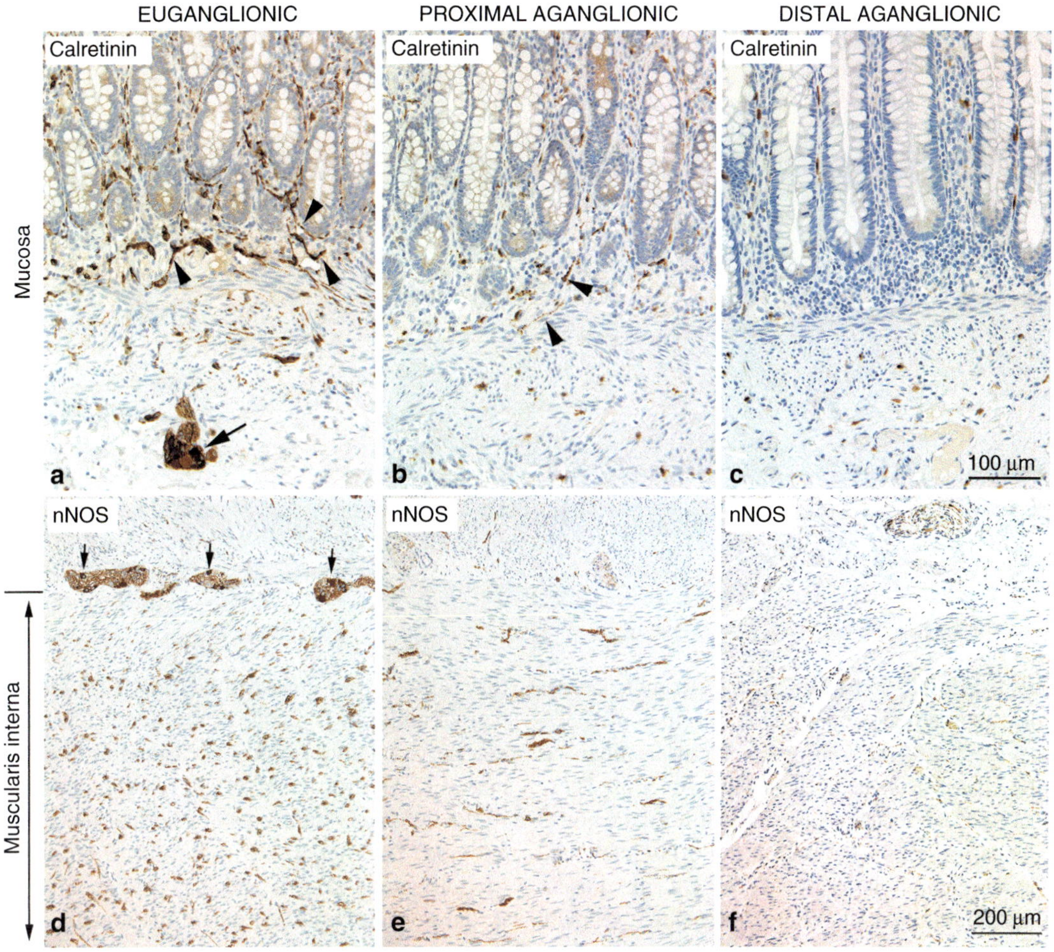

Fig. 17.2 Calretinin and nNOS immunoreactive innervation in the ganglionic, proximal aganglionic, and distal aganglionic segments of a HSCR resection specimen. (**a**–**c**) Calretinin-immunoreactive nerves (arrowheads) and submucosal ganglion cells (arrow) are present in the mucosa of the euganglionic bowel (**a**). Similar, but less dense innervation exists in the proximal aganglionic segment (**b**, arrowheads), but calretinin-immunoreactive mucosal innervation is absent in the more distal aganglionic segment (**c**). Immunoreactive mast cells are present at all three sites. (**d**–**f**) Similarly, nNOS-immunoreactive nerves are present in the muscularis interna of the euganglionic and proximal aganglionic segments but virtually absent in the aganglionic segment. These nNOS-positive fibers are projections of inhibitory motor neurons with cell bodies in the myenteric plexus (arrows in **d**)

cally because these nerves are sampled even in shallow rectal biopsies and are consistently absent in aganglionic bowel more than 2 cm downstream from the ganglionic segment [29, 37]. It is important to validate immunohistochemistry approaches with appropriate controls, as some commercially available antibodies work better than others and/or require different labeling conditions (e.g., Phox2B) [9, 39].

The caliber of extrinsic nerves in the aganglionic segment is increased, a phenomenon referred to as "nerve hypertrophy," although individual neurites are probably more numerous rather than significantly enlarged. These changes are graded—more dramatic in the distal rectum and gradually less dramatic more proximally, probably because large nerves trunks are more prevalent closer to their origins in pelvic autonomic ganglia [52]. In the aganglionic rectum, nerve hypertrophy occurs through the entire thickness of the bowel wall but, with traditional hematoxylin and eosin (H&E)-stained sections, is most obvious in the myenteric and submucosal plexuses (Fig. 17.3). Immunohistochemical studies have shown that innervation in the aganglionic rectosigmoid colon differs between ssHSCR and lsHSCR [50, 61]. In

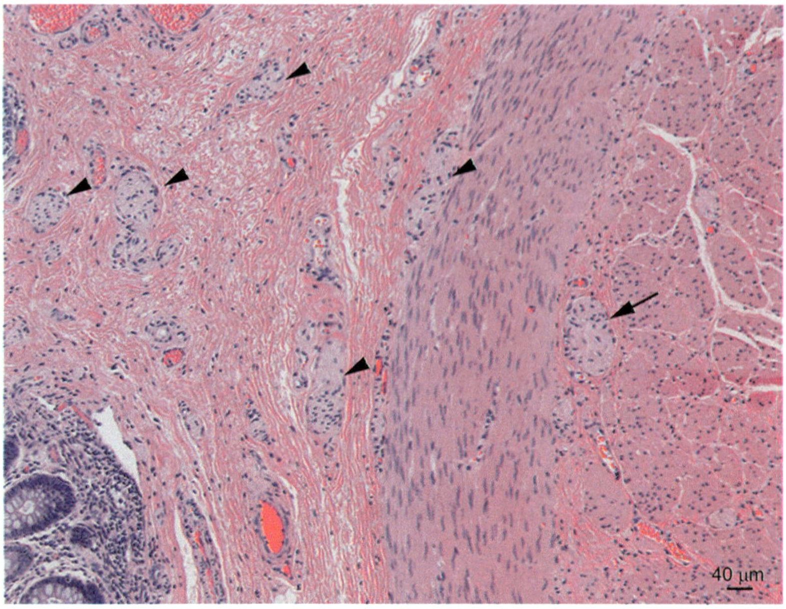

Fig. 17.3 Abnormal innervation in aganglionic rectum. In addition to an absence of ganglion cells, large nerves are present in the submucosa (arrowheads) and myenteric (arrow) plexuses

both ssHSCR and lsHSCR, hypertrophic nerves of presumed pelvic autonomic origin course perpendicular to the long axes of muscle fibers as they pass through the muscularis interna. These nerves are oriented centripetally toward the bowel lumen, primarily between muscle fascicles, and predominate in lsHSCR. In ssHSCR, the muscularis interna in the proximal aganglionic segment also contains nerves that run parallel to the serosal surface (Fig. 17.1). The latter are intrinsic neurons which project for a short distance into the aganglionic segment from the transition zone. Thus, in long-segment HSCR, the ascending extrinsic nerves and descending intrinsic nerves do not overlap significantly, and an intervening gap exists in which the muscularis propria and submucosa contain almost no nerves [50].

Ultrastructural and immunohistochemical analyses support the extrinsic nature of hypertrophic nerves in the aganglionic segment. Except as discussed below, normal myenteric and submucosal nerves differ from extra-enteric nerves in several respects (Fig. 17.4). Distinctive features of extrinsic nerves include a prominent nerve growth factor receptor-positive and glucose transporter 1 (Glut1)-positive perineurium [26], presence of occasional myelinated fibers [102], a compact arrangement of nonmyelinating Schwann cells with an antigenically different form of GFAP that differs from enteric glial cells [25], endoneurial collagen [7], and expression of a peripheral nerve laminin isoform not found in intrinsic nerves [2]. Extrinsic nerves are readily identified in the mesentery and serosa of normal bowel. In addition, occasional extrinsic nerves penetrate the muscularis externa and may be encountered in the myenteric plexus, where they merge with the intrinsic components of the enteric nervous system (Fig. 17.4). Finally, some nerves with extrinsic features are normal in the myenteric and submucosal plexuses of the distal rectum. These are sparse and, in neonates, are restricted to the terminal rectum, but their caliber, density, and proximal extent increase with age [31].

Submucosal nerve hypertrophy is a useful diagnostic finding and is assessed subjectively by most experienced pathologists. In the rectal submucosa of infants less than 6 months of age, it is very unusual to encounter a nerve more than 40 μm wide, except in HSCR [58]. However, nerve caliber is age dependent, and this “40 μm rule” cannot be relied upon at older ages [31].

The graded nature of nerve hypertrophy is very evident in longer-segment aganglionosis. Aganglionic bowel proximal to the sigmoid, or especially left colon, often lacks submucosal nerve hypertrophy, although occasional large myenteric nerves persist in these areas. It has been observed

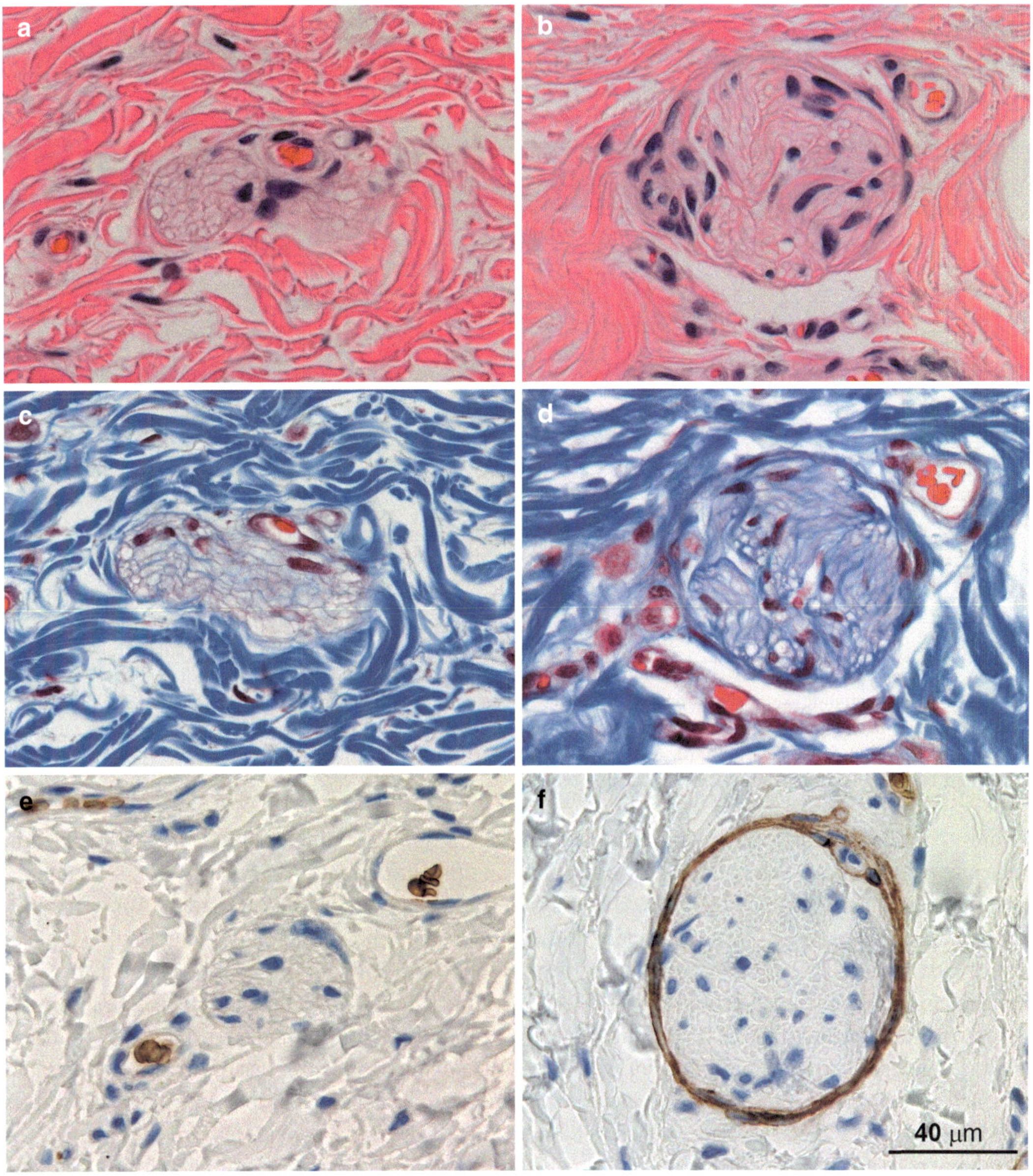

Fig. 17.4 Comparative histology and immunohistochemistry of normal intrinsic submucosal nerves in ganglionic rectum (**a**, **c**, **e**) versus extrinsic submucosal innervation in aganglionic rectum (**b**, **d**, **f**). Most of the submucosal nerves in ganglionic rectum, especially in young infants, have intrinsic features including a "loose" arrangement of nerve fibers (**a**), paucity of intraneural collagen (blue in **c**), and absent Glut-1-immunoreactive perineurium (**e**). In contrast, nerves in the aganglionic rectal submucosa have more compact and regularly spaced nerve fibers (**b**), abundant intraneural collagen (blue in **d**), and conspicuous Glut-1-positive perineurium (**f**). All figures are taken at the same magnification. **a**, **b** (H&E); **c**, **d** (Mallory trichrome); **e**, **f** (Glut-1 immunohistochemistry)

paradoxically that some patients with very long-segment disease (e.g., total colonic aganglionosis) may have no or only distal, rectal nerve hypertrophy; therefore, this submucosal nerve hypertrophy is not universally present in rectal biopsies from all HSCR patients [50, 52, 61]. One might speculate that it is because neurogenesis in pelvic autonomic ganglia is also impaired in these individuals, as has been observed in murine models of pan-intestinal aganglionosis [35].

Although distal rectal aganglionosis with or without contiguous proximal aganglionic bowel

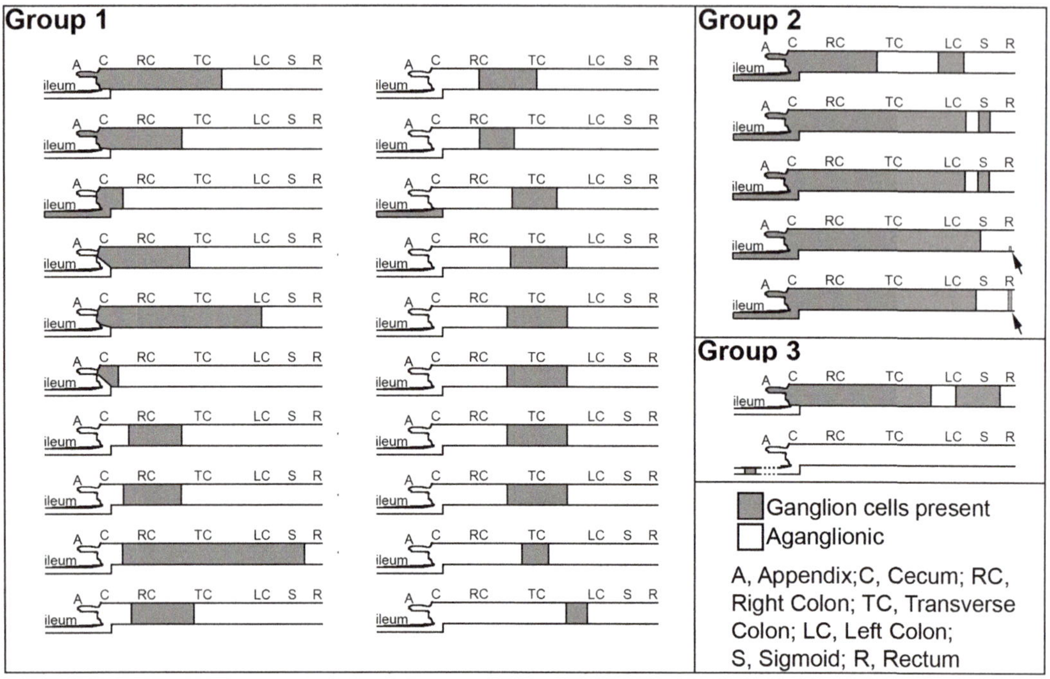

Fig. 17.5 Diagrammatic representation of SS-HSCR cases described in the English literature (reference numbers provided to the left of each diagram). The 27 reported cases can be subdivided into group 1 (ileocecal + rectal aganglionosis), group 2 (ganglionic ileum and right colon with distal skip segments), and group 3 (others). (From: Coe et al. [13] with permission)

is most common, occasionally skip areas exist in which myenteric and/or submucosal ganglion cells interrupt the aganglionic segment [13, 32]. Skip areas have been described most commonly in the colon with a second proximal aganglionic segment centered in the cecum/appendix region and extending into the distal ileum (Fig. 17.5). Proximal aganglionic segments restricted to portions of the colon or small intestine appear to be rare but include the potential for a distal rectal skip area which, if biopsied, may pose a diagnostic dilemma [13].

17.2.2 Transition Zone

The histopathological transition zone in HSCR refers to ganglionic but neuroanatomically abnormal bowel situated immediately proximal to the aganglionic segment [30, 33]. It is to be distinguished from the funnel-shaped gross anatomic transition zone, which often occurs at or near the proximal end of the aganglionic segment, because correlation between the gross and microscopic is imperfect. Many secondary microanatomic changes occur proximal to the aganglionic segment due to bowel distension and/or inflammation, but are not considered diagnostic features of the transition zone per se. Rather, the histopathologic transition zone is defined specifically based on primary neuroanatomical malformations, which like aganglionosis are thought to impair normal bowel motility. The distinction is important because incomplete resection of the transition zone (transition zone pull-through) is considered an explanation for persistent obstructive symptoms after HSCR pull-through surgery [19, 46]. However, it is important to acknowledge that the clinical significance of transition zone pull-through is largely inferred from retrospective analysis of patients with postoperative symptoms and not based on well-controlled prospective analyses of patient with and without complete resection of the transition zone [33].

The most consistently recognized neuropathological features of the transition zone are *partial circumferential aganglionosis*, *myenteric hypoganglionosis*, and *submucosal nerve hypertrophy* [30]. One or more of these findings in ganglionic bowel proximal to the aganglionic segment are considered sufficient to diagnose transition zone and justification for additional surgery to excise the affected intestine.

Partial circumferential aganglionosis reflects the irregular nature of the interface between ganglionic and aganglionic bowel, whereby the "leading edge" of ganglion cells along part of the circumference is more distal than that in another part. The pattern of paint drippings on the external surface of a used paint can is a visual metaphor for the manner in which ganglion cells are distributed farther down some portions of the intestinal wall. The cumulative data from several studies suggest that in ssHSCR, partial circumferential aganglionosis typically occupies a segment less than 3 cm long, proximal to the circumferentially aganglionic colon [30]. In most cases, the circumferential distributions of myenteric and submucosal ganglion cells are closely aligned such that areas with ganglion cells in one plexus overlie ganglion cells in the other. However, in a significant subset of patients, deviations of 1–2 cm are present. When this occurs, myenteric ganglion cells are usually more distal than submucosal ganglion cells, but the reverse is observed occasionally [30].

Partial circumferential aganglionosis of the distal transition zone has important diagnostic and surgical implications. A biopsy of the ganglionic wall in an area of partial circumferential aganglionosis can have normal histology, but should not lead to the erroneous conclusion that the entire circumference has the same appearance. In very short-segment disease, the presence of ganglion cells in a biopsy of this type may falsely exclude HSCR. This is also important during surgery; the presence of normal ganglia in a leveling biopsy does not exclude transition zone. Additional intraoperative measures are required to reduce the likelihood of transition zone pull-through (see below).

Myenteric hypoganglionosis is a second neuropathological finding in the transition zones of most HSCR patients. The density of ganglion cells in the myenteric plexus normalizes gradually between the aganglionic and normoganglionic segments [34, 79]. In short-segment HSCR, normalization is usually achieved within a 5 cm segment proximal to the circumferentially aganglionic segment [30, 34]. Resolution of mild or moderately severe hypoganglionosis is problematic and requires formal neuronal counts of reasonably large intestinal samples with robust normative data and significant interobserver variability [79]. In practice, therefore, most pathologists strive to exclude moderate-to-severe myenteric hypoganglionosis, which is recognized by lengthy (e.g., contiguous one-eighth of circumference) stretches of the myenteric plexus occupied principally by ganglia composed of individual ganglion cells or ganglion cell doublets (Fig. 17.6a). These hypoplastic ganglia are sandwiched tightly between the muscularis interna and externa and lack the generous neuropil (glia and nerve processes) found in normal myenteric ganglia. Moderate-to-severe myenteric hypoganglionosis is usually found in the distalmost 1–2 cm border that outlines the proximal aganglionic segment.

The third widely accepted feature of the transition zone is *submucosal nerve hypertrophy* [14, 34]. Large extrinsic nerves of identical origin as that of those in the aganglionic segment do not respect the boundary between ganglionic and aganglionic bowel. Rather, these nerves extend into the myenteric and submucosal plexuses of the transition zone, primarily in short-segment or colonic HSCR (Fig. 17.6b). The transition zone in longer segment disease is generally not affected, because of the pelvic origin and graded nature of hypertrophic nerves in the aganglionic segment. The large nerves have similar extrinsic properties (e.g., Glut1-immunoreactive perineurium) to those in the aganglionic segment [26]. Although they are found in both the myenteric and submucosal plexus, recognition of abnormal myenteric extrinsic innervation is more difficult because some extrinsic innervation of the myenteric plexus is normal. Assessment of submucosal nerve hypertrophy is also challenging, in part because the caliber of submucosal nerves is age and site dependent (e.g., rectum bigger than more proximal colon) [31]. However, proximal to the rectum of an infant less than 6 month of age, when most pull-through resections are performed, it is very uncommon to encounter a submucosal nerve >40 μm in width and exceptional to identify more than two such nerves in a single 400x field [31].

In ssHSCR, submucosal nerve hypertrophy, like myenteric hypoganglionosis, seldom extends more than 5 cm proximal to the circumferentially

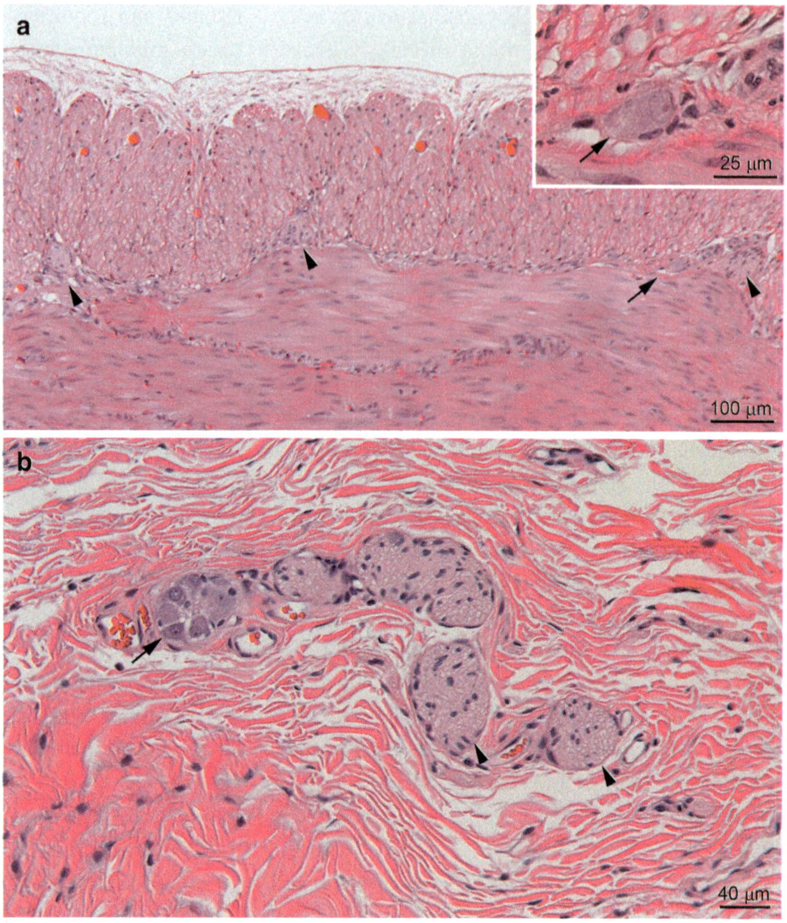

Fig. 17.6 Histological features of transition zone. (**a**) Myenteric hypoganglionosis denotes a long stretch of myenteric plexus in which ganglia (arrow) are sparse and composed of only one or two ganglion cell bodies with scant surrounding neuropil (inset). (**b**) Large nerves (arrowheads) are typically present in the adjacent plexus, especially if the transition zone is distal to the splenic flexure

aganglionic segment. Therefore, in most patients with ssHSCR, resection of >5 cm of ganglionic bowel along with the aganglionic segment will avoid a transition zone pull-through. In practice, this means that resection should be performed at least 5 cm proximal to a ganglionic leveling biopsy for ssHSCR. For lsHSCR, rigorous studies of the transition zone in a large series of patients have not been published. However, anecdotal data suggests that myenteric hypoganglionosis is likely to span more than 5 cm in longer segment disease [30].

17.2.3 "Normoganglionic" Proximal Bowel

The normo- or euganglionic bowel in HSCR disease refers to a contiguous segment of bowel between the esophagus and the proximal end of the transition zone. None of the histological features of transition zone (partial circumferential aganglionosis, myenteric hypoganglionosis, or submucosal nerve hypertrophy) are present in the normoganglionic segment. This definition of "normality" does not exclude microscopic changes that may be resolved in routine H&E-stained sections or by other techniques, but which are not widely accepted as either causes of dysmotility and/or are secondary to distal obstruction and passive distension (Table 17.1). The truth is that histology and immunohistochemistry are relatively insensitive and indirect approaches to assess enteric neuromuscular function, and dysfunction of "normoganglionic" bowel is frequently postulated when a patient has persistent post-pull-through symptoms with no other explanation irrespective of whether neuropathology is found.

Table 17.1 Various histopathological and/or immunohistochemical alterations reported in bowel from HSCR patients

Cell type	Alteration	Reference
Innervation	Complete or near-complete loss of nitrergic innervation (nNOS- or NADPH-diaphorase-positive nerves) in the aganglionic segment	[8, 65]
	Reduced percentage of calretinin- and tyrosine hydroxylase-immunoreactive myenteric ganglion cells in the transition zone	[39]
	Absent neurofilament immunoreactivity in myenteric plexus in the ganglionic bowel of a subset of patients who did poorly after pull-through surgery	[40]
	Reduced expression of a variety of neuropeptides with increased expression of neuropeptide Y in the muscular layers of the aganglionic segment	[45, 63, 84]
	Increased polysialic neural cell adhesion molecule (putative marker of immature neurons) in ganglionic bowel	[57]
	Choline acetyltransferase immunoreactivity highlights large nerves in aganglionic segment, but not mucosal innervation	[74]
	FABP7 (immature glial marker) is absent in aganglionic bowel and labels nerves in ganglionic bowel of Hirschsprung patients more strongly than normal controls	[85]
	Reduced nerves that express specific markers (e.g., PGP9.5, Tuj1) in the mucosa of the aganglionic segment and transition zone	[4, 104]
Extracellular matrix	Reduced nidogen in muscularis externa and muscularis mucosae	[67]
	Increased fibronectin, tenascin, laminin, and collagen IV expression in aganglionic and transition zones	[67, 68, 69, 70]
	Peripheral nerve pattern of laminin expression in aganglionic and transition zones	[2]
Smooth muscle	Altered immunoreactivity of cytoskeletal proteins in muscularis propria of ganglionic and/or aganglionic bowel	[102]
	Reduced rho-kinase expression in smooth muscle of aganglionic segment	[17]
Interstitial cells of Cajal	Loss of CD117-immunoreactive interstitial cells of Cajal in aganglionic and/or ganglionic segments (conflicting data on this subject)	[16, 97, 105]
	Downregulated neuroligin and heme oxygenase in interstitial cells of Cajal of aganglionic segment > transition zone	[72, 100]
	Deficiency of platelet-derived growth factor receptor-alpha-positive cells in Hirschsprung disease colon	[64]
Vessels	Submucosal arterial fibromuscular dysplasia in aganglionic and ganglionic segments	[83, 88]
Inflammatory cells	Eosinophilic periganglionitis +/− myositis in aganglionic and ganglionic segments	[48]
	Increased mast cells in aganglionic segment and transition zone	[42]
Mucosal epithelium	Decreased expression of markers of goblet cell differentiation in aganglionic and ganglionic segments	[60]
	Altered colonic epithelial cell expression of interleukin-36 and its receptor in aganglionic and ganglionic segments	[94]
	Increased expression of nitric oxide synthase-inhibitory protein in the epithelium of aganglionic and ganglionic segments	[92]
	Increased enteroendocrine cells in aganglionic segment but decreased in ganglionic segment with enterocolitis	[77, 78]
Multiple cell types	Altered expression of membrane channel proteins in a variety of cell types in aganglionic and/or ganglionic segments	[15, 90, 91, 93]
	Decreased expression of enzymes involved in hydrogen sulfide metabolism by numerous cell types in aganglionic and ganglionic segments	[95]

17.3 Secondary Pathological Changes

The most obvious anatomic consequence of congenital aganglionosis is distension of upstream ganglionic bowel. Massive distension or megacolon is relatively common, particularly if diagnosis and treatment are delayed. In some cases, the discordance in size between the dilated ganglionic and spastic aganglionic bowel is so great that pull-through and anastomosis is not possible. When such a mismatch exists, diversion for several weeks to months allows for constriction of the dilated segment prior to definitive surgery. The distended segment is also thick-walled due to hypertrophy of the muscularis propria, an adaptation that increases the contractile force required to overcome spasticity of the aganglionic segment. Thickness of the muscular tunics is due to both myocyte enlargement and proliferation, as evidenced by abundant mitotic figures in the muscularis interna of the distal ganglionic segments of neonates (Fig. 17.7a).

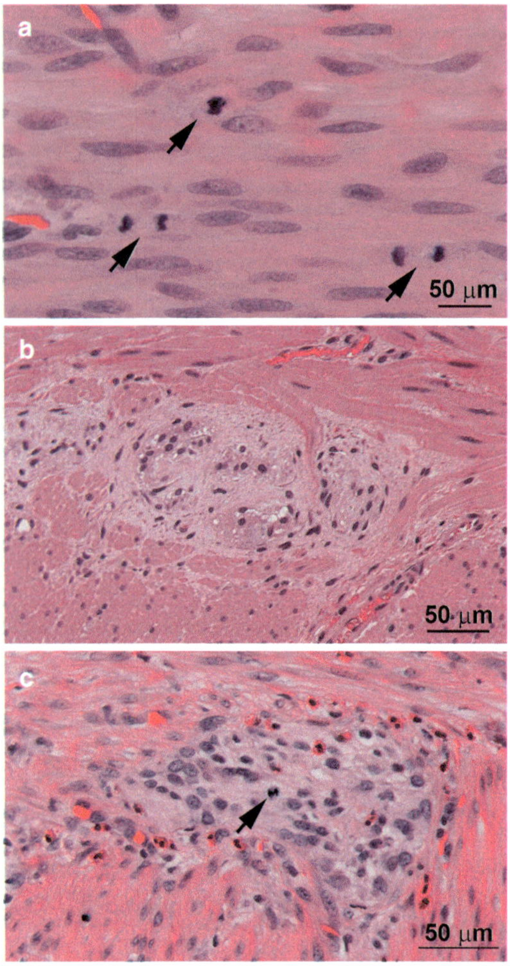

Fig. 17.7 Non-specific histopathological findings in HSCR. (**a**) Mitotic figures (arrows) in the muscularis propria likely represent a response to distal obstruction and will lead to muscular hypertrophy. (**b**) Gangliosclerosis (fibrosis within and around myenteric ganglia) is occasionally observed proximal to the aganglionic segment, particularly with longstanding distension. (**c**) Eosinophilic inflammation within and around myenteric ganglia is common, but has not been shown to be clinically significant. In this example, a mitotic figure (arrow) is present with the ganglia, likely in an enteric glial cell

Distension can damage the bowel wall and lead to mural fibrosis or perforation. Frequent sites of perforation include the cecum or, in patients with total colonic aganglionosis, the distal ileum. The pathogenesis of perforation is different from intestinal atresia-associated aganglionosis, whereby the entire bowel downstream from the site of atresia is aganglionic. Atresia in these cases is thought to occur during the first trimester and interrupt the cranial-to-caudal migration of neural progenitors in the gut wall. Although unusual, discrete zones of muscular atrophy and intramuscular fibrosis occur, presumably due to stretch and physical trauma to the muscularis propria. A more common, but somewhat subtle, alteration is fibrosis around the myenteric plexus. Collagen, sometimes hyalinized, is deposited and expands the space between myenteric ganglia/nerves and adjacent smooth muscle (Fig. 17.7b). In some cases, gangliosclerosis, fibrous dissociation of an individual ganglion, is observed. These patterns of mural fibrosis occur proximal to the aganglionic segment, as expected if they are due to distension.

Intestinal inflammation is another acquired change in HSCR. Two nonexclusive types of inflammation predominate. The first, and potentially most serious, is enterocolitis. Hirschsprung-associated enterocolitis is a mucosa-based process. The earliest change is active inflammation in the mucosa, which may progress to crypt abscesses, ulceration, and transmural necrosis +/− perforation in severe cases [86]. Enterocolitis can occur in the ganglionic or aganglionic bowel, is often multifocal or patchy, and may proceed or follow surgery. A histopathological staging system for Hirschsprung-associated enterocolitis has been proposed [86].

Eosinophilic inflammation is also common in HSCR [30, 48]. In contrast with allergic eosinophilic gastroenteritis, the eosinophils in HSCR are typically in the muscularis propria and/or in and around ganglia (Fig. 17.7c). Eosinophilic inflammation is patchy and can occur in aganglionic or ganglionic bowel. Despite an intimate relationship between eosinophils and smooth muscle cells or ganglion cells, histopathological signs of myocyte or neuronal injury are usually not present. In contrast with Hirschsprung-associated enterocolitis, Hirschsprung-associated eosinophilic inflammation is not known to cause any physiologic alteration and is not known to persist after the obstructive aganglionic segment is resected.

Vascular pathology is also common in the resected bowel of HSCR patients. Specifically, arteries in the submucosa, muscularis propria, or serosa frequently exhibit adventitial changes termed "fibromuscular dysplasia" [83]. Early and late phases of fibromuscular dysplasia have been described [88]. The early phase is only observed neonatally and is characterized by aggregated myofibroblasts (smooth muscle actin-positive, desmin-negative) in a myxedematous matrix of the adventitia (Fig. 17.8). Lymphohistiocytic inflammation is occasionally admixed with the myofibroblasts. Myofibroblasts mature into smooth muscle (smooth muscle actin- and

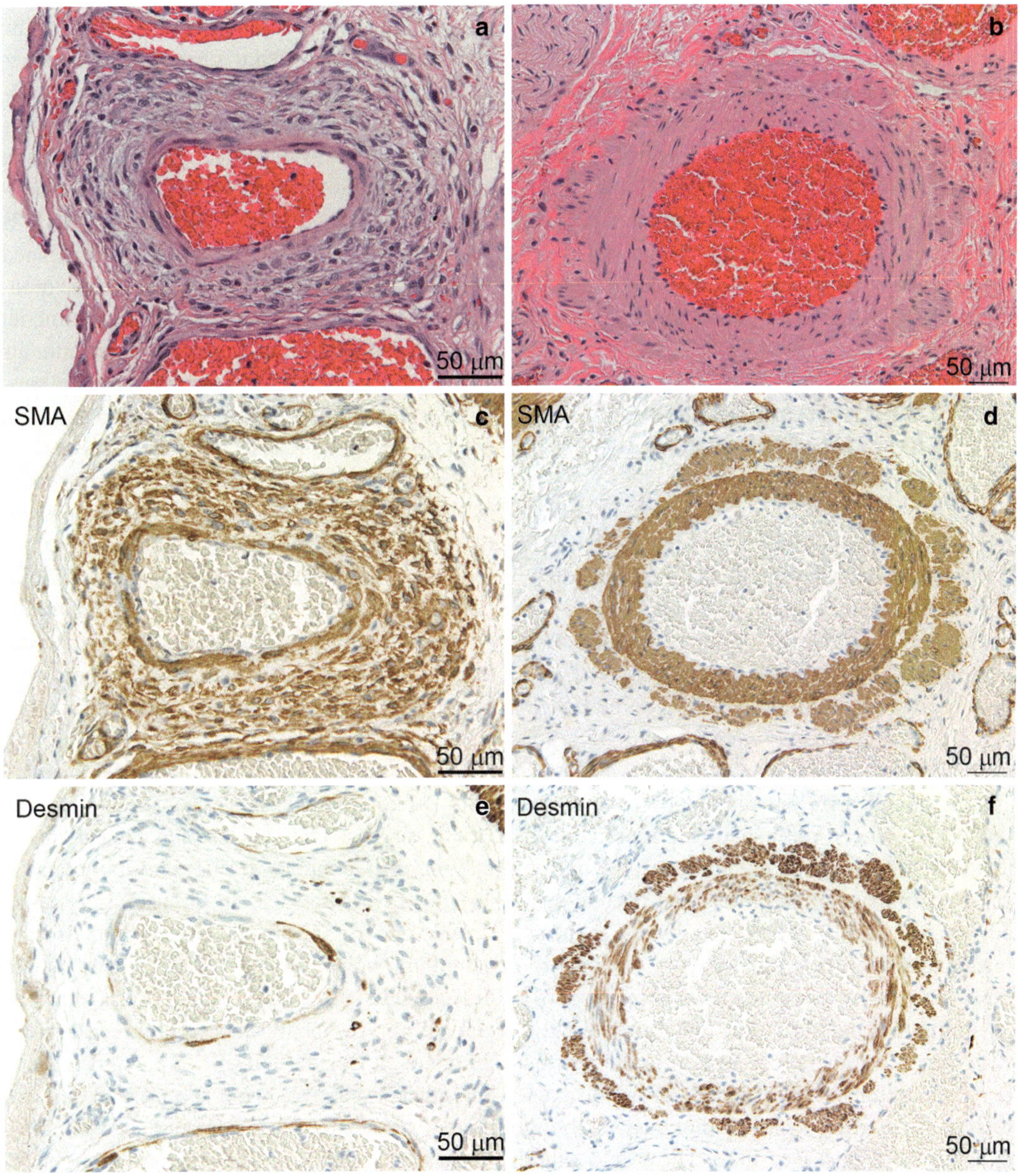

Fig. 17.8 Adventitial fibromuscular dysplasia. Immature (**a**, **c**, **e**) and mature (**b**, **d**, **f**) stages of adventitial fibromuscular dysplasia are illustrated. The immature stage is characterized by crowded myofibroblasts (**a**), which express smooth muscle actin (**c**), and not desmin (**e**). In the mature stage, the adventitia contains closely packed smooth muscle cells (**b**), which express both smooth muscle actin (**d**) and desmin (**f**)

desmin-positive), which probably persist indefinitely (Fig. 17.8). Adventitial fibromuscular dysplasia was originally believed to be specific to HSCR and confined to the transition zone [83] but has more recently been observed in other contexts with bowel stenosis and/or distension, including the aganglionic segment of HSCR [88].

A host of other alterations have been reported in the aganglionic and/or ganglionic bowel of patients with HSCR. These include quantitative differences in the density of various cell populations (e.g., enteroendocrine cells and mast cells), immunohistochemically distinct nerve processes (e.g., muscular nitrergic innervation, mucosal PGP 9.5-positive nerves), CD117-positive interstitial cells of Cajal, and others (Table 17.1). Although most of these reported changes are statistically significant, their functional relevance remains unproven, and they are generally regarded as not useful diagnostically.

17.4 Hirschsprung Disease-Associated Intestinal Neuronal Dysplasia

Intestinal neuronal dysplasia type B (IND-B) is discussed elsewhere in this text. This controversial histopathological phenotype has been considered by some to be an isolated neuropathological cause of dysmotility, as well as a finding in the ganglionic bowel of some HSCR patients, where it may increase the risk for postoperative obstructive symptoms [38, 41, 76]. Although different diagnostic criteria for IND-B have been published, the most consistent feature is a pattern of submucosal ganglion cell hyperplasia with a larger-than-normal proportion of giant ganglia. Diagnosis requires formal ganglion cell counts from frozen sections stained by enzyme histochemistry [54] or alternative methods that must be validated with large numbers of appropriate controls [80]. Quantitative assessment of giant ganglia is affected by section thickness, staining methods, and observer bias. These and other problems associated with the histopathological diagnosis are discussed in detail elsewhere [27, 38, 54]. Because of these issues, HSCR-associated IND-B is diagnosed with regularity in some parts of the world and virtually never diagnosed in others [43, 49, 81, 87]. A recent study supporting the existence of HSCR-associated IND-B used different methods and independently validated control data [80]. However, the approach required was laborious and impractical for routine practice.

The pathogenesis of IND-B is unclear [73]. It has been suggested that IND-B is a non-specific response to downstream obstructive processes and/or inflammation, as similar patterns of IND-B-like submucosal hyperganglionosis occur proximal to stenosis in intestinal atresia, necrotizing enterocolitis, fibrosing colonopathy, and experimental animal models [89]. Alternatively, IND-B has been regarded as a genetically determined malformation, in part because some murine models have IND-B-like pathology. One such model is *endrb*$^{s/+}$ mice [98]. The heterozygous animals have ganglion cell hyperplasia, but no symptoms, whereas mice homozygous for the same mutation have distal aganglionosis. The apparent genetic link between the two phenotypes in this model is viewed by some as strong evidence that IND-B, and presumably Hirschsprung-associated IND-B, is a primary developmental disorder [73]. However, the data at present are inconclusive, and it remains unclear whether submucosal hyperganglionosis proximal to the aganglionic segment in HSCR is a primary malformation or an acquired adaptation.

The few published studies that have mapped IND-B-like submucosal hyperganglionosis in HSCR suggest that the histological phenotype may be discontinuous, occurs only in neonates, and is not restricted to the transition zone, as defined above [56, 80]. It is likely that affected ganglionic bowel is not, nor necessarily should be, resected in many patients. Spontaneous clinical improvement has been observed in most infants with isolated IND-B [54], and it is probable that excessive giant submucosal ganglia regress after surgery for HSCR, as well [55]. Regardless, no compelling information exists to support more aggressive surgery for a patient with IND-B-like submucosal hyperganglionosis.

17.5 Miscellaneous Alterations in Hirschsprung Disease

Many other changes have been reported in the bowel of Hirschsprung patients (Table 17.1). These include light microscopic alterations in mucosal epithelial cells, smooth muscle, vessels, matrix components, and inflammatory cells. Most of the reported changes are quantitative or semiquantitative differences in cell number or immunohistochemical staining intensity. Speculation aside, none of the findings listed in Table 17.1 have proven to be specific for HSCR or prognostically significant. Many of these changes are likely secondary in nature. These findings are seldom referred to in surgical pathology reports because they have no established clinical significance.

17.6 Diagnosis of Hirschsprung Disease

Clinical, radiological, and manometric features of HSCR, including common and atypical presentations, are discussed elsewhere in this book, as are methods of rectal biopsy. The text that follows addresses the histopathological and other laboratory approaches used to diagnose or exclude aganglionosis. Most of these are applicable to either suction biopsies or incisional biopsies, which are obtained to determine whether a patient will require surgery. Less commonly, the diagnosis is established from a surgical resection specimen, such as bowel distal to intestinal atresia or perforation.

17.6.1 Suction Rectal Biopsy

In an exhaustive review of the literature, Friedmacher and Puri found the mean diagnostic sensitivity and specificity of rectal suction biopsies were 97% and 99%, respectively [20]. However, a universally accepted standardized approach to the pathological evaluation of rectal biopsies for HSCR does not exist. Instead, multiple effective strategies have evolved, most of which use some combination of conventional H&E-based histopathology with or without routine ancillary enzymatic and/or immunohistochemistry. Valid comparisons of the different approaches are difficult to conduct or interpret because the most important variable with each approach is technical and interpretational experience. It is likely that accurate diagnosis is equally likely with any of the commonly used approaches, provided the laboratory is adept with the specific techniques and the pathologist understands the methodological limitations and can confidently recognize diagnostic versus atypical results.

By definition, a distal rectal biopsy from a patient with HSCR should be aganglionic. With H&E-stained sections alone, confident identification of aganglionosis in a suction biopsy requires generous histological sampling of an adequate sample of submucosa. An adequate suction biopsy is usually 2–3 mm in greatest dimension, surfaced entirely by colonic mucosa (not anal or transitional epithelium), and 50% or more submucosa. For laboratories that use formalin-fixed paraffin-embedded tissues, adequacy is usually achieved by routinely cutting 50–75 H&E-stained sections (4–5 μm thick). The overwhelming majority of sections should contain some submucosa, and one-third or more of the cut surface should be submucosa in the majority of sections. If no ganglion cell is identified and overt submucosal nerve hypertrophy is present, the diagnosis is established. Conversely, if an unequivocal ganglion cell is present and hypertrophic nerves are not, HSCR is effectively excluded. Unfortunately, many biopsies lack these unequivocal diagnostic findings or have atypical features that require additional study.

One common challenge associated with suction rectal biopsies is inadequate or borderline-adequacy of submucosal tissue. Submucosal ganglia are concentrated near the muscularis propria and, to a lesser degree, superficially near the muscularis mucosae. A superficial suction biopsy will miss deep ganglia. Furthermore, in the distal rectum, submucosal ganglia are normally less numerous and may be excluded from a small biopsy, which is also less likely to sample enlarged submucosal nerves. In a laboratory dependent on H&E staining and without access to ancillary approaches (see below), it is appropriate to exhaust the tissue block to maximize submucosal evaluation. In the event that the biopsy remains inadequate, it may be necessary to rebiopsy the patient, perhaps by a full-thickness incisional/forceps biopsy.

Suction biopsies are very helpful and are a routine at many centers to obtain biopsies at multiple distances above the dentate line. In practice, these distances are only estimates because the dentate line is not visualized directly, but rather the distance between the anal verge and the biopsy port on the barrel of the instrument is known. Biopsies from 1, 2, and 3 cm rostral to the dentate line are ideal, although some groups prefer 2, 3, and 4 cm. One value of multiple biopsies is simply additional submucosa in which to survey for ganglion cells and hypertrophic nerves. Biopsies at different distances improve the odds that if the most caudal biopsy is actually anal mucosa ("too low"), one or both of the more proximal biopsies will be from the distal rectum. Multiple biopsies also provide useful topographic information and facilitate the diagnosis of vssHSCR, as when diagnostic features of aganglionosis are present in the distal biopsies, but ganglion cells, often with hypertrophic nerves, are present in the most proximal biopsies.

Traditionally clinicians have been taught not to biopsy the distal 1–2 cm of rectum because the normal paucity of ganglion cells in this region may lead to a false-positive diagnosis of HSCR. The original paper by Aldridge and Campbell which led to this practice was based on a limited sampling strategy of cadaveric specimens [1]. In practice, with exhaustive sectioning of suction rectal biopsies, aganglionosis in low biopsies has not been proven to be a diagnostic problem, especially with attention to the presence or absence of nerve hypertrophy and the application of exhaustive sections and ancillary staining methods. Arguably of more concern is the potential to miss clinically significant very short-segment disease, if biopsies are obtained too far above the anorectal junction.

The challenge posed by nondiagnostic H&E findings have led to the development of histochemical approaches to visualize changes in mucosal innervation that correlate strongly with aganglionosis (Table 17.2). Acetylcholinesterase (AChE) enzyme histochemistry was the first such method to be widely applied. AChE is expressed in cholinergic nerves including the mucosal projections from extrinsic nerves, which are thicker and more densely distributed in the aganglionic rectum (Fig. 17.9). The method requires frozen sections because the enzymatic activity is lost after formalin fixation and paraffin embedding. In some centers, all biopsies are frozen for AChE histochemistry; additional frozen sections from the same biopsy may be stained with H&E and/or other histochemical stains (e.g., lactate dehydrogenase, succinate dehydrogenase) to facilitate identification of ganglion cells [51]. In these laboratories, confidence in frozen section, and particularly AChE histochemistry, interpretation is sufficient to diagnose or exclude HSCR without complementary paraffin section-based pathology [5]. Limitations associated with this approach include introduction and maintenance of a method that is only applied in one clinical setting, as opposed to formalin-fixed paraffin-based H&E and immunohistochemical approaches

Table 17.2 Ancillary diagnostic approaches to Hirschsprung disease

Acetylcholinesterase enzyme histochemistry	Calretinin immunohistochemistry	Choline transporter immunohistochemistry
Frozen sections	Formalin-fixed paraffin sections	Formalin-fixed paraffin sections
Unique reagents and methodology	Routine in most laboratories	Routine in most laboratories
Manual processing	Can be done with automated immunostainer	Can be done with automated immunostainer
Abnormal innervation equates with gain of histochemical staining	Abnormal innervation equates with loss of immunoreactivity	Abnormal innervation equates with gain of immunoreactivity
Usually easy to interpret but requires regular practice	Usually easy to interpret without much practice	Often requires considerable practice to interpret correctly

which are routine in every pathology laboratory. Reliance on frozen tissue also requires special and relatively expedient handling of the biopsy, which may be problematic in some settings.

Rather than rely solely on frozen sections, most laboratories utilize H&E-stained paraffin sections and complement the H&E analysis with either AChE histochemistry from a separately frozen biopsy (or portion of biopsy) or paraffin-based immunohistochemistry. Calretinin immunohistochemistry is an extremely valuable diagnostic adjunct. Calretinin is a calcium-binding protein that is expressed by the majority of submucosal ganglion cells. Calretinin immunohistochemistry labels the perikarya of these cells and their lengthy nerve processes, including numerous small nerves in the muscularis propria and lamina propria. In aganglionic bowel that is devoid of submucosal ganglion cells, calretinin-immunoreactive mucosal nerves are completely absent, which multiple studies have shown to be a very specific and highly sensitive diagnostic finding (Fig. 17.9) [18, 24, 37].

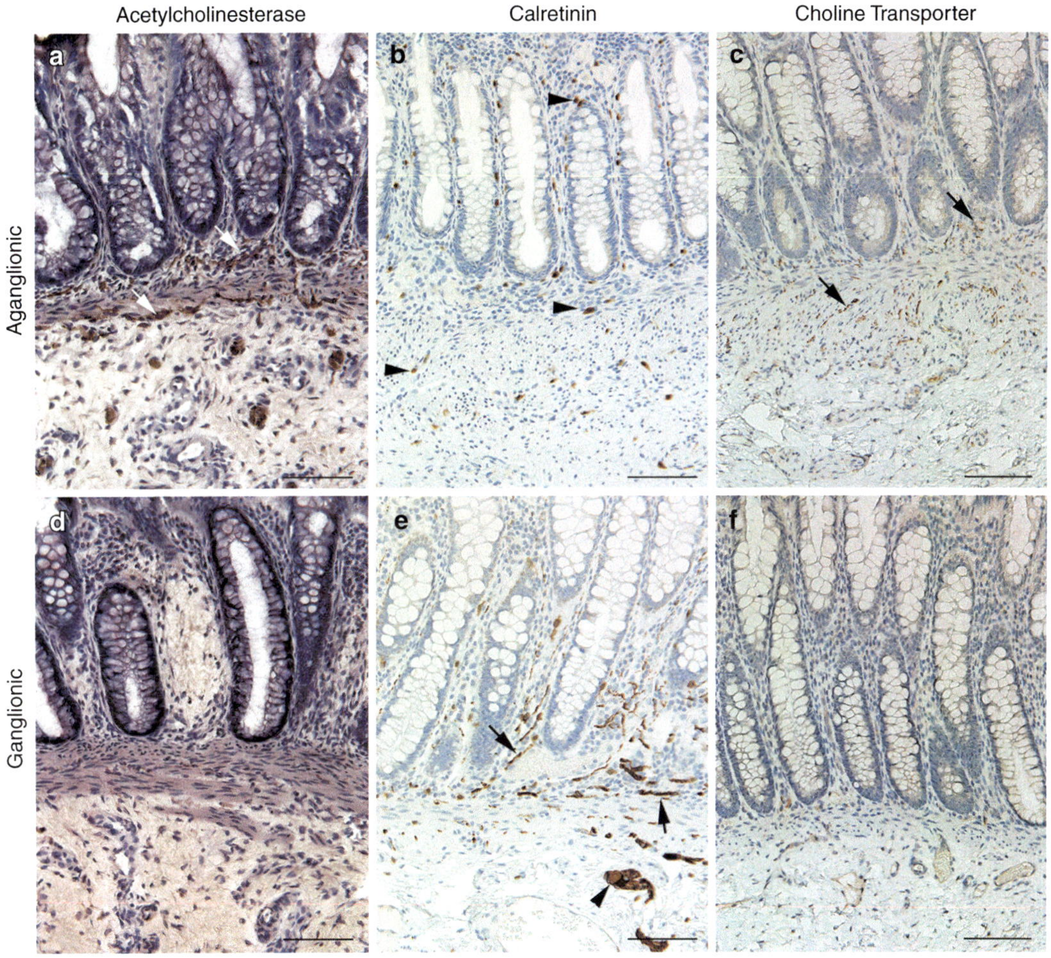

Fig. 17.9 Diagnostically useful ancillary stains. Aganglionic rectal mucosa (**a**–**c**) typically shows an increased density of cholinergic nerves, which can be visualized by AChE histochemistry (brown-stained fibers as indicated by white arrows in **a**) or ChT immunohistochemistry (arrows in **c**), along with absent calretinin-immunoreactive mucosal innervation (**b**). Oval brown areas in **b** (arrowheads) are mast cells. In contrast, normal ganglionic mucosa (**d**–**f**) contains few or no visible AChE- (**d**) or ChT-positive (**f**) nerves and abundant calretinin-immunoreactive nerves (arrows in **e**). An immunoreactive submucosal ganglion cell is present in **b** (arrowhead). Scale bar = 100 μm

Several caveats for use and interpretation of calretinin immunohistochemistry need to be kept in mind. First, calretinin is expressed in the cytoplasm of mast cells, which sometimes extend short processes that may mimic neurites. In general, the labeling in mast cells is less intense and less punctate than in neurites; calretinin in mucosal neurites often has a beaded granular appearance (Fig. 17.10a). Second, calretinin is expressed in a subset of extrinsic nerves and is retained by the large submucosal nerves characteristic of aganglionic distal rectum (Fig. 17.10b). Therefore, the complete absence of calretinin immunoreactive innervation in aganglionic bowel refers only to the mucosa, not deeper portions of the bowel wall; calretinin immunohistochemistry should not be used on seromuscular biopsies to establish a diagnosis of aganglionosis, although it is normally expressed in the soma of a small minority of myenteric ganglion cells. Third, submucosal ganglia from the transition zone send calretinin-immunoreactive neurites downstream to the proximal 1–2 cm of the aganglionic segment. The presence of these nerves is seldom a diagnostic issue, because rectal biopsies usually are taken farther downstream. However, in vssHSCR, a suction biopsy may sample aganglionic bowel with transition zone-derived calretinin-positive mucosal nerves [29]. In this situation, inability to document ganglion cells, the presence of hypertrophic submucosal nerves, +/− abnormal AChE, or choline transporter-positive innervation may lead to the correct diagnosis. In some instances, an incisional strip or full-thickness biopsy may be required to confidently diagnose vssHSCR. Another rare situation in which calretinin immunostaining can yield discordant results is a distal skip area, whereby a lengthy aganglionic segment is interrupted by a patch of ganglionic bowel (skip area) in the distal rectum [13]. Fourth, calretinin immunoreactivity, at least with some antibodies, appears to be lost after tissue freeze-thaw prior to formalin fixation and paraffin embedding [47]. Finally, diagnosis rests on loss of calretinin immunoreactivity. Therefore, it is important to run a

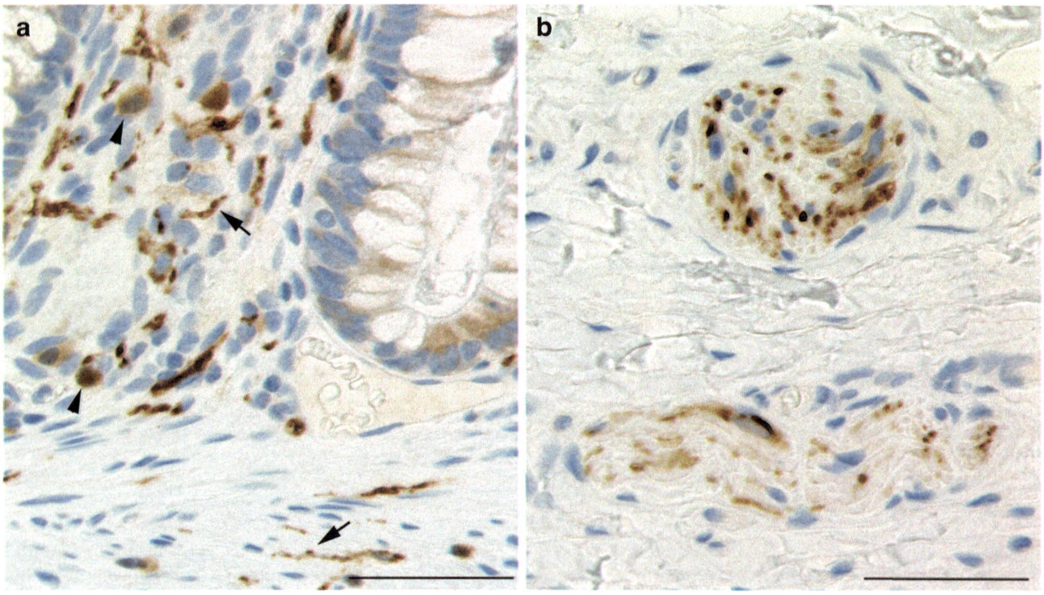

Fig. 17.10 Interpretation of calretinin immunohistochemistry. (**a**) Immunoreactive nerves (arrows) typically have a granular or beaded appearance, in contrast with the more homogeneous immunoreactivity found in mast cells (arrowheads). (**b**) Calretinin is retained in large submucosal nerves in aganglionic bowel and should not be misinterpreted as retained immunoreactive mucosal innervation. Scale bar = 50 μm

positive control, ideally a sample of bowel with normal innervation on the same slide as the patient's biopsy and to pay attention to mast cell and hypertrophic nerve immunoreactivity as indices of technical proficiency.

In principle, immunohistochemistry specific for AChE could replace AChE histochemistry, particularly if the method worked with FFPE sections. To date, such antibodies have been effective in frozen sections, but not after paraffin embedding. However, immunostaining for the choline transporter protein (ChT), another marker of cholinergic nerves, has been proposed as a surrogate for AChE [36]. Like AChE histochemistry, ChT immunohistochemistry demonstrates larger and more numerous nerves in the mucosa of aganglionic bowel (Fig. 17.9), a finding that is particularly useful with biopsies from patients with vssHSCR, because calretinin may be misleading in this context. Abnormal mucosal innervation in aganglionic biopsies is sometimes, but less consistently, resolved with other more general markers of enteric nerves, such as PGP9.5 or S100 [75].

Numerous other immunohistochemical markers have been suggested as potentially useful for diagnosis of HSCR [28]. These include individual [11] and multi-antibody panels [3]. Most of these highlight ganglion cell bodies +/− nerve processes, and it is not necessary or cost-efficient to apply such immunostains in place of H&E-staining. They are only useful when unable to unequivocally exclude ganglion cells in a particular H&E-stained section, which is a rare situation for an experienced pathologist. In such situations, it is possible to remove the coverslip, destain the slide, and immunostain the equivocal cell(s). The Hu C/D antigen, a selective marker of all enteric ganglion cell bodies [21], works well (Fig. 17.11).

17.6.2 Incisional Rectal Biopsy

Incisional rectal biopsies refer to either longitudinal strips of superficial and deep submucosa or full-thickness biopsies that include muscularis propria and myenteric plexus. In contrast with suction biopsies, these require examination under anesthe-

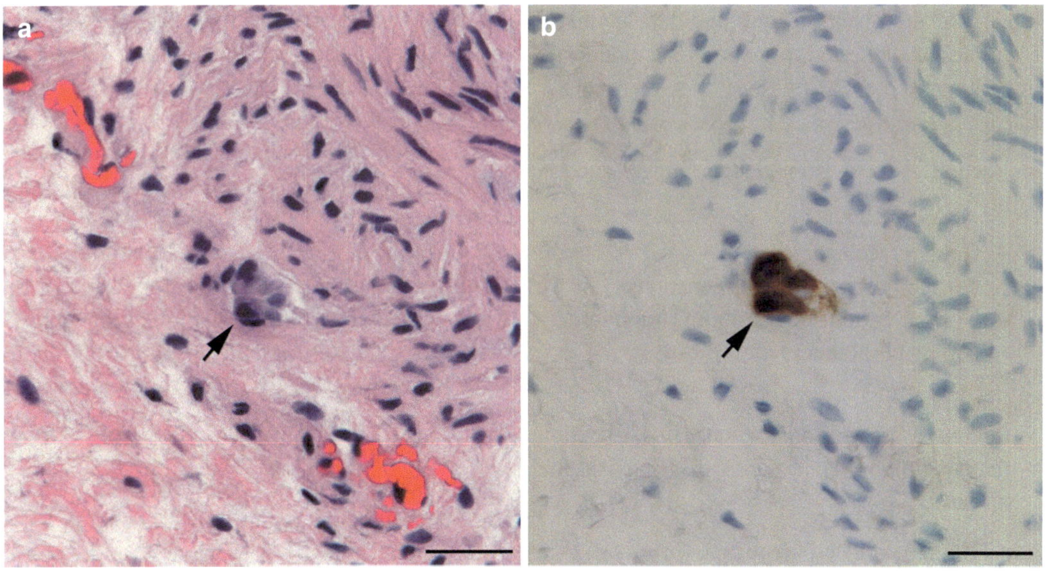

Fig. 17.11 Confirmation of ganglion cells with Hu C/D immunolabeling. (**a**) Cytologically immature ganglion cells (arrow) may be difficult to confidently identify in H&E-stained sections. (**b**) After the slide is destained and Hu C/D immunolabeling is performed, strong perikaryal immunoreactivity confirms their neuronal identities. Scale bar = 25 μm

sia and are done with direct visualization of the dentate line, so the location is precise. Incisional biopsies may be advantageous in older patients (>1 year) because suction biopsies yield a smaller proportion of the submucosa as the patient grows and the submucosa becomes more fibrotic [96]. They are also used to confirm or exclude vssHSCR, when suction rectal biopsy findings are equivocal. Incisional biopsy is also part of the evaluation of some post-pull-through patients who continue to have serious obstructive symptoms [12, 44].

Since incisional biopsies are much larger and deeper than suction rectal biopsies, fewer H&E-stained sections are generally required. Typically, two slides with two ribbons per slide are sufficient. In other respects, the diagnostic findings and use of calretinin immunohistochemistry and/or AChE histochemistry for HSCR are identical to suction biopsies.

17.6.3 Rectal Biopsy Report

Surgical pathology reports from rectal biopsies should, at a minimum, include the location and type of each biopsy, whether or not a ganglion cell or submucosal nerve hypertrophy was identified, and the results of any ancillary staining. Examples of suggested formats for the diagnostic lines in a report are as follows:

Example 1:
Rectum, "1 cm from dentate line," suction biopsy:

- Ganglion cells present.
- No submucosal nerve hypertrophy.
- Normal pattern of calretinin-immunoreactive mucosal innervation.

Example 2:
Rectum, "1 cm from dentate line," suction biopsy: findings consistent with Hirschsprung disease

- No ganglion cell identified.
- Abundant hypertrophic submucosal nerves.
- Absent calretinin-immunoreactive mucosal innervation.

17.6.4 Other Diagnostic Laboratory Tests

Histology remains the accepted method to diagnose HSCR. The search for replacement or complementary nonhistological techniques has yielded some interesting published data, but no practical alternative. Given that increased AChE-positive innervation is nearly always present in the mucosa and superficial submucosa of aganglionic rectum, biochemical quantification of acetylcholinesterase activity in suction biopsies has been investigated with conflicting published results [10, 59, 103]. While mean AChE activity values, particularly if normalized to non-specific cholinesterase activity, from aganglionic biopsies are significantly higher than those from ganglionic biopsies, the range of values observed in individual patients limits the diagnostic utility of this approach.

More recently, investigators from China have touted changes in the levels of various serum components as diagnostically useful biomarkers. These include reduced glutamate and elevated gamma-amino butyric acid (GABA) [99, 106] and three peptide markers, distinguished by their mass-charge ratios as revealed by mass spectrometry [101]. As with AChE quantification, none of these putative blood tests have been widely adopted.

As described elsewhere in this text (see Chap. 7), HSCR is a complex genetic disorder with alterations in many specific genes that act as risk factors. For some patients, particularly those with syndromic features (e.g., Mowat-Wilson syndrome), molecular genetic testing may establish the etiology and help with genetic counseling and some aspects of clinical management. However, the diagnosis of HSCR per se is not affected significantly by molecular genetic results, in part because the penetrance of aganglionosis is often variable, even in many syndromes, and cannot be predicted accurately based on mutational analysis, particularly in patients with isolated aganglionosis.

17.7 Intraoperative Surgical Pathology

An early step in the operative management of HSCR is to localize distal ganglionic bowel so that either a primary pull-through or a diverting ostomy can be performed proximal to the aganglionic segment and transition zone. A strong partnership between surgeon and pathologist is essential. A small biopsy of the bowel wall, either full-thickness or seromuscular (muscularis propria and myenteric plexus), is obtained by the surgeon. A typical biopsy may be only 3–5 mm in greatest dimension, but a larger piece usually leads to a faster intraoperative diagnosis. If possible, the pathologist orients the tissue so that it is frozen perpendicular to the serosal surface, thereby yielding sections that traverse both layers of the muscularis propria and any intervening ganglia. Use of a dissection microscope can facilitate orientation. Frozen sections are cut at 5–8 μm and stained with H&E (some pathologists prefer Diff-Qwik). Rapid AChE staining is done in some centers, in part to exclude intestinal neuronal dysplasia type B (discussed above), but this is not considered standard of care in most parts of the world.

Myenteric ganglion cells are readily identified with a well-oriented, appropriately cut and stained, frozen section. The density of myenteric ganglia is such that ganglion cells should be identified with <10 sections. However, if the tissue is misoriented, additional sections may be required. The presence or absence of ganglion cells does not exclude transition zone because only a tiny portion of the circumference is sampled. A biopsy of aganglionic bowel will often, but not always, contain large myenteric nerves. Therefore, the diagnosis rests entirely on finding or excluding ganglion cells. Since the transition zone in ssHSCR is typically <5 cm, it is advisable to resect 5 cm or more proximal to a ganglionic biopsy site.

In the intraoperative search for the transition zone, the process of biopsy and frozen section interpretation may have to be repeated at many successive more proximal sites, which can tax the patience of everyone involved. It is tempting to try to establish a diagnosis of total colonic aganglionosis with frozen sections of the appendix, but this practice is to be discouraged for two reasons. First, aganglionosis of the appendix does not always correlate with aganglionosis of the entire large intestine. A skip area with intact innervation may be present downstream from the appendix and may encompass a significant length of colon that does not need to be resected [13]. Second, appendicostomy for anterograde enemas is sometimes used to manage severe chronic constipation after a pull-through procedure, but is not an option after appendectomy.

Once the resection or ostomy site has been determined, it is prudent for the pathologist to perform an intraoperative frozen section of the proximal resection/ostomy site margin to exclude histologic features of transition zone (partial circumferential aganglionosis, myenteric hypoganglionosis, submucosal nerve hypertrophy) (Fig. 17.12). This frozen section of the full circumference ("donut")

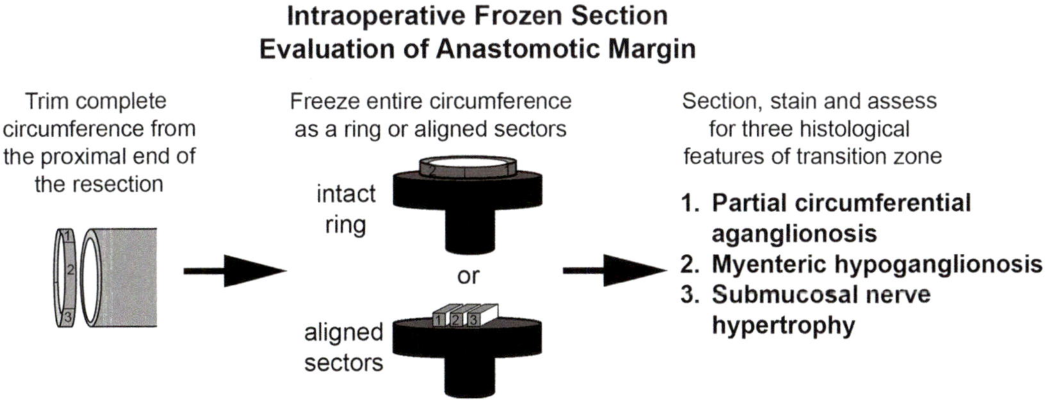

Fig. 17.12 Recommended procedure for frozen section analysis of anastomotic margin to reduce likelihood of a transition zone pull-through

encompasses a generous amount of tissue that can be difficult to freeze in a well-oriented manner. One trick is to divide the donut into pieces and arrange full-thickness sectors of the circumference one against the other like books on a shelf. Aligned in this manner, they support one another upright as they are frozen.

17.8 Resection Specimens

A variety of types of bowel resections are performed on HSCR patients. All eventually include resection of the aganglionic and some proximal ganglionic bowel up to the site of "anal" anastomosis between ganglionic bowel and the distalmost rectum. In one-stage procedures, the resection is typically received as a single length of rectum +/− more contiguous proximal intestine. In multistage procedures, the latter is collected along with one or more separate segments of intestine, often including an ostomy takedown. It is important for the pathologist to understand the surgical history and to be certain about the proximal-most margin, which corresponds most closely to the distal end of ganglionic bowel used to create the anal anastomosis. In two-stage procedures, the latter is the proximal margin of an end-ostomy takedown.

When examining HSCR resection specimens, the surgical pathologist has a minimum of three goals: confirm distal aganglionosis, exclude features of transition zone or other significant pathology at the proximal-most margin, and ascertain the approximate length of the aganglionic segment. Other findings such as the length of the transition zone may have academic value, but are not known to affect prognosis or familial recurrence risks, unless the proximal margin is affected.

Gross examination should begin with measurements of specimen length and diameter or circumference, noting the distance between obvious transitions in the latter measurements and the proximal or distal margin. If a mucosal sleeve is present distally (Soave procedure), the length should be noted. The positions of intraoperative biopsy sites should also be recorded. The bowel should be opened longitudinally and the mucosal surface inspected. Sometimes sites of rectal biopsies are apparent if the pull-through was performed less than a week after diagnosis. It is very helpful to fix the bowel flat for several hours prior to sampling for permanent sections.

A simple approach used by many pathologists to sample resection specimens is illustrated in Fig. 17.13. A full-circumference section from the distal rectal margin is submitted, which should confirm aganglionosis. A full-circumference section from the proximal-most margin is used to exclude features of transition zone. Ideally, this was done intraoperatively with frozen sections, in which case permanent sections from any remaining frozen tissue should be evaluated. In addition, it is helpful to submit a full-circumference section immediately downstream from the frozen proximal margin to provide an optimally oriented and fixed histological sample with no freeze artifact. Finally, the longitudinal strip provides a reasonable indication of the point of transition between ganglionic and aganglionic bowel, at least on one side of the specimen. The options of a second strip from the opposite side of the circumference or closely spaced transverse sections help define this often irregular border, but neither is essential. To conserve resources, most pathologists embed more than one segment of the longitudinal strip together and use ink or some other method to identify each piece and orient their proximal ends. For short resections, a full-length longitudinal strip can be "jelly-rolled" and fit in a single cassette. Pieces that correspond to intraoperative biopsy sites should be documented in the gross description so that correlation between biopsy results and the distribution of ganglion cells in the resection specimen can be drawn.

Microscopic evaluation should explicitly state which sections contain ganglion cells in the myenteric, submucosal, or both plexuses, whether features of transition zone are present, and whether any other histopathology is evident. The presence or absence of active inflammation or other mucosal changes that may indicate enterocolitis should be stated. Careful consideration should be afforded to

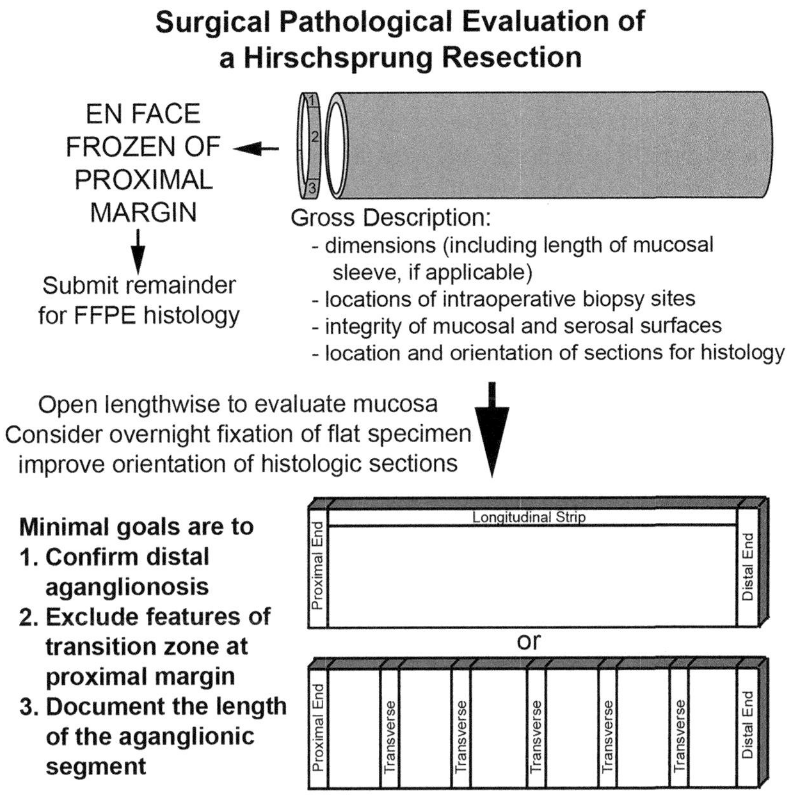

Fig. 17.13 Recommended procedure to process and histologically sample a Hirschsprung disease resection specimen. FFPE formalin fixation and paraffin embedding

mention of submucosal ganglion cell hyperplasia or other features that might suggest intestinal neuronal dysplasia, given controversy with regard to its diagnostic criteria and clinical significance. Other microscopic findings which may be of interest, but have no well-established clinical utility, include eosinophilic ganglionic or muscular infiltrates, muscular hypertrophy +/− mitotic activity, ectopic ganglia in the muscularis propria or serosa, and more (Table 17.1).

In addition to gross and microscopic descriptions, diagnostic lines should be constructed which include the information shown in the following examples:

Example 1:
Rectosigmoid colon, Soave pull-through resection (14 cm): Hirschsprung disease with the following features:

- Aganglionosis (distal 7 cm).
- No significant neuromuscular pathology at the proximal margin.

Example 2:

A. Terminal ileum (9 cm) and colon, swenson resection (68 cm): Hirschsprung disease with the following features:
   - Distal ileal (3 cm) and total colonic aganglionosis.
   - No significant neuromuscular pathology at the ileal margin.

B. End ileostomy takedown (2 cm): enterocutaneous fistula with no diagnostic alteration; no significant neuromuscular pathology at the proximal margin.

17.9 Postoperative Diagnosis of Transition Zone Pull-Through

Many patients with HSCR continue to have obstructive symptoms after definitive surgery. Potential anatomic etiologies are strictures or torsion around the anastomosis site, skip areas with retained proximal aganglionic bowel, inadequate resection of distal aganglionic rectum (retained long aganglionic segment), and transition zone pull-through. Some of these etiologies are diagnosed or suspected based on a combination of physical and imaging results; confirmatory biopsies (e.g., proximal aganglionosis is patient with a skip area) may be required. However, transition zone pull-through is a histopathologic diagnosis.

Identification of one or more histological feature of transition zone at the proximal-most surgical margin of the patient's resection specimen is the gold standard for the diagnosis of transition zone pull-through. Therefore, every effort should be made to review the original pathology slides, especially those corresponding to the proximal margin. In some instances, this may not be practical (e.g., patient operated on in a different country). If the original pathology is not available, a full-thickness neorectal biopsy may be helpful. In this setting, biopsy is also valuable to exclude a long segment of residual aganglionic rectum.

Anorectal examination under anesthesia is part of the workup for post-pull-through patients with significant dysmotility [12, 44], at which time rectal biopsy can be performed. Use of suction rectal biopsies should be discouraged as these patients are often several years old and diagnosis of transition zone is challenging enough with a generous tissue sample versus the small amount of submucosa present in a suction rectal biopsy from an older patient [96].

If a true full-thickness biopsy of pulled through normally innervated bowel is obtained with both layers of muscularis propria and intervening myenteric plexus, normal ganglia with multiple ganglion cells should be present. Aganglionosis suggests either incomplete resection of the proximal aganglionic segment (complete or partial circumferential aganglionosis) or a biopsy or residual distal native rectum inferior to the anastomosis site. Sometimes obvious fibrosis and/or smooth muscle hyperplasia in the submucosa indicates that the biopsy is close to or within the anastomosis site, in which case the biopsy may be inadequate to exclude transition zone pull-through. In an older patient, native rectum usually will have abundant huge submucosal and myenteric nerves, as opposed to proximal aganglionic segment in which abnormal nerves may be present, but are not as prominent. Calretinin-immunoreactive mucosal innervation is likely to be present and lush in proximal aganglionic segment close to the transition zone but absent or sparse in aganglionic distal native rectum after a pull-through procedure. Myenteric hypoganglionosis (ganglia composed only of one or two ganglion cells without accompanying neuropil) may be interpreted as evidence for transition zone pull-through, but equivocal hypoganglionosis is a problem due to the small amount of myenteric plexus typically sampled.

Many biopsies designated "full-thickness" by the surgeon do not contain the entire muscularis propria or myenteric plexus. In this case, the only histologic feature of transition zone that can be evaluated is submucosal nerve hypertrophy, recognition of which is complicated by age- and possibly surgery-related changes in nerve caliber. In contrast with young infants, it is common to encounter nerves >40 μm in the distal native rectum or post-pull-through neorectum of a child over 1 year of age [31]. The density and caliber of large nerves have to be significantly greater than expected to diagnose transition zone pull-through on this basis alone.

17.10 Conclusion and Future Directions

Surgical pathology and familiarity with normal and HSCR-related enteric neuroanatomy are essential elements in the diagnosis and management of patients with HSCR. Many of the requisite pathology skills are somewhat unique to this disorder, and therefore experience and practice are particularly important. In clinical laboratories that handle a high volume of rectal biopsies, accurate and reliable diagnosis is the norm. In other settings, diagnosis can be problematic but may have improved since introduction of calretinin immunohistochemistry. The search for simple, less labor-intensive, less invasive, and inexpensive diagnostic methods continues [22, 101]. Perhaps in the future, a blood test or another type of automated assay will replace the contemporary histological approach.

The pathology of HSCR is far more complex than distal intestinal aganglionosis, and unfortunately, many patients continue to have dysmotility after HSCR surgery. Some of this morbidity may be avoided through intraoperative recognition and complete resection of the histopathologic transition zone, but the possibility must be considered that anatomically subtle, but physiologically significant, primary or secondary neuromuscular alterations exist in the ganglionic bowel of HSCR. Routine histopathology and the limited number of immunohistochemical methods that have worked their way into contemporary HSCR pathology resolve only tiny aspects of the diverse and complicated network of neurons in the enteric nervous system. Many vital aspects of normal enteric neuromuscular biology remain opaque, including a wide variety of neuronal subtypes with varied neurotransmitters and receptors, an intricate network of neuronal projections, pacemaker activity maintained by interstitial cells of Cajal, and the responses and adaptations of smooth muscle cells that ultimately mediate propulsive events. Advancement in the care of patients with HSCR will probably require more in-depth analysis of some or all of these components.

Acknowledgments The author thanks Dr. Annie Samraj for her thoughts and editorial comments.

References

1. Aldridge RT, Campbell PE. Ganglion cell distribution in the normal rectum and anal canal: a basis for the diagnosis of Hirschsprung's disease by anorectal biopsy. J Pediatr Surg. 1968;3:475–89.
2. Alpy F, Ritie L, Jaubert F, Becmeur F, Mechine-Neuville A, Lefebvre O, et al. The expression pattern of laminin isoforms in Hirschsprung disease reveals a distal peripheral nerve differentiation. Hum Pathol. 2005;36:1055–65.
3. Bachmann L, Besendorfer M, Carbon R, Lux P, Agaimy A, Hartmann A, et al. Immunohistochemical panel for the diagnosis of Hirschsprung's disease using antibodies to MAP2, calretinin, GLUT1 and S100. Histopathology. 2015;66(6):824–35.
4. Badizadegan K, Thomas AR, Nagy N, Ndishabandi D, Miller SA, Alessandrini A, et al. Presence of intramucosal neuroglial cells in normal and aganglionic human colon. Am J Physiol Gastrointest Liver Physiol. 2014;307(10):G1002–12.
5. Bagdzevicius R, Gelman S, Gukauskiene L, Vaicekauskas V. Application of acetylcholinesterase histochemistry for the diagnosis of Hirschsprung's disease in neonates and infants: a twenty-year experience. Medicina (Kaunas). 2011;47(7):374–9.
6. Barshack I, Fridman E, Goldberg I, Chowers Y, Kopolovic J. The loss of calretinin expression indicates aganglionosis in Hirschsprung's disease. J Clin Pathol. 2004;57(7):712–6.
7. Baumgarten HG, Holstein AF, Stelzener F. Nervous elements in the human colon of Hirschsprung's disease. Virchows Arch (Pathol Anat). 1973;358:113–36.
8. Bealer JF, Natuzzi ES, Buscher C, Ursell PC, Flake AW, Adzick NS, et al. Nitric oxide synthase is deficient in the aganglionic colon of patients with Hirschsprung's disease. Pediatrics. 1994;93(4):647–51.
9. Bielle F, Freneaux P, Jeanne-Pasquier C, Maran-Gonzalez A, Rousseau A, Lamant L, et al. PHOX2B immunolabeling: a novel tool for the diagnosis of undifferentiated neuroblastomas among childhood small round blue-cell tumors. Am J Surg Pathol. 2012;36(8):1141–9.
10. Bonham JR, Dale G, Scott DJ, Wagget J. A 7-year study of the diagnostic value of rectal mucosal acetylcholinesterase measurement in Hirschsprung's disease. J Pediatr Surg. 1987;22(2):150–2.
11. Chisholm KM, Longacre TA. Utility of peripherin versus MAP-2 and calretinin in the evaluation of Hirschsprung disease. Appl Immunohistochem Mol Morphol. 2016;24(9):627–32.
12. Chumpitazi BP, Nurko S. Defecation disorders in children after surgery for Hirschsprung disease. J Pediatr Gastroenterol Nutr. 2011;53(1):75–9.
13. Coe A, Avansino JR, Kapur RP. Distal rectal skip-segment Hirschsprung disease and the potential for false-negative diagnosis. Pediatr Dev Pathol. 2016;19(2):123–31.
14. Coe A, Collins MH, Lawal T, Louden E, Levitt MA, Pena A. Reoperation for Hirschsprung disease: pathology of the resected problematic distal pull-through. Pediatr Dev Pathol. 2012;15:30–8.
15. Coyle D, Doyle B, Murphy JM, O'Donnell AM, Gillick J, Puri P. Expression of connexin 26 and connexin 43 is reduced in Hirschsprung's disease. J Surg Res. 2016;206(1):242–51.
16. Coyle D, Kelly DA, O'Donnell AM, Gillick J, Puri P. Use of anoctamin 1 (ANO1) to evaluate interstitial cells of Cajal in Hirschsprung's disease. Pediatr Surg Int. 2016;32(2):125–33.
17. Coyle D, O'Donnell AM, Corcionivoschi N, Gillick J, Puri P. Rho-kinase expression in Hirschsprung's disease. Pediatr Surg Int. 2015;31(11):1077–85.

18. de Arruda Lourencao PL, Takegawa BK, Ortolan EV, Terra SA, Rodrigues MA. A useful panel for the diagnosis of Hirschsprung disease in rectal biopsies: calretinin immunostaining and acetylcholinesterase histochesmistry. Ann Diagn Pathol. 2013;17(4):352–6.
19. Friedmacher F, Puri P. Residual aganglionosis after pull-through operation for Hirschsprung's disease: a systematic review and meta-analysis. Pediatr Surg Int. 2011;27(10):1053–7.
20. Friedmacher F, Puri P. Rectal suction biopsy for the diagnosis of Hirschsprung's disease: a systematic review of diagnostic accuracy and complications. Pediatr Surg Int. 2015;31(9):821–30.
21. Ganns D, Schrodl F, Neuhuber W, Brehmer A. Investigation of general and cytoskeletal markers to estimate numbers and proportions of neurons in the human intestine. Histol Histopathol. 2006;21(1):41–51.
22. Gao H, He X, Wu M, Zhang Z, Wang D, Lv L, et al. Proteomic analysis of differentially expressed proteins between stenotic and normal colon segment tissues derived from patients with Hirschsprung's disease. Protein J. 2011;30(2):138–42.
23. Garrett JR, Howard ER, Nixon HH. Autonomic nerves in rectum and colon in Hirschsprung's disease. Arch Dis Child. 1969;44:405–17.
24. Holland SK, Ramalingam P, Podolsky RH, Reid-Nicholson MD, Lee JR. Calretinin immunostaining as an adjunct in the diagnosis of Hirschsprung disease. Ann Diagn Pathol. 2011;15(5):323–8.
25. Jessen KR, Thorpe R, Mirsky R. Molecular identity, distribution and heterogeneity of glial fibrillary acidic protein: an immunoblotting and immunohistochemical study of Schwann cells, satellite cells, enteric glia and astrocytes. J Neurocytol. 1984;13(2):187–200.
26. Kakita Y, Oshiro K, O'Briain DS, Puri P. Selective demonstration of mural nerves in ganglionic and aganglionic colon by immunohistochemistry for glucose transporter-1: prominent extrinsic nerve pattern staining in Hirschsprung disease. Arch Pathol Lab Med. 2000;124(9):1314–9.
27. Kapur RP. Neuronal dysplasia: a controversial pathological correlate of intestinal pseudo-obstruction. Am J Med Genet. 2003;122A(4):287–93.
28. KapurRP.Canwestoplooking?Immunohistochemistry and the diagnosis of Hirschsprung disease. Am J Clin Pathol. 2006;126(1):9–12.
29. Kapur RP. Calretinin-immunoreactive mucosal innervation in very short-segment Hirschsprung disease: a potentially misleading observation. Pediatr Dev Pathol. 2014;17(1):28–35.
30. Kapur RP. Histology of the transition zone in Hirschsprung disease. Am J Surg Pathol. 2016;40(12):1637–46.
31. Kapur RP. Submucosal nerve diameter of greater than 40 mum is not a valid diagnostic index of transition zone pull-through. J Pediatr Surg. 2016;51(10):1585–91.
32. Kapur RP, deSa DJ, Luquette M, Jaffe R. Hypothesis: pathogenesis of skip areas in long-segment Hirschsprung's disease. Pediatr Pathol Lab Med. 1995;15(1):23–37.
33. Kapur RP, Kennedy AJ. Transitional zone pull through: surgical pathology considerations. Semin Pediatr Surg. 2012;21(4):291–301.
34. Kapur RP, Kennedy AJ. Histopathologic delineation of the transition zone in short-segment Hirschsprung disease. Pediatr Dev Pathol. 2013;16(4):252–66.
35. Kapur RP, Livingston R, Doggett B, Sweetser DA, Siebert JR, Palmiter RD. Abnormal microenvironmental signals underlie intestinal aganglionosis in Dominant megacolon mutant mice. Dev Biol. 1996;174:360–9.
36. Kapur RP, Raess PW, Hwang S, Winter C. Choline transporter immunohistochemistry: an effective substitute for acetylcholinesterase histochemistry to diagnose Hirschsprung disease with formalin-fixed paraffin-embedded rectal biopsies. Pediatr Dev Pathol. 2017;20(4):308–20.
37. Kapur RP, Reed RC, Finn LS, Patterson K, Johanson J, Rutledge JC. Calretinin immunohistochemistry versus acetylcholinesterase histochemistry in the evaluation of suction rectal biopsies for Hirschsprung disease. Pediatr Dev Pathol. 2009;12(1):6–15.
38. Kapur RP, Reyes-Mugica M. Intestinal neuronal dysplasia type B: an updated review of a problematic diagnosis. Arch Pathol Lab Med. 2019;143(2):235–43.
39. Kawai H, Satomi K, Morishita Y, Murata Y, Sugano M, Nakano N, et al. Developmental markers of ganglion cells in the enteric nervous system and their application for evaluation of Hirschsprung disease. Pathol Int. 2014;64(9):432–42.
40. Kluck P, Ten Kate FJ, Van der Kamp AW, Tibboel D, Molenaar JC. Pathologic explanation for postoperative obstipation in Hirschsprung's disease revealed with monoclonal antibody staining. Am J Clin Pathol. 1986;86(4):490–2.
41. Kobayashi H, Hirakawa H, Surana R, O'Briain DS, Puri P. Intestinal neuronal dysplasia is a possible cause of persistent bowel symptoms after pull-through operation for Hirschsprung disease. J Pediatr Surg. 1995;30(2):253–9.
42. Kobayashi H, Yamataka A, Fujimoto T, Lane GJ, Miyano T. Mast cells and gut nerve development: implications for Hirschsprung's disease and intestinal neuronal dysplasia. J Pediatr Surg. 1999;34(4): 543–8.
43. Lake BD. Intestinal neuronal dysplasia. Why does it only occur in parts of Europe? Virchows Arch. 1995;426(6):537–9.
44. Langer JC, Rollins MD, Levitt M, Gosain A, Torre L, Kapur RP, et al. Guidelines for the management of postoperative obstructive symptoms in children with Hirschsprung disease. Pediatr Surg Int. 2017;33(5):523–6.
45. Larsson LT. Hirschsprung's disease--immunohistochemical findings. Histol Histopathol. 1994;9(3):615–29.
46. Lawal TA, Chatoorgoon K, Collins MH, Coe A, Pena A, Levitt MA. Redo pull-through in Hirschprung's

disease for obstructive symptoms due to residual aganglionosis and transition zone bowel. J Pediatr Surg. 2011;46(2):342–7.
47. Lim KH, Wan WK, Lim TKH, Loh AHL, Nah SA, Chang KTE. Primary diagnosis of Hirschsprung disease – calretinin immunohistochemistry in rectal suction biopsies, with emphasis on diagnostic pitfalls. World J Pathol. 2014;3:14–22.
48. Lowichik A, Weinberg AG. Eosinophilic infiltration of the enteric neural plexuses in Hirschsprung's disease. Pediatr Pathol Lab Med. 1997;17:885–91.
49. Martucciello G, Pini Prato A, Puri P, Holschneider AM, Meier-Ruge W, Jasonni V, et al. Controversies concerning diagnostic guidelines for anomalies of the enteric nervous system: a report from the fourth International Symposium on Hirschsprung's disease and related neurocristopathies. J Pediatr Surg. 2005;40(10):1527–31.
50. Matsuda H, Hirato J, Kuroiwa M, Nakazato Y. Histopathological and immunohistochemical study of the enteric innervations among various types of aganglionoses including isolated and syndromic Hirschsprung disease. Neuropathology. 2006;26(1):8–23.
51. Meier-Ruge W, Bruder E. Pathology of chronic constipation in pediatric and adult coloproctology. Pathobiology. 2005;72(1–2):1–106.
52. Meier-Ruge W, Hunziger O, Tobler H-J, Walliser C. The pathophysiology of aganglionosis of the entire colon (Zuelzer-Wilson syndrome): morphometric investigations of the extent of sacral parasympathetic innervation of the circular muscles of the aganglionic colon. Beitr Path Bd. 1972;147:228–36.
53. Meier-Ruge WA, Bruder E, Holschneider AM, Lochbuhler H, Piket G, Posselt HG, et al. Diagnosis and therapy of ultrashort Hirschsprung's disease. Eur J Pediatr Surg. 2004;14(6):392–7.
54. Meier-Ruge WA, Bruder E, Kapur RP. Intestinal neuronal dysplasia type B: one giant ganglion is not good enough. Pediatr Dev Pathol. 2006;9(6):444–52.
55. Meyrat BJ, Laurini RN. Plasticity of the enteric nervous system in patients with intestinal neuronal dysplasia associated with Hirschsprung's disease: a report of three patients. Pediatr Surg Int. 2003;19(11):715–20.
56. Meyrat BJ, Lesbros Y, Laurini RN. Assessment of the colon innervation with serial biopsies above the aganglionic zone before the pull-through procedure in Hirschsprung's disease. Pediatr Surg Int. 2001;17(2–3):129–35.
57. Miyahara K, Kato Y, Seki T, Arakawa A, Lane GJ, Yamataka A. Neuronal immaturity in normoganglionic colon from cases of Hirschsprung disease, anorectal malformation, and idiopathic constipation. J Pediatr Surg. 2009;44(12):2364–8.
58. Monforte-Munoz H, Gonzales-Gomez I, Rowland JM, Landing BH. Increased submucosal nerve trunk caliber in aganglionosis. A "positive" and objective finding in suction biopsies and segmental resections in Hirschsprung's disease. Arch Pathol Lab Med. 1998;122:721–5.
59. Moore SW, Johnson G. Acetylcholinesterase in Hirschsprung's disease. Pediatr Surg Int. 2005;21:255–63.
60. Nakamura H, Tomuschat C, Coyle D, O'Donnel AM, Lim T, Puri P. Altered goblet cell function in Hirschsprung's disease. Pediatr Surg Int. 2018;34(2):121–8.
61. Narayanan SK, Soundappan SS, Kwan E, Cohen RC, Charlton A, Cass DT. Aganglionosis with the absence of hypertrophied nerve fibres predicts disease proximal to rectosigmoid colon. Pediatr Surg Int. 2016;32(3):221–6.
62. Neilson IR, Yazbeck S. Ultrashort Hirschsprung's disease: myth or reality. J Pediatr Surg. 1990;25:1135–8.
63. O'Donnell A, Puri P. Deficiency of purinergic P2Y receptors in aganglionic intestine in Hirschsprung's disease. Pediatr Surg Int. 2008;24(1):77–80.
64. O'Donnell AM, Coyle D, Puri P. Deficiency of platelet-derived growth factor receptor-alpha-positive cells in Hirschsprung's disease colon. World J Gastroenterol. 2016;22(12):3335–40.
65. O'Kelly TJ, Davies JR, Tam PK, Brading AF, Mortensen NJ. Abnormalities of nitric-oxide-producing neurons in Hirschsprung's disease: morphology and implications. J Pediatr Surg. 1994;29(2):294–9; discussion 9–300
66. Okamoto E, Satani M, Kuwata K. Histologic and embryologic studies on the innervation of the pelvic viscera in patients with Hirschsprung's disease. Surg Gynecol Obstet. 1982;155(6):823–8.
67. Parikh DH, Leibl M, Tam PK, Edgar D. Abnormal expression and distribution of nidogen in Hirschsprung's disease. J Pediatr Surg. 1995;30(12):1687–93.
68. Parikh DH, Tam PK, Van Velzen D, Edgar D. Abnormalities in the distribution of laminin and collagen type IV in Hirschsprung's disease. Gastroenterology. 1992;102(4 Pt 1):1236–41.
69. Parikh DH, Tam PK, Van Velzen D, Edgar D. The extracellular matrix components, tenascin and fibronectin, in Hirschsprung's disease: an immunohistochemical study. J Pediatr Surg. 1994;29(10):1302–6.
70. Parikh DH, Tam PKH, Lloyd DA, VanVelzen D, Edgar DH. Quantitative and qualitative analysis of the extracellular matrix protein, laminin, in Hirschsprung's disease. J Pediatr Surg. 1992;27:991–6.
71. Park S-Y, Min H, Chi JG, Park KW, Yang H-R, Seo JK. Immunohistochemical studies of pediatric intestinal pseudo-obstruction: bcl2, a valuable biomarker to detect immature ganglion cells. Am J Surg Pathol. 2005;29:1017–24.
72. Piotrowska AP, Solari V, de Caluwe D, Puri P. Immunocolocalization of the heme oxygenase-2 and interstitial cells of Cajal in normal and aganglionic colon. J Pediatr Surg. 2003;38(1):73–7.
73. Puri P, Gosemann JH. Variants of Hirschsprung disease. Semin Pediatr Surg. 2012;21(4):310–8.

74. Ratcliffe EM, deSa DJ, Dixon MF, Stead RH. Choline acetyltransferase (ChAT) immunoreactivity in paraffin sections of normal and diseased intestines. J Histochem Cytochem. 1998;46(11):1223–31.
75. Sams VR, Bobrow LG, Happerfield L, Keeling J. Evaluation of PGP9.5 in the diagnosis of Hirschsprung's disease. J Pathol. 1992;168(1):55–8.
76. Schmittenbecher PP, Sacher P, Cholewa D, Haberlik A, Menardi G, Moczulski J, et al. Hirschsprung's disease and intestinal neuronal dysplasia – a frequent association with implications for the postoperative course. Pediatr Surg Int. 1999;15(8):553–8.
77. Soeda J, O'Briain DS, Puri P. Mucosal neuroendocrine cell abnormalities in the colon of patients with Hirschsprung's disease. J Pediatr Surg. 1992;27(7):823–7.
78. Soeda J, O'Briain DS, Puri P. Regional reduction in intestinal neuroendocrine cell populations in enterocolitis complicating Hirschsprung's disease. J Pediatr Surg. 1993;28(8):1063–8.
79. Swaminathan M, Kapur RP. Counting myenteric ganglion cells in histologic sections: an empirical approach. Hum Pathol. 2010;41(8):1097–108.
80. Swaminathan M, Oron AP, Chatterjee S, Piper H, Cope-Yokoyama S, Chakravarti A, et al. Intestinal neuronal dysplasia-like submucosal ganglion cell hyperplasia at the proximal margins of Hirschsprung disease resections. Pediatr Dev Pathol. 2015;18(6):466–76.
81. Taguchi T, Ieiri S, Miyoshi K, Kohashi K, Oda Y, Kubota A, et al. The incidence and outcome of allied disorders of Hirschsprung's disease in Japan: results from a nationwide survey. Asian J Surg. 2017;40(1):29–34.
82. Taguchi T, Obata S, Ieiri S. Current status of Hirschsprung's disease: based on a nationwide survey of Japan. Pediatr Surg Int. 2017;33(4):497–504.
83. Taguchi T, Suita S, Hirata Y, Hirose R, Yamada T, Toyohara T. Abnormally shaped arteries in the intestine of children with Hirschsprung's disease: etiological considerations related to ischemic theory. J Pediatr Gastroenterol Nutr. 1994;18:200–4.
84. Tam PK. An immunochemical study with neuron-specific-enolase and substance P of human enteric innervation – the normal developmental pattern and abnormal deviations in Hirschsprung's disease and pyloric stenosis. Gastroenterology. 1986;90(6):1901–6.
85. Tani G, Tomuschat C, O'Donnell AM, Coyle D, Puri P. Increased population of immature enteric glial cells in the resected proximal ganglionic bowel of Hirschsprung's disease patients. J Surg Res. 2017;218:150–5.
86. Teitelbaum DH, Caniano DA, Qualman SJ. The pathophysiology of Hirschsprung's-associated enterocolitis: importance of histologic correlates. J Pediatr Surg. 1989;24(12):1271–7.
87. Terra SA, de Arruda Lourencao PL, G Silva M, A Miot H, Rodrigues MAM. A critical appraisal of the morphological criteria for diagnosing intestinal neuronal dysplasia type B. Mod Pathol. 2017;30(7):978–85.
88. Thaker AI, Kapur RP. Colonic adventitial fibromuscular dysplasia: a nonspecific arteriopathy associated with Hirschsprung disease and other obstructive disorders. Pediatr Dev Pathol. 2018;21(4):363–70. https://doi.org/10.1177/1093526617739772.
89. Toledo de Arruda Lourencao PL, Terra SA, Ortolan EV, Rodrigues MA. Intestinal neuronal dysplasia type B: a still little known diagnosis for organic causes of intestinal chronic constipation. World J Gastrointest Pharmacol Ther. 2016;7(3):397–405.
90. Tomuschat C, O'Donnell AM, Coyle D, Dreher N, Kelly D, Puri P. Altered expression of a two-pore domain (K2P) mechano-gated potassium channel TREK-1 in Hirschsprung's disease. Pediatr Res. 2016;80(5):729–33.
91. Tomuschat C, O'Donnell AM, Coyle D, Dreher N, Kelly D, Puri P. Altered expression of ATP-sensitive K(+) channels in Hirschsprung's disease. J Pediatr Surg. 2016;51(6):948–52.
92. Tomuschat C, O'Donnell AM, Coyle D, Dreher N, Kelly D, Puri P. NOS-interacting protein (NOSIP) is increased in the colon of patients with Hirschsprungs's disease. J Pediatr Surg. 2017;52(5):772–7.
93. Tomuschat C, O'Donnell AM, Coyle D, Puri P. Reduced expression of voltage-gated Kv11.1 (hERG) K(+) channels in aganglionic colon in Hirschsprung's disease. Pediatr Surg Int. 2016;32(1):9–16.
94. Tomuschat C, O'Donnell AM, Coyle D, Puri P. Altered expression of IL36gamma and IL36 receptor (IL1RL2) in the colon of patients with Hirschsprung's disease. Pediatr Surg Int. 2017;33(2):181–6.
95. Tomuschat C, O'Donnell AM, Coyle D, Puri P. Reduction of hydrogen sulfide synthesis enzymes cystathionine-beta-synthase and cystathionine-gamma-lyase in the colon of patients with Hirschsprungs's disease. J Pediatr Surg. 2018;53(3):525–30.
96. Vadva Z, Nurko S, Hehn R, Vargas SO. Rectal suction biopsy in patients with previous anorectal surgery for Hirschsprung disease. J Pediatr Gastroenterol Nutr. 2017;65(2):173–8.
97. Vanderwinden J-M, Rumessen JJ, Liu H, Descamps D, De Laet M-H, Vanderhaeghen J-J. Interstitial cells of Cajal in human colon and in Hirschsprung's disease. Gastroenterology. 1996;111:901–10.
98. von Boyen GBT, Krammer H-J, Suss A, Dembowski C, Ehrenreich H, Wedel T. Abnormalities of the enteric nervous system in heterozygous endothelin B receptor deficient (spotting lethal) rats resembling intestinal neuronal dysplasia. Gut. 2002;51(3):414–9.
99. Wang J, Du H, Mou YR, Niu JY, Zhang WT, Yang HC, et al. Abundance and significance of neuroligin-1 and glutamate in Hirschsprung's disease. World J Gastroenterol. 2015;21(23):7172–80.
100. Wang J, Mou Y, Zhang Q, Zhang F, Yang H, Zhang W, et al. Expression and significance of neuroligins in myenteric cells of Cajal in Hirschsprung's disease. PLoS One. 2013;8(6):e67205.
101. Wang JX, Qin P, Liu QL, Yang HY, Fan YZ, Yu JK, et al. Detection and significance of serum

protein marker of Hirschsprung disease. Pediatrics. 2007;120(1):e56–60.
102. Wedel T, Holschneider AM, Krammer H-J. Ultrastructural features of nerve fascicles and basal lamina abnormalities in Hirschsprung disease. Eur J Pediatr Surg. 1999;9:75–82.
103. Wells FE, Addison GM. Acetylcholinesterase activity in rectal biopsies: an assessment of its diagnostic value in Hirschsprung's disease. J Pediatr Gastroenterol Nutr. 1986;5(6):912–9.
104. Wendelschafer-Crabb G, Neppalli V, Jessurun J, Hodges J, Vance K, Saltzman D, et al. Mucosal nerve deficiency in chronic childhood constipation: a postmigration defect? J Pediatr Surg. 2009;44(4):773–82.
105. Yamataka A, Kato Y, Tibboel D, Murata Y, Sueyoshi N, Fujimoto T, et al. A lack of intestinal pacemaker (c-kit) in aganglionic bowel of patients with Hirschsprung's disease. J Pediatr Surg. 1995;30:441–4.
106. Yang H, Niu J, Wang J, Zhang F, Zhang Q, Zhang W, et al. The down-regulation of neuroligin-2 and the correlative clinical significance of serum GABA over-expression in Hirschsprung's disease. Neurochem Res. 2014;39(8):1451–7.

18 Total Colonic Aganglionosis and Very-Long-Segment Hirschsprung's Disease

Samuel William Moore

Contents

18.1 Introduction

Hirschsprung's disease (HSCR) would appear to be part of a spectrum of conditions producing a functional intestinal obstruction and which has aganglionosis of the intermyenteric plexuses in a segment of bowel as a common feature. Although over 75% involves only the rectum and sigmoid colon, the length of the aganglionic segment varies, and long segments (L-HSCR) occur [1]. L-HSCR can probably be divided into colonic aganglionosis, total colonic aganglionosis (TCA), and very-long-segment HSCR (Zuelzer's disease/syndrome) [2]; there are also reports of total bowel aganglionosis [3, 4] which may or may not be familial.

TCA is an uncommon form of HSCR occurring in approximately 2–13% of cases [5, 6] and has long been recognized as presenting particular problems in diagnosis [7, 8] and management [9–12].

TCA has been defined as aganglionosis extending from the anus to at least the ileocecal valve but no more than 50 cm proximal to the ileocecal valve [13] (Fig. 18.1). This differenti-

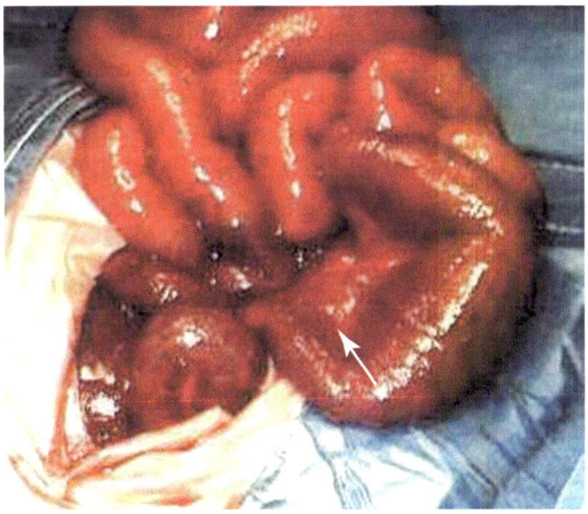

Fig. 18.1 Operative picture of a transition zone (TZ) in the terminal ileum in a familial case. His brother had exactly the same TZ site

S. W. Moore (✉)
Division of Pediatric Surgery, Faculty of Medicine and Health Sciences, University of Stellenbosch, Stellenbosch, South Africa
e-mail: swm@sun.ac.za

P. Puri (ed.), *Hirschsprung's Disease and Allied Disorders*, https://doi.org/10.1007/978-3-030-15647-3_18

ates it from the extended intestinal form, as well as the very rare form of aganglionosis which may stretch from the duodenum to the anus [14, 15], namely, total or near-total aganglionosis or Zuelzer's disease. TCA and extended intestinal aganglionosis are regarded as special problem areas in HSCR but it is not yet completely clear whether separation of these two entities is justified in terms of pathogenesis and biology.

Although being regarded as a special problem in HSCR, TCA and extended intestinal aganglionosis may prove difficult to diagnose, posing certain difficult management problems. Clinically, TCA appears to represent a different spectrum of disease.

Although TCA shares the common feature of aganglionosis with other forms of HSCR, there are a number of differences, which require explanation, if its ubiquitous clinical features are to be understood. Firstly, the mode of presentation is often much later than expected considering the length of the aganglionic segment. One would expect TCA to present early on, which is not always the case. Secondly, there is evidence of significant enteric nervous system (ENS) disruption in TCA that differs from short-segment HSCR (S-HSCR). Solari and Puri [16] have reported a markedly reduced peripherin immunoreactivity, as well as a lack of myenteric interstitial cells of Cajal (ICC-MY) in the smooth muscle layer, and a markedly reduced number of Nicotinamide adenine dinucleotide phosphate (NADPH)-positive nerve trunks in TCA samples. In addition, a moderate hypoplasia of extramural sympathetic innervation has also been reported [16]. This suggests a distinct difference in innervation that is not easily explained, based on increased gene penetrance alone. It is possible that the immature ganglion cells may still be open to being influenced by processes which may still continue after birth such as apoptosis or, alternatively, death of enteric nervous system (ENS) cells [17]. Therefore some degree of postnatal ENS plasticity may contribute to and possibly explain the histological differences observed in this and other studies [16]. The presence of ghost cells in two of our cases might also suggest some ongoing apoptotic process, since DNA migrates from the nucleus in apoptotic cells. This hypothesis appears more logical when the numbers of molecular and cellular changes that underlie ENS development are considered [18–20]. Support for this hypothesis also comes from experiments showing early death of neural crest cells in the Sox10(Dom)/Sox10(Dom) experimental murine animal [17] and suggests a genetic cause. Thirdly, although the genetics of TCA are not yet completely understood, the RET proto-oncogene appears to be the most important of the candidate susceptibility genes, as opposed to the more complicated etiology of the recto-sigmoid disease. Other modifying genetic influences may well play a part in determining the final phenotypic expression. It would appear that the genetic profile in TCA might offer essential clues regarding the reasons for such a long aganglionic segment in these patients. Although the endothelin-B receptor (EDNRB) gene, which provides instructions for making a protein called endothelin receptor type-B connection, remains intriguing [17], other genes such as glial cell line-derived neurotrophic factor (GDNF)/Neurturin (NTN) may well play a part [21].

18.1.1 Etiology

It is generally accepted that HSCR is a genetic condition resulting from aberrant colonization of the enteric nervous system (ENS) neuroblasts during development [22]. HSCR is characterized as a sex-linked heterogonous disorder with variable severity and incomplete penetrance [23], giving rise to a variable pattern of inheritance. The variability observed in the penetrance and severity of Hirschsprung's disease suggests a role for modifier genes with possible interaction with the central RET proto-oncogene variations (see the section on genetic associations). This is of particular relevance in the subject of total colonic aganglionosis and other extended forms of HSCR.

18.1.2 Diagnosis of TCA

The diagnosis of TCA requires careful physical examination, along with some special tests, to

Table 18.1 Clinical, radiological, and histopathological feature of 22 patients with TCA

Symptom	No. of patients
Failure to pass meconium	22
Intestinal obstruction	10
Enterocolitis	2
Failure to thrive	2
Family history	9
MEN association	2
Radiology: normal	1
Stricture sigmoid	2
Histology: unclear	5
Histology revised >1 month	3

help diagnose Hirschsprung's disease. The clinical, radiological, and histopathological features are depicted in Table 18.1 [24].

18.1.3 Clinical Features of TCA

TCA does not infrequently differ clinically from other HSCR phenotypes, and this may lead to misdiagnosis [24]. Although TCA shares the common feature of aganglionosis with HSCR, there are a number of differences which require explanation, if its ubiquitous clinical features are to be understood. The first issue relates to whether TCA merely represents a long form of HSCR or a different expression of the disease. Alternatively, it may represent different pathophysiologic mechanisms that may continue to be active after birth. Exploration of these pathophysiologic mechanisms could contribute to understanding the late presentation of TCA patients who present later than anticipated considering the severity of disease.

The first issue relates to the mode of presentation that is often much later than expected considering the length of the aganglionic segment.

We previously reported nine (27%) of those with TCA presenting outside the NN period (eight presenting >6 months and two (2%) >12 months) [25], in keeping with other studies [25–29]. There are also a number of reports of TCA presenting as late as adolescence and early adulthood [27–29]. This therefore suggests an exceptional pathophysiology, which differs from the more common shorter-segment forms of HSCR.

Infants with TCA usually begin having symptoms during the first 24–48 hours of life. While infants may experience a range of symptoms, the following are the most common:

- Delay in onset of bowel movement in the first 48 hours of life
- Gradual abdominal distention
- Onset of vomiting
- Small, watery stools
- Possible signs of fever and sepsis (occasionally an overwhelming infection)
- Constipation that increases over time
- Transition zone may/may not be seen at surgery (Fig. 18.1)

Although extensive disease would suggest a severe clinical picture, with early presentation, and although most present within the first few weeks of life [30], a number of late-presenting TCA cases have been reported [27–29], even as adolescents and adults, suggesting that the process may differ from the more common form of short-segment Hirschsprung's disease (HSCR).

18.1.4 Special Investigations

Special investigations include both radiological and histological evaluations.

18.1.4.1 Radiological Features

Special radiological investigations include an abdominal X-ray and a contrast enema.

Abdominal X-Ray

A plain abdominal radiograph may show an obstructive pattern of abdominal bowel gas and multiple air-fluid levels in TCA. The presence of small bowel obstruction without colonic distension suggests a possible TCA diagnosis if other clinical and radiological features are present.

Contrast Enema

A contrast enema assists in evaluating abnormalities in the large intestine (colon). It may show an abnormal featureless colon often described as a "lead pipe" picture. There is usually no transition zone, a normal recto-sigmoid ratio index, and possible reflux of contrast into a dilated ileum [31]. The identification of a transitional zone may be difficult with false transition zones being reported in the sigmoid [10]. The sensitivity and specificity of a contrast enema in the diagnosis of standard HSCR are reported as being 76% and 97%, respectively [32] (Fig. 18.2). However, the diagnosis of TCA on contrast enema may be misleading, and difficulties in interpretation may be encountered, particularly in newborn infants. A lack of consistency in the radiological findings has been observed in this group for a long time [10] as it may be influenced by the length of small bowel involvement. The identification of a transition zone on contrast enema may be as low as 25% in TCA [33]. Early studies suggested that the retention of barium >24 hours was strongly suggestive [10, 34]. In a more recent study [35], three types of radiological pictures were observed in TCA, namely, the presence of a microcolon as well as the question mark-shaped colon and the lack of features in an otherwise normal colon.

Our own study showed that retention of barium on delayed film was observed in most cases. A featureless microcolon may be present, or alternatively, a normal-sized colon with abnormal irregular contractions may be observed, and it may be associated with shortening of the colon and lack of redundancy. However, the TCA colon may appear normal on contrast studies and the diagnosis of TCA must be entertained if clinical symptoms of obstruction persist in the absence of any other known causes.

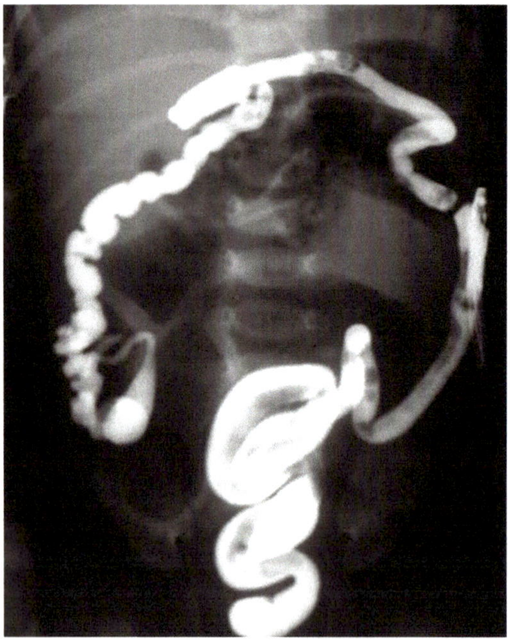

Fig. 18.2 Contrast enema in a patient with TCA. Note the microcolon and an otherwise normal (unused) colon. The background small bowel obstruction provides the clue of a TCA

18.1.4.2 Histological Features

A rectal biopsy is required to establish the diagnosis of Hirschsprung's disease and aganglionosis. The HSCR diagnosis is confirmed if no ganglion cells are seen. If total colonic Hirschsprung's disease is suspected, multiple biopsies are carried out to determine the extent of the disease. These biopsies may be performed at the time of ileostomy as full-thickness biopsies of the intestinal wall.

Whereas histological diagnosis proved to be generally reliable on rectal biopsy in the majority of HSCR cases, there may be differences in the histological features of TCA.

In our patient sample [24], difficulties were experienced in interpreting the histology in 4 of the 22 TCA cases studied (18%). In two of these, the transition zone was mistaken for frozen section due to the presence of abnormal cells, leading to reoperation in those patients. These findings are not unusual, as abnormal bowel innervation and ganglion cells have been reported in TCA, also being associated with a moderate hypoplasia of extramural sympathetic innervation [16]. The histological differences reported by Solari and Puri [16] included a markedly reduced peripherin immunoreactivity in TCA samples, a lack of myenteric interstitial cells of Cajal (ICCs-MY) in the smooth muscle layer, and a markedly reduced number of NADPH-positive nerve trunks. These observations, along with degenerating ganglion cells observed in our study, suggest that a hypothesis of involvement of possible alternative signaling pathways is not without scientific basis. In addition, the presence of a long hypoganglionic segment and increased immaturity of cells reported in some animal models [36] has not been proven, although suspected in humans, which may have an influence on post-surgical outcome.

18.1.5 Risk Factors for TCA

Some cases of Hirschsprung's disease are linked to a genetic (inherited) cause. There is an increased chance (3–12%) of recurrence in a family with HSCR. The increased HSCR risk is higher if one of the parents has the condition, especially if the mother is affected.

On the genetic front, Edery et al. [37] presented strong evidence that both short-segment and long-segment types are fundamentally the same disorder caused by mutations in the RET gene. Although the role of RET in short-segment disease has proved to be more complicated, RET mutations remain the main cause of long-segment disease. It is interesting that both long-segment and short-segment HSCR can occur in the same family and is associated with increased penetrance in the longer form.

Iwashita et al. [38] introduced five HSCR mutations into the extracellular domain of human RET cDNA and concluded that sufficient levels of RET expression on the cell surface are required for migration of ganglia toward the distal portion of the colon or for full differentiation. Hofstra et al. [39] pointed out that mutations of the RET, GDNF, EDNRB, and Endothelin 3 (EDN3) genes may be responsible for dominant, recessive, or polygenic patterns of inheritance. Mutations in RET, GDNF, EDNRB, EDN3, and SOX10 have all been shown to lead to long-segment Hirschsprung's disease and syndromic HSCR but fail to explain the transmission of the much more common short-segment form (S-HSCR).

In addition to an increased HSCR risk, there is a significantly increased incidence of TCA in families which have recurrence of aganglionosis in family members [6]. In our series, we reported TCA and Zuelzer's disease in three families with increasing gene penetrance [24]. Thus it is not unexpected, and cases with more extensive involvement are more likely to be because of familial inheritance [40] [Fig. 18.3a, b] shows the significantly ($p < 0.01$) higher prevalence in familial vs. non-familial cases].

18.2 Developmental Etiology of Hirschsprung's Disease

One of the areas of advancing knowledge is in our understanding of how the enteric nervous system forms during fetal development. Hirschsprung's disease results from a disturbance of the normal ENS development resulting in the lack of normal ganglion cells in the myenteric plexuses. As a result, there is a functional loss of coordinated peristalsis, leading to a functional intestinal obstruction, as occurs in HSCR.

The ENS originates from neural crest-derived cells that undergo aboral migration in the gut following the vagal pathways. The role of a second sacral inflow of neural cells [41] appears to be uncertain. Early studies showed that the migration of neuroblasts in the vagal trunk begins at about week 5 of embryonic life and progresses down the gut and reaches the rectum by week 12 [42]. The more recent work of Fu et al. [43] showed an earlier migration of vagal neuroblasts, which colonize the entire gut in a rostrocaudal manner between week 4 and week 7 of embryonic life.

As they migrate, the enteric neuroblasts undergo key developmental processes such as migration, proliferation, survival, and differentiation, differentiating into at least 14 different classes of cells that make up the ENS [44, 45]. These neuroblasts then form definable intramural ganglia collections by perpendicular migrations within the gut wall [41]. The ENS then develops into the complex interconnecting network of neurons and glial cells that regulate motility, sensory response, secretion, and blood flow within the Gastro-intestinal tract (GIT) [46]. This development of the ENS relies on coordinated interactions between neural crest-derived neuroblasts, the controlling signaling pathways, and developmental processes (e.g., maturation, survival) to coordinate a normal ENS development. They are under the molecular control of a number of interdependent signaling pathways, transcription, and neurotrophic factors that interact with the extra-

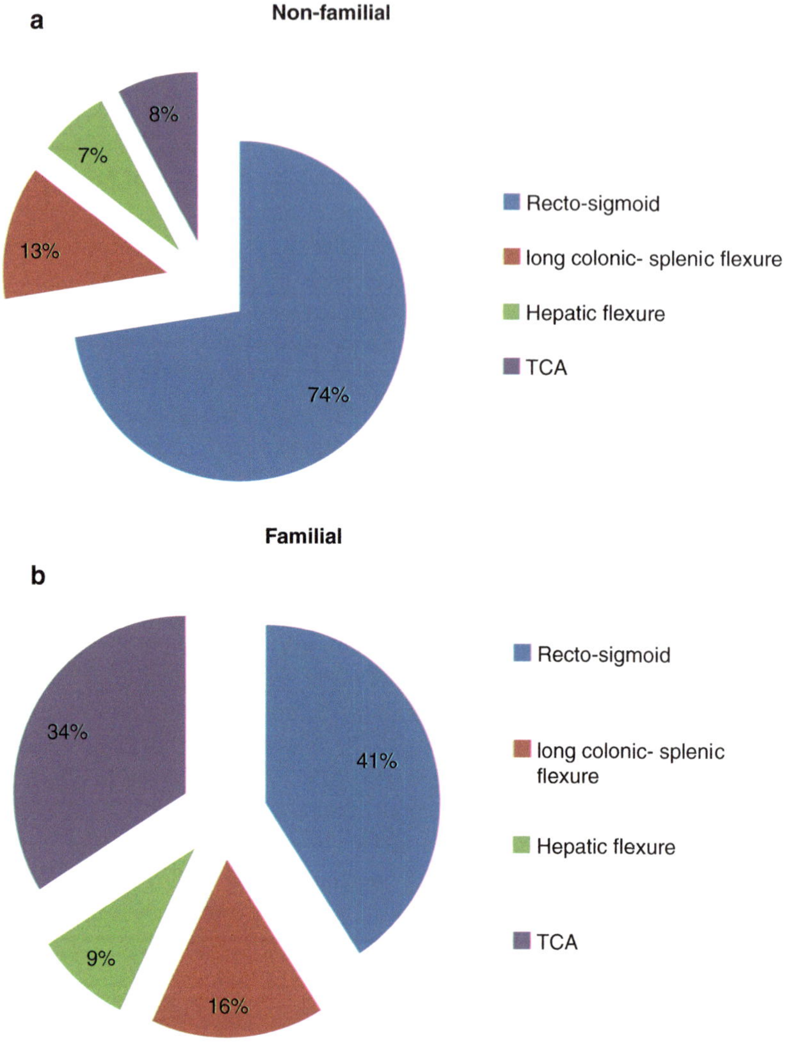

Fig. 18.3 (**a**) Pie graph showing the proportion of patients with TCA as opposed to other aganglionic lengths in non-familial cases. (**b**) Pie graph showing the significant ($p < 0.05$) TCA increase in familial cases as opposed to other aganglionic lengths

cellular matrix components to form a functional ENS. Defective molecular signaling during this developmental process results in maldevelopment and functional conditions such as Hirschsprung's disease.

18.3 Genetic Associations of TCA

There is strong evidence of a genetic connection in TCA and an association exists between TCA and an increased risk of recurrence in families [6, 47]. A previous study showed a significant 15–21% recurrence in families with long-segment aganglionosis, particularly in patients with TCA ($p < 0.01$) [6]. The risk of recurrence reaches more than 50% prevalence in patients with ultra-long-segment aganglionosis (Zuelzer's disease) (Fig. 18.4). In addition, a progression of the length of segment to TCA and Zuelzer's disease was reported in succeeding generations in certain affected families. A complex segregation analysis of data on 487 probands and their families concluded that the sex ratio decreased and the recurrence risk to siblings increased as the length of aganglionosis increased [23].

Although the genetic profile of TCA is not yet completely clear, RET has been identified as the main susceptibility gene of TCA as opposed to the more involved pathogenesis of short-segment aganglionosis [48].

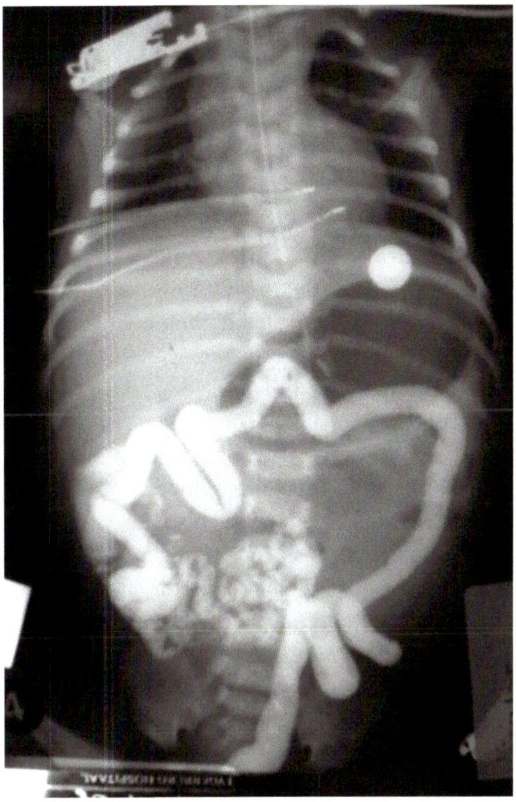

Fig. 18.4 Contrast enema of a patient with extensive small bowel aganglionosis in addition to TCA. Note the small caliber of the ileum proximal to the cecum

The first report, linking a mutation of the rearranged during transfection (RET) gene by Martucciello et al. [49], identified TCA in a patient with a proximal deletion of chromosome 10q, del(10)(q11.21q21.2). This report was followed up in a study by Lyonnet et al. [50], who reported genetic linkage analysis of 15 non-syndromic long-segment HSCR patients, making use of a high-density genetic map of microsatellite DNA markers, indicating a likely location for a HSCR locus between D10S208 and D10S196. This suggested a dominant gene mapping to 10q11.2, a region already mapped for other neural crest defects. An association between total colonic aganglionosis and a 10q deletion, del (10) (q11.2q21.2), was then reported [51]. Further homozygous pathogenic RET variants have been associated with total colonic aganglionosis in some cases [21, 52]. Shimotake et al. [53] then reported a RET mutation in the terminal tyrosine kinase (TK) region in a child with total colonic aganglionosis.

Having said that the RET proto-oncogene mutations are the most likely pathogenetic mechanisms in TCA, current research and animal models suggest possible additional modifying signaling pathways involved in its pathogenesis. Examples of this include EDNRB [54, 55] and patients with Phosphate repressible alkaline phosphatase 2 B (PHOX2B) mutations [56], Glial cell drived neurotrophic factor (GDNF) and NTN [21], and SOX10 [57]. In our own study [24] RET variations were detected in 82% of TCA patients as opposed to 33% of patients with s-HSCR, with multiple genetic RET variations in 28% (5/22). Genetic variations included exon 2 Single nucleotide polymorphism (SNP) but less in short-segment HSCR (S-HSCR). One patient had an isolated RET A45 variation with no other abnormalities. Intronic RET variations occurred in introns 6 (2), viz., [IVS6 + 56delG], and intron 16 (two patients) [IVS16-38delG]. A cysteine radical mutation (C620R) (two patients) was related to Multiple endocrine neoplasia 2 (MEN) in a family. In contrast to S-HSCR, genetic variations in TCA aggregated to the important tyrosine kinase (intracellular) region in five patients suggesting a possible pathogenetic link. EDNRB variations occurred in seven patients (32%) all within exon 4 of the gene [24].

Potential disease-related RET gene mutations include genetic variations in the exon 17–21 tyrosine kinase area, which suggest the possibility of disrupted downstream signaling pathways from vital gene recruitment sites as possible TCA contributing factors. It is not yet clear whether TCA merely represents a long form of HSCR or a different expression of the disease, but its nature suggests a different pathophysiology from the more common forms of HSCR.

The following table shows the results of analysis of the RET proto-oncogene in 22 patients with TCA [24] (Table 18.2).

Table 18.2 RET gene variations in HSCR patients and controls

	A45	G691S	C620 W	L769	S904	R928	P973L
S-HSCR ($n = 69$)	50 (73%)	0	0	33 (48%)	37 (50%)	11 (8%)	0
L-HSCR ($n = 21$)	13 (62%)	0	0	10 (50%)	13 (62%)	5 (25%)	0
TCA ($n = 22$)	7 (32%)	1	2 (9%)	7 (32%)	2 (9%)	6 (27%)	1 (4%)
Controls ($n = 60$)	24 (40%)	0	0	12 (20%)	9 (15%)	0	0

18.3.1 Intronic Variations

- IVS6 + 56delG(he) 2 TCA; 2 S-HSCR
- IVS16-38delG(he) 1 TCA
- IVS10-2A/G(he) S-HSCR
- IVS19-9C/T(he) S-HSCR

Identified genetic variations in TCA include deletions, frameshifts, and missense mutations as well as a number of significant SNP variations. Transmitted RET mutations occurred in 5 of 16 kindreds (30%). Splice RET mutation (IVS1) plus variants of exon 17 (973L) affected children with identical TCA. In a three-generation family, variations in RET exon 6, 13, and 18 (928) affected three male children with increasing penetration to recur as total intestinal aganglionosis.

There is, however, increasing evidence that disturbance of downstream RET-related signaling pathways influences the HSCR phenotypic expression. It is interesting that although potential disease-related RET mutations were present in the majority of TCA patients investigated in our study [24], the RET genetic variation appeared to be less consistent. In five of them, the extent of RET gene variations was combined with a clustering of genetic variations to the tyrosine kinase (TK) intracellular portion of the RET gene (particularly exons 17–21). As far as we are aware, this was the first linking of these sites to extensive aganglionosis and TCA. There are cases of HSCR with the only RET mutation being in the TK region, which suggests that the position of the RET genetic variations may be as important as their extent in order to understand the pathogenetic mechanisms involved.

These sites in the intracellular TK region appear to be vital to the RET tyrosine kinase function as well as downstream signaling due to the number of signaling molecules that interact there [e.g., Shc, Src, FRS2, IRS1, Gab1/2, and Enigma]. In addition, the intracellular portion of the RET gene is activated by binding to a ligand complex formed by the glial cell line-derived neurotrophic factor (GDNF) [58] and its ligand co-receptor, the GDNF-family receptor-alpha (GFR alpha) receptors. GDNF has not only been shown to stimulate the differentiation of neuronal cells during development but also appears to prevent cellular apoptosis, protecting against neurodegeneration [59]. Gene variation at or close to this site may therefore interfere with vital functions leading to more extensive disease.

Because of the involved nature of the genetic background to HSCR and TCA, the hypothesis has been advanced that although RET is central to its cause, other genes interact with related signaling pathways which determine the eventual phenotypic expression [60]. In addition, the relevance of individual variations has brought the whole field of bioinformatics into play, and there is much to do to show how the various genetic mutation/variation affects.

A further issue is whether the genetic profile offers clues as to the reasons for the different pathogenesis in patients with TCA. In general, HSCR is widely regarded as a genetic, sex-modified, multifactorial condition with variable severity and incomplete penetrance of a number of genes (at least nine). RET and EDNRB remain the two major susceptibility genes, with RET being the most important in TCA. Although potential disease-related RET mutations were present in the majority of patients investigated in this study, the genetic variation appeared to be more severe in five, suggesting that increased gene penetrance may account for many TCA phenotypes. There is, however, increasing evidence that disturbances of downstream RET-related signaling pathways may influence the phenotypic expression. It is in this context that further signaling modification by aberrant downstream pathways remains a strong possibility.

The genetics of TCA are not completely clear although the RET proto-oncogene has been identified as the main susceptibility gene, being associated with the first classic description of RET in association with HSCR [49]. Heterogeneity of RET proto-oncogene has also been well established in autosomal dominant forms of HSCR [61].

The position of the genetic variations on the RET gene may also influence other signaling pathways creating the resultant phenotype. Other animal knockout (KO) models mostly have total intestinal aganglionosis, although TCA has been reported in the Dominant megacolon mouse (Dom) along with a long hypoganglionic transition zone [62].

In a fairly recent study, the clustering of genetic variations to the intracellular portion of the RET gene (particularly exons 17–21) suggests the possible involvement of other signaling pathways that bind to receptors on those sites. In keeping with the histological findings of degenerating cells and "ghost" cells, this suggests some ongoing apoptotic process, since apoptotic cells are thought to result in migration of DNA from the nucleus.

In addition to what is known, new previously unknown mechanisms are currently being identified, whereby the recruitment of phosphotyrosine-binding domain-containing adaptor proteins appear to mediate different downstream RET-related functions [63]. These appear to act by relocating RET receptor complexes to lipid rafts, thereby promoting downstream signaling and RET-mediated cellular functions. Experimental with fairly minor genetic variations in this region have been shown to redirect adaptor protein pathways which may lead to a decrease in cell survival [63]. As a result, the fact that genetic variation in this area may well lead to the non-survival and subsequent apoptosis or degeneration of cells could form a hypothesis for TCA pathogenesis and a potential reason for the late degenerative cellular features of cells noted in certain TCA cases.

18.4 Animal Models of TCA

Animal models have made major contributions to our understanding of HSCR by both the study of the developmental processes that contribute to ENS development in animal models and the study of ENS changes in Hirschsprung's disease.

Historically, there are a number of good examples of animal models of HSCR. These include both murine [e.g., the lethal spotting mouse (point mutation EDN3), piebald lethal mice (SL) (absent EDNRB)] and rodent [e.g., spotting lethal rat (301 bp EDNRB del) and Dominant megacolon (Dom) (point mutation SOX10)]. Although early animal models had limited aganglionic lengths [64, 65], the spotting lethal rat showed two lengths of aganglionosis, i.e., mid-colon and TCA. These animals had autosomal recessive inheritance. The spotting lethal rat has an endothelin-B receptor (EDNRB) gene deletion that prevents functional EDNRB receptor expression. Since then, numerous knockout (KO) models have been developed which include the RET ligands GDNF, GFRα1-2, and Neurturin, those affecting the endothelin pathway (e.g., EDN3, ECE-1, and EDNRB) and the hedgehog pathways (Indian Hedgehog pathway (IHH) and Sonic Hedgehog pathway (SHH)). Those gene knockout models affecting the RET ligands GDNF and GFRα tended to produce total intestinal aganglionosis along with those related to SOX10, PHOX 2B, and PAX3. Only the sl rodent model (EDNRB −/−) produced TCA fairly consistently.

Nagahama et al. [66, 67] investigated those sl rats which had a constricted segment of intestine extending from the dilated distal ileum to the rectum, very similar to TCA in humans. Furthermore, histologic evaluation of these rats showed a paucity of myenteric and submucosal nerve fibers in the affected intestine, while bundles of irregular nerve fibers without ganglion cells were present in the circular muscle layer of the mid- to distal colon [66, 68].

Ultrastructural electron microscopy confirmed these findings in this animal model [67]. One of the interesting features of this particular strain of rodent is that, in the sl model, groups of ganglion cells may be visualized on NADPH immunostaining in the distal "aganglionic" bowel, usually associated with increased nerve fibers. Genetic mutations in these animal models result in developmental defects in neural crest cell migration, differentiation, or survival. Even in the ileum, the cells remain immature [36]. Transgenic expression has been shown to be able to prevent aganglionosis in these animals [55]. More severe ENS defects are associated with double SOX10 mutants, but no apoptosis, cell proliferation, or overall neuronal or glial differentiation defects in neural crest cells were observed. Increased apoptosis was observed in non-ENS vagal neural crest cells [69].

The PHOX2B transcription factor appears to be an essential component of the normal development of the autonomic nervous system, being essential for normal neurogenesis. Among other things, it regulates RET expression. Malfunction of PHOX2B gene results in a Hirschsprung-like phenotype.

It is well known that a balanced, coordinated interaction between Sox10 and EDNRB has been shown to be necessary for normal ENS development. The development of the ENS in the colon appears to be specifically related to EDN3 activity [70]. In a study on 14 HSCR patients, Oue and Puri [71] identified both altered EDN3 and EDNRB mRNA levels in 2 of the 14 cases. In six cases, EDN3 mRNA expression was reduced in the aganglionic segment, and EDNRB mRNA expression was reduced but did not differ from controls in the remaining four cases.

Kapur [17] concluded from studies on the Dom animal model that the underlying defect is an increase in neural crest cell apoptosis early in their development rather than defects in the enteric microenvironment, as the Sox10(Dom)/Sox10(Dom) intestine has been shown to support wild-type neural crest cell colonization and neuronal differentiation.

This suggests difference in the genetic mechanisms in the pathogenesis of aganglionosis, as well as the role of apoptosis in TCA (possibly Sox10 related).

It has been shown recently that diminished RET expression compromises neuronal survival in the colon and causes intestinal aganglionosis in mice suggesting once again that apoptotic mechanisms may be important [72].

18.5 Treatment of TCA

TCA has long been recognized as presenting particular problems in diagnosis and management [24]. In terms of management, TCA can be divided into separate clinical groups. The more frequent total colonic aganglionosis (TCA) type, where the aganglionosis extends from the anus to <50 cm beyond the ileocecal valve into the small bowel, is one group which is easier to manage and can expect reasonable outcome. A second longer type where total colonic and extensive small bowel aganglionosis (TCSA) exists is much more challenging as it may involve a very long segment of aganglionosis (sometimes referred to as Zuelzer's disease).

Although the initial management of HSCR usually involves rectal irrigations, which assist in treating the obstruction and preventing enterocolitis, this does not always work for patients with TCA. Most patients therefore require an intestinal defunctioning stoma (ileostomy), surgically performed in ganglionated bowel. Decompression is important, as patients with TCA are more likely to develop enterocolitis.

It is widely accepted that surgery is the best treatment in all cases of Hirschsprung's disease including TCA. However, the length of the affected segment has a major influence on the surgical approach. As in other HSCR forms, definitive surgery involves the identification and removal of the aganglionic segment and the normally innervated intestine being identified and pulled down to be surgically attached to the anus. However, in TCA, anastomotic modification may be required, depending on the length of intestinal involvement.

A number of special problems may present themselves due to the length of the bowel involved. As a result, many different surgical techniques have been utilized for TCA [12, 73, 74] with outcomes mostly related to the type of surgical technique performed. Many surgeons now accept a modification of the Duhamel procedure as the best option in TCA in terms of long-term function [75].

18.6 An Extended Transition Zone?

Many of the HSCR animal models demonstrate an extended transition zone or region of hypoganglionosis. TCA has been reported in the Dominant megacolon mouse (Dom) along with a long hypoganglionic transition zone [62]. These cells may also remain immature beyond an age when they should be mature [36]. This is also reported in the murine-16 animal model of DS-HSCR [76]. The presence of a long hypoganglionic segment and increased immaturity of cells reported in these animal models [36] has not been proven, although suspected in humans, and this may have an influence on postsurgical outcome.

18.6.1 TCA Outcome

Many different surgical techniques have been utilized for TCA [12, 73, 74] with outcomes mostly related to the type of surgical technique performed. In the main, the outcome in the more frequent form with a limited small bowel involvement is acceptable.

A modification of the Duhamel procedure is widely regarded as the best option in these cases of TCA in terms of long-term function [75]. Tsuji et al. [73] reported on the long-term outcome of 48 patients managed over a 17-year period (1980 to 1996). Mortality was 6% (3/48), two being due to associated major congenital anomalies. Of the 41 patients who underwent a pull-through procedure in this series, 27 could be followed up in terms of outcome and function. A permanent stoma was necessary in six patients (two with Down's syndrome). Ten patients underwent anal dilatations and six had an additional sphincterotomy. A further two required resection of the side-to-side anastomosis for intractable diarrhea. The number of the stools per day, although initially high, was noted to decrease with time. Fecal incontinence improved with time, and at 10 and 15 years, the rate of incontinence was considerably improved. Growth and development were delayed, with 25% of patients being below the second percentile for body weight at 5 years, 20% at 10 years, and 63% at 15 years. Similar long-term follow-up reports were produced by Escobar et al. [75], Menezes et al. [77], and Yeh et al. [78], and they also reported good long-term follow-up results in 36, 58, and 9 patients, respectively.

Despite acceptable overall results, a mortality of up to 22% has been reported, mostly in patients with extensive disease and associated anomalies. Enterocolitis remains a problem as it may persist after surgery, in up to 55.4% in the early stages. Although the risk of enterocolitis decreases with age, caregivers should always be alert to its signs and symptoms, due to its dangers.

Most cases require some dietary adjustments and/or medication to control stool frequency, especially in the early stages. Patients with total colonic Hirschsprung's disease have an ileostomy for many months and sometimes years. These patients need to be followed closely for growth and watched carefully for dehydration. Patients can lose water and sodium through ileostomy and often need to take an oral sodium supplement.

Weight gain may remain a clinical problem in the long term. Nevertheless, up to 83% of patients were reported as exhibiting weight gain of at least 25% of their expected weight in the long term. Short bowel syndrome developed in up to 22%, because of the long aganglionic segment.

Only 53% of patients who were old enough for evaluation had early continence and normal bowel control. This was associated with an average 5.2 bowel movements per day. The continence rate improved in most studies as the stool frequency reduced to a mean of approximately 3.4 stools per day by 15 years. Should problems continue, an additional surgical technique, the Kimura colon patch graft, has been shown to be of value for "ileostomy diarrhea" and extended aganglionosis or hypoganglionosis [79].

18.7 Genetic Counseling and Prevention

Genetic factors are known to be implicated in HSCR pathogenesis. However, the pattern of inheritance remains unclear and variable. Mendelian inheritance occurs, with autosomal dominant, recessive, and multigenic patterns all being reported. This is not entirely surprising as HSCR is known to be a complex condition involving a multifactorial and multigenic etiology.

Pedigree analysis alone is a particularly difficult basis for genetic counseling in a multifactorial condition such as HSCR and may depend on a number of unrelated factors such as small family size, poor history, and the possibility of adoption into a family. Despite recent advances in understanding its molecular background, practical therapeutic interventions are still very limited. Should a major genetic defect be detected in a particular family, the door is open for fetal genetic testing and evaluation of risk.

Acknowledgments This work is based on the research supported in part by the National Research Foundation and the Medical Research Council of South Africa.

References

1. Kaiser G, Bettex M. Disorders and congenital malformations associated with Hirschsprungs disease. In: Holschneider AM, editor. Hirschsprung's disease. 1st ed. Stuttgart: Hipokrates-Verlag; 1982. p. 49–53.
2. Zuelzer WW, Wilson JL. Functional intestinal obstruction on a congenital neurogenic basis in infancy. Am J Dis Child. 1948;75:40–64.
3. Caniano DA, Ormsbee HS, Polito W, Sun CC, Baronne FC, Hill JL. Total intestinal aganglionosis. J Pediatr Surg. 1985;20:456–60.
4. Moore SW. Total colonic aganglionosis and Hirschsprung's disease: a review. Pediatr Surg Int. 2015;31(1):1–9.
5. Cass D, Myers N. Total colonic aganglionosis: 30 years experience. Pediatr Surg Int. 1987;2:68–75.
6. Moore SW, Rode H, Millar AJ, Albertyn R, Cywes S. Familial aspects of Hirschsprungs disease. Eur J Pediatr Surg. 1991;1:97–107.
7. Davies MR, Cywes S, Rode H. The manometric evaluation of the rectosphincteric reflex in total colonic aganglionosis. J Pediatr Surg. 1981;16(5):660–3.
8. Festen C, Severijnen RS, vd Staak F, Rieu PN. Total colonic aganglionosis: treatment and follow-up. Z Kinderchir. 1988;4:153–5.
9. Bodian M, Carter CO, Ward BCH. Hirschsprungs disease. Lancet. 1951;i:302–9.
10. Louw JH. Total colonic aganglionosis. Can J Surg. 1971;21:397–405.
11. Freeman NV. Long segment Hirschsprungs disease. Proc Roy Soc Med. 1971;64:30–2.
12. Martin LW. Surgical management of total colonic aganglionosis. Ann Surg. 1972;176:343–6.
13. Hoehner JC, Ein SH, Shandling B, Kim PC. Long-term morbidity in total colonic aganglionosis. J Pediatr Surg. 1998;33(7):961–5.
14. Senyuz OF, Buyukunal C, Danismend N, Erdogan E, Ozbay G, Soylet Y. Extensive intestinal aganglionosis. J Pediatr Surg. 1989;24(5):453–6.
15. Sharif K, Beath SV, Kelly DA, McKiernan P, van Mourik I, Mirza D, et al. New perspective for the management of near-total or total intestinal aganglionosis in infants. J Pediatr Surg. 2003;38(1):25–8.
16. Solari V, Ennis S, Yoneda A, Wong L, Messineo A, Hollwarth ME, et al. Mutation analysis of the RET gene in total intestinal aganglionosis by wave DNA fragment analysis system. J Pediatr Surg. 2003;38(3):497–501.
17. Kapur RP. Hirschsprung disease and other enteric dysganglionoses. Crit Rev Clin Lab Sci. 1999;36(3):225–73.
18. Meyrat BJ, Laurini RN. Plasticity of the enteric nervous system in patients with intestinal neuronal dysplasia associated with Hirschsprung's disease: a report of three patients. Pediatr Surg Int. 2003;19(11):715–20.
19. Turrigiano GG, Nelson SB. Homeostatic plasticity in the developing nervous system. Nat Rev Neurosci. 2004;5(2):97–107.
20. von Boyen GB, Krammer HJ, Suss A, Dembowski C, Ehrenreich H, Wedel T. Abnormalities of the enteric nervous system in heterozygous endothelin B receptor deficient (spotting lethal) rats resembling intestinal neuronal dysplasia. Gut. 2002;51(3):414–9.
21. Inoue K, Shimotake T, Iwai N. Mutational analysis of RET/GDNF/NTN genes in children with total colonic aganglionosis with small bowel involvement. Am J Med Genet. 2000;93(4):278–84.
22. Meijers J, van der Sanden MP, Tibboel D, van der Kamp AW, Luider TM, Molenaar JC. Colonization characteristics of enteric neural crest cells: embryological aspects of Hirschsprung's disease. J Pediatr Surg. 1992;27(7):811–4.
23. Badner JA, Sieber WK, Garver KL, Chakravarti A. A genetic study of Hirschsprung disease. Am J Hum Genet. 1990;46:568–80.
24. Moore SW. Total colonic aganglionosis and Hirschsprung's disease: shades of the same or different? Pediatr Surg Int. 2009;25(8):659–66.
25. Moore SW, Albertyn R, Cywes S. Clinical outcome and long term quality of life after surgical correction of Hirschsprungs disease. J Pediatr Surg. 1996;31(11):1496–502.

26. Anupama B, Zheng S, Xiao X. Ten-year experience in the management of total colonic aganglionosis. J Pediatr Surg. 2007;42(10):1691–6.
27. Lefebvre MP, Leape LL, Pohl DA, Safaii H, Grand RJ. Total colonic aganglionosis initially diagnosed in an adolescent. Gastroenterology. 1984;87(6):1364–6.
28. Lall A, Agarwala S, Bhatnagar V, Gupta AK, Mitra DK. Total colonic aganglionosis: diagnosis and management in a 12-year-old boy. J Pediatr Surg. 1999;34(9):1413–4.
29. Myers MB, Bradburn D, Vela R, Payzant A, Karlin S. Total aganglionic colon in an adult: first reported case. Ann Surg. 1966;163(1):97–102.
30. Ikeda K, Goto S. Additional anomalies in Hirschsprungs disease: an analysis based on a nationwide survey in Japan. Z Kinderchir. 1986;41:279–81.
31. Hayakawa K, Hamanaka Y, Suzuki M, Nakatsu M, Nishimura K, Tanaka M, et al. Radiological findings in total colon aganglionosis and allied disorders. Radiat Med. 2003;21(3):128–34.
32. De Lorijn F, Reitsma JB, Voskuijl WP, Aronson DC, Ten Kate FJ, Smets A, et al. Diagnosis of Hirschsprung's disease: a prospective, comparative accuracy study of common tests. J Pediatr. 2005;146(6):787–92.
33. Jamieson DH, Dundas SE, Belushi SA, Cooper M, Blair GK. Does the transition zone reliably delineate aganglionic bowel in Hirschsprung's disease? Pediatr Radiol. 2004;34(10):811–5.
34. Berdon WE, Koontz P, Baker D. The diagnosis of colonic and terminal ileal aganglionosis. Am J Roentgenol Radium Therapy, Nucl Med. 1964;91:680–9.
35. Stranzinger E, Dipietro MA, Teitelbaum DH, Strouse PJ. Imaging of total colonic Hirschsprung disease. Pediatr Radiol. 2008;38(11):1162–70.
36. Horigome F, Seki T, Kobayashi H, Ozaki T, Yamataka A. Developmental anomalies of the enteric nervous system in normoganglionic segments of bowel from rats with total colonic aganglionosis. Pediatr Surg Int. 2007;23(10):991–5.
37. Edery P, Eng C, Munnich A, Lyonnet S. RET in human development and oncogenesis. BioEssays. 1997;19(5):389–95.
38. Iwashita T, Murakami H, Asai N, Takahashi M. Mechanism of ret dysfunction by Hirschsprung mutations affecting its extracellular domain. Hum Mol Genet. 1996;5(10):1577–80.
39. Hofstra RM, Fattoruso O, Quadro L, Libroia A, Verga U, Colantuoni V, et al. A novel point mutation in the intracellular domain of the ret protooncogene in a family with medullary thyroid carcinoma. J Clin Endocrinol Metab. 1997;82(12):4176–8.
40. Passarge E. Dissecting Hirschsprung disease. Nat Genet. 2002;1:11–2.
41. Burns AJ, Thapar N. Advances in ontogeny of the enteric nervous system. Neurogastroenterol Motil. 2006;18(10):876–87.
42. Okamoto E, Ueda T. Embryogenesis of intramural ganglia of the gut and its relationship to Hirschsprungs disease. J Pediatr Surg. 1967;2:437–43.
43. Fu M, Lui VC, Sham MH, Cheung AN, Tam PK. HOXB5 expression is spatially and temporarily regulated in human embryonic gut during neural crest cell colonization and differentiation of enteric neuroblasts. Dev Dyn. 2003;228(1):1–10.
44. Le DN, Teillet MA. Origin of intramural ganglionic system cells of the digestive tract of bird embryos. C R Acad Sci Hebd Seances Acad Sci D. 1971;273(16):1411–4.
45. Le DN. Migration and differentiation of neural crest cells. Curr Top Dev Biol. 1980;16:31–85.
46. Anderson RB, Stewart AL, Young HM. Phenotypes of neural-crest-derived cells in vagal and sacral pathways. Cell Tissue Res. 2006;23(1):11–25.
47. Ehrenpreiss TH. Hirschsprungs disease. Chicago: Year Book Medical Publishers; 1970. p. 57–61.
48. Hofstra RM, Wu Y, Stulp RP, Elfferich P, Osinga J, Maas SM, et al. RET and GDNF gene scanning in Hirschsprung patients using two dual denaturing gel systems. Hum Mutat. 2005;15(5):418–29.
49. Martuciello G, Bicocci MP, Dodero P, Lerone M, Silengo-Cirillo M, Puliti A, et al. Total colonic aganglionosis associated with interstitial deletion of the long arm of chromosome 10. Pediatr Surg Int. 1992;7(4):308–10.
50. Lyonnet S, Bolino A, Pelet A, Abel L, Nihoul-Fekete C, Briard M, et al. A gene for HSCR maps to the proximal long arm of chromosome 10. Nat Genet. 1993;4:346–50.
51. Fewtrell MS, Tam PK, Thomson AH, Fitchett M, Currie J, Huson SM, et al. Hirschsprung's disease associated with a deletion of chromosome 10 (q11.2q21.2): a further link with the neurocristopathies? J Med Genet. 1994;31(4):325–7.
52. So MT, Leon TY, Cheng G, Tang CS, Miao XP, Cornes BK, et al. RET mutational spectrum in Hirschsprung disease: evaluation of 601 Chinese patients. PLoS One. 2011;6(12):e28986.
53. Shimotake T, Go S, Inoue K, Tomiyama H, Iwai N. A homozygous missense mutation in the tyrosine E kinase domain of the RET proto-oncogene in an infant with total intestinal aganglionosis. Am J Gastroenterol. 2001;96(4):1286–91.
54. Ceccherini I, Zhang AL, Matera I, Yang G, Devoto M, Romeo G, et al. Interstitial deletion of the endothelin-B receptor gene in the spotting lethal (sl) rat. Hum Mol Genet. 1995;4(11):2089–96.
55. Gariepy CE, Williams SC, Richardson JA, Hammer RE, Yanagisawa M. Transgenic expression of the endothelin-B receptor prevents congenital intestinal aganglionosis in a rat model of Hirschsprung disease. J Clin Invest. 1998;102(6):1092–101.
56. Ou-Yang MC, Yang SN, Hsu YM, Ou-Yang MH, Haung HC, Lee SY, et al. Concomitant existence of total bowel aganglionosis and congenital central hypoventilation syndrome in a neonate with PHOX2B gene mutation. J Pediatr Surg. 2007;42(2):e9–11.
57. Tomiyama H, Shimotake T, Ono S, Kimura O, Tokiwa K, Iwai N. Relationship between the type of RET/GDNF/NTN or SOX10 gene mutations and long-term results after surgery for total colonic agangli-

onosis with small bowel involvement. J Pediatr Surg. 2001;36(11):1685–8.
58. Jing S, Wen D, Yu Y, et al. GDNF-induced activation of the *RET* protein tyrosine kinase is mediated by *GDNFR-alpha*, a novel receptor for *GDNF*. Cell. 1996;85:1113–24.
59. Bordeaux MC, Forcet C, Granger L, Corset V, Bidaud C, Billaud M, et al. The RET proto-oncogene induces apoptosis: a novel mechanism for Hirschsprung disease. EMBO J. 2000;19(15):4056–63.
60. Moore SW. Genetic impact on the treatment & management of Hirschsprung disease. J Pediatr Surg. 2017;52(2):218–22.
61. Luo Y, Barone V, Seri M, Bolino A, Bocciardi R, Ceccherini I, et al. Heterogeneity of mutations of the RET proto-oncogene in autosomal dominant HSCR. Eur J Hum Genet. 1994;2:272–80.
62. Lane PW, Liu HM. Association of megacolon with a new dominant spotting gene (Dom) in the mouse. J Hered. 1984;75(6):435–9.
63. Stenqvist A, Lundgren T, Smith MJ, Hermanson O, Pawson T, Ernfors P. Subcellular receptor redistribution and enhanced microspike formation by a Ret receptor preferentially recruiting Dok. Neurosci Lett. 2008;435(1):11–6.
64. Derrick EH, St George-Grambauer BM. Megacolon in mice. J Pathol Bacteriol. 1957;73:569–71.
65. Lane PW. Association of megacolon with 2 recessive spotting genes in the mouse. J Hered. 1966;57:29–31.
66. Nagahama M, Ozaki T, Hama K. A study of the myenteric plexus of the congenital aganglionosis rat (spotting lethal). Anat Embryol (Berl). 1985;171(3):285–96.
67. Nagahama M, Semba R, Tsuzuki M, Ozaki T. Distribution of peripheral nerve terminals in the small and large intestine of congenital aganglionosis rats (Hirschsprung's disease rats). Pathol Int. 2001;51(3):145–57.
68. Nagahama M, Tsutsui Y, Kuwahara A, Akagawa K. Immunohistochemical demonstration of neuron specific antigen, HPC-1 in the enteric nervous system of the Guinea-pig distal colon. Neurosci Lett. 1993;160(1):37–40.
69. Stanchina L, Baral V, Robert F, Pingault V, Lemort N, Pachnis V, et al. Interactions between Sox10, Edn3 and Ednrb during enteric nervous system and melanocyte development. Dev Biol. 2006;295(1):232–49.
70. Kenny SE, Hofstra RM, Buys CH, Vaillant CR, Lloyd DA, Edgar DH. Reduced endothelin-3 expression in sporadic Hirschsprung disease. Br J Surg. 2000;87:580–5.
71. Oue T, Puri P. Altered endothelin-3 and endothelin-B receptor mRNA expression in Hirschsprung's disease. J Pediatr Surg. 1999;34(8):1257–60.
72. Uesaka T, Nagashimada M, Yonemura S, Enomoto H. Diminished Ret expression compromises neuronal survival in the colon and causes intestinal aganglionosis in mice. J Clin Invest. 2008;118(5):1890–8.
73. Tsuji H, Spitz L, Kiely EM, Drake DP, Pierro A. Management and long-term follow-up of infants with total colonic aganglionosis. J Pediatr Surg. 1999;34(1):158–61.
74. Goto S, Gunter M, Scherer LR, Bloch T, Grosfeld JL. Surgical treatment of total colonic aganglionosis: efficacy of aganglionic patch enteroplasty in the rat. J Pediatr Surg. 1986;21(7):601–7.
75. Escobar MA, Grosfeld JL, West KW, Scherer LR, Rouse TM, Engum SA, et al. Long-term outcomes in total colonic aganglionosis: a 32-year experience. J Pediatr Surg. 2005;40(6):955–61.
76. Leffler A, Wedel T, Busch LC. Congenital colonic hypoganglionosis in murine trisomy 16--an animal model for Down's syndrome. Eur J Pediatr Surg. 1999;9(6):381–8.
77. Menezes M, Pini PA, Jasonni V, Puri P. Long-term clinical outcome in patients with total colonic aganglionosis: a 31-year review. J Pediatr Surg. 2008;43(9):1696–9.
78. Yeh YT, Tsai HL, Chen CY, Wang JB, Chin TW, Wei CF, et al. Surgical outcomes of total colonic aganglionosis in children: a 26-year experience in a single institute. J Chin Med Assoc. 2014;77(10):519–23.
79. Nishijima E, Kimura K, Tsugawa C, Muraji T. The colon patch graft procedure for extensive aganglionosis: long-term follow-up. J Pediatr Surg. 1998;33(2):215–9.

19 Hirschsprung's Disease in Adolescents and Adults

Shilpa Sharma and Devendra K. Gupta

Contents

19.1 Introduction

Hirschsprung's disease (HD), being a congenital disorder, is usually diagnosed in the neonatal period or early childhood. However, due to certain factors, it may remain undiagnosed for years and then present as an acute condition in adolescence or adulthood. The first case of HSCR in an adult was reported in 1950 by Rosin [1]. Since then there have been anecdotal case reports [2–11]. A review in 1983 reported less than 300 cases over a 50-year period, at an average age of 24 years at diagnosis, the oldest being 74 years in age [12]. More cases have been identified now with 2 large series of 50 cases from Mayo clinic and 90 cases from the Association of Coloproctology of Great Britain and Ireland [13, 14]. As the age advances, the problems associated with suspecting or narrowing down the diagnosis to HSCR increase as the differential diagnosis of constipation in older age groups is large and one would always try to rule out the commoner causes first. The definition of adult HSCR has been described as those cases in which the diagnosis is established when the patient is over 10 years of age [2, 3]. Adult HSCR has been more commonly seen in men than women with a male to female ratio of 133 to 42 [9]. There has been a relatively high incidence of cases documented in Africa [15, 16]. This seems to be due to poor awareness and scarcity of resources to establish a diagnosis. Other reasons for delayed presentation include illiteracy, ignorance, inadequate access to specialized centers, poverty, and long distances to travel for medical help [17].

S. Sharma (✉) · D. K. Gupta
Department of Pediatric Surgery, All India Institute of Medical Sciences, New Delhi, India

P. Puri (ed.), *Hirschsprung's Disease and Allied Disorders*,
https://doi.org/10.1007/978-3-030-15647-3_19

19.2 Symptoms

The most common symptom of HSCR is chronic constipation. However, the diagnosis of HSCR may be missed over years when, instead of seeking medical help, the parents or patient self-medicates with the chronic use of laxatives, low residue diet, antispasmodics, and other medications. Thus the symptoms are attenuated and the diagnosis is delayed. The frequency of defecation ranges from once per week to once every 2 months. The patients of HSCR may accommodate with this for prolonged periods of time. Some patients with mild symptoms may even go undiagnosed into adulthood, as the colonic region proximal to the distally obstructed segment may assume a compensatory role [5]. Though the patients may be managing with the use of cathartic agents, at some point, the dilated proximal colonic segment may decompensate secondary to the distal obstruction and patients may experience rapidly worsening constipation or even acute obstruction. In some instances, the constipation in older cases may even improve over the years through use of enemas, giving a false sense of security [18]. Cases have been reported who underwent stoma formation for intestinal obstruction, yet the diagnosis of HSCR was not made until late in adulthood when the patient wanted to have the stoma closed [18]. The authors have managed a case that presented at the age of 11 years with a history of constipation since 1.5 months of age. The child was worked up and was diagnosed as HSCR with a rectal biopsy and barium enema (Fig. 19.1). The child was kept on rectal washouts as a preparation for a primary pull-through. However, the child developed sigmoid volvulus mandating emergency laparotomy. The bowel was further prepared on table. The aganglionic segment was resected, and a primary Scott Boley's pull-through was done (Fig. 19.2) [19].

On rare occasions, patients with adult HSCR present with acute intestinal obstruction necessitating a laparotomy. In such situations, the diagnosis can only be established if there is a suspicion of HSCR due to a history of chronic constipation, and an intraoperative frozen section biopsy of the colon and rectum is done if a dilated colon is observed without any identifiable obstructive cause. Some patients may also have growth retardation and/or asymmetrically distended abdomen with visible peristalsis [20]. Few cases may present with symptoms in adulthood for the first time [21]. The authors have managed a lady who presented at the age of 35 years with 25 kg weight [17] (Fig. 19.3).

Adult HSCR may also present with fecal impaction and megacolon [14]. Fortunately,

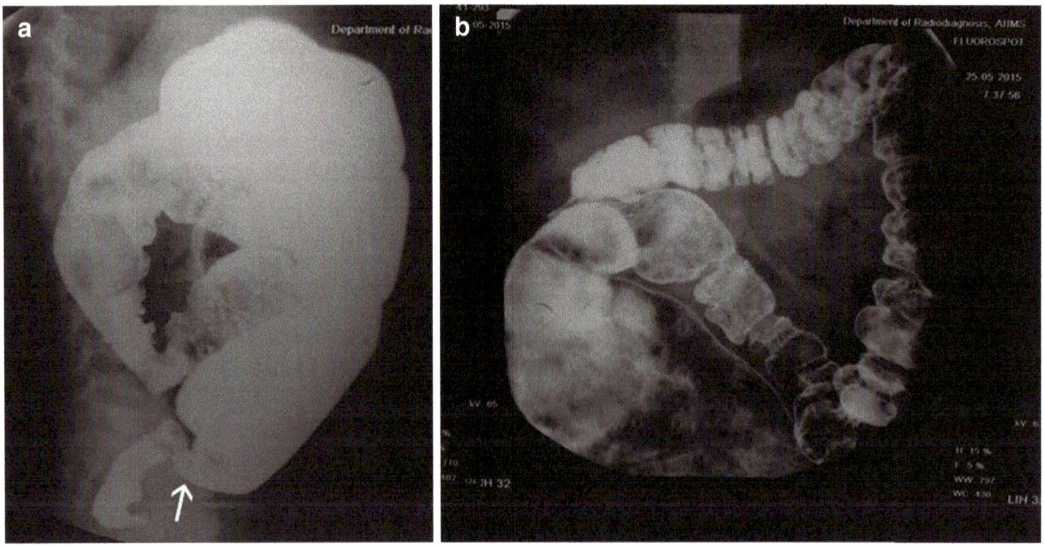

Fig. 19.1 Barium enema in an 11-year-old boy showing (**a**) reversed rectosigmoid ratio (arrow) and (**b**) distended sigmoid occupying the right side of the abdomen

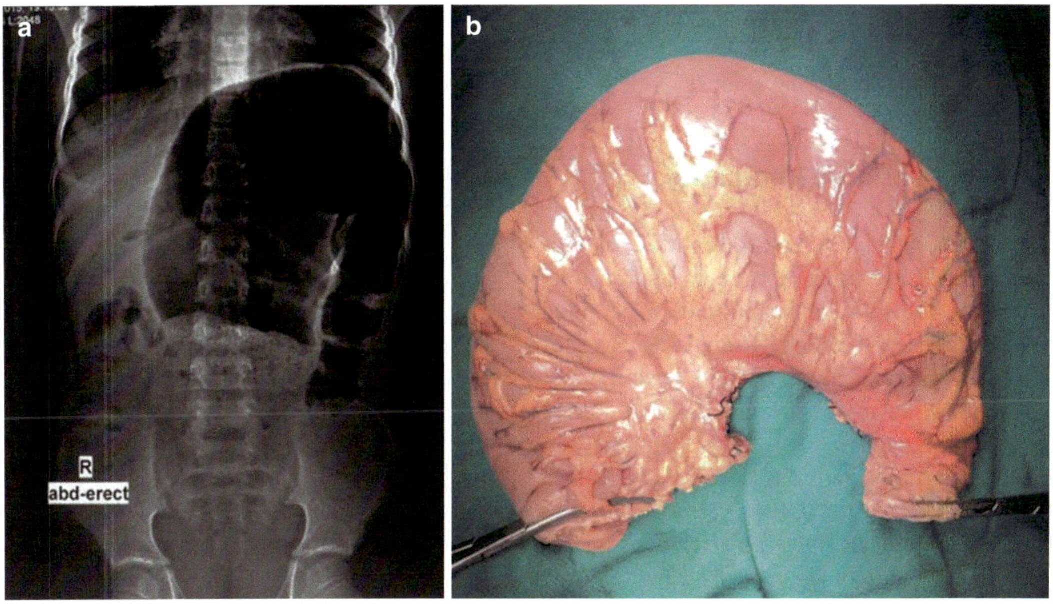

Fig. 19.2 (**a**) Skiagram of the abdomen showing a dilated sigmoid with air fluid level. (**b**) Operative photograph showing the resected sigmoid volvulus and aganglionic distal segment

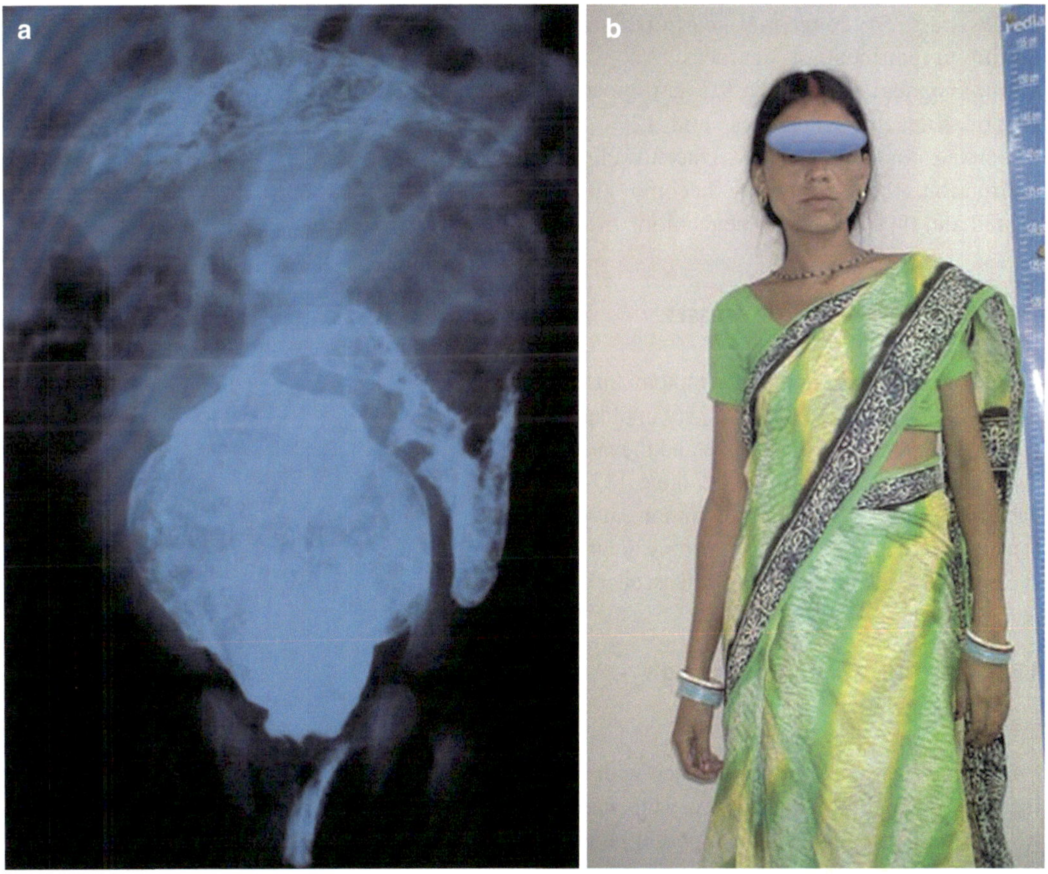

Fig. 19.3 (**a**) Barium enema of a young lady with dilated sigmoid colon with impacted stool. (**b**) Clinical picture of the lady with poor weight gain

enterocolitis is not a common complication among adult patients [22]. Adult HSCR may rarely be diagnosed during autopsy.

19.3 Associated Anomalies

In the cases of adult HSCR reported, associated anomalies have not been appreciable. However, Down's syndrome should be ruled out in all cases of HSCR. Though 2% cases of anorectal malformation (ARM) have HSCR, the median delay for the diagnosis of HSCR from initial diagnosis of ARM is 8 months, and hence these cases are diagnosed early and do not reach the adult HSCR age [23]. A prospective observational study on 106 consecutive HSCR patients looking for associated anomalies identified them in up to 58% patients, including 43% ophthalmologic issues (mostly refraction anomalies), 9% visual impairment, 21% congenital anomalies of the kidney and urinary tract, 5% congenital heart disease, 5% hearing impairment or deafness, 2% central nervous system anomalies, 9% chromosomal abnormalities or syndromes, and 12% other associated anomalies [24]. Due to chronic obstruction, the bowel may become grossly dilated and thus become a megacolon.

19.4 Differential Diagnosis

Constipation is the common symptom that has innumerable causes. As HSCR is rare in older age groups, the other common causes and the needful investigation for that should be done [25–32]. Table 19.1 outlines the various common causes of constipation. There can be many wrong diagnoses in cases of HSCR presenting in adolescence [33].

19.5 Types of Hirschsprung's Disease

Late diagnosis is especially associated with short segment or zonal forms of disease. Thus the two types of HSCR that have been reported in adults include:

Table 19.1 Causes of constipation in adults

1.	Habitual constipation
2.	Peripheral diabetes mellitus
3.	Neurogenic disorders
4.	Hypothyroidism
5.	Hyperparathyroidism
6.	Autonomic neuropathy
7.	Chagas disease
8.	Intestinal pseudo-obstruction
9.	Malignancy
10.	Central multiple sclerosis
11.	Spinal cord injury
12.	Hirschsprung's disease
13.	Parkinson disease
14.	Electrolyte imbalance (hypercalcemia, hypokalemia, hypomagnesemia)
15.	Medications: opioids, anticholinergics, antacids, anticonvulsants, antihypertensives, supplements (iron, calcium)
16.	Anorectal conditions: fissures, hemorrhoids, rectal prolapse, rectocele
17.	Diverticulitis
18.	Amyloidosis
19.	Scleroderma
20.	Chronic renal failure, uremia
21.	Pregnancy

1. Classical short segment HSCR
2. Ultrashort segment HSCR

In a series of 90 cases, ultrashort segment HSCR was found in 5.6% patients, rectal involvement in 54.4%, rectosigmoid in 38.9%, and total aganglionosis of the colon in 1.1% [14].

19.6 Investigations

X-ray of the abdomen An erect X-ray of the abdomen typically shows massive distension of the proximal region of the colon, with a small narrowed distal segment. Multiple air fluid levels may be seen in cases with obstructive symptoms.

Barium enema It may show the classical three zones in cases of rectosigmoid HSCR. Barium enema is diagnostic in more than 80% of the cases [14]. However, in ultrashort segment variety, there may not be any visible distinction in the bowel calibers [34].

Rectal biopsy A rectal biopsy is the gold standard for diagnosis showing aganglionosis in the myenteric plexus and hypertrophied nerve endings [35]. A suction biopsy or seromuscular biopsy may be done to establish the diagnosis. However, a full-thickness biopsy may be warranted in doubtful cases. A myectomy may be diagnostic as well as therapeutic in cases of ultrashort segment HSCR. A 60 mm full-thickness strip biopsy with estimation of acetylcholinesterase activity was useful in cases with diagnostic uncertainty in adult HSCR [14].

Anorectal physiology In a series of 90 cases of adult HSCR, 36.2% had a positive, but weak, rectoanal inhibitory reflex.

Acetylcholinesterase staining It was positive in 85.7%, but full-thickness strip biopsy was positive in 100% of equivocal cases of adult HSCR [14].

CT scan It is a useful imaging tool providing the opportunity to not only view the dilated colon and the transition zones but also to definitively exclude other diseases which can also cause chronic constipation in adults, such as colorectal cancer.

19.7 Surgical Treatment

A surgical intervention is almost always indicated to prevent complications and remove the symptoms. The primary aim of surgery in Hirschsprung's disease is to resect the aganglionic segment of bowel and relieve the obstruction. A variable length of dilated proximal colon is also resected. Several procedures, initially developed for the pediatric population, have been applied to older children and adults. In the initial series, there were many cases of anterior resection [13].

19.7.1 Various Procedures Adopted in Adult HSCR

1. *Anterior resection*
2. *Swenson's abdominoanal prolapse technique*: In the Swenson abdominoanal prolapse technique, the rectal aganglionic segment is resected, and a low colorectal or coloanal anastomosis is performed.
3. *Duhamel procedure*: The retrorectal pull-through procedure described by Duhamel leaves the rectum in place and bypasses the aganglionic zone by descending the proximal bowel in the retrorectal space, followed by an anastomosis to the posterior wall of the distal rectum. This is the procedure of choice for older children and adults diagnosed with HSCR with limited degree of megacolon and is performed in most patients [14].
4. *Soave's endorectal pull-through*: It also avoids rectal dissection by stripping the aganglionic mucosa and submucosa off the rectum and pulling the healthy proximal bowel through the rectal sleeve.
5. *Posterior anorectal myectomy*: It has lower morbidity and complication rates. A strip of extramucosal rectal wall is resected through a transanal approach, relieving the spasm of the aganglionic segment. However, the aganglionic segment remains in continuity, possibly leading to recurrence of symptoms and further surgery in up to 50% of patients.

A colostomy may be done followed by a pull-through later [36]. Staged surgical resection and subsequent reanastomosis provides a good outcome. A loop "leveling" colostomy should be avoided due to its grotesque size and tendency to retract or prolapse [36]. When a diverting ostomy is required, it should be an ileostomy rather than a colostomy because its subsequent closure will not endanger the marginal artery, which, if divided, could compromise the blood supply to the pulled-through colon [36]. Rectal tube decompression can often adequately prepare a patient for a primary pull-through procedure. A one-stage approach has been found to be feasible when treating adult HSCR due to the relatively healthier nutritional status of adult HSCR patients and the ability to use a Gastrointestinal Anastomosis (GIA) stapling device. Several applications of the stapling instrument are required in the Duhamel procedure to fully divide the septum between the aganglionic rectum anteriorly and the normal colon posteriorly [36].

Laparoscopy Though, theoretically, laparoscopy can be used to establish a diagnosis and also do a pull-through, its use has not been reported extensively in adult HSCR. This may be due to the fact that the diagnosis is not often thought of and is difficult to establish. In a report on 39 patients managed by the Duhamel procedure, one-third of the patients underwent at least one abdominal surgical procedure before the correct diagnosis was made [37].

19.7.2 Complications

The natural course leads to a massive megacolon with risks of denutrition, fecal impaction, intestinal perforation, respiratory failure (as a consequence of major abdominal distension), and necrotizing enterocolitis with septic shock and death [11, 12].

The complications include anastomotic leak that has been commonly reported after anterior resection and Soave's procedure. In serious cases, this leak can lead to sepsis and mortality [36]. The incidence of anastomotic dehiscence was 13% in a series following Soave's procedure. Impotence has been reported following Swenson's procedure [34]. Recurrent megacolon may require resection of an additional segment of colon [34]. The least complications have been reported using Duhamel's procedure.

19.8 Outcome and Follow-Up

The outcome of adult HSCR has been favorable. However, when the presentation is with intestinal obstruction, the outcome may be poor. A preliminary stoma may be indicated to prevent complications in cases with a massively dilated bowel. Duhamel's procedure has had excellent results with adult HSCR [37]. Thirty-six out of thirty-nine patients of HSCR who underwent Duhamel pull-through had excellent functional results [37]. A good or satisfactory functional outcome was achieved with a modified Duhamel procedure in another series in 96.7% [14]. The long-term functional outcome after resection depends on the degree of preoperative megacolon. The megacolon limited to the sigmoid colon was associated with a good outcome in 89.7% cases, but with more proximal dilatation, good outcome was seen in only 66.7% ($p < 0.05$) [14]. Resolution of constipation and good fecal continence can be expected in 80–91% of patients [14]. Results following myectomy have not been satisfactory with minimal to no relief of symptoms [34, 38].

19.9 Future Directions

Constipation is a common problem. In cases where the duration of symptoms dates back to childhood, a suspicion of HSCR should be kept, and directed investigations should be done. In patients presenting with abdominal complications, a pediatric surgeon who is well versed with this anomaly should be consulted, and seromuscular biopsies from different levels should be taken. The gold standard of diagnosis remains a rectal biopsy. Once the diagnosis is established, the colon can be decompressed with rectal washouts and prepared for a single-stage pull-through procedure. To date, the progression for adolescent or adult patients is not fully clarified due to the small number of reported cases [39].

References

1. Rosin JD, Bargen JA, Wargh JM. Congenital megacolon of a man 54 years of age. Report of a case. Proc Staff Meet Mayo Clin. 1950;25:710–5.
2. Fairgrieve J. Hirschsprung's disease in adults. Br J Surg. 1963;50:506–14.
3. Barnes PR, Lennard-Jones JE, Howley PR, Todd IP. Hirschsprung's disease and idiopathic megacolon in adults and adolescents. Gut. 1986;27:534–41.
4. Lesser PB, El-Nahas AM, Lukl P, Andrew P, Schuler JG, Filtzer HS. Adult-onset Hirschsprung's disease. JAMA. 1979;242:747–8.
5. Natsikas NB, Sbarounis CN. Adult Hirschsprung's disease: an experience with the Duhamel-Martin procedure with special reference to obstructed patients. Dis Colon Rectum. 1987;30:204–6.
6. Chen F, Winston JH 3rd, Jain SK, Frankel WL. Hirschsprung's disease in a young adult: report of a case and review of the literature. Ann Diagn Pathol. 2006;10:347–51.
7. Suita S, Taguchi T, Ieiri S, Nakatsuji T. Hirschsprung's disease in Japan: analysis of 3852 patients based

on a nationwide survey in 30 years. J Pediatr Surg. 2005;40:197–201.
8. Fu CG, Muto T, Masaki T, Nagawa H. Zonal adult Hirschsprung's disease. Gut. 1996;39:765–7.
9. Miyamoto M, Egami K, Maeda S, Ohkawa K, Tanaka N, Uchida E, Tajiri T. Hirschsprung's disease in adults: report of a case and review of the literature. J Nippon Med Sch. 2005;72:113–20.
10. Wheatley MJ, Wesley JR, Coran AG, et al. Hirschsprung's disease in adolescents and adults. Dis Colon Rectum. 1990;33:622e629.
11. Yüksel I, Ataseven H, Ertuğrul I, Başar O, Saşmaz N. Adult segmental Hirschsprung disease. South Med J. 2009;102:184–5.
12. Rich AJ, Lennard TW, Wilsdon JB. Hirschsprung's disease as a cause of chronic constipation in the elderly. Br Med J. 1983;287:1777–8.
13. McCready RA, Beart RW Jr. Adult Hirschsprung's disease: results of surgical treatment at Mayo Clinic. Dis Colon Rectum. 1980;23:401–7.
14. Vorobyov GI, Achkasov SI, Biryukov OM. Clinical features diagnostics and treatment of Hirschsprung's disease in adults. Colorect Dis. 2010;12:1242–8.
15. Bakari AA, Gali BM, Ibrahim AG, Nggada HA, Ali N, Dogo D. Congenital aganglionic megacolon in Nigerian adults: two case reports and review of the literature. Niger J Clin Pract. 2011;14:249–52.
16. Arowolo OA, Lawal OO, Adisa AO, Adetiloye VA, Afolabi AI, Sowande OA. Adulthood Hirschsprung's disease: a report of 4 cases in Ile-Ife. Nigeria. Afr J Med Med Sci. 2013;42:277–82.
17. Sharma S, Gupta DK. Hirschsprung's disease presenting beyond infancy: surgical options and postoperative outcome. Pediatr Surg Int. 2012;28:5–8.
18. Qiu JF, Shi YJ, Hu L, Fang L, Wang HF, Zhang MC. Adult Hirschsprung's disease: report of four cases. Int J Clin Exp Pathol. 2013;6:1624–30.
19. Ranjan A, Jain V, Sharma S, Gupta DK. Sigmoid volvulus: an uncommon complication of Hirschsprung's disease. BMJ Case Rep. 2016;2016:bcr2016214693.
20. Shitta AH, Ugwu BT, Peter SD, Ozoilo KN, Adighije PF, Omolabake BI. Hirschsprung's disease in an adult: a case report. J West Afr Coll Surg. 2014;4:121–6.
21. Chatzoulis G, Milias S, Kostogloudis N, Christopoulos C, Chatzoulis K, Pantelidou V, Mourelatos K, Ploumis A. Hirschsprung disease in adulthood: an alternative surgical approach using a U-shaped circular anastomosis. Hell J Surg. 2013;85:390–4.
22. Chatelain D, Manaouil C, Marc B, Ricard J, Brevet M, Montpellier D. Adult Hirschsprung's disease diagnosed during forensic autopsy. J Forensic Sci. 2006;51:1160–3.
23. Hofmann AD, Puri P. Association of Hirschsprung's disease and anorectal malformation: a systematic review. Pediatr Surg Int. 2013;29:913–7.
24. Pini Prato A, Rossi V, Mosconi M, Holm C, Lantieri F, Griseri P, et al. A prospective observational study of associated anomalies in Hirschsprung's disease. Orphanet J Rare Dis. 2013;8:184.
25. Doig CM. Childhood constipation and late-presenting Hirschsprung's disease. J R Soc Med. 1984;77(Suppl 3):3–5.
26. Talley NJ, Fleming KC, Evans JM, et al. Constipation in an elderly community: a study of prevalence and potential risk factors. Am J Gastroenterol. 1996;91:19e25.
27. Meier-Ruge WA, Bruder E. Pathology of chronic constipation in pediatric and adult coloproctology. Pathobiology. 2005;72:1–102.
28. Chitkara DK, Bredenoord AJ, Cremonini F, Delgado-Aros S, Smoot RL, El-Youssef M, Freese D, Camilleri M. The role of pelvic floor dysfunction and slow colonic transit in adolescents with refractory constipation. Am J Gastroenterol. 2004;99:1579–84.
29. Youssef NN, Sanders L, Di Lorenzo C. Adolescent constipation: evaluation and management. Adolesc Med Clin. 2004;15:37–52.
30. Brandt LJ, Prather CM, Quigley EM, et al. Systematic review on the management of chronic constipation in North America. Am J Gastroenterol. 2005;100:S1e22.
31. Rao SS, Ozturk R, Laine L. Clinical utility of diagnostic tests for constipation in adults: a systematic review. Am J Gastroenterol. 2005;100:1605–15.
32. McCrea GL, Miaskowski C, Stotts NA, et al. Pathophysiology of constipation in the older adult. World J Gastroenterol. 2008;14:2631–8.
33. Powell RW. Hirschsprung's disease in adolescents. Misadventures in diagnosis and management. Am Surg. 1989;55:212–8.
34. Kim HJ, Kim AY, Lee CW, Yu CS, Kim JS, Kim PN, Lee MG, Ha HK. Hirschsprung disease and hypoganglionosis in adults: radiologic findings and differentiation. Radiology. 2008;247:428–34.
35. Tomita R, Ikeda T, Fujisaki S, et al. Hirschsprung's disease and its allied disorders in adults: histological and clinical studies. Hepatogastroenterology. 2003;50:1050–3.
36. Ricketts RR, Pettitt BJ. Management of Hirschsprung's disease in adolescents. Am Surg. 1989;55:219–25.
37. Elliot MS, Todd IP. Adult Hirschsprung's disease: results of the Duhamel procedure. Br J Surg. 1985;72:884–5.
38. Wu JS, Schoetz DJ Jr, Coller JA, Veidenheimer MC. Treatment of Hirschsprung's disease in the adult. Report of five cases. Dis Colon Rectum. 1995;38:655–9.
39. Martins MR, dos Santos CHM, Falcão GR. Late diagnosis of Hirschsprung's disease. J Coloproctol. 2015;35:178–81.

Variants of Hirschsprung's Disease 20

Florian Friedmacher and Prem Puri

Contents

F. Friedmacher
Department of Pediatric Surgery, The Royal London Hospital, Whitechapel, London, UK

National Children's Research Centre, Our Lady's Children's Hospital, Crumlin, Dublin, Ireland

P. Puri (✉)
National Children's Research Centre, Our Lady's Children's Hospital, Crumlin, Dublin, Ireland

Conway Institute of Biomolecular and Biomedical Research, School of Medicine & Medical Science, University College Dublin, Dublin, Ireland
e-mail: prem.puri@ncrc.ie

P. Puri (ed.), *Hirschsprung's Disease and Allied Disorders*,
https://doi.org/10.1007/978-3-030-15647-3_20

20.1 Introduction

There are a number of infants and young children who present with clinical symptoms similar to Hirschsprung's disease (HSCR) despite the presence of ganglion cells in rectal biopsies. Over the years, various terms such as "*chronic idiopathic intestinal pseudo-obstruction*", "*intestinal hypoperistalsis syndrome*" or "*pseudo-HSCR*" have been used to describe these conditions [1, 2]. At present, there are only a few articles in the literature that have attempted to standardize the terminology of HSCR and allied intestinal disorders [3, 4]. In 1997, Puri et al. [5, 6] suggested that "*variant HSCR*" may be a more appropriate description for this heterogeneous group of functional bowel disorders (Box 20.1) in patients who suffer from chronic constipation and abdominal distension despite a ganglionic rectal biopsy. Specific histological and immunohistochemical staining methods combined with anorectal manometry studies are required to delineate between the different variants of HSCR [7]. Although the initial diagnostic workup and subsequent management can be challenging, the majority of these patients will have a satisfactory long-term outcome.

Box 20.1 Variants of Hirschsprung's Disease

Intestinal neuronal dysplasia (IND)
Intestinal ganglioneuromatosis (GNM)
Isolated hypoganglionosis (HG)
Immature ganglia (IG)
Absence of the argyrophil plexus (AP)
Internal anal sphincter achalasia (IASA)

20.2 Intestinal Neuronal Dysplasia

In 1971, intestinal neuronal dysplasia (IND) was first described by William A. Meier-Ruge as a hyperplastic malformation of the enteric plexus [8]. Shortly afterwards, Puri et al. [9] reported a case of rectosigmoid aganglionosis that was associated with IND of the descending and transverse colon. IND can be classified into two clinical and histologically distinct subtypes [10]: IND type A (IND A), which occurs in less than 5% of all IND cases, is characterized by congenital aplasia or hypoplasia of the sympathetic innervation. Patients with IND A typically present in the neonatal period with abdominal distension, intestinal obstruction, and episodes of diarrhea with hemorrhagic stools. IND type B (IND B) is defined by hyperplasia of the parasympathetic submucosal plexus and accounts for over 95% of all IND cases. Typical histological features of IND B are hyperganglionosis, giant ganglia, ectopic ganglion cells, and increased activity of acetylcholinesterase (AChE) in the lamina propria and around submucosal blood vessels [6]. IND occurring in association with HSCR is invariably IND B.

20.2.1 Pathogenesis of Intestinal Neuronal Dysplasia

Controversy remains regarding the existence of IND as a distinct histopathological entity

[3, 11–13]. Some authors suggested that the observed changes may be either a variant of normal bowel development or a secondary acquired phenomenon caused by congenital obstruction or inflammation [14, 15]. An underlying autoimmune mechanism has also been proposed for IND [16]. Furthermore, there may be an additional genetic component, as several familial cases of IND have been found [17, 18]. The strongest evidence that IND is a real entity actually came from two different *Hox11L1* knockout mouse models [19, 20]. In both cases, homozygous mutant mice developed megacolon at the age of 3–5 weeks. Histological and immunohistochemical evaluation revealed hyperplasia of ganglia similar to the phenotype observed in human IND. Another animal model resulting in a phenotype similar to IND was reported in rats with a heterozygous mutation of the endothelin B receptor (*Ednrb*) showing features of hyperganglionosis, giant ganglia, and hypertrophied nerve fiber strands in the submucosal plexus [21]. However, mutational screening of *HOX11L1* and *EDNRB* genes in human patients with IND demonstrated no mutations in these genes [22–24].

20.2.2 Epidemiology of Intestinal Neuronal Dysplasia

IND occurs with an estimated incidence of approximately 1 in every 7,500 newborns [25]. However, the frequency of isolated IND cases seems to be highly varying with reported rates ranging between 0.3% and 40% of all rectal biopsies [15, 26, 27]. IND proximal to an aganglionic colon segment is not uncommon and has been suggested as a possible cause of persistent bowel problems after pull-through operation for HSCR [28]. Some authors have found IND in up to 44% of their patients with HSCR, while others have rarely observed this combination [29–33]. The high variability of patient's age, specimen type, and applied staining methods has resulted in considerable confusion in the published literature regarding the accurate diagnostic criteria [34].

20.2.3 Clinical Presentation of Intestinal Neuronal Dysplasia

Most patients with IND present with chronic constipation with or without abdominal distension, thus clinically resembling HSCR, but with a normal contrast enema examination of the colon [35]. It has been shown that intestinal obstruction is the most characteristic clinical feature of IND in infants and young children [36]. Furthermore, there appears to be a high incidence of associated congenital anomalies, ranging from 25% to 30% [37]. The most common ones are anorectal malformations, megacystis, intestinal malrotation, congenital short bowel, hypertrophic pyloric stenosis, necrotizing enterocolitis, and Down syndrome [38, 39].

20.2.4 Diagnosis of Intestinal Neuronal Dysplasia

Rectal suction biopsy is the method of choice for the diagnosis of IND. It is essential to include a sufficient amount of submucosal tissue in the biopsy specimens. Previously, the diagnosis of IND was based on qualitative criteria, thus resulting in a high interobserver variation [40, 41]. Therefore, the debate about the existence of IND as a distinct histopathological entity remains controversial, mainly due to the lack of consensus in diagnostic criteria [14, 42]. Initially, IND was diagnosed on the basis of AChE immunohistochemistry of nerve fibers in rectal suction biopsies [43, 44] (Fig. 20.1a, b). However, as AChE activity in the lamina propria mucosae has been shown to be an age-dependent phenomenon that disappears on maturation of the submucosal plexus [45–47], more specific staining techniques were required to assess the enteric nervous system in more detail [48]. Enzyme histochemistry for lactate dehydrogenase, succinate dehydrogenase, and nitric oxide synthase has been suggested by Meier-Ruge et al. [49–51] to evaluate and diagnose IND B quantitatively. Various other neuronal and glial markers such as nicotinamide adenine dinucleotide phosphate diaphorase (NADPH-d)

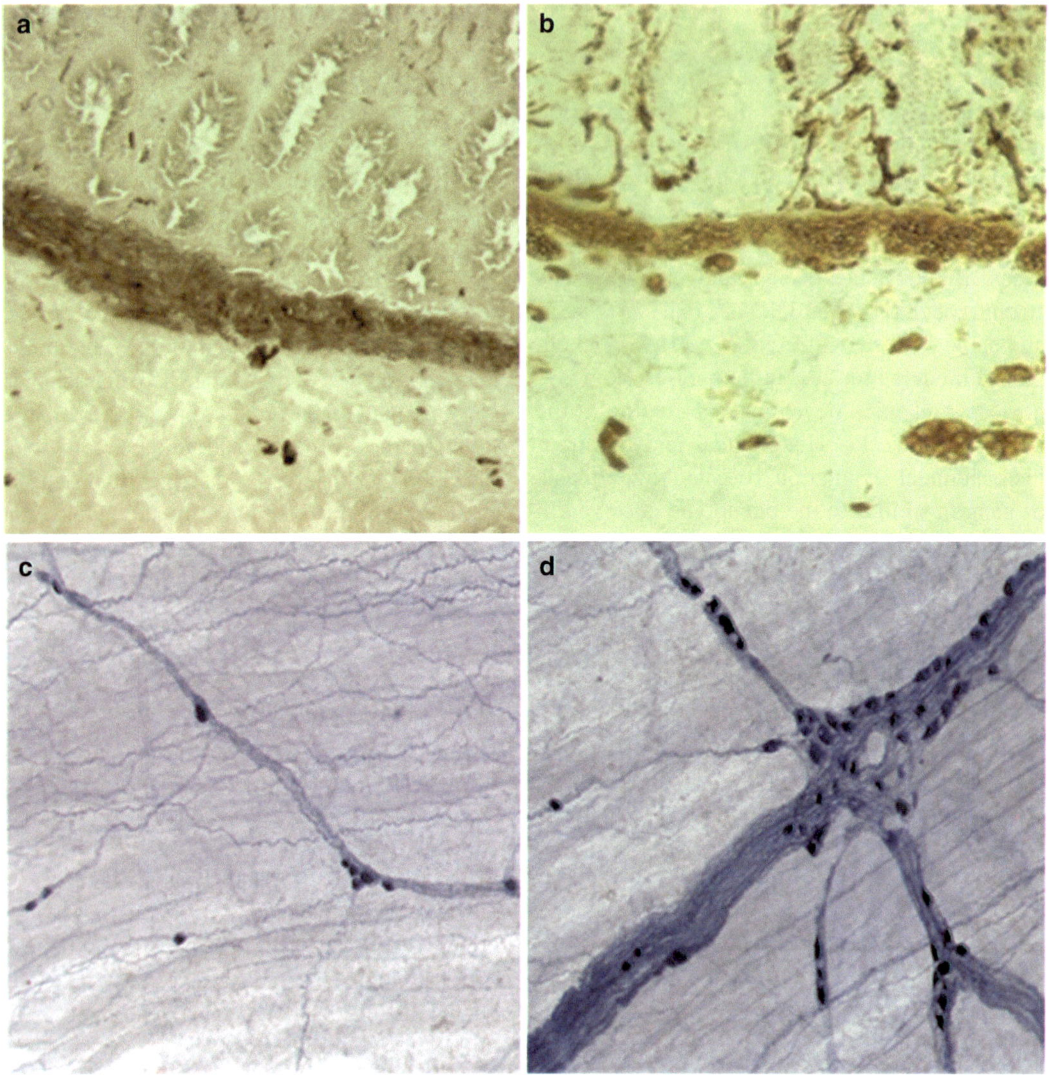

Fig. 20.1 AChE immunohistochemistry of a normal rectal suction biopsy (**a**). Rectal suction biopsy from a patient with IND showing hyperganglionosis, giant ganglia, and increased AChE activity in the lamina propria (**b**). NADPH-d staining of a normal submucosal plexus (**c**). Submucosal plexus of a patient with IND showing giant ganglia (**d**)

(Fig. 20.1c, d), neural cell adhesion molecule (NCAM), neuron-specific enolase (NSE), cathepsin D, protein gene product 9.5 (PGP9.5), S-100 protein, peripherin, synaptophysin, and cuprolinic blue have also been used [52–55]. Cuprolinic blue staining has been proposed as it stains the whole population of ganglion cells [55, 56], but only their cell bodies and not their axons, which makes differentiation between the individual cell types relatively easy. In addition, a defective innervation of the neuromuscular junction within the affected bowel segment of patients with IND has been identified [57]. Abnormal submucosal vasculature is a further histological finding in isolated IND and IND associated with HSCR, which may also be a useful diagnostic feature [58]. Furthermore, a reduced number of c-Kit-positive interstitial cells of Cajal (ICCs) have been demonstrated in the myenteric plexus and muscle layers of IND cases [59, 60]. More recently, a marked reduction in the expression of phosphatase and tensin homolog (PTEN) has been discovered in the submucosal and myenteric plexuses of patients with IND, which may explain the observed motility dysfunction [61]. Due to the age-dependent AChE expression and discrepancy of applied staining techniques, the most commonly used diagnostic criteria at present are (1) more than 20% of 25 submucosal ganglia must be giant ganglia containing 9 or more ganglion cells and (2) the patient must be older than 1 year as before that age, giant ganglia may be misinterpreted due to the fact that immature ganglia (IG) often have an incomplete differentiation in nerve cells [62–64]. The majority of patients with IND do not display any specific radiological features on contrast enema studies other than rectosigmoid distension. The rectosphincteric reflex has often been shown to be present, absent, or atypical in these patients [37].

20.2.5 Management of Intestinal Neuronal Dysplasia

In the first instance, the management of IND B should be conservative, consisting of laxatives and enemas [65]. Most patients have been shown to respond well to this treatment strategy. However, if bowel symptoms persist longer than six months of conservative bowel management, surgical treatment options should be considered [66]. Internal sphincter myectomy has been performed by several authors with satisfactory results, whereas others recommend injection of botulinum toxin into the anal sphincter [6]. Resection of the affected bowel segment and pull-through procedure is rarely indicated in infants and children with IND, but in adolescent or adult patients, that is often the only successful therapeutic option [37, 67]. The indication for surgery should not be determined on the basis of histopathological findings alone; instead, the decision must be based on the individual patient's clinical symptoms [68].

20.2.6 Outcome of Intestinal Neuronal Dysplasia

In general, a team of experienced pediatric surgeons and gastroenterologists is essential for the long-term follow-up of patients with IND and chronic constipation [69]. In 2001, authors from Ireland reported functional outcomes in 33 patients with IND [70]: 64% had a good response to conservative management with normal bowel habits and did not require any surgical intervention. However, 36% of their patients underwent internal sphincter myectomy after failed conservative treatment. Seven out of these 12 patients had normal bowel habits after surgery, and 2 were able to stay clean with regular enemas. Three patients continued having persistent constipation after myectomy and subsequently required resection of their redundant and dilated sigmoid colon, which resulted in normal bowel habits. Schärli et al. [32] achieved satisfactory results in 90% of their patients within 6 months after internal sphincter myectomy.

20.3 Intestinal Ganglioneuromatosis

Intestinal ganglioneuromatosis (GNM) is characterized by a diffuse proliferation of nerve fibers with significant hyperplasia of submucosal and myenteric ganglion cells causing thickening of the bowel wall [71]. This extremely rare condition leads to chronic bowel obstruction and is frequently associated with multiple endocrine neoplasia type 2B (MEN 2B), neurofibromatosis 1, or Cowden syndrome [72].

20.3.1 Pathogenesis of Intestinal Ganglioneuromatosis

The pathogenesis of intestinal GNM is linked with complex hyperplasia of peptidergic, cholinergic, and probably adrenergic nerve fibers and neurons [73]. Transmural GNM mainly originates from the myenteric plexus, while mucosal GNM predominantly affects the submucosal plexus and is often associated with neurofibromatosis [73]. Furthermore, mutation analysis in patients with MEN 2B identified a *de novo* germline Met918Thr mutation in exon 16 of the *rearranged during transfection (RET)* proto-oncogene [74], suggesting a clear genetic component to this condition. In addition, a recent experimental study in mice revealed that deletion of the *Pten* gene on chromosome 10 disrupts the development of the enteric nerve system resulting in a phenotype similar to human intestinal GNM [75].

20.3.2 Epidemiology of Intestinal Ganglioneuromatosis

Although the exact incidence of intestinal GNM is unknown, it has been reported that the frequently associated MEN 2B syndrome occurs in approximately 1:4,000,000 live births [74]. Conversely, it can be estimated that intestinal GNM is present in nearly 90% of patients with MEN 2B [76].

20.3.3 Clinical Presentation of Intestinal Ganglioneuromatosis

The vast majority of patients with intestinal GNM present with severe chronic constipation and abdominal distension due to intestinal obstruction [76, 77]. Constipation may also alternate with episodes of diarrhea [78, 79]. The similarity of the gastrointestinal symptoms between patients with HSCR, IND, and MEN 2B-associated intestinal GNM has suggested that these three conditions could be the result of mutations affecting the same domain of the *RET* proto-oncogene [26]. Despite the fact that gastrointestinal dysmotility is a common initial presentation of patients with MEN 2B, the rarity of this syndrome often delays the diagnosis. Further findings are mucosal neuromas of the lips and tongue, as well as medullated corneal nerve fibers, distinctive facies with enlarged lips, and an asthenic "marfanoid" body habitus [74].

20.3.4 Diagnosis of Intestinal Ganglioneuromatosis

Intestinal GNM is mainly diagnosed on the basis of clinical presentation and histological analysis of rectal suction or open full-thickness biopsies showing massive proliferation of submucosal and myenteric plexuses comprising thick nerve trunks with scattered mature neurons, giant ganglia with often 15–40 nerve cells, and a high AChE activity [80–83]. Unlike neurofibromatosis, which occurs more commonly in the small intestine, intestinal GNM appears to be largely limited to the colon and rectum [84]. Although AChE immunohistochemistry has been suggested to show the typical submucosal and myenteric changes in intestinal GNM (i.e., increased thickness of nerve fibers), it can easily be appreciated in standard hematoxylin and eosin-stained paraffin sections [85]. NSE, synaptophysin, and S-100 protein immunostaining have also been used to evaluate and diagnose intestinal GNM [73]. It has been demonstrated that the submucosal hyperplasia can be extensive, but not as prominent as the one described in the myenteric plexus [85, 86]. As intestinal GNM is frequently associated with MEN 2B, the diagnosis should prompt additional molecular, endocrinological, and oncological investigations [87, 88]. In general, a mutational analysis of the *RET* proto-oncogene is strongly recommended in all patients with intestinal GNM and MEN 2B as well as their family members [79].

20.3.5 Management of Intestinal Ganglioneuromatosis

Surgical resection of the affected bowel segment is not always mandatory in patients with MEN 2B-associated intestinal GNM [89]. It has been shown that in most cases the gastrointestinal symptoms can be managed with daily laxatives and enemas [90]. However, some patients eventually require surgery for severe intestinal obstruction or stricture formation [91]. Furthermore, all patients with intestinal GNM who carry MEN 2B mutations should undergo a prophylactic total thyroidectomy to prevent development of medullary thyroid carcinoma [76, 83].

20.3.6 Outcome of Intestinal Ganglioneuromatosis

Early diagnosis and treatment of patients with MEN 2B-associated intestinal GNM is crucial for long-term survival. Thus, a yearly follow-up with monitoring of basal plasma calcitonin and carcinoembryonic antigen levels for possible tumor recurrence is strongly recommended [83]. In addition, continued surveillance of the adrenal glands with abdominal ultrasonography and urine analysis of catecholamine metabolites including metanephrine, normetanephrine, dopamine, and vanillylmandelic acid is required as patients with MEN 2B have at least a 50% risk of developing a pheochromocytoma [82].

20.4 Isolated Hypoganglionosis

Isolated hypoganglionosis (HG) is a very rare entity that has been classified as a hypogenetic type of intestinal innervation disorders. The clinical presentation of patients with isolated HG is similar to those with classical HSCR with non-specific symptoms of severe constipation or bowel obstruction [5, 92]. It has been demonstrated that congenital and acquired HG are two separate entities with different clinical features and histological findings [93]. At present, there are only a few cases in the published literature as isolated HG is one of the rarest subtypes of intestinal innervation disorders, and there remains controversy regarding it as a distinct isolated histopathological entity [14].

20.4.1 Pathogenesis of Isolated Hypoganglionosis

The pathogenesis and the genetic basis of isolated HG are still largely unknown. Although various mutational analyses of the *RET* gene have been performed, neither causative missense mutation nor neutral substitutions were found [94, 95]. Some cases of isolated HG were reported to exhibit deficient expression of c-Kit-positive ICCs within the myenteric plexus and the smooth muscle layer [96], which may contribute to the observed motility dysfunction in the hypoganglionic bowel segment [60]. A lack or reduced expression of NCAM-positive nerve fibers within the lamina propria, muscularis mucosae, as well as circular and longitudinal muscle layers of patients with isolated HG has also been described [92, 97, 98].

20.4.2 Epidemiology of Isolated Hypoganglionosis

Reports of finding isolated HG in rectal biopsies are rare, ranging between 0.3% and 6.4% [27, 29, 33]. Since 1978, there have been a total number of 92 cases published in the English literature, and 32% of them were diagnosed in the newborn period [99]. However, the median age at diagnosis was 4.8 years, which was most likely due to the fact that in several cases the diagnosis was not made until the patients were adolescents.

20.4.3 Clinical Presentation of Isolated Hypoganglionosis

Severe chronic constipation with intestinal obstruction and enterocolitis is the most common presenting symptom of isolated HG, thus resembling clinical features of HSCR. The median age at diagnosis is considerably higher in patients with isolated HG compared to patients with HSCR, which is generally diagnosed during the newborn period. Enterocolitis of the newborn has been reported to be the most serious and potentially life-threatening complication of isolated HG [99].

20.4.4 Diagnosis of Isolated Hypoganglionosis

There is an ongoing debate whether isolated HG represents an extreme form of intestinal dysganglionosis or solely a developmental abnormality of the enteric nervous system that leads to severe constipation [14]. Hence, the precise diagnosis of isolated HG remains difficult, and a consensus in diagnostic criteria still needs to be established. In general, a full-thickness biopsy is required for the definitive diagnosis of isolated HG [100–103]. The vast majority of reported cases have been analyzed by immunohistochemical staining showing sparse and small myenteric ganglia, absent or low AChE activity in the lamina propria, as well as hypertrophy of muscularis mucosae and circular muscle [104]. Meier-Ruge et al. [105] discovered significant histopathological differences between resected bowel specimens from patients with isolated HG and normal bowel tissue by using AChE immunohistochemistry. They showed a 40% reduction in the number of nerve cells, accompanied by a doubled distance between ganglia and a three times smaller plexus area in the hypoganglionic bowel segment. These observations currently form the basis for the histopathological diagnosis of isolated HG. It has also been suggested that the size of the myenteric plexus may be an indicator of clinical severity [106]. Therefore, various neuronal markers have been introduced to facilitate the diagnosis of isolated HG. NADPH-d staining has been used to determine the muscular nitrergic innervation and differentiation of mature from immature ganglia in patients with isolated HG, demonstrating a reduced number of positive nerve fibers in the muscularis mucosae with absent or sparse submucosal and myenteric ganglion cells [107] (Fig. 20.2a–d). Additionally, c-Kit staining has been employed to investigate the expression of ICCs and thus intestinal pacemaker activity, which is markedly decreased or even absent in patients with isolated HG [59, 96, 108].

20.4.5 Management of Isolated Hypoganglionosis

The management of isolated HG is similar to that of HSCR. According to the literature, most patients undergo resection of the affected bowel segment with subsequent pull-through procedure [99, 109].

20.4.6 Outcome of Isolated Hypoganglionosis

The postoperative outcome after resection of the hypoganglionic segment usually is good [110]. Typical complications of isolated HG are enterocolitis, chronic constipation, overflow encopresis, and the need for redo pull-through operation due to residual hypoganglionosis [37]. An overall mortality rate of 8% has recently been reported with the majority of patients who died being newborns suffering from severe enterocolitis [37].

20.5 Immature Ganglia

Immature ganglia are normally found in rectal biopsies from premature infants presenting with functional bowel obstruction. Not surprisingly, delayed maturation of ganglion cells in the submucosal and myenteric plexuses has been reported to be the most common cause of chronic constipation during the first year of life [88].

20.5.1 Pathogenesis of Immature Ganglia

A combination of large (i.e., fully mature) and small (i.e., immature) ganglion cells can be found at birth [111]. In the early postnatal period, ganglion cells in the submucosal plexus are generally less developed than the ones in the myenteric plexus [112]. It has further been demonstrated that this immaturity is a physiological, age-dependent phenomenon and maturation of IG strongly correlates with the age of the patient [3, 112]. Strong evidence supporting this theory has arisen from several animal studies showing postnatal maturation of the submucosal and myenteric plexuses [113–115]. Hence, the finding of IG on rectal biopsy may be a reliable indicator of transient functional immaturity of the bowel [111].

20.5.2 Epidemiology of Immature Ganglia

Strong epidemiological data on the incidence of IG is unfortunately lacking. In 1997, Ure et al. [33] reported four (2.8%) cases of immature ganglion cells in their cohort of 141 patients with intestinal neuronal malformations. More recently, Puri et al. [37] discovered 10 (5.6%) cases of IG in bowel specimens of 178 patients with variants of HSCR.

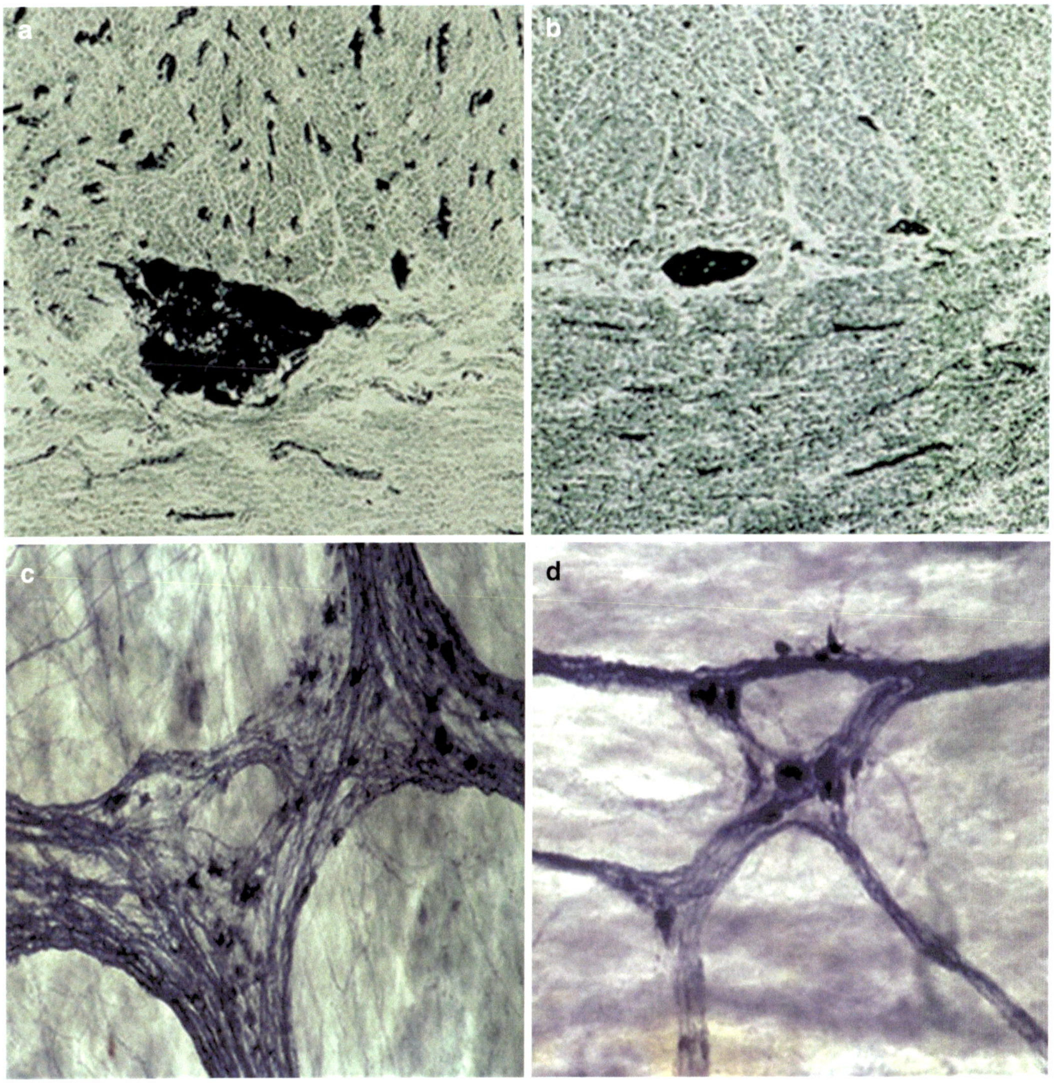

Fig. 20.2 NADPH-d staining in whole-mount preparation of a normal myenteric plexus (**a**, **c**). Myenteric plexus of a patient with isolated HG showing a markedly reduced number of ganglion cells (**b**, **d**)

20.5.3 Clinical Presentation of Immature Ganglia

The typical patient with IG is usually a premature infant who presents with a history of chronic constipation or functional bowel obstruction resembling HSCR. Further clinical features may include slow-transit peristalsis and insufficient defecation [116].

20.5.4 Diagnosis of Immature Ganglia

In general, the diagnosis of IG can be made from rectal suction biopsies. The ganglion cells appear very small and have a less significant nucleus with an inconspicuous nucleolus [112, 117] (Fig. 20.3a, b). However, it is often not possible with AChE immunohistochemistry to distinguish between these small ganglion cells and the sup-

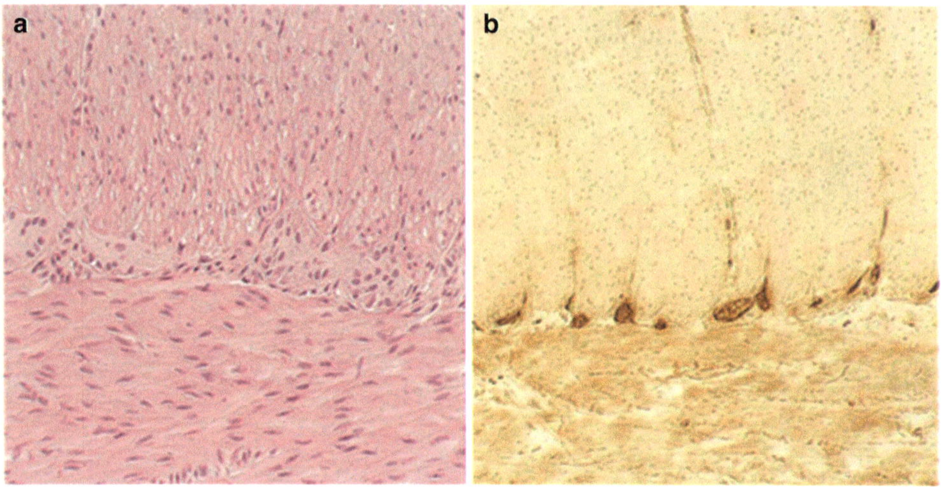

Fig. 20.3 Hematoxylin and eosin staining (**a**) and AChE immunohistochemistry (**b**) in a patient with IG showing immature ganglion cells

porting enteric glial cells. Therefore, NADPH-d and NCAM stainings have been suggested as neuronal markers to show the small ganglion cells more clearly [5, 104]. Enzyme histochemistry for succinate and lactate dehydrogenase is also commonly used to determine IG demonstrating an absent or rather weak positive reaction [3, 49]. In addition, cathepsin D has been recommended to assess the maturation of immature ganglion cells in more detail [53]. Another helpful biomarker to detect IG is the apoptosis regulator B-cell lymphoma 2 [118], which clearly differentiates immature small neurons from enteric glial cells and satellite cells.

20.5.5 Management of Immature Ganglia

The management of patients with IG is conservative with use of laxatives and enemas [5, 6].

20.5.6 Outcome of Immature Ganglia

The vast majority of patients with IG can successfully be managed with conservative treatment until their ganglion cells are fully mature [3, 6].

20.6 Absence of the Argyrophil Plexus

Deficiency of argyrophil cells in the myenteric plexus, which is also known as absence of the argyrophil plexus (AP), is a rare cause of constipation and functional bowel obstruction in infants and children.

20.6.1 Pathogenesis of Absence of the Argyrophil Plexus

There are two distinct subtypes of nerve cells in the myenteric plexus, which can be distinguished by their affinity for silver stains: (1) *argyrophil* cells and (2) *argentaffin* cells. Argyrophil cells normally comprise between 5% and 20% of the total number of myenteric neurons [119]. The processes of these cells along with extrinsic and parasympathetic fibers form a complex neuronal network within the myenteric plexus, which is involved in the regulation of gastrointestinal peristalsis and transit time. Argyrophil cells coordinate the activation of argentaffin cells, which in turn secrete specific neurotransmitters and ultimately cause contraction or relaxation of muscle fibers within the bowel wall [119]. A distinct time lag has been demonstrated between the developments of both cell types with argyrophil cells appearing earlier than argentaffin cells [120]. It has further been shown that there is a caudocranial gradient in the differentiation of these neuron cells in the human bowel [120, 121]. Therefore, it is suspected that the disruption of this differentiation process may lead to an absence of the AP.

20.6.2 Epidemiology of Absence of the Argyrophil Plexus

There is a paucity of published data on the incidence of this very rare condition. Puri et al. found three cases with absence of the AP in their series of 178 patients with functional bowel disorders [37]. Familial cases in the offspring of consanguineous parents and recurrence in siblings suggest that the absence of the AP may be inherited in an autosomal-recessive manner [119, 122].

20.6.3 Clinical Presentation of Absence of the Argyrophil Plexus

The clinical symptoms of patients with absence of the AP are highly similar to HSCR presenting with severe constipation, moderate abdominal distension, and lack of peristalsis [122].

20.6.4 Diagnosis of Absence of the Argyrophil Plexus

The absence of argyrophil cells and their neuronal processes can only be demonstrated by using silver impregnation of full-thickness biopsies (Fig. 20.4a, b), whereas conventional hematoxylin and eosin staining, AChE immunohistochemistry, and histochemistry with other neuronal markers fail to show this abnormality [5, 104, 123].

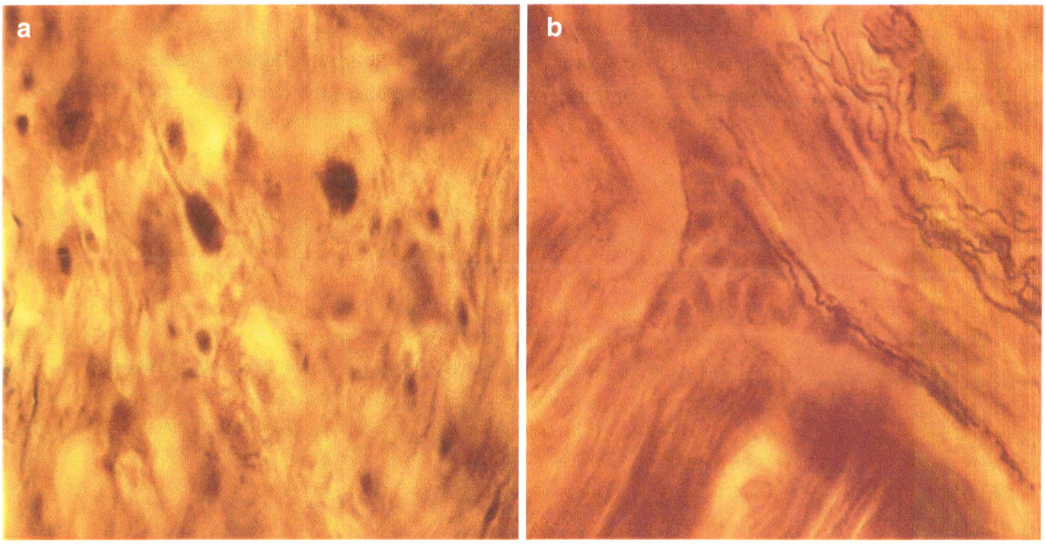

Fig. 20.4 Silver staining showing normal AP (**a**) and absence of argyrophil cells (**b**) in a patient with absence of the AP

20.6.5 Management of Absence of the Argyrophil Plexus

Most patients with absence of the AP can be managed conservatively with laxatives and enemas, but in some cases internal sphincter myectomy or formation of a colostomy may be necessary due to severe chronic constipation [5, 124].

20.6.6 Outcome of Absence of the Argyrophil Plexus

Conservative and surgical treatment of patients with absence of the AP usually results in a satisfactory outcome [5, 124].

20.7 Internal Anal Sphincter Achalasia

Internal anal sphincter achalasia (IASA) is a disorder with clinical presentation similar to HSCR [125–127] but with the presence of ganglion cells in rectal biopsies. Previously, IASA was referred to as ultrashort-segment HSCR, which is characterized by an aganglionic segment of 1–3 cm above the pectinate line, normal AChE activity in the lamina propria, and increased AChE activity in the muscularis mucosae [128]. Thus, several authors have suggested that IASA is a more accurate term for this pathological entity as many patients with absence of the rectosphincteric reflex on anorectal manometry actually showed presence of ganglion cells combined with normal AChE activity in rectal biopsies [129–131].

20.7.1 Pathogenesis of Internal Anal Sphincter Achalasia

Despite attempts of numerous investigators to determine the pathophysiological mechanisms of IASA in more detail, the exact pathogenesis remains unclear. Fujimoto et al. [132] suggested that age-related changes in the developing intramuscular innervation of the internal anal sphincter (IAS) may form the basis for the observed motility dysfunction. In 1995, by analyzing NADPH-d activity (Fig. 20.5a, b), a group from Ireland reported absent or a marked reduction of nitrergic innervation within the IAS of patients with IASA as the underlying pathomechanism leading to spasm or increased tone [133]. Additionally, a defective

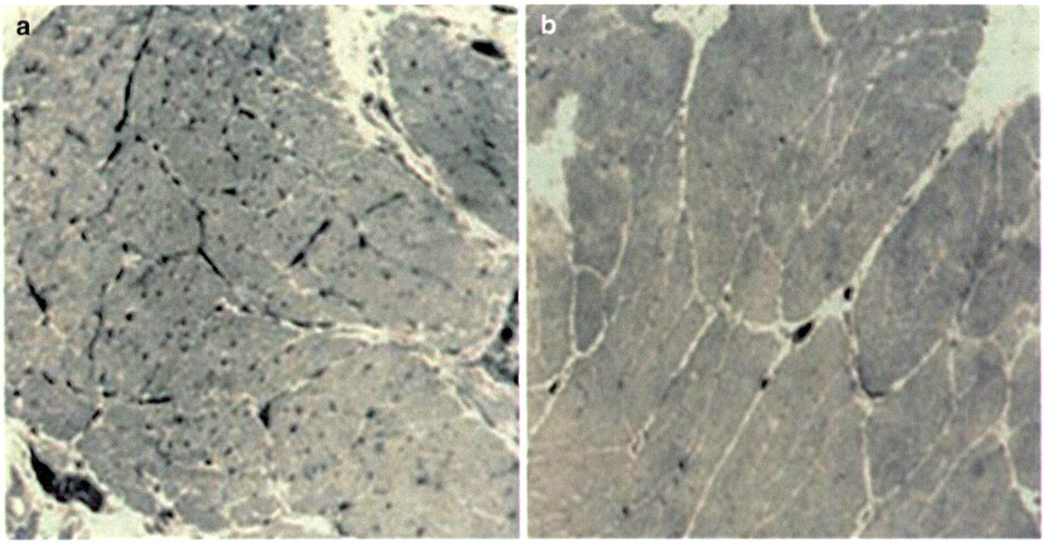

Fig. 20.5 NADPH-d staining of normal IAS (**a**). Reduced NADPH-d-positive innervations (**b**) in a patient with IASA

innervation of the neuromuscular junction of the IAS with decreased expression of PGP9.5 and synapsin-1 has been identified [134]. In 1996, Kobayashi et al. [97] further demonstrated absent to markedly reduced NADPH-d and NCAM activity in the IAS of patients with IASA. More recently, a reduced number of c-Kit-positive ICCs have been found in the IAS of patients with IASA [135]. The deficiency in nitrergic innervation and ICCs may explain the impaired IAS relaxation in patients with IASA [136].

20.7.2 Epidemiology of Internal Anal Sphincter Achalasia

A total number of 395 cases with IASA have been reported in the literature since 1973 [137]. However, the exact incidence of IASA is unknown.

20.7.3 Clinical Presentation of Internal Anal Sphincter Achalasia

The clinical presentation of IASA is in most cases similar to that of HSCR. Patients with IASA usually suffer from chronic and severe constipation with or without soiling. Approximately one-third of these patients have a history of abdominal distension and failure of laxative therapy [128, 129].

20.7.4 Diagnosis of Internal Anal Sphincter Achalasia

The diagnosis of IASA is based on clinical symptoms combined with the finding of absence of the rectosphincteric reflex on rectal balloon inflation with marked increased rhythmic activity on anorectal manometry (Fig. 20.6a, b), presence of

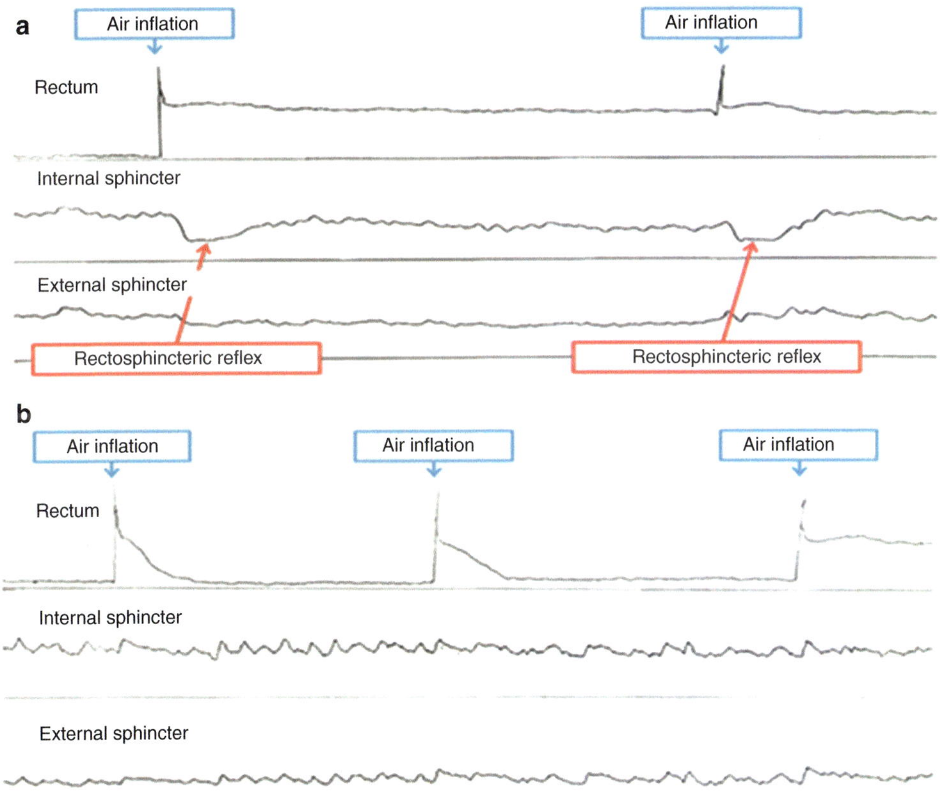

Fig. 20.6 Anorectal manometry showing evidence of the rectosphincteric reflex in a normal IAS (**a**). Absence of the rectosphincteric reflex on rectal balloon inflation with marked increased rhythmic activity of the IAS (**b**) in a patient with IASA

ganglion cells and normal AChE activity in rectal biopsies, as well as reduction of nitrergic innervation within the IAS.

20.7.5 Management of Internal anal Sphincter Achalasia

Traditionally, posterior IAS myectomy has been recommended for the treatment of IASA [138–140]. More recently, intrasphincteric injection of botulinum toxin has been introduced as a therapeutic alternative [141–146].

20.7.6 Outcome of Internal Anal Sphincter Achalasia

The vast majority of patients with IASA have regular bowel movements after treatment irrespective of the therapeutic approach [37, 138]. However, a recent meta-analysis indicated that posterior IAS myectomy appears to be a more effective treatment option resulting in a better functional outcome compared to intrasphincteric botulinum toxin injection [137]. The rate of transient fecal incontinence, nonresponse, and subsequent surgical procedures was significantly higher after injection of botulinum toxin, whereas long-term improvements were significantly more frequent following IAS myectomy. Interestingly, no differences were found in the postoperative use of laxatives or enemas, postoperative soiling, as well as constipation between both procedures.

20.8 Conclusions

Conditions that clinically resemble HSCR, despite the presence of ganglion cells on rectal biopsies, can be diagnosed by providing an adequate biopsy specimen and employing a variety of histological techniques. The two most common disorders in variant HSCR are IND and IASA. The majority of patients with IND can be successfully managed by conservative treatment or IAS myectomy. Pull-through operation is rarely indicated in the management of IND. IASA, which is characterized by nitrergic nerve depletion, can be diagnosed by anorectal manometry and successfully treated by either IAS myectomy or intrasphincteric Botox injection.

References

1. Ravitch MM. Pseudo Hirschsprung's disease. Ann Surg. 1958;147:781–95.
2. Bentley JFR, Nixon HH, Ehrenpreis TH, Spencer B, Lister L, Duhamel B, et al. Seminar on pseudo-Hirschsprung's disease and related disorders. Arch Dis Child. 1966;41:143–55.
3. Holschneider AM, Meier-Ruge W, Ure BM. Hirschsprung's disease and allied disorders - a review. Eur J Pediatr Surg. 1994;4:260–6.
4. Schärli AF. Standardization of terminology of dysganglionoses. Pediatr Surg Int. 1995;10:440.
5. Puri P. Variant Hirschsprung's disease. J Pediatr Surg. 1997;32:149–57.
6. Puri P, Rolle U. Variant Hirschsprung's disease. Semin Pediatr Surg. 2004;13:293–9.
7. Friedmacher F, Puri P. Classification and diagnostic criteria of variants of Hirschsprung's disease. Pediatr Surg Int. 2013;29:855–72.
8. Meier-Ruge W. Casuistic of colon disorder with symptoms of Hirschsprung's disease. Verh Dtsch Ges Pathol. 1971;55:506–10.
9. Puri P, Lake BD, Nixon HH, Mishalany H, Claireaux AE. Neuronal colonic dysplasia: an unusual association of Hirschsprung's disease. J Pediatr Surg. 1977;12:681–5.
10. Fadda B, Maier WA, Meier-Ruge W, Schärli A, Daum R. Neuronal intestinal dysplasia. Critical 10-years' analysis of clinical and biopsy diagnosis. Z Kinderchir. 1983;38:305–11.
11. Lake BD. Intestinal neuronal dysplasia. Why does it only occur in parts of Europe? Virchows Arch. 1995;426:537–9.
12. Lumb PD, Moore L. Back to the drawing board. Intestinal neuronal dysplasia type B: not a histological entity yet. Virchows Arch. 1998;432:99–102.
13. Sacher P, Briner J, Hanimann B. Is neuronal intestinal dysplasia (NID) a primary disease or a secondary phenomenon? Eur J Pediatr Surg. 1993;3:228–30.
14. Martucciello G, Pini Prato A, Puri P, Holschneider AM, Meier-Ruge W, Jasonni V, et al. Controversies concerning diagnostic guidelines for anomalies of the enteric nervous system: a report from the fourth International Symposium on Hirschsprung's disease and related neurocristopathies. J Pediatr Surg. 2005;40:1527–31.
15. Milla PJ, Smith VV. Intestinal neuronal dysplasia. J Pediatr Gastroenterol Nutr. 1993;17:356–7.
16. Hirobe S, Doody DP, Ryan DP, Kim SH, Donahoe PK. Ectopic class II major histocompatibility antigens in Hirschsprung's disease and neuronal intestinal dysplasia. J Pediatr Surg. 1992;27:357–62.
17. Kobayashi H, Mahomed A, Puri P. Intestinal neuronal dysplasia in twins. J Pediatr Gastroenterol Nutr. 1996;22:398–401.

18. Moore SW, Kaschula ROC, Cywes S. Familial and genetic-aspects of neuronal intestinal dysplasia and Hirschsprungs disease. Pediatr Surg Int. 1993;8:406–9.
19. Hatano M, Aoki T, Dezawa M, Yusa S, Iitsuka Y, Koseki H, et al. A novel pathogenesis of megacolon in Ncx/Hox11L.1 deficient mice. J Clin Invest. 1997;100:795–801.
20. Shirasawa S, Yunker AM, Roth KA, Brown GA, Horning S, Korsmeyer SJ. Enx (Hox11L1)-deficient mice develop myenteric neuronal hyperplasia and megacolon. Nat Med. 1997;3:646–50.
21. von Boyen GB, Krammer HJ, Süss A, Dembowski C, Ehrenreich H, Wedel T. Abnormalities of the enteric nervous system in heterozygous endothelin B receptor deficient (spotting lethal) rats resembling intestinal neuronal dysplasia. Gut. 2002;51:414–9.
22. Gath R, Goessling A, Keller KM, Koletzko S, Coerdt W, Müntefering H, et al. Analysis of the RET, GDNF, EDN3, and EDNRB genes in patients with intestinal neuronal dysplasia and Hirschsprung disease. Gut. 2001;48:671–5.
23. Costa M, Fava M, Seri M, Cusano R, Sancandi M, Forabosco P, et al. Evaluation of the HOX11L1 gene as a candidate for congenital disorders of intestinal innervation. J Med Genet. 2000;37:E9.
24. Fava M, Borghini S, Cinti R, Cusano R, Seri M, Lerone M, et al. HOX11L1: a promoter study to evaluate possible expression defects in intestinal motility disorders. Int J Mol Med. 2002;10:101–6.
25. Granero Cendón R, Millán López A, Moya Jiménez MJ, López Alonso M, De Agustín Asensio JC. Intestinal neuronal dysplasia: association with digestive malformations. Cir Pediatr. 2007;20:166–8.
26. Martucciello G, Caffarena PE, Lerone M, Mattioli G, Barabino A, Bisio G, et al. Neuronal intestinal dysplasia: clinical experience in Italian patients. Eur J Pediatr Surg. 1994;4:287–92.
27. Meier-Ruge W. Epidemiology of congenital innervation defects of the distal colon. Virchows Arch A Pathol Anat Histopathol. 1992;420:171–7.
28. Kobayashi H, Hirakawa H, Surana R, O'Briain DS, Puri P. Intestinal neuronal dysplasia is a possible cause of persistent bowel symptoms after pull-through operation for Hirschsprung's disease. J Pediatr Surg. 1995;30:253–7.
29. Montedonico S, Cáceres P, Muñoz N, Yáñez H, Ramírez R, Fadda B. Histochemical staining for intestinal dysganglionosis: over 30 years experience with more than 1,500 biopsies. Pediatr Surg Int. 2011;27:479–86.
30. Schmittenbecher PP, Sacher P, Cholewa D, Haberlik A, Menardi G, Moczulski J, et al. Hirschsprung's disease and intestinal neuronal dysplasia - a frequent association with implications for the postoperative course. Pediatr Surg Int. 1999;15:553–8.
31. Hanimann B, Inderbitzin D, Briner J, Sacher P. Clinical relevance of Hirschsprung-associated neuronal intestinal dysplasia (HANID). Eur J Pediatr Surg. 1992;2:147–9.
32. Schärli AF. Neuronal intestinal dysplasia. Pediatr Surg Int. 1992;7:2–7.
33. Ure BM, Holschneider AM, Schulten D, Meyer-Ruge W. Clinical impact of intestinal neuronal malformations: a prospective study in 141 patients. Pediatr Surg Int. 1997;12:377–82.
34. Csury L, Peña A. Intestinal neuronal dysplasia: myth or reality? Literature review. Pediatr Surg Int. 1995;10:441–6.
35. Schärli AF, Meier-Ruge W. Localized and disseminated forms of neuronal intestinal dysplasia mimicking Hirschsprung's disease. J Pediatr Surg. 1981;16(2):164–70.
36. Montedonico S, Acevedo S, Fadda B. Clinical aspects of intestinal neuronal dysplasia. J Pediatr Surg. 2002;37:1772–4.
37. Puri P, Gosemann JH. Variants of Hirschsprung disease. Semin Pediatr Surg. 2012;21:310–8.
38. Martucciello G, Torre M, Pini Prato A, Lerone M, Campus R, Leggio S, et al. Associated anomalies in intestinal neuronal dysplasia. J Pediatr Surg. 2002;37:219–23.
39. Pini Prato A, Rossi V, Fiore M, Avanzini S, Mattioli G, Sanfilippo F, et al. Megacystis, megacolon, and malrotation: a new syndromic association? Am J Med Genet A. 2011;155A:1798–802.
40. Koletzko S, Jesch I, Faus-Kebetaler T, Briner J, Meier-Ruge W, Müntefering H, et al. Rectal biopsy for diagnosis of intestinal neuronal dysplasia in children: a prospective multicentre study on interobserver variation and clinical outcome. Gut. 1999;44:853–61.
41. Lumb PD, Moore L. Are giant ganglia a reliable marker of intestinal neuronal dysplasia type B (IND B)? Virchows Arch. 1998;432:103–6.
42. Kapur RP. Neuronal dysplasia: a controversial pathological correlate of intestinal pseudo-obstruction. Am J Med Genet A. 2003;122A:287–93.
43. Meier-Ruge WA, Brönnimann PB, Gambazzi F, Schmid PC, Schmidt CP, Stoss F. Histopathological criteria for intestinal neuronal dysplasia of the submucosal plexus (type B). Virchows Arch. 1995;426:549–56.
44. Kobayashi H, Hirakawa H, Puri P. What are the diagnostic criteria for intestinal neuronal dysplasia? Pediatr Surg Int. 1995;10:459–64.
45. Coerdt W, Michel JS, Rippin G, Kletzki S, Gerein V, Müntefering H, et al. Quantitative morphometric analysis of the submucous plexus in age-related control groups. Virchows Arch. 2004;444:239–46.
46. Smith VV. Intestinal neuronal density in childhood: a baseline for the objective assessment of hypo- and hyperganglionosis. Pediatr Pathol. 1993;13:225–37.
47. Cord-Udy CL, Smith VV, Ahmed S, Risdon RA, Milla PJ. An evaluation of the role of suction rectal biopsy in the diagnosis of intestinal neuronal dysplasia. J Pediatr Gastroenterol Nutr. 1997;24:1–6.
48. Meyrat BJ, Laurini RN. Plasticity of the enteric nervous system in patients with intestinal neuronal dysplasia associated with Hirschsprung's disease: a report of three patients. Pediatr Surg Int. 2003;19:715–20.
49. Meier-Ruge WA, Bruder E. Pathology of chronic constipation in pediatric and adult coloproctology. Pathobiology. 2005;72:1–102.

50. Meier-Ruge WA, Schmid PC, Stoss F. Intestinal neuronal dysplasia and its morphometric evidences. Pediatr Surg Int. 1995;10:447–53.
51. Meier-Ruge WA, Longo-Bauer CH. Morphometric determination of the methodological criteria for the diagnosis of intestinal neuronal dysplasia (IND B). Pathol Res Pract. 1997;193:465–9.
52. Krammer HJ, Meier-Ruge W, Sigge W, Eggers R, Kühnel W. Histopathological features of neuronal intestinal dysplasia of the plexus submucosus in whole mounts revealed by immunohistochemistry for PGP 9.5. Eur J Pediatr Surg. 1994;4:358–61.
53. Tatekawa Y, Kanehiro H, Kanokogi H, Nakajima Y, Nishijima E, Muraji T, et al. The evaluation of meconium disease by distribution of cathepsin D in intestinal ganglion cells. Pediatr Surg Int. 2000;16:53–5.
54. Kobayashi H, Miyano T, Yamataka A, Lane GJ, Fujimoto T, Puri P. Use of synaptophysin polyclonal antibody for the rapid intraoperative immunohistochemical evaluation of functional bowel disorders. J Pediatr Surg. 1997;32:38–40.
55. Wester T, O'Briain S, Puri P. Morphometric aspects of the submucous plexus in whole-mount preparations of normal human distal colon. J Pediatr Surg. 1998;33:619–22.
56. Wester T, O'Briain DS, Puri P. Notable postnatal alterations in the myenteric plexus of normal human bowel. Gut. 1999;44:666–74.
57. Kobayashi H, Hirakawa H, Puri P. Is intestinal neuronal dysplasia a disorder of the neuromuscular junction? J Pediatr Surg. 1996;31:575–9.
58. Rolle U, Piotrowska AP, Puri P. Abnormal vasculature in intestinal neuronal dysplasia. Pediatr Surg Int. 2003;19:345–8.
59. Rolle U, Piaseczna-Piotrowska A, Puri P. Interstitial cells of Cajal in the normal gut and in intestinal motility disorders of childhood. Pediatr Surg Int. 2007;23:1139–52.
60. Yamataka A, Ohshiro K, Kobayashi H, Fujiwara T, Sunagawa M, Miyano T. Intestinal pacemaker C-KIT+ cells and synapses in allied Hirschsprung's disorders. J Pediatr Surg. 1997;32:1069–74.
61. O'Donnell AM, Puri P. A role for Pten in paediatric intestinal dysmotility disorders. Pediatr Surg Int. 2011;27:491–3.
62. Bruder E, Meier-Ruge WA. Intestinal neuronal dysplasia type B: how do we understand it today? Pathologe. 2007;28:137–42.
63. Meier-Ruge WA, Ammann K, Bruder E, Holschneider AM, Schärli AF, Schmittenbecher PP, et al. Updated results on intestinal neuronal dysplasia (IND B). Eur J Pediatr Surg. 2004;14:384–91.
64. Meier-Ruge WA, Bruder E, Kapur RP. Intestinal neuronal dysplasia type B: one giant ganglion is not good enough. Pediatr Dev Pathol. 2006;9:444–52.
65. Ure BM, Holschneider AM, Meier-Ruge W. Neuronal intestinal malformations: a retro- and prospective study on 203 patients. Eur J Pediatr Surg. 1994;4:279–86.
66. Puri P, Wester T. Intestinal neuronal dysplasia. Semin Pediatr Surg. 1998;7:181–6.
67. Stoss F, Meier-Ruge W. Experience with neuronal intestinal dysplasia (NID) in adults. Eur J Pediatr Surg. 1994;4:298–302.
68. Puri P. Intestinal neuronal dysplasia. Semin Pediatr Surg. 2003;12:259–64.
69. Schmittenbecher PP, Gluck M, Wiebecke B, Meier-Ruge W. Clinical long-term follow-up results in intestinal neuronal dysplasia (IND). Eur J Pediatr Surg. 2000;10:17–22.
70. Gillick J, Tazawa H, Puri P. Intestinal neuronal dysplasia: results of treatment in 33 patients. J Pediatr Surg. 2001;36:777–9.
71. Charagundla SR, Levine MS, Torigian DA, Campbell MS, Furth EE, Rombeau J. Diffuse intestinal ganglioneuromatosis mimicking Crohn's disease. AJR Am J Roentgenol. 2004;182:1166–8.
72. Matthews MA, Adler BH, Arnold MA, Kumar S, Carvalho R, Besner GE. Diffuse intestinal ganglioneuromatosis in a child. J Pediatr Surg. 2013;48:1129–33.
73. D'Amore ESG, Manivel JC, Pettinato G, Niehans GA, Snover DC. Intestinal ganglioneuromatosis: mucosal and transmural types. A clinicopathological and immunohistochemical study of 6 cases. Hum Pathol. 1991;22:276–86.
74. Moline J, Eng C. Multiple endocrine neoplasia type 2: an overview. Genet Med. 2011;13:755–64.
75. Puig I, Champeval D, De Santa Barbara P, Jaubert F, Lyonnet S, Larue L. Deletion of Pten in the mouse enteric nervous system induces ganglioneuromatosis and mimics intestinal pseudoobstruction. J Clin Invest. 2009;119:3586–96.
76. O'Riordain DS, Obrien T, Crotty TB, Gharib H, Grant CS, van Heerden JA. Multiple endocrine neoplasia type 2B: more than an endocrine disorder. Surgery. 1995;118:936–42.
77. Dunzendorfer T, Lee VW, Levine S, Morenas AD, Beazley RM, Chipkin S. Refractory constipation and megacolon in MEN 2b. Dig Dis Sci. 1996;41:2233–7.
78. Carney JA, Go VL, Sizemore GW, Hayles AB. Alimentary-tract ganglioneuromatosis: a major component of the syndrome of multiple endocrine neoplasia type 2b. N Engl J Med. 1976;295:1287–91.
79. de Krijger RR, Brooks A, van der Harst E, Hofstra RM, Bruining HA, Molenaar JC, et al. Constipation as the presenting symptom in de novo multiple endocrine neoplasia type 2B. Pediatrics. 1998;102:405–8.
80. Plenat F, Vignaud JM, Floquet J, Leroux P, Briquel N, Morali A, et al. Intestinal ganglioneuromatosis: histochemical, histoenzymological and ultrastructural study of a case. Ann Pathol. 1984;4:131–6.
81. DeSchryver-Kecskemeti K, Clouse RE, Goldstein MN, Gersell D, O'Neal L. Intestinal ganglioneuromatosis. A manifestation of overproduction of nerve growth factor? N Engl J Med. 1983;308:635–9.
82. Smith VV, Eng C, Milla PJ. Intestinal ganglioneuromatosis and multiple endocrine neoplasia type 2B: implications for treatment. Gut. 1999;45:143–6.
83. Torre M, Martucciello G, Ceccherini I, Lerone M, Aicardi M, Gambini C, et al. Diagnostic and therapeutic approach to multiple endocrine neoplasia type 2B in pediatric patients. Pediatr Surg Int. 2002;18:378–83.

84. Shekitka KM, Sobin LH. Ganglioneuromas of the gastrointestinal tract: relation to Von Recklinghausen disease and other multiple tumor syndromes. Am J Surg Pathol. 1994;18:250–7.
85. Yin M, King SK, Hutson JM, Chow CW. Multiple endocrine neoplasia type 2B diagnosed on suction rectal biopsy in infancy: a report of 2 cases. Pediatr Dev Pathol. 2006;9:56–60.
86. Sonsino E, Nabarra B, Andrianarison I, Weisgerber G, Navarro J, Bocquet L. Histological and ultrastructural study of intestinal ganglioneuromatosis. The multiple endocrine neoplasms type IIb syndrome. Ann Anat Pathol (Paris). 1979;24:29–44.
87. Demos TC, Blonder J, Schey WL, Braithwaite SS, Goldstein PL. Multiple endocrine neoplasia (MEN) syndrome type IIB: gastrointestinal manifestations. AJR Am J Roentgenol. 1983;140:73–8.
88. Feichter S, Meier-Ruge WA, Bruder E. The histopathology of gastrointestinal motility disorders in children. Semin Pediatr Surg. 2009;18:206–11.
89. Unruh A, Fitze G, Janig U, Bielack S, Lochbühler H, Coerdt W. Medullary thyroid carcinoma in a 2-month-old male with multiple endocrine neoplasia 2B and symptoms of pseudo-Hirschsprung disease: a case report. J Pediatr Surg. 2007;42:1623–6.
90. Cohen MS, Phay JE, Albinson C, DeBenedetti MK, Skinner MA, Lairmore TC, et al. Gastrointestinal manifestations of multiple endocrine neoplasia type 2. Ann Surg. 2002;235:648–54.
91. Brauckhoff M, Gimm O, Weiss CL, Ukkat J, Sekulla C, Brauckhoff K, et al. Multiple endocrine neoplasia 2B syndrome due to codon 918 mutation: clinical manifestation and course in early and late onset disease. World J Surg. 2004;28:1305–11.
92. Kobayashi H, Yamataka A, Lane GJ, Miyano T. Pathophysiology of hypoganglionosis. J Pediatr Gastroenterol Nutr. 2002;34:231–5.
93. Taguchi T, Masumoto K, Ieiri S, Nakatsuji T, Akiyoshi J. New classification of hypoganglionosis: congenital and acquired hypoganglionosis. J Pediatr Surg. 2006;41:2046–51.
94. Do MY, Myung SJ, Park HJ, Chung JW, Kim IW, Lee SM, et al. Novel classification and pathogenetic analysis of hypoganglionosis and adult-onset Hirschsprung's disease. Dig Dis Sci. 2011;56:1818–27.
95. Inoue K, Shimotake T, Tomiyama H, Iwai N. Mutational analysis of the RET and GDNF gene in children with hypoganglionosis. Eur J Pediatr Surg. 2001;11:120–3.
96. Rolle U, Yoneda A, Solari V, Nemeth L, Puri P. Abnormalities of C-Kit-positive cellular network in isolated hypoganglionosis. J Pediatr Surg. 2002;37:709–14.
97. Kobayashi H, Hirakawa H, Puri P. Abnormal internal anal sphincter innervation in patients with Hirschsprung's disease and allied disorders. J Pediatr Surg. 1996;31:794–9.
98. Kobayashi H, Li Z, Yamataka A, Lane GJ, Miyano T. Overexpression of neural cell adhesion molecule (NCAM) antigens on intestinal smooth muscles in hypoganglionosis: is hypoganglionosis a disorder of the neuromuscular junction? Pediatr Surg Int. 2003;19:190–3.
99. Dingemann J, Puri P. Isolated hypoganglionosis: systematic review of a rare intestinal innervation defect. Pediatr Surg Int. 2010;26:1111–5.
100. Zhang HY, Feng JX, Huang L, Wang G, Wei MF, Weng YZ. Diagnosis and surgical treatment of isolated hypoganglionosis. World J Pediatr. 2008;4:295–300.
101. Wedel T, Roblick UJ, Ott V, Eggers R, Schiedeck TH, Krammer HJ, et al. Oligoneuronal hypoganglionosis in patients with idiopathic slow-transit constipation. Dis Colon Rectum. 2002;45:54–62.
102. Watanabe Y, Ito F, Ando H, Seo T, Kaneko K, Harada T, et al. Morphological investigation of the enteric nervous system in Hirschsprung's disease and hypoganglionosis using whole-mount colon preparation. J Pediatr Surg. 1999;34:445–9.
103. Bruder E, Meier-Ruge WA. Hypoganglionosis as a cause of chronic constipation. Pathologe. 2007;28:131–6.
104. Puri P, Fujimoto T. Diagnosis of allied functional bowel disorders using monoclonal antibodies and electronmicroscopy. J Pediatr Surg. 1988;23:546–54.
105. Meier-Ruge WA, Brunner LA, Engert J, Heminghaus M, Holschneider AM, Jordan P, et al. A correlative morphometric and clinical investigation of hypoganglionosis of the colon in children. Eur J Pediatr Surg. 1999;9:67–74.
106. Kubota A, Yamauchi K, Yonekura T, Kosumi T, Oyanagi H, Mushiake S, et al. Clinicopathologic relationship of hypoganglionosis. J Pediatr Surg. 2001;36:898–900.
107. Miyazaki E, Ohshiro K, Puri P. NADPH-diaphorase histochemical staining of suction rectal biopsies in the diagnosis of Hirschsprung's disease and allied disorders. Pediatr Surg Int. 1998;13:464–7.
108. Yamataka A, Fujiwara T, Nishiye H, Sunagawa M, Miyano T. Localization of intestinal pacemaker cells and synapses in the muscle layers of a patient with colonic hypoganglionosis. J Pediatr Surg. 1996;31:584–7.
109. Munakata K, Okabe I, Morita K. Hypoganglionosis. Pediatr Surg Int. 1992;7:8–11.
110. Schärli AF, Sossai R. Hypoganglionosis. Semin Pediatr Surg. 1998;7:187–91.
111. Burki T, Kiho L, Scheimberg I, Phelps S, Misra D, Ward H, et al. Neonatal functional intestinal obstruction and the presence of severely immature ganglion cells on rectal biopsy: 6 year experience. Pediatr Surg Int. 2011;27:487–90.
112. Smith B. Pre- and postnatal development of the ganglion cells of the rectum and its surgical implications. J Pediatr Surg. 1968;3:386–91.
113. Montedonico S, Sri Paran T, Pirker M, Rolle U, Puri P. Developmental changes in submucosal nitrergic neurons in the porcine distal colon. J Pediatr Surg. 2006;41:1029–35.
114. Sri Paran T, Rolle U, Puri P. Postnatal development of the mucosal plexus in the porcine small and large intestine. Pediatr Surg Int. 2006;22:997–1001.

115. Sri Paran T, Rolle U, Puri P. Postnatal changes in enteric plexus axonal thickness. Pediatr Surg Int. 2008;24:1365–7.
116. Bughaighis AG, Emergy JL. Functional obstruction of the intestine due to neurological immaturity. Prog Pediatr Surg. 1971;3:37–52.
117. Venugopal S, Mancer K, Shandling B. The validity of rectal biopsy in relation to morphology and distribution of ganglion cells. J Pediatr Surg. 1981;16:433–7.
118. Park SH, Min H, Chi JG, Park KW, Yang HR, Seo JK. Immunohistochemical studies of pediatric intestinal pseudo-obstruction: bcl2, a valuable biomarker to detect immature enteric ganglion cells. Am J Surg Pathol. 2005;29:1017–24.
119. Tanner MS, Smith B, Lloyd JK. Functional intestinal obstruction due to deficiency of argyrophil neurones in the myenteric plexus: familial syndrome presenting with short small bowel, malrotation, and pyloric hypertrophy. Arch Dis Child. 1976;51:837–41.
120. Singh I. The prenatal development of enterochromaffin cells in the human gastro-intestinal tract. J Anat. 1963;97:377–87.
121. Lolova IS, Davidoff MS, Itzev DE. Histological and immunocytochemical data on the differentiation of intestinal endocrine cells in human fetus. Acta Physiol Pharmacol Bulg. 1998;23:61–71.
122. Auricchio A, Brancolini V, Casari G, Milla PJ, Smith VV, Devoto M, et al. The locus for a novel syndromic form of neuronal intestinal pseudoobstruction maps to Xq28. Am J Hum Genet. 1996;58:743–8.
123. Garvey W, Fathi A, Bigelow F, Carpenter B, Jimenez C. A new method for demonstrating argyrophil cells of the pancreas and intestines. Stain Technol. 1989;64:87–91.
124. Puri P, Lake BD, Nixon HH. Adynamic bowel syndrome: report of a case with disturbance of the cholinergic innervation. Gut. 1977;18:754–9.
125. Bentley JF. Faecal soiling and anal achalasia. Arch Dis Child. 1978;53:185–6.
126. Fadda B, Welskop J, Müntefering H, Meier-Ruge W, Engert J. Achalasia of the anal sphincter: Enzyme-histotopochemical studies of internal sphincter muscle biopsies. Pediatr Surg Int. 1987;2:81–5.
127. Davidson M, Bauer CH. Studies of distal colonic motility in children. IV. Achalasia of the distal rectal segment despite presence of ganglia in the myenteric plexuses of this area. Pediatrics. 1958;21:746–61.
128. De Caluwé D, Yoneda A, Akl U, Puri P. Internal anal sphincter achalasia: outcome after internal sphincter myectomy. J Pediatr Surg. 2001;36:736–8.
129. Doodnath R, Puri P. Internal anal sphincter achalasia. Semin Pediatr Surg. 2009;18:246–8.
130. Lake BD, Puri P, Nixon HH, Claireaux AE. Hirschsprung's disease: an appraisal of histochemically demonstrated acetylcholinesterase activity in suction rectal biopsy specimens as an aid to diagnosis. Arch Pathol Lab Med. 1978;102:244–7.
131. Neilson IR, Yazbeck S. Ultrashort Hirschsprung's disease: myth or reality. J Pediatr Surg. 1990;25:1135–8.
132. Fujimoto T, Puri P, Miyano T. Abnormal peptidergic innervation in internal sphincter achalasia. Pediatr Surg Int. 1992;7:12–7.
133. Hirakawa H, Kobayashi H, O'Briain DS, Puri P. Absence of NADPH-diaphorase activity in internal anal sphincter (IAS) achalasia. J Pediatr Gastroenterol Nutr. 1995;20:54–8.
134. Oue T, Puri P. Altered intramuscular innervation and synapse formation in internal sphincter achalasia. Pediatr Surg Int. 1999;15:192–4.
135. Piotrowska AP, Solari V, Puri P. Distribution of interstitial cells of Cajal in the internal anal sphincter of patients with internal anal sphincter achalasia and Hirschsprung disease. Arch Pathol Lab Med. 2003;127:1192–5.
136. de Lorijn F, de Jonge WJ, Wedel T, Vanderwinden JM, Benninga MA, Boeckxstaens GE. Interstitial cells of Cajal are involved in the afferent limb of the rectoanal inhibitory reflex. Gut. 2005;54:1107–13.
137. Friedmacher F, Puri P. Comparison of posterior internal anal sphincter myectomy and intrasphincteric botulinum toxin injection for treatment of internal anal sphincter achalasia: a meta-analysis. Pediatr Surg Int. 2012;28:765–71.
138. Hecker WC, Holschneider A, Fendel H, Schauer A, Meister P, Beige H. Chronic constipation in children due to achalasia of the internal anal sphincter. Dtsch Med Wochenschr. 1973;98:2334–40.
139. Heikkinen M, Lindahl H, Rintala RJ. Long-term outcome after internal sphincter myectomy for internal sphincter achalasia. Pediatr Surg Int. 2005;21:84–7.
140. Doodnath R, Puri P. Long-term outcome of internal sphincter myectomy in patients with internal anal sphincter achalasia. Pediatr Surg Int. 2009;25:869–71.
141. Langer JC, Birnbaum E. Preliminary experience with intrasphincteric botulinum toxin for persistent constipation after pull-through for Hirschsprung's disease. J Pediatr Surg. 1997;32:1059–61.
142. Minkes RK, Langer JC. A prospective study of botulinum toxin for internal anal sphincter hypertonicity in children with Hirschsprung's disease. J Pediatr Surg. 2000;35:1733–6.
143. Messineo A, Codrich D, Monai M, Martellossi S, Ventura A. The treatment of internal anal sphincter achalasia with botulinum toxin. Pediatr Surg Int. 2001;17:521–3.
144. Ciamarra P, Nurko S, Barksdale E, Fishman S, Di Lorenz C. Internal anal sphincter achalasia in children: clinical characteristics and treatment with Clostridium botulinum toxin. J Pediatr Gastroenterol Nutr. 2003;37:315–9.
145. Irani K, Rodriguez L, Doody DP, Goldstein AM. Botulinum toxin for the treatment of chronic constipation in children with internal anal sphincter dysfunction. Pediatr Surg Int. 2008;24:779–83.
146. Koivusalo AI, Pakarinen MP, Rintala RJ. Botox injection treatment for anal outlet obstruction in patients with internal anal sphincter achalasia and Hirschsprung's disease. Pediatr Surg Int. 2009;25:873–6.

Megacystis Microcolon Intestinal Hypoperistalsis Syndrome

21

Prem Puri and Hiroki Nakamura

Contents

21.1 Introduction

Megacystis microcolon intestinal hypoperistalsis syndrome (MMIHS) is a rare congenital and generally fatal cause of functional intestinal obstruction in the newborn [2]. This syndrome is characterized by massive abdominal distension caused largely by a dilated non-obstructed urinary bladder, microcolon, and decreased or absent intestinal peristalsis [2]. Usually incomplete intestinal rotation and shortened small bowel are associated factors. MMIHS represents the most severe form of functional intestinal obstruction in the newborn and is generally associated with a fatal outcome [2, 29].

P. Puri (✉)
National Children's Research Centre, Our Lady's Childrens Hospital, University College Dublin, Dublin, Ireland
e-mail: prem.puri@ncrc.ie

H. Nakamura
National Children's Research Centre, Our Lady's Children's Hospital, Crumlin, Dublin, Ireland
e-mail: hinakamu@juntendo.ac.jp

21.2 Pathogenesis

MMIHS was first described by Berdon et al. in 1976 in a series of five female neonates. The etiology of this syndrome has not fully been understood. Several hypotheses have been proposed to explain the pathogenesis of MMIHS: genetic [9–11, 18], neurogenic [8, 20, 35], myogenic [5, 27, 28, 31], and hormonal [14].

Familial occurrence of MMIHS has been reported. The first insights into the genetic basis of MMIHS appeared to come from transgenic mice lacking certain nicotinic acetylcholine receptor (ηAChR) subunits, which showed some of the phenotypic features of MMIHS, thus suggesting a basis for this condition. Xu et al. [42] produced a MMIHS phenotype in beta 4/alpha 3 (two of the seven neuronal nicotinic acetylcholine receptor subunits) knockout mice. The alpha 3 and beta 4 subunits have been localized to human chromosome 15. Richardson et al. [30] carried out in situ hybridization and immunocytochemistry studies to determine whether alpha 3 mRNA or alpha 3 subunit protein was expressed in the resected specimens of small bowel from patients

P. Puri (ed.), *Hirschsprung's Disease and Allied Disorders*,
https://doi.org/10.1007/978-3-030-15647-3_21

with MMIHS. They found a lack of α3 ηAChR staining in most MMIHS tissues, thus suggesting that the absence of functional α3 subunit containing ηAChR may provide a possible explanation for the underlying pathogenesis of MMIHS.

It has been suggested that MMIHS is inherited in an autosomal recessive manner as consanguinity between parents and recurrence in siblings is frequently seen [23]. However, since most cases of MMIHS occur sporadically, it has been hypothesized that locus heterogeneity exists and that the genetic etiology of sporadic and familial MMIHS cases may differ. In recent years, using whole-exome sequencing, a powerful tool used to identify disease genes, four genes have been found to be involved in the pathogenesis of MMIHS. De novo variants in the ACTG2 gene are implicated in the autosomal-dominant form of MMIHS, whereas homozygous variants in MYH11, MYLK, and LMOD1 cause a recessive form of the disease. Heterozygous missense variants in the *ACTG2* gene have been reported as a cause of sporadic MMIHS cases in several independent studies [36, 37, 39], while a homozygous missense variant in *MYH11* was identified in a newborn patient with consanguineous parents [6], and homozygous variants in *MYLK* were found in three MMIHS patients from two consanguineous families [9]. *ACTG2* is the main actin isoform expressed in smooth muscle cells (SMCs), and changes affecting its structure lead to severe disruption of smooth cell development and function. The *MYH11* gene is a highly specific contractile gene for smooth muscle linages. Mice with homozygous deletion of *MYH11* show several smooth muscle cell abnormalities including a large and thin-walled bladder and abnormal intestinal movement, the typical features of MMIHS. The *MYLK* gene is an important kinase required for myosin activation and subsequent interaction with actin filaments, and its absence leads to impairment of smooth muscle cell contraction. The *LMOD1* gene is involved in the smooth muscle cytoskeletal-contractile coupling, and loss of *LMOD1* results in a reduction of filamentous actin, elongated cytoskeletal dense bodies, and impaired intestinal smooth muscle cell contractility.

21.2.1 Epidemiology

Between 1976 and 2018, 450 patients with the diagnosis of MMIHS have been reported in the literature [24]. The overall female to male ratio of MMIHS cases was 2.3:1, suggesting a female predominance in this condition. It has been reported that male MMIHS patients seem to have a shorter life span than affected females. This has been suggested to be most likely due to a more severe disorder in males compared with females [17, 43]. Familial occurrence of MMIHS has been frequently reported. There were 56 (12.4%) cases in which familial MMIHS was confirmed, 25 families with multiple siblings, and 3 families with a single affected infant. Seven further confirmed index cases of MMIHS had a probable afflicted sibling, and one of the sibling pairs had a probable third affected sibling. The probable cases suffered intrauterine death or died in the early neonatal period with evidence of bladder and bowel pathology consistent with MMIHS but without a confirmed diagnosis. Of the 25 families with multiple siblings, 22 families had two siblings with confirmed MMIHS and 3 families had 3 children each with MMIHS. Consanguinity between parents was confirmed in 30 (6.7%) cases (18 siblings and 12 individual cases) (Tables 21.1 and 21.2).

21.2.2 Diagnosis

21.2.2.1 Prenatal Diagnosis

The literature on the prenatal diagnosis of MMIHS is not extensive. A recent review of the diagnosis of MMIHS reported that 25% of cases were diagnosed prenatally [37]. The most frequent finding was an enlarged bladder in 88%, with hydronephrosis seen in 57% [4, 8, 13, 37, 40]. Normal amniotic fluid volume was revealed in 59%, increased volume in 33%, and decreased volume in 7%. Oligohydramnios changed to polyhydramnios at the end of the third trimester [34]. Serial obstetric ultrasonography showed that the earliest finding in MMIHS is an enlarged

Table 21.1 Cases in siblings with MMIHS and consanguinity

Author	Year	Number of siblings		Consanguinity
Winter	1986		2	+
Penman	1989		2	+
Gakmak	1989		3	+
Anneren	1991		2	+
Moreno	2016		2	+
Halim	2016		2	+
Halim	2017	Family 1	3	+
		Family 2	2	+

Table 21.2 Individual cases with MMIHS and consanguinity

Author	Year	Number of individual case	Consanguinity
Kirtane	1984	1	+
Mc. Namara	1994	1	+
Junior	1996	1	+
Al Harbi	1999	1	+
White	2000	1	+
Narayanan	2007	1	+
Melek	2009	1	+
Hiradfar	2013	1	+
Gauthier	2015	1	+
Garcia	2015	1	+
Halim	2016	1	+
Halim	2017	1	+

bladder, detectable from 16 weeks of gestational age (Fig. 21.1). A later finding is hydronephrosis, caused by the functional obstruction of the bladder. Usually polyhydramnios develops late, appearing during the third trimester.

More recently, Rosenblatt et al. [32] reported prenatal diagnosis of MMIHS by biochemical analysis of fetal urine. They retrospectively performed biochemical analysis of fetal urine samples collected from patients who presented prenatally with megabladder detected at the second-trimester or third-trimester routine ultrasound examination. Mean fetal urine β2-microglobulin was significantly higher in end-stage renal failure than in MMIHS and the control group. Fetal urine profiles (e.g., median sodium, median calcium, and median phosphorus) differed significantly between MMIHS and the control group.

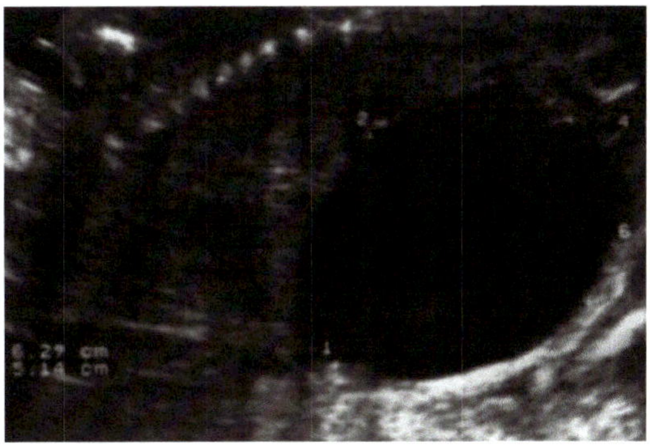

Fig. 21.1 Large fetal bladder seen on a longitudinal abdominal ultrasound image at 22 weeks of gestation. The fetus is in the prone position

21.2.2.2 Postnatal Diagnosis

The clinical presentation of MMIHS is similar to that of other severe neonatal intestinal obstructions. The most prominent and frequent finding is abdominal distension, which is a consequence of the massively enlarged urinary bladder with or without upper urinary tract dilatation. Most patients are not able to void spontaneously and require catheterization or vesicostomy. Other frequently reported clinical features include bile-stained vomiting, failure to pass meconium, and absent or decreased bowel sounds.

21.2.3 Radiological Findings

Radiological evaluation usually suggests the diagnosis of MMIHS. Plain abdominal films show either dilated small bowel loops or a gasless abdomen with evident gastric bubble. An enlarged urinary bladder was present in all reported cases which had cystography or ultrasonography (Fig. 21.2). Cystography may also show vesicoureteral reflux [8, 12, 26] and a urachal remnant [29]. Ultrasonography detected unilateral or bilateral hydronephrosis in 46% of patients [41]. Barium enema showed microcolon in all patients in whom this study was done (Fig. 21.3); Puri et al. [29] reported 53% of patients with MMIHS had malrotation.

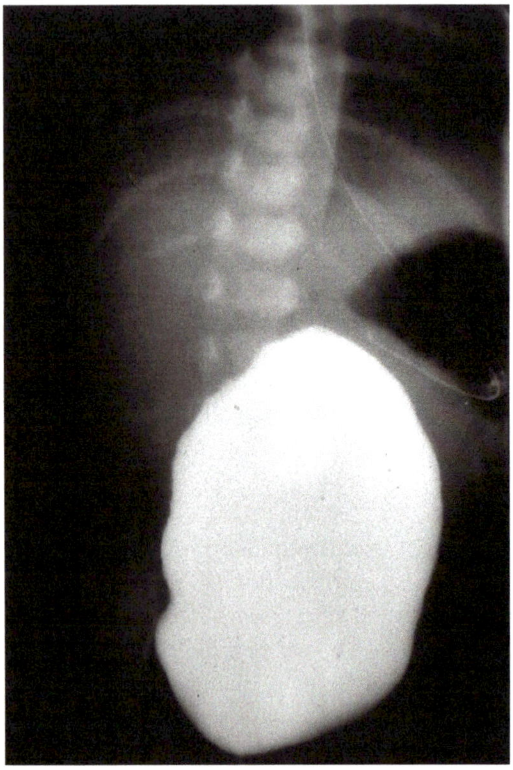

Fig. 21.2 Voiding cystourethrogram showing a massively enlarged bladder in a MMIHS patient

21.2.4 Surgical or Autopsy Findings

Megacystis (Fig. 21.4) and microcolon were the two most frequent findings at surgery or autopsy and were present in all patients. Although surgical management was not mentioned in several reports, over 70% of patients underwent one or more surgical procedures [29]. Different kinds of interventions were performed: gastrostomy, jejunostomy, ileostomy, cecostomy, segmental resection of the jejunum and ileum, lysis of adhesions, and internal sphincter myectomy. Surgical manipulation of the gastrointestinal tract generally has been unsuccessful, and in most patients, total parenteral nutrition (TPN) was required [29]. Wymer et al. [41] reported urologic management in 73 cases with MMIHS and found that 30% (22/73) of the patients received vesicostomy while the remaining patients managed with clean intermittent catheterization.

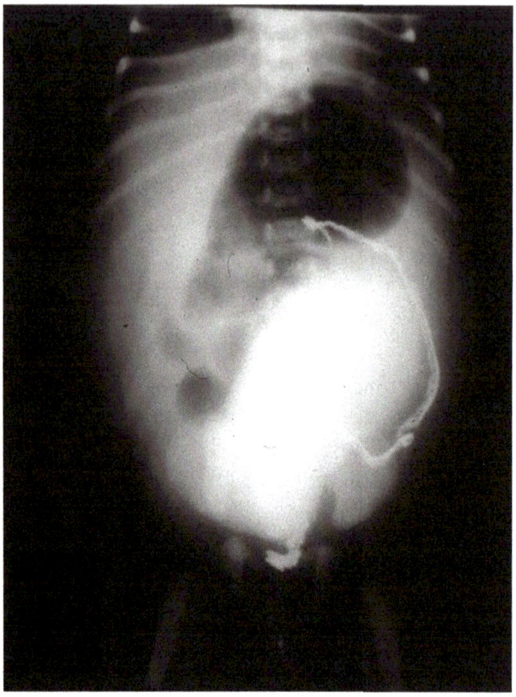

Fig. 21.3 A contrast enema showing microcolon in a MMIHS patient

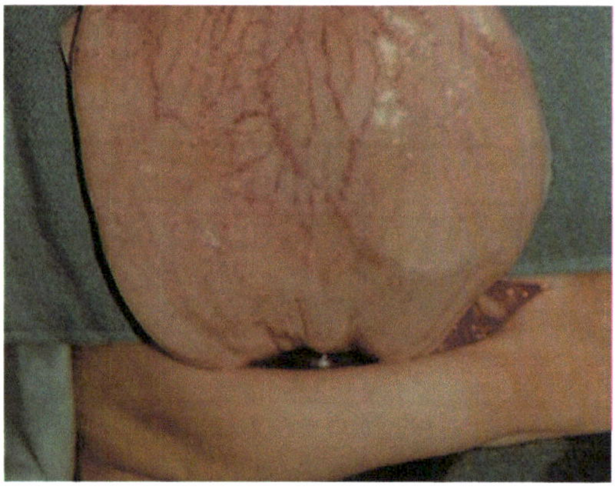

Fig. 21.4 Operative photograph of a massively dilated urinary bladder in MMIHS

21.2.5 Histological Findings

Puri et al. [29] reviewed the histological studies of the myenteric and submucous plexuses which have been reported in 93 out of 182 patients in their review. In 72 patient's the ganglion cells were normal in appearance and number. Young et al. [43] found one patient with diffuse hypoganglionosis, and Vezina et al. [38] found aganglionic zones together with hyperganglionic zones in another patient. Immature ganglion cells were found by Manco and Osterdahl [22] in one patient. Kirtane et al. [15] found two patients with immature ganglion cells and hypoganglionosis. Krook [19] found both aganglionic zones and immature zones throughout the bowel. In four patients [14, 33], hyperganglionosis was evident. Bindl et al. [3] reported neuronal intestinal dysplasia type B in one patient. Observations on the nerve fibers in the intestinal plexuses were reported for 26 patients. In 15 the appearance was normal, in 9 the nerve fibers were observed to be increased, and in 2 they were decreased. Taguchi et al. [35] noted an abnormal peptidergic innervation caused by a decrease in vasoactive intestinal polypeptide and peptide histidine methionine fibers and an increase in substance P and leucine-enkephalin fibers. At autopsy, neonatal axonal dystrophy was found in a patient with previous findings of hypertrophic nerve bundles and dystrophic neuritis in rectal biopsy [1]. Kobayashi et al. [16] observed hyperganglionosis of the submucous and myenteric plexuses and giant ganglia and ectopic ganglia throughout the entire gastrointestinal tract in two patients. Acetylcholinesterase staining and neural cell adhesion molecule (NCAM) staining of the uterus in one patient demonstrated a large number of ganglioneuromas [16]. Piotrowska et al. [27] reported an absence of ICCs in the bowel and bladder of patients with MMIHS.

The majority of reports do not mention the histological findings in the muscle layers of the bowel and bladder wall. Nevertheless, some authors found significant abnormalities in smooth muscle cells including thinning of the longitudinal muscle, connective tissue proliferation, and absence or deficiency of α-smooth muscle actin and other contractile and cytoskeletal proteins in the smooth muscle layers of MMIHS bowel and bladder [27, 31]. In 1983, Puri et al. reported findings using electron microscopy in MMIHS and showed vacuolar degenerative changes in the center of smooth muscle cells (SMCs) with abundant connective tissue between SMCs in the bowel and bladder of these patients. Several subsequent reports have confirmed evidence of hollow visceral myopathy in MMIHS (Fig. 21.5) [27, 28, 31].

21.2.6 Management

MMIHS is the most severe form of functional intestinal obstruction in the newborn and is generally a fatal condition. Treatment usually involves targeting both gastrointestinal and genitourinary deficits associated with the condition. Most patients are maintained on long-term TPN which may lead to serious complications such as catheter-associated sepsis and liver failure. Surgical interventions have been performed frequently in MMIHS patients such as gastrostomy, jejunostomy, ileostomy, and colostomy. The need for surgical intervention should be carefully evaluated and the intervention individualized since most exploration might not be helpful and probably not necessary. MMIHS patients are not able to void spontaneously and, therefore, would require either a vesicostomy or clean intermittent catheterization.

Recently, intestinal and multivisceral transplantation was introduced as a valuable therapeutic alternative for children with irreversible intestinal and total parenteral nutrition failure [21]. In a review, data from 12 MMIHS patients, who underwent multivisceral transplant surgery to date, were obtained [7]. The majority received liver, pancreas, small bowel, and colon transplants. Loinaz et al. reported a 3-year survival of 50% in their series [21]. The authors further reported that all survivors tolerated enteral feedings and showed adequate gastric emptying. In contrast, bladder function did not improve, and catheterization had to be continued after transplantation [21].

21.2.7 Outcome

The management of patients with MMIHS is frustrating as the outcome is generally fatal. These patients are mainly maintained on total parenteral nutrition (TPN), which leads to further comorbid-

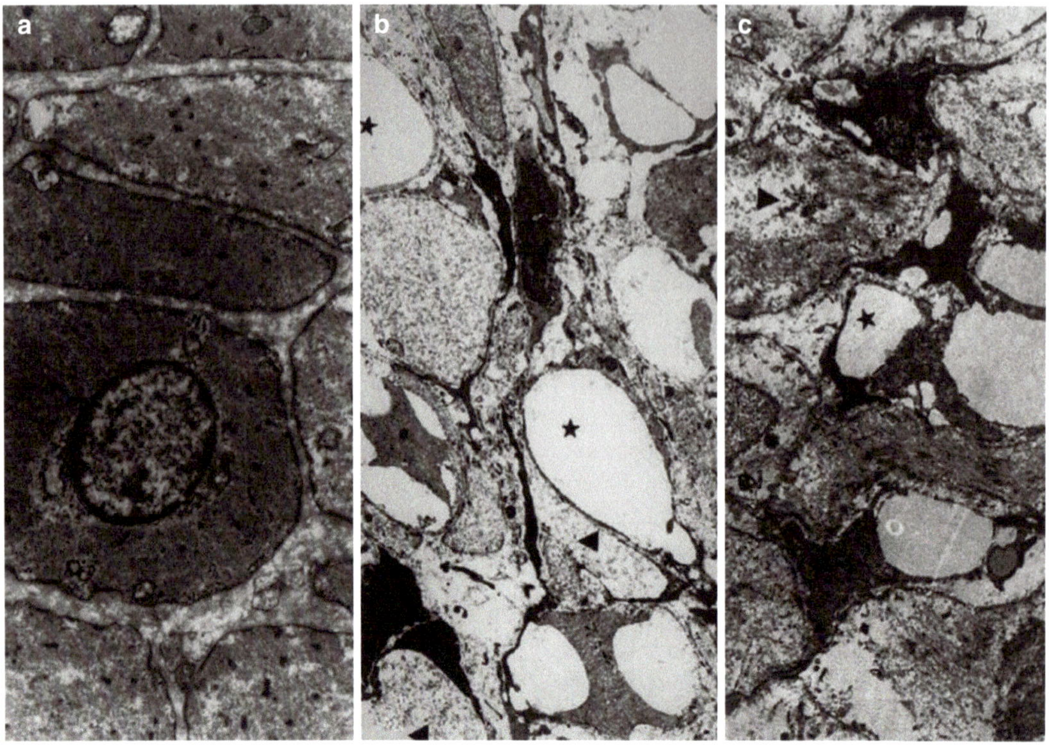

Fig. 21.5 (a–c) Electron microscopy. (a) Smooth muscle cells from normal ileum. (b) Ileum from a patient with MMIHS showing vacuolar changes in the center of smooth muscle cells. (c) Vacuolar degeneration of smooth muscle cells in the urinary bladder from the same patient (*asterisks* vacuolated cells, *arrowheads* excessive collagen between smooth muscles) (×6800)

ities, such as catheter sepsis, dyslipidemia, TPN-associated liver disease, and eventually chronic liver failure. In recent years, survival in MMIHS has improved due to more specialized care, innovations in TPN, and introduction of multivisceral transplantation. A large review by Gosemann et al. [7] found that the survival rate of patients with MMIHS increased from 13% to 55% when comparing patients diagnosed from 1976 to 2004 to those diagnosed from 2005 to 2011, respectively. However, as regards the long-term outcome, only 67 (15%) of the 450 reported cases were alive, the oldest being 24 years old [25]. The majority of survivors are either maintained by TPN or have undergone multivisceral transplantation.

21.2.8 Conclusion

MMIHS is the rarest and most severe form of functional intestinal obstruction in the newborn. The major features of this congenital and usually lethal anomaly are abdominal distension, bile-stained vomiting, and absent or decreased bowel peristalsis. Abdominal distension is a consequence of the distended, unobstructed urinary bladder with or without upper urinary tract dilatation. Most patients with MMIHS are not able to void spontaneously and require either clean intermittent catheterization or vesicostomy. Surgical intervention of the gastrointestinal tract has generally been unsuccessful [29]. The majority of long-term survivors are either maintained by TPN or have undergone multivisceral transplantation.

References

1. al-Rayess M, Ambler MW. Axonal dystrophy presenting as the megacystis-microcolon-intestinal hypoperistalsis syndrome. Pediatr Pathol. 1992;12(5):743–50.
2. Berdon WE, Baker DH, Blanc WA, Gay B, Santulli TV, Donovan C. Megacystis-microcolon-intestinal hypoperistalsis syndrome: a new cause of intestinal obstruction in the newborn. Report of radiologic find-

ings in five newborn girls. AJR Am J Roentgenol. 1976;126(5):957–64.
3. Bindl L, Emons D, Haverkamp F, Fahnenstich H, Kowalewski S, Meier-Ruge W. Megacystis microcolon intestinal hypoperistalsis syndrome: a neuropathy? Z Kinderchir. 1989;44(4):249–52.
4. Buinoiu N, Panaitescu A, Demetrian M, Ionescu S, Peltecu G, Veduta A. Ultrasound prenatal diagnosis of typical megacystis, microcolon, intestinal hypoperistalsis syndrome. Clin Case Rep. 2018;6(5):855–8.
5. Ciftci AO, Cook RC, van Velzen D. Megacystis microcolon intestinal hypoperistalsis syndrome: evidence of a primary myocellular defect of contractile fiber synthesis. J Pediatr Surg. 1996;31(12):1706–11.
6. Gauthier J, Ouled Amar Bencheikh B, Hamdan FF, Harrison SM, Baker LA, Couture F, et al. A homozygous loss-of-function variant in MYH11 in a case with megacystis-microcolon-intestinal hypoperistalsis syndrome. Eur J Hum Genet. 2015;23(9):1266–8.
7. Gosemann JH, Puri P. Megacystis microcolon intestinal hypoperistalsis syndrome: systematic review of outcome. Pediatr Surg Int. 2011;27(10):1041–6.
8. Granata C, Puri P. Megacystis-microcolon-intestinal hypoperistalsis syndrome. J Pediatr Gastroenterol Nutr. 1997;25(1):12–9.
9. Halim D, Brosens E, Muller F, Wangler MF, Beaudet AL, Lupski JR, et al. Loss-of-function variants in MYLK cause recessive megacystis microcolon intestinal hypoperistalsis syndrome. Am J Hum Genet. 2017;101(1):123–9.
10. Halim D, Hofstra RM, Signorile L, Verdijk RM, van der Werf CS, Sribudiani Y, et al. ACTG2 variants impair actin polymerization in sporadic megacystis microcolon intestinal hypoperistalsis syndrome. Hum Mol Genet. 2016;25(3):571–83.
11. Halim D, Wilson MP, Oliver D, Brosens E, Verheij JB, Han Y, et al. Loss of LMOD1 impairs smooth muscle cytocontractility and causes megacystis microcolon intestinal hypoperistalsis syndrome in humans and mice. Proc Natl Acad Sci U S A. 2017;114(13):E2739–E47.
12. Hoehn W, Thomas GG, Mearadji M. Urologic evaluation of megacystis-microcolon-intestinal hypoperistalsis syndrome. Urology. 1981;17(5):465–6.
13. Hsu CD, Craig C, Pavlik J, Ninios A. Prenatal diagnosis of megacystis-microcolon-intestinal hypoperistalsis syndrome in one fetus of a twin pregnancy. Am J Perinatol. 2003;20(4):215–8.
14. Jona JZ, Werlin SL. The megacystis microcolon intestinal hypoperistalsis syndrome: report of a case. J Pediatr Surg. 1981;16(5):749–51.
15. Kirtane J, Talwalker V, Dastur DK. Megacystis, microcolon, intestinal hypoperistalsis syndrome: possible pathogenesis. J Pediatr Surg. 1984;19(2):206–8.
16. Kobayashi H, O'Briain S, Puri P. New observation of the pathogenesis of megacystis microcolon intestinal hypoperistalsis syndrome. Presentation at the Meeting of the American Pediatric Surgical Association, Boca Raton. 1995.
17. Kohler M, Pease PW, Upadhyay V. Megacystis-microcolon-intestinal hypoperistalsis syndrome (MMIHS) in siblings: case report and review of the literature. Eur J Pediatr Surg. 2004;14(5):362–7.
18. Korğalı EÜ, Yavuz A, Şimşek CEÇ, Güney C, Kurtulgan HK, Başer B, et al. Megacystis microcolon intestinal hypoperistalsis syndrome in which a different de novo actg2 gene mutation was detected: a case report. Fetal Pediatr Pathol. 2018;37(2):109–16.
19. Krook PM. Megacystis-microcolon-intestinal hypoperistalsis syndrome in a male infant. Radiology. 1980;136(3):649–50.
20. Kubota M, Ikeda K, Ito Y. Autonomic innervation of the intestine from a baby with megacystis microcolon intestinal hypoperistalsis syndrome: II. Electrophysiological study. J Pediatr Surg. 1989;24(12):1267–70.
21. Loinaz C, Rodriguez MM, Kato T, Mittal N, Romaguera RL, Bruce JH, et al. Intestinal and multivisceral transplantation in children with severe gastrointestinal dysmotility. J Pediatr Surg. 2005;40(10):1598–604.
22. Manco LG, Osterdahl P. The antenatal sonographic features of megacystis-microcolon-intestinal hypoperistalsis syndrome. J Clin Ultrasound. 1984;12(9):595–8.
23. Mc Laughlin D, Puri P. Familial megacystis microcolon intestinal hypoperistalsis syndrome: a systematic review. Pediatr Surg Int. 2013;29(9):947–51.
24. Nakamura H, O'Donnell AM, Puri P. Consanguinity and its relevance for the incidence of megacystis microcolon intestinal hypoperistalsis syndrome (MMIHS): systematic review. Pediatr Surg Int. 2019;35(2):175–80.
25. Okada M, Sato M, Ogura M, Kamei K, Matsuoka K, Ito S. Central venous catheter infection-related glomerulonephritis under long-term parenteral nutrition: a report of two cases. BMC Res Notes. 2016;9:196.
26. Patel R, Carty H. Megacystis-microcolon-intestinal hypoperistalsis syndrome: a rare cause of intestinal obstruction in the newborn. Br J Radiol. 1980;53(627):249–52.
27. Piotrowska AP, Rolle U, Chertin B, De Caluwe D, Bianchi A, Puri P. Alterations in smooth muscle contractile and cytoskeleton proteins and interstitial cells of Cajal in megacystis microcolon intestinal hypoperistalsis syndrome. J Pediatr Surg. 2003;38(5):749–55.
28. Puri P, Lake BD, Gorman F, O'Donnell B, Nixon HH. Megacystis-microcolon-intestinal hypoperistalsis syndrome: a visceral myopathy. J Pediatr Surg. 1983;18(1):64–9.
29. Puri P, Shinkai M. Megacystis microcolon intestinal hypoperistalsis syndrome. Semin Pediatr Surg. 2005;14(1):58–63.
30. Richardson CE, Morgan JM, Jasani B, Green JT, Rhodes J, Williams GT, et al. Megacystis-microcolon-intestinal hypoperistalsis syndrome and the absence of the alpha3 nicotinic acetylcholine receptor subunit. Gastroenterology. 2001;121(2):350–7.
31. Rolle U, O'Briain S, Pearl RH, Puri P. Megacystis-microcolon-intestinal hypoperistalsis syndrome:

evidence of intestinal myopathy. Pediatr Surg Int. 2002;18(1):2–5.
32. Rosenblatt J, Dreux S, Spaggiari E, Morin C, Allaf B, Valat AS, et al. Prenatal diagnosis of megacystis microcolon intestinal hypoperistalsis syndrome by biochemical analysis of fetal urine. Prenat Diagn. 2018;38(8):585–90.
33. Shalev J, Itzchak Y, Avigad I, Hertz M, Straus S, Serr DM. Antenatal ultrasound appearance of megacystis microcolon intestinal hypoperistalsis syndrome. Isr J Med Sci. 1983;19(1):76–8.
34. Stamm E, King G, Thickman D. Megacystis-microcolon-intestinal hypoperistalsis syndrome: prenatal identification in siblings and review of the literature. J Ultrasound Med. 1991;10(10):599–602.
35. Taguchi T, Ikeda K, Shono T, Goto S, Kubota M, Kawana T, et al. Autonomic innervation of the intestine from a baby with megacystis microcolon intestinal hypoperistalsis syndrome: I. Immunohistochemical study. J Pediatr Surg. 1989;24(12):1264–6.
36. Thorson W, Diaz-Horta O, Foster J 2nd, Spiliopoulos M, Quintero R, Farooq A, et al. De novo ACTG2 mutations cause congenital distended bladder, microcolon, and intestinal hypoperistalsis. Hum Genet. 2014;133(6):737–42.
37. Tuzovic L, Tang S, Miller RS, Rohena L, Shahmirzadi L, Gonzalez K, et al. New insights into the genetics of fetal megacystis: ACTG2 mutations, encoding gamma-2 smooth muscle actin in megacystis microcolon intestinal hypoperistalsis syndrome (Berdon syndrome). Fetal Diagn Ther. 2015;38(4):296–306.
38. Vezina WC, Morin FR, Winsberg F. Megacystis-microcolon-intestinal hypoperistalsis syndrome: antenatal ultrasound appearance. AJR Am J Roentgenol. 1979;133(4):749–50.
39. Wangler MF, Gonzaga-Jauregui C, Gambin T, Penney S, Moss T, Chopra A, et al. Heterozygous de novo and inherited mutations in the smooth muscle actin (ACTG2) gene underlie megacystis-microcolon-intestinal hypoperistalsis syndrome. PLoS Genet. 2014;10(3):e1004258.
40. White SM, Chamberlain P, Hitchcock R, Sullivan PB, Boyd PA. Megacystis-microcolon-intestinal hypoperistalsis syndrome: the difficulties with antenatal diagnosis. Case report and review of the literature. Prenat Diagn. 2000;20(9):697–700.
41. Wymer KM, Anderson BB, Wilkens AA, Gundeti MS. Megacystis microcolon intestinal hypoperistalsis syndrome: case series and updated review of the literature with an emphasis on urologic management. J Pediatr Surg. 2016;51(9):1565–73.
42. Xu W, Gelber S, Orr-Urtreger A, Armstrong D, Lewis RA, Ou CN, et al. Megacystis, mydriasis, and ion channel defect in mice lacking the alpha3 neuronal nicotinic acetylcholine receptor. Proc Natl Acad Sci U S A. 1999;96(10):5746–51.
43. Young LW, Yunis EJ, Girdany BR, Sieber WK. Megacystis-microcolon-intestinal hypoperistalsis syndrome: additional clinical, radiologic, surgical, and histopathologic aspects. AJR Am J Roentgenol. 1981;137(4):749–55.

Degenerative Hollow Visceral Myopathy Mimicking Hirschsprung's Disease

22

Robin Brown, Alp Numanoglu, Dirk von Delft, and Heinz Rode

Contents

22.1 Introduction

Intestinal motility is a highly coordinated process and depends on smooth muscle contractility, the pacemaker activity evoked by the interstitial cells of Cajal, and the summation of the effects of the enteric and autonomic nervous systems on gut function. Crippling gastrointestinal dysfunction can result from a variety of abnormalities, involving these elements individually or in combination.

The pathological abnormalities underlying chronic idiopathic intestinal pseudo-obstruction (CIIP) can be classified into four major groups: myopathies, neuropathies (inflammatory, degenerative, or immune-mediated), mesenchymopathies (changes in the interstitial cells of Cajal network), and idiopathic. Alternatively, they may

This is an updated version of the chapter contributed by Heinz Rode, Robin Brown, and Alp Numanoglu for book Hirschsprungs Disease and Allied Disorders: Third Edition in 2008. The updates in this chapter were solely done by Dirk von Delft, Alp Numanoglu, and Robin Brown.

R. Brown · A. Numanoglu (✉) · D. von Delft · H. Rode
Division of Paediatric Surgery, Red Cross War Memorial Children's Hospital, Cape Town, South Africa

Faculty of Health Sciences, University of Cape Town, Cape Town, South Africa
e-mail: profbrown@paedsurgeon.co.za; Alp.Numanoglu@uct.ac.za; dirk.vondelft@uct.ac.za

P. Puri (ed.), *Hirschsprung's Disease and Allied Disorders*, https://doi.org/10.1007/978-3-030-15647-3_22

be secondary to systemic diseases involving the intestinal smooth muscle, endocrine disorders, drugs, and toxins or other miscellaneous causes. Secondary pseudo-obstruction syndromes in pediatric patients are uncommon compared to their occurrence in adults. Refinements in morphological techniques have improved our understanding of them.

CIIP is a clinicopathological syndrome characterized by ineffective prograde intestinal propulsion and recurrent symptoms of bowel obstruction in the absence of mechanical occlusion [1–6]. These disorders can lead to malnutrition and a protracted debilitating illness with impaired life expectancy. The disorders may differ in genetic transmission as well as pattern and distribution of involvement within the gastrointestinal tract and there may be concomitant extraintestinal manifestations. They may cause functional abnormalities without a discernible morphological diagnosis or, alternatively, may cause mechanical obstruction with changes easily recognizable on routine light microscopy of biopsied tissue.

Hollow visceral myopathy (HVM) constitutes part of CIIP. These disorders usually manifest during adolescence or early adulthood, although infants and children may be similarly affected with significant morbidity and mortality [2, 4, 7–17]. Symptoms tend to be more severe and prognosis worse in the primary myopathies [6, 7].

It is probable that many of these disorders were previously reported in the pediatric literature under a variety of different titles, viz., pseudo-Hirschsprung's disease, segmental small-bowel dilatation, hypo- or adynamic bowel syndrome, megaduodenum, idiopathic megacolon, and megacystis-microcolon-intestinal hypoperistalsis syndrome.

22.2 Classification

The disorders can be classified according to heredity, age at presentation, or morphological characteristics. A modified and practical classification based on clinical and morphological features is presented in Table 22.1 [1, 2, 8, 9, 16, 17]. Various pathological subtypes of HVM are increasingly being recognized with H&E staining, Smith's silver staining, and electron microscopy. This classification reflects our current understanding of these disorders, although a significant number of children with pseudo-obstruction have no demonstrable primary disease or identifiable histological changes in the affected viscera and are idiopathic.

Table 22.1 Hollow visceral myopathy

1. Familial visceral myopathy	*Autosomal dominant*
	Autosomal recessive with ophthalmoplegia
	Autosomal recessive with total bowel involvement
2. Sporadic visceral myopathy	*Infantile*
	Childhood
3. Degenerative leiomyopathy	
4. Muscle disease	*Myotonic dystrophy*
	Progressive muscular dystrophy
	Progressive systemic sclerosis miscellaneous
5. Idiopathic	

Adapted from Krishnamurthy and Schuffler [2]

22.3 Etiology

A specific etiological factor has not been identified, and no genetic defect is known. The disorders may be caused by genetic aberrations, abnormal protein synthesis, toxins, autoimmune disorder, or other factors.

The patterns of inheritance in familial visceral myopathy (FVM) are varied and may be autosomal dominant with high or low penetrance. The absence of demonstrable male-to-male transmission in some kindreds excludes the possibility of a sex-linked dominant mode of transmission [8–10, 14, 18–20]. The clinical expression of the disease amongst families with dominant inheritance usually starts after the first decade of life and asymptomatic, but affected members are not uncommon. Symptoms are less severe than amongst those patients with autosomal recessive inheritance. Gastrointestinal lesions in patients within the same family are similar. In 15 reported families, the inheritance pattern was autosomal dominant in 8, and autosomal recessive in

7, although sex-linked dominance could not be excluded in 4 [20, 21]. The genetic aberration is unknown but has been linked to a defect in synthesis of a contractile protein resulting in the degeneration of smooth muscle fibers [22].

Individuals affected by either FVM or mitochondrial myopathy manifest many common features, including intestinal pseudo-obstruction as well as extraintestinal neurological manifestations, ophthalmoplegia, leukoencephalopathy, polyneuropathy, dementia, and seizures, suggesting that a mitochondrial DNA mutation could be the molecular lesion in FVM [23].

In HVM, a deficiency of smooth muscle alpha actin within the circular muscle coat has also been implicated as an etiological factor [24]. There is additional evidence that the pronounced fibrosis has its origin in the transformation of smooth muscle fibers from a purely contractile to a myofibroblast collagen synthetic phenotype [25]. The etiology of sporadic cases is uncertain. Spontaneous mutations, pre- or postnatal acquired diseases, or exposure to a common environmental agent cannot be excluded.

Although the etiology of degenerative leiomyopathy (DL) remains obscure, the morphological and functional defects are considered postnatal events. It appears to be region-specific and presents usually after a number of years, suggesting that the disease is acquired rather than congenital. A smooth muscle toxin is the most likely pathogen, supported by the geographical distribution in ethnic groups from rural areas in southern, central, and eastern Africa [26]. Alternatively, it may present as a "burn-out" autoimmune disorder [27]. There is no association with other congenital abnormalities, and the predilection for specific geographical regions suggests cultural–environmental causes [28].

22.4 Diagnosis

The diagnosis of HVM should be contemplated in children with the typical clinical presentation, aided by radiological findings and supplemented by other special investigations including manometry, scintigraphy, and histology [5]. An underlying mechanical obstruction must be excluded. Histological confirmation is mandatory for the diagnosis.

22.4.1 Clinical

Although varied, the predominant feature of HVM is that of intestinal obstruction which may present at any age [3–5, 8, 11, 13, 17]. No sign or symptom is pathognomonic of pseudo-obstruction. The location of the affected bowel and the fact that it may be diffusely involved is more important than the underlying cause [6]. A family history must always be sought, as it supports the diagnosis of pseudo-obstruction and may determine the pattern of inheritance for genetic counseling. An intrauterine diagnosis can be suspected if the fetus is noted to have megacystis in conjunction with dilated loops of bowel [8]. The longitudinal muscle layer is predominantly involved in HVM, and this could reflect an insult at a specific time within the first trimester of pregnancy. Symptoms may fluctuate markedly in frequency and severity and may be present for years before pseudo-obstruction is established, with myopathy usually presenting earlier than a neuropathy [8, 9, 29].

Nonspecific symptoms of gastrointestinal involvement include dysphagia, nausea, vomiting, colicky abdominal pain, and constipation or diarrhea [8]. Unfortunately, these overlap with many other conditions which may obscure the true nature of the disease. On examination, malnutrition and weight loss are evident, together with abdominal distension, present in 85% of the series of Vargas et al. (Fig. 22.1) [8]. Loops of bowel

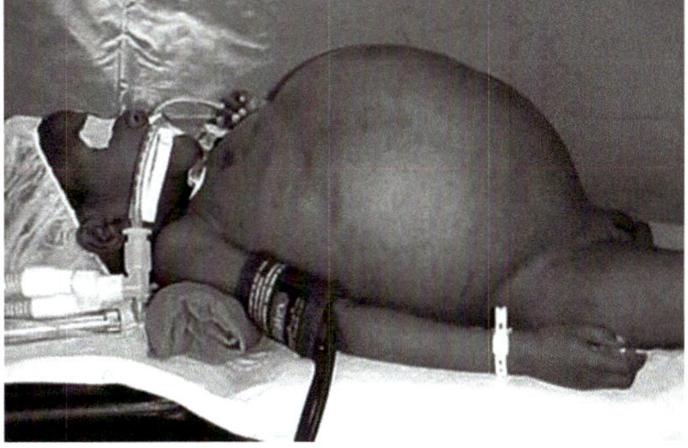

Fig. 22.1 Marked abdominal distension in a 3-year-old girl presenting with degenerative leiomyopathy

may be visible or palpable, and bowel sounds may be absent or even hyperactive. A succussion splash may be elicited [3, 11]. Anal sphincter tone is normal on rectal examination. Progressive symptomatic episodes of intestinal obstruction occur with increasing frequency and severity, necessitating further investigations to establish a diagnosis for treatment and counseling.

22.4.2 Radiology

22.4.2.1 Abdominal Radiographs

These are essential to exclude a mechanical cause of intestinal obstruction [3, 8, 30]. They reveal dilated loops of small and/or large bowel, which may be gross and featureless and contain air-fluid levels. Colonic dilatation is often misdiagnosed as cecal or sigmoid volvulus (Figs. 22.2 and 22.3). Fecal loading is present in 50% of patients; however, the findings are nonspecific and may be absent in up to 20% of patients, especially if there has been preceding gaseous evacuation of the colon and an empirical trial of pharmacological management [18].

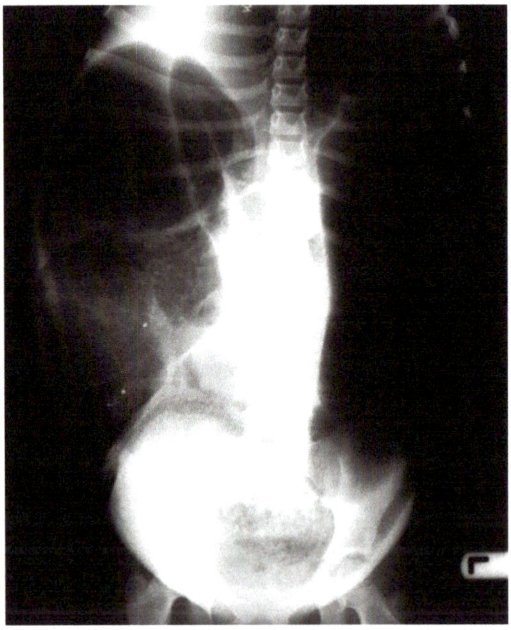

Fig. 22.2 Plain abdominal radiograph showing gross and featureless distension of bowel, air-fluid levels, and fecal loading

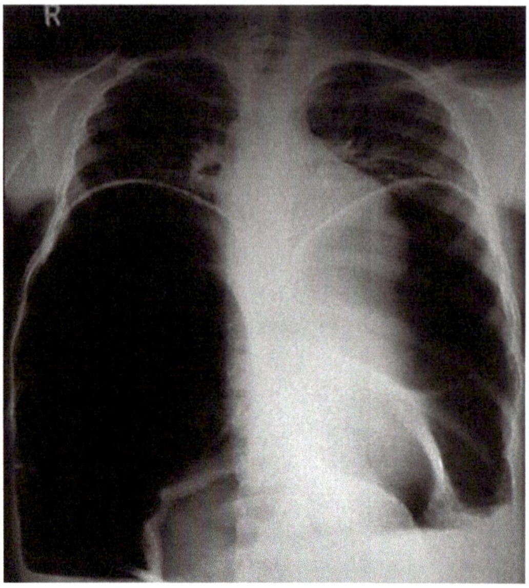

Fig. 22.3 Chest radiograph showing gross bowel distension, diaphragmatic elevation, and decreased lung volumes

22.4.2.2 Contrast Radiology

A contrast medium rather than Gastrografin should be used for this investigation, as the hygroscopic action of large volumes of intraluminal Gastrografin in a small child can result in hypovolemia. Generalized dilatation of the entire intestine favors the diagnosis of HVM (or neuropathy) [30]. The dilatation may be associated with abnormal peristalsis and hypocontractility, delay in gastric emptying with or without gastroesophageal reflux in the presence of a normal lower esophageal sphincter, megaesophagus and megaduodenum, valvular "packing" in the small intestine because of circular muscle fibrosis and an enlarged redundant colon with a loss of haustral patterns, and retention of contrast for more than 24 hours (Fig. 22.4). Bowel dilatation is an absolute requirement for diagnosis and radiological deterioration can be demonstrated (Fig. 22.5). Malrotation of the bowel must be excluded [8].

22.4.2.3 Transit Studies

These will confirm delay in gastric emptying and slow intestinal transit as well as a decrease in motility. In addition to radio-opaque markers,

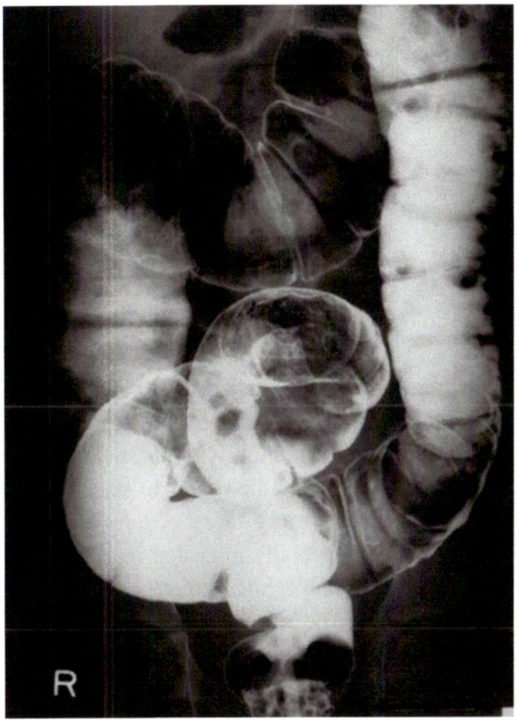

Fig. 22.4 Barium enema showing distension of the colon, haustrations appear to be present deficient haustral markings, and redundancy

the breath hydrogen technique and sulfasalazine absorption and organic dyes have been used [31].

22.4.3 Manometry

Prolonged (>6 hours) manometric readings of the various anatomical regions of the intestine offer a valuable means of diagnosing HVM as well as differentiating it from other forms of pseudo-obstruction [4, 5, 19, 29, 32]. It shows hypomotility with low-amplitude coordinated contractions in myopathy, compared to normal-amplitude uncoordinated contractions in neuropathy [31]. It was 95–100% accurate in the diagnosis of pseudo-obstruction in the series of Vargas et al. and Boige et al., supporting its use as a screening procedure for pseudo-obstruction [8, 33]. Manometric abnormalities correlate with both the extent of the pathological process and the prognosis [5, 34].

Esophageal peristalsis is uncoordinated with low-amplitude waves or absent contractions and with normal or high lower esophageal sphincter pressures. Antroduodenal motility is

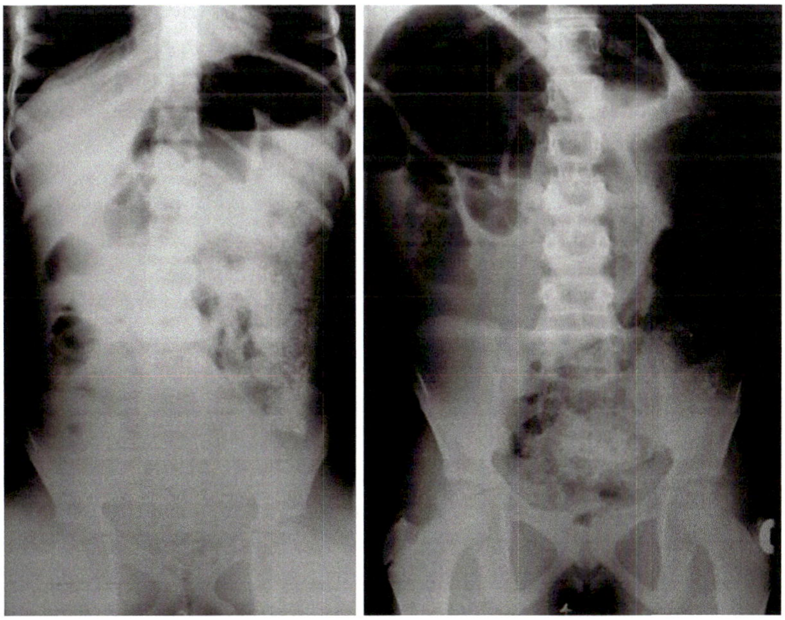

Fig. 22.5 Plain abdominal radiographs taken at presentation and 3 years later showing progressive bowel dilatation associated with clinical deterioration

coordinated with poor propagation while the phasic waves of the migrating motor complex (MMC) are infrequent, with low amplitude and coordinated or absent contractions [19, 29, 32, 34]. This distinguishes it from a visceral neuropathy and can be explained on the basis of bowel damage, weak contractions, and grossly dilated intestine [29]. The presence of a normal migrating complex may predict successful enteral feeding. Disordered foregut motility can be detected in relatives of patients with HVM and may precede other manifestations of the disease by months or even years [18]. Colonic contractions are absent in the decompensation phase of the disease. The biliary tree has low-amplitude phasic contractions with low basal sphincter of Oddi pressures [29]. Anorectal manometry shows a normal rectosphincteric inhibitory reflex. The rectum may be so dilated that the rectal balloon volume is insufficient to elicit a relaxation reflex response.

22.4.4 Scintigraphy

Radioisotopes allow accurate quantification of the pattern and efficacy of propulsion of intestinal contents along the bowel lumen. Technetium-99 is the most widely used radioisotope, as it is easily obtained and cheap, and the radiation dosage is low. For longer studies, indium-111 and iodine-131 have been used. Prolonged small-bowel and colonic transit times are commonly seen in visceral myopathy and accumulation or "clumping" of radioactivity may identify the functionally most impaired segments of the dilated bowel [5, 35].

22.4.5 Electrogastrography

This technique is similar to electrocardiography and measures gastrointestinal electrical activity via surface electrodes attached to the abdominal wall [36]. The surface electrogastrography (EGG) can assess gastric emptying and shows a low-amplitude trace in a myopathy, compared to a tachygastria in children with idiopathic pseudo-obstruction and a neuropathy. The severity of the dysmotility cannot be assessed with the present technique, but ongoing investigations may lead to advances in this noninvasive method [37].

22.4.6 Histology

It is essential to confirm the diagnosis of HVM [38]. Endoscopic mucosal biopsies are inadequate for histological assessment. DL should be diagnosed on full-thickness rectal biopsies performed after careful preparation and decompression of the distal bowel. At exploratory laparotomy or laparoscopy, full-thickness biopsies of an adequate size (2 × 2 cm), taken from the stomach, small bowel, and large bowel, are necessary. A laparotomy or laparoscopy is especially indicated in children in whom a congenital or mechanical cause for the obstruction has to be excluded. This was necessary in two-thirds of the patients in the series of Vargas et al. [8]. Histological methods should include a large variety of techniques including H&E, Smith's silver and Meier-Ruge staining, immunocytochemical staining, and electron microscopy [2–4, 28, 38]. Normal histology may not exclude HVM. In 9 of 20 patients in the series of Smith and Milla from Great Ormond Street Hospital, London, abnormalities were not detected on routine paraffin sections but required further special studies, i.e., electron microscopy, immunohistochemistry, and histochemistry [27]. Fortunately laparoscopy has replaced laparotomy and the added problem of postoperative adhesive obstruction can now be minimized. Noninvasive techniques, e.g., laparoscopic biopsy, may decrease the incidence of postoperative adhesions [39].

22.5 Pathology

The pathology can be localized to a segment of bowel, or it may be more extensive, affecting the entire gastrointestinal tract. The most important histological features—smooth muscle cell vacuolar degeneration and fibrosis—are easily recognizable on routine light microscopy. Although the target area is predominantly the smooth muscle layer, nonspecific changes may be observed in all layers of the intestinal wall [21, 27, 28].

22.5.1 Macroscopy

At surgery the bowel may be distended, thin-walled, and redundant and lack haustrations (Fig. 22.6). The colon is predominantly involved, and the dilatation usually extends proximally into the small bowel, duodenum, stomach, and esophagus to varying degrees. The bladder may also become megacystic. The presence of early esophageal and duodenal involvement favors a diagnosis of chronic intestinal pseudo-obstruction syndrome over DL.

22.5.2 Microscopy

22.5.2.1 Muscular Layer

Visceral myopathy is characterized by specific alterations in the muscularis propria (Figs. 22.7 and 22.8) [2, 28, 38]. The pathology varies from mild to severe, with the most extensive changes affecting the clinically diseased bowel. Muscle layers are thin and attenuated with muscle cell degeneration, muscle cell loss, amorphous debris, and extracellular edema. There is an increase in fibrous tissue with replacement of muscle fibers by collagen fibers surrounding both residual muscle cell fragments and areas of dropout, imparting a vacuolated appearance. These fibrotic changes are most prominent in the longitudinal muscle layer, whereas extracellular edema is most obvious within the circular muscle layer. Enlargement, irregularity, and hyperchromia of the smooth muscle nuclei have been reported in two adult patients with FVM in association with hypertrophy of the muscularis mucosa [21]. Severity of involvement is not uniform, with clusters of apparently well-preserved muscle fibers interspersed amongst degenerated muscle fibers [38]. Inflammatory foci are occasionally seen within the muscle layers.

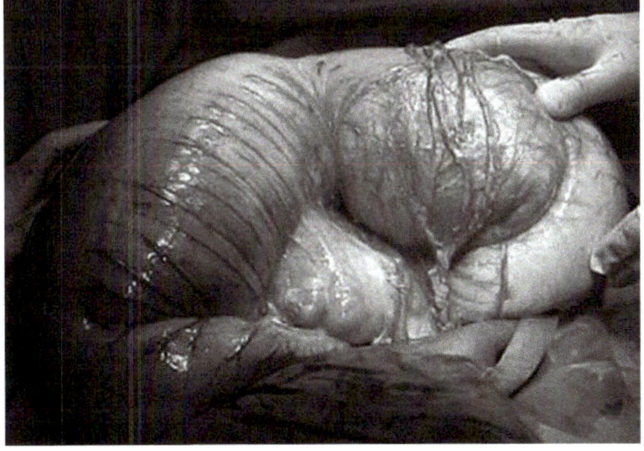

Fig. 22.6 Operative picture of massively distended colon

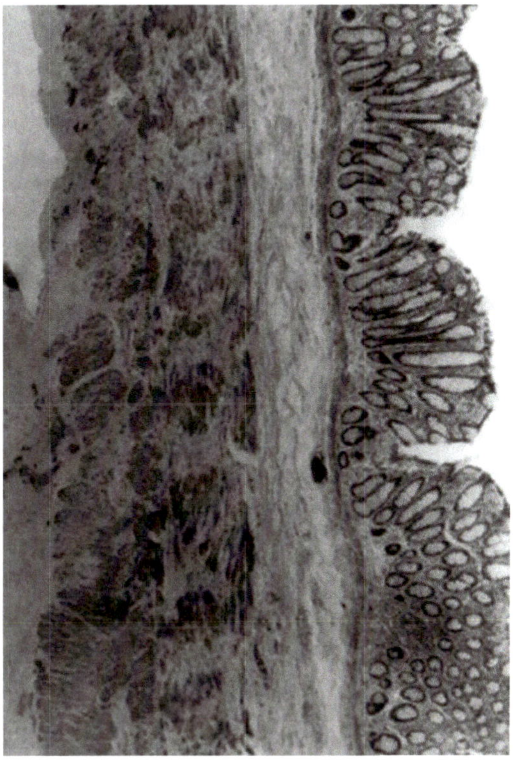

Fig. 22.7 Full-thickness colonic wall in degenerative leiomyopathy showing thickened and partly fibrosed muscularis mucosa, with extensive degeneration and loss of smooth muscle in circular and longitudinal layers associated with fibrous replacement together with subserosal fibrosis (H&E, × 16)

22.5.2.2 Neuronal Plexus

The myenteric plexus in HVM remains morphologically intact and no damage is evident on histology.

22.5.2.3 Mucosal Lesions

Mild to severe damage and inflammation of the mucosal architecture may be present and probably reflect mucosal insult from the underlying stasis syndrome [18, 28, 38]. These changes may be similar to those in celiac disease or progressive systemic sclerosis.

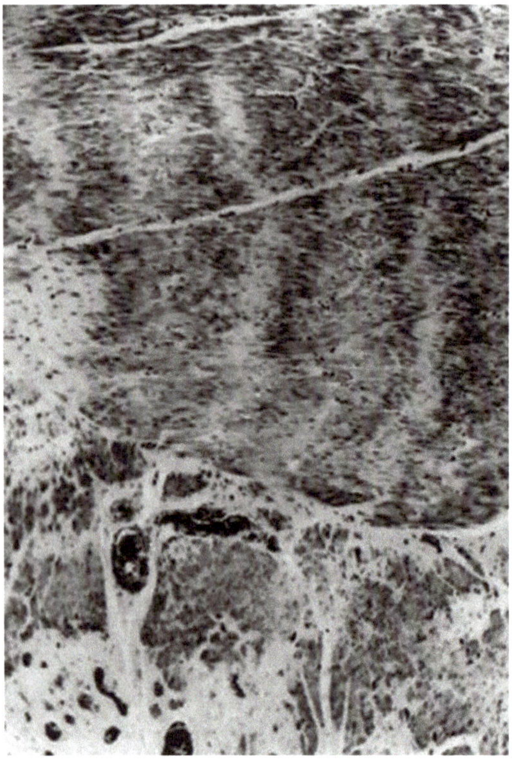

Fig. 22.8 Degenerative leiomyopathy showing circular and longitudinal layers of muscularis propria. There is regular alignment of nuclei and cytoplasm of smooth muscle cells with intervening fibrosis in the circular layer. In the longitudinal layer, the smooth muscle is degenerate and being replaced by connective tissue (H&E, × 40)

22.5.2.4 Ultrastructure

The muscularis propria is predominantly affected with loss of internal structure. The earliest changes consist of smooth muscle cells appearing more electrolucent with disorganization, loss of myofilaments, and mitochondrial swelling (Fig. 22.9). In established disease, damaged cells have discontinuous plasma membranes with loss of alignment of contractile elements, vacuolated mitochondria, and clear cytoplasm. In advanced disease, muscle cells show degeneration with replacement by fibrosis and collagen. The intracellular spaces are filled with edema, muscle debris and collagen, and there is no evidence of vasculitis or inflammation [2, 28, 38].

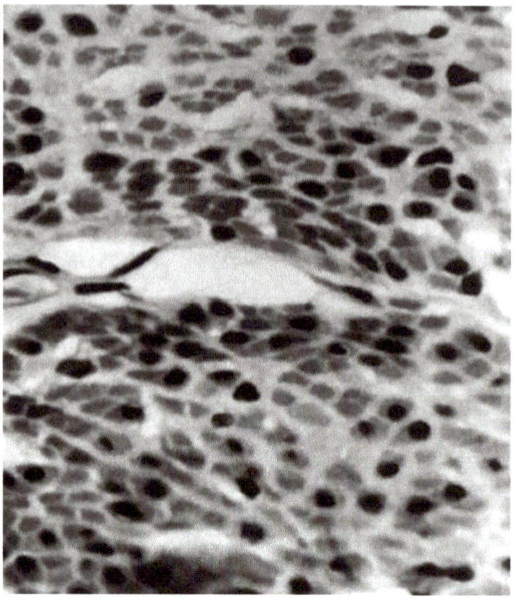

Fig. 22.9 Degenerative leiomyopathy showing vacuolation of smooth muscle cells with pyknotic nuclei in smooth muscle of circular layer (H&E, × 400)

22.6 Extraintestinal Lesions

Megacystis is present in 33–86% of patients with HVM and is easily demonstrated by sonography or cystography [9, 10, 14, 40]. Histologically, the bladder wall is either normal or thickened and partly replaced with mature collagen. Extraintestinal lesions may include external ophthalmoplegia [16, 19]. Autonomic and peripheral neuropathy are seen in neuropathic and not myopathic diseases.

22.7 Specific Disorders of Smooth Muscle

22.7.1 Familial Visceral Myopathy

Three types of FVM have been identified (Table 22.2) with two modes of transmission and variable expression of gastrointestinal involvement, symptoms, and response to treatment and associated extraintestinal manifestations [2, 9].

Table 22.2 Familial visceral myopathy

Type 1		Type 2	Type 3
Mode of transmission	Autosomal dominant	Autosomal recessive	Autosomal recessive
Pathology	Degeneration and fibrosis of muscularis propria; myenteric plexus normal	Indistinguishable from type 1	Indistinguishable from type 1
Intestinal lesions	Esophageal dilatation; megaduodenum and dilatation of proximal jejunum; redundant colon	Gastric atony and dilatation; dilatation of entire small bowel; multiple diverticula	Dilatation of the entire intestinal tract
Clinical manifestations			
Age of onset	After first decade of life	Teenager	Adult life
Symptomatic	<50%	>75%	Most
Symptoms	Pseudo-obstruction; variable expression	Pseudo-obstruction; malnutrition	Pseudo-obstruction; malnutrition
Treatment	Symptomatic relief with medication and surgery	Recalcitrant	Recalcitrant
Prognosis	Moderate	Poor	Poor
Extraintestinal manifestations	Megacystis; ophthalmoplegia	Ophthalmoplegia; ptosis	None observed

Adapted from Refs. [2, 9, 14]

Histologically, intestinal smooth muscle degeneration and increased fibrosis are indistinguishable throughout the various types, raising doubt about the specificity of bowel involvement in the subgroups [20].

22.7.2 Sporadic Visceral Myopathy

The pathological features are identical to those of FVM in adolescents and adults, but with more severe symptoms, earlier onset, and a worse outcome (Table 22.3). The etiology is unknown and the possibility of genetic transmission unlikely, as only 4 of 170 family members were affected in one study [10]. The entire gastrointestinal tract and bladder may be affected, and it has been reported in infants with megacystis-microcolon-intestinal hypoperistalsis syndrome [41].

22.7.3 Degenerative Leiomyopathy

DL is a distinct entity indigenous to young Africans from southern, central, and eastern Africa [17, 26, 28, 42].

In only one instance has a family history with affected siblings been reported. DL is characterized by a long history of increasing abdominal distension with massive megacolon presenting in older children (mean age 9.5 years) [17]. The disease primarily affects the distal bowel, but it may extend proximally into the small bowel, stomach, and esophagus and may also affect the urinary tract. The accumulation of intraluminal fluid and bacterial overgrowth probably accounts for malabsorption and progressive clinical deterioration.

Although the etiology of the condition remains unknown, the morphological and functional defects are considered to be postnatal events. A smooth muscle toxin or an autoimmune disorder could be implicated in the pathogenesis [26, 27]. Comorbidity with pulmonary tuberculosis has been seen in 50% of patients in the past [17].

Histologically, the presence of interstitial and intracellular edema of the muscularis propria, the absence of vacuolated mitochondria, and pattern of submembrane cytoplasmic translucency on electron microscopy separate DL from other forms of HVM. The degenerative changes tend to be distributed focally or in alternating waves along the longitudinal axis of the muscle. Muscle cell cytoplasm is homoge-

Table 22.3 Hollow visceral myopathy and degenerative leiomyopathy

Infantile		Childhood	Degenerative leiomyopathy	Idiopathic (unclassified)
Mode of transmission	Sporadic	Sporadic	Geographic distribution; sporadic	Mixed
Pathology	Visceral myopathy	Visceral myopathy	Visceral myopathy with blood vessel changes	No demonstrable abnormalities
Intestinal lesions	Gastric, small-bowel, and colon dilatation	Gastric and small bowel dilatation	Predominantly distal bowel; whole gastrointestinal tract may be involved	Dilatation of gastrointestinal tract distal to esophagus
Clinical manifestations				
Sex distribution	72% female	75% male	Equal	60% female
Age of onset	Within 1–3 weeks	First year of life	Early childhood (9.5 years)	Newborn to 4 months
Symptomatic	100%	100%	100%	100%
Symptoms	Pseudo-obstruction; emaciation	Pseudo-obstruction; malnutrition	Pseudo-obstruction; malnutrition	Pseudo-obstruction
Treatment	Recalcitrant	Symptomatic relief	Recalcitrant	Recalcitrant
Prognosis	Fatal	Moderate	Unremitting; progressive deterioration	60% mortality
Extraintestinal manifestations	Urinary tract dilatation 86%	None observed	Urinary tract dilatation small muscular arteries of other viscera 50%; pulmonary tuberculosis	Megacystis
References	[2, 9, 16, 41]	[26, 32]	[17, 26]	[13]

neous and eosinophilic with shrunken and pyknotic nuclei, and 25% will have a pre-dominant lymphocyte inflammatory cell infiltration in the muscularis propria, which could represent a response to an infective agent.

Although the myenteric plexus appears morphologically normal, ganglion cells are displaced centripetally in more than 50% of patients, with an excess of thick stubby acetylcholinesterase-positive nerve fibers in the muscularis propria. In 29 of 35 children (83%) in the study of Moore et al., there was a raised vasoactive intestinal peptide (VIP) level in the intestine, and in 7 of this group there was hyperplasia of the myenteric plexus [26]. This increased VIP level may cause neurogenic inhibition of the smooth muscle or it may be expressed as a reaction to neurotoxic damage to the bowel. Often encountered at autopsy are diffuse structural lesions affecting the small muscular arteries of the bowel, bronchioli, spleen, liver, and kidneys causing fibrotic stenosis of the lumina. This histological pattern separates DL from other muscular lesions occurring in mixed connective tissue diseases of childhood (Fig. 22.10) [43].

22.8 Differential Diagnosis

The majority of causes of secondary pseudo-obstruction can be excluded by a careful clinical history and appropriate investigations; however, many of these are rarely seen in pediatric patients. These include visceral neuropathies, progressive muscular dystrophy, progressive systemic sclerosis, myotonic dystrophy, generalized leiomyositis, celiac disease, malrotation, toxins, pharmacological agents, and diffuse lymphoid infiltration [2, 3, 8, 41, 44–47].

22.9 Treatment

Due to the progressive unremitting course of HVM together with the lack of understanding of its etiology, treatment consists at present of dietary manipulation and symptomatic relief with medication, reserving surgery for diagnostic and palliative roles [3, 4, 8, 11, 17].

Because of the erratic response, therapy may be difficult to evaluate, although it tends to be better earlier on in the disease process

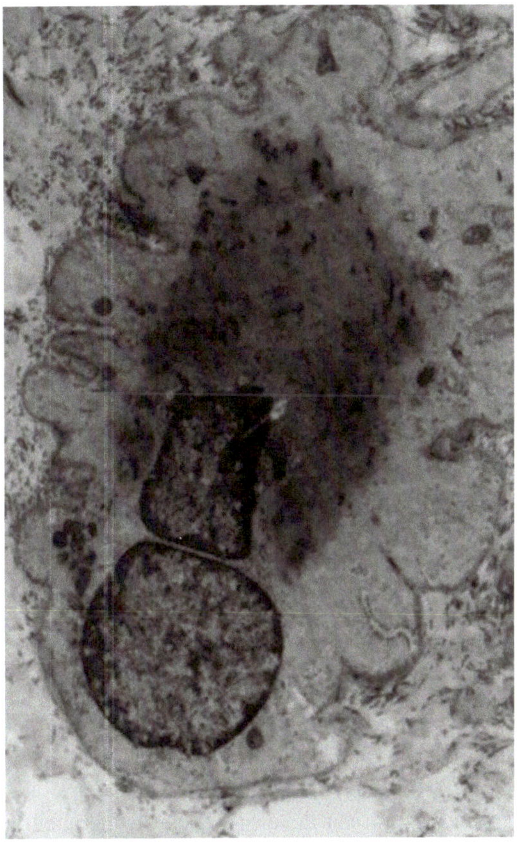

Fig. 22.10 Electron micrograph in degenerative leiomyopathy showing a transverse section of a smooth muscle cell with indentation of sarcolemmal membrane, peripheral rarefaction, central condensation of fibrils with accumulation of spindly densities, and an indented nucleus. The cell is surrounded by much glycosylated aminoglycans and collagen fibers (×10,080)

and in familial types. All forms of therapy confer incomplete and temporary benefit only. As DL may present in theory as a "burnt-out" autoimmune disorder, its progression may be arrested with steroids and immunosuppressive treatment [27].

22.9.1 Medical

22.9.1.1 Gastrointestinal Rest

Nasogastric tube decompression, restricted oral intake, intravenous fluids, colonic lavage, and decompression by rectal tube or colonoscopy are the most effective means of managing the acute attack. This reduces the gas and fluid load, thereby decreasing the diameter of the intestine with symptomatic relief.

22.9.1.2 Dietary Management

Nutritional therapy plays an important role and initially includes a low residue diet and the avoidance of spicy or gas-producing foods. An elemental or semi-elemental diet may be required and administered as a bolus or continuous drip infusion via a nasogastric or nasoduodenal tube or gastrostomy [48]. This may be supplemented or even replaced by parenteral nutrition. Oral intake should be encouraged despite the presence of obstructive symptoms, but prolonged and even permanent intravenous feeding often becomes necessary. Limited amounts of enteral feeding, however, are desirable to prevent cholestatic jaundice and to maintain bowel mucosal integrity.

22.9.1.3 Pharmacological Agents

The empirical use of broad-spectrum non-absorbable antibiotics may reduce bacterial overgrowth in the proximal intestine, thereby reducing symptoms such as pain, distension, and diarrhea [3].

Prokinetic drugs are used to encourage prograde peristalsis. Cholinergic drugs increase intestinal activity, and some success has been obtained using Rae's mixture (which contains pyridostigmine 2.5 g. magnesium sulfate 260 g, liquid paraffin 1000 ml, Aq chloroform conc. 15 ml, water 2000 ml). Erythromycin and subcutaneous octreotide, a somatostatin analog, which induces propagating phase 3 MMCs during fasting, can be of benefit [49]. Tegaserod is a promotility agent like cisapride, without its cardiac toxicity, and can also be used [49]. Children with an absent MMC, megaduodenum, and small-bowel dilatation respond less favorably to prokinetic agents and require more parenteral nutritional support [15].

22.9.2 Surgical

This should be reserved for patients only if there is potential benefit. Early laparoscopic placement of a Mic-Key Gastrostomy device into the dilated colon for use as an Antegrade

Continent Enema provides significant symptomatic relief and aids in evacuation of colonic gas and leads to significant nutritional improvement.

22.9.2.1 Management

Because HVM is a generalized alimentary disorder, surgical intervention is confined to a palliative role [8, 17]. Surgery must be tailored as the disease can affect many parts of the digestive or other organ systems. Procedures may include intestinal diversion, decompression gastrostomy, tapering duodenoplasty, duodenojejunostomy, limited small-bowel resection, subtotal or total colectomy, ileostomy, cecostomy, or colostomy [18]. In practice, many of these bring only temporary or no relief. Surgery is also unlikely to protect renal function or restore normal micturition.

Application of the Malone Antegrade Continence Enema (MACE) principle provides significant symptomatic relief and improves quality of life. Since adequate bowel decompression and evacuation of stool and flatus is possible with the "MACE," patients are able to eat sufficiently to meet nutritional requirements. Early intervention has led to significant improvement in general health, weight gains, and decreased mortality. The "MACE" principle can be achieved by a laparoscopically placed skin level gastrostomy device such as the Mic-Key button.

Laparotomy and colectomy should be avoided or should be reserved for patients who have a perforated bowel or where laparoscopy seems impossible [50, 51].

Mechanical obstruction may subsequently develop due to adhesions, cecal or colonic volvulus, or rarely strictures [17, 52]. Substantial numbers of operations in these patients are therefore for complications of previous surgery. Other postsurgical complications include wound infection, bowel perforation, peritonitis, and the short bowel syndrome. These are not infrequently the ultimate cause of mortality [3, 10, 17]. Exploratory laparotomy should therefore be avoided except where the patient is incapacitated by symptoms and fails to respond to medical therapy or where unequivocal evidence of mechanical obstruction exists.

22.10 Prognosis

HVM has a poor prognosis with the prospect of increasing obstructive symptoms, malnutrition, and deterioration [3, 8, 17]. Emaciation, overwhelming sepsis, parenteral nutrition complications, and surgical complications are the most frequent causes of death. Small-bowel transplantation is only indicated if there are life-threatening complications due to irreversible gut failure. These children may need a multivisceral transplant [53].

22.11 Conclusion

HVM is a long-term illness with a variable natural history. Radiographic examination, intestinal manometry, and full-thickness histology will confirm the diagnosis and extent of disease and allow the rational development of a therapeutic program. This should include pharmacological stimulation of intestinal motor function, preservation of adequate nutritional status, maximum symptom relief, and goal-directed surgical intervention. Unfortunately, the long-term prognosis is guarded, with the disease impacting significantly on the life of the patient with frequent hospital admissions, bowel dysfunction, dietary restrictions, chronic empirical medication, and failed surgery.

Acknowledgments We acknowledge Professors R.O.C. Kaschula and A. Bosenberg and Mr. M. Emms for allowing reproduction of the figures and legends.

References

1. Maldonado JE, Gregg JA, Green PA, Brown AL. Chronic idiopathic intestinal pseudo-obstruction. Am J Med. 1970;49:203–12.
2. Krishnamurthy S, Schuffler MD. Pathology of neuromuscular disorders of the small intestine and colon. Gastroenterology. 1987;93:610–39.

3. Schuffler MD, Rohrmann CA, Chaffee RG, Brand DL, Delaney JH, Young JH. Chronic intestinal pseudo-obstruction. A report of 27 cases and review of the literature. Medicine. 1981;60:173–95.
4. Schuffler MD. Chronic intestinal pseudo-obstruction: progress and problems (editorial). J Pediatr Gastroenterol Nutr. 1990;10:157–60.
5. Rudolph CD. Diagnosis of pseudo-obstruction in children. Am J Gastroenterol. 1993;88:802–6.
6. Di Lorenzo C. Pseudo-obstruction: current approaches. Gastroenterology. 1999;116:980–7.
7. Koletzko S. Other intestinal motility disorders. In: Walker WA, Durie PR, Hamilton JR, Walker Smith JA, Watkins JB, editors. Pediatric gastrointestinal disease. Patho-physiology, diagnosis, management. Philadelphia: BC Decker; 2000. p. 849–62.
8. Vargas JH, Sachs P, Ament ME. Chronic intestinal pseudo-obstruction syndrome in pediatrics. J Pediatr Gastroenterol Nutr. 1988;7:323–32.
9. Anuras S, Mitros FA, Milano A, Kuminsky R, Decanio R, Green JB. A familial visceral myopathy with dilatation of the entire gastrointestinal tract. Gastroenterology. 1986;90:385–90.
10. Schuffler MD, Pagon RB, Schwartz R, Bill AH. Visceral myopathy of the gastrointestinal and genitourinary tracts in infants. Gastroenterology. 1988;94:892–8.
11. Byrne WJ, Cipel L, Euler AR, Halpin TC, Ament ME. Chronic idiopathic intestinal pseudo-obstruction syndrome in children – clinical characteristics and prognosis. J Pediatr. 1977;90:585–9.
12. Shaw A, Shaffer H, Teja K, Kelly T, Grogan E, Bruni C. A perspective for pediatric surgeons: chronic idiopathic intestinal pseudo-obstruction. J Pediatr Surg. 1979;14:719–27.
13. Anuras S, Mitros FA, Soper RT, Pringle KC, Maves BV, Younoszai MK, et al. Chronic intestinal pseudo-obstruction in young children. Gastroenterology. 1986;91:62–70.
14. Faulk DL, Anuras S, Gardner GD, Mitros FA, Summer RW, Christensen J. A familial visceral myopathy. Ann Intern Med. 1978;89:600–6.
15. Hyman PE, DiLorenzo C, McAdams L, Flores AF, Tomosasa T, Garvey TQ. Predicting the clinical response to cisapride in children with chronic intestinal pseudo-obstruction. Am J Gastroenterol. 1993;88:832–6.
16. Ghosh S, Eastwood MA. Primary chronic intestinal pseudo-obstruction: an update. Postgrad Med J. 1994;70:65–7.
17. Rode H, Moore SW, Kaschula ROC, Brown RA, Cywes S. Degenerative leiomyopathy in children. A clinico-pathological study. Pediatr Surg Int. 1992;7:23–9.
18. Schuffler MD, Lowe MC, Bill AH. Studies of idiopathic intestinal pseudoobstruction. 1. Hereditary hollow visceral myopathy: clinical and pathological studies. Gastroenterology. 1977;73:327–38.
19. Anuras S, Mitros FA, Nowak TV, Ionasescu VV, Gurll NJ, Christensen J, et al. A familial visceral myopathy with external ophthalmoplegia and autosomal recessive transmission. Gastroenterology. 1983;84:346–53.
20. Jones SC, Dixon MF, Lintott DJ, Axon ATR. Familial visceral myopathy. A family with involvement of four generations. Dig Dis Sci. 1992;37:464–9.
21. Fitzgibbons PL, Chandrasoma PT. Familial visceral myopathy. Evidence of diffuse involvement of intestinal smooth muscle. Am J Surg Pathol. 1987;11:846–54.
22. Ionasescu V, Ionasescu R, Anuras S, Christensen J. Alterations in synthesis of contractile proteins in fresh and cultured stomach smooth muscle in familial visceral myopathy. Gastroenterology. 1981;80:1182.
23. Lowsky R, Davidson G, Wolman S, Jeejeebhoy KN, Hegele RA. Familial visceral myopathy associated with a mitochondrial myopathy. Gut. 1993;34:279–83.
24. Smith VV, Lake BD, Kamm MA, Nicholls RJ. Intestinal pseudo-obstruction with deficient smooth muscle α-actin. Histopathology. 1992;21:535–42.
25. Martin JE, Benson M, Swash M, Salih V, Gray A. Myofibroblasts in hollow visceral myopathy: the origin of gastrointestinal fibrosis? Gut. 1993;34:999–1001.
26. Moore SW, Schneider JW, Kaschula ROC. Non-familial visceral myopathy: clinical and pathologic features of degenerative leiomyopathy. Pediatr Surg Int. 2002;18:6–12.
27. Smith VV, Milla PJ. Histological phenotypes of enteric smooth muscle disease causing functional intestinal obstruction in childhood. Histopathology. 1997;31:112–22.
28. Kaschula ROC, Cywes S, Katz A, Louw JH. Degenerative leiomyopathy with massive megacolon. Perspect Pediatr Pathol. 1987;11:193–213.
29. Di Lorenzo C, Flores AF, Reddy SN, Snape WJ Jr, Bazzocchi G, Hyman PE. Colonic manometry in children with chronic intestinal pseudo-obstruction. Gut. 1993;34:803–7.
30. Schuffler MD, Rohrmann CA Jr, Templeton FE. The radiologic manifestations of idiopathic intestinal pseudo-obstruction. Am J Roentgenol. 1976;127:729–36.
31. Rudolf CD, Hyman PE, Altshuler SM, Christensen J, Colletti RB, Cucchiara S, Di Lorenzo C, Flores AF, Hillemeier AC, McCallum RW, Vanderhoof JA. Diagnosis and treatment of chronic intestinal pseudo-obstruction in children: report of consensus workshop. J Pediatr Gastroenterol Nutr. 1997;24:102–12.
32. Cucchiara S, Annese V, Minella R, Franco MT, Iervolino M, Emiliano M, et al. Antroduodenojejunal manometry in the diagnosis of chronic idiopathic intestinal pseudo-obstruction in children. J Pediatr Gastroenterol Nutr. 1994;18:294–305.
33. Boige N, Faure C, Cargill G, Mashako LMN, Cordeiro-Ferreira G, Viarme F, et al. Manometrical

evaluation in visceral neuropathies in children. J Pediatr Gastroenterol Nutr. 1994;19:71–7.
34. Hyman PE, McDiarmid SV, Napolitano J, Abrams CE, Tomomasa T. Antroduodenal motility in children with chronic intestinal pseudo-obstruction. J Pediatr. 1988;112:899–905.
35. Kamm MA. The small intestine and colon: scintigraphic quantitation of motility in health and disease. Eur J Nucl Med. 1992;19:902–12.
36. Devane SP, Ravelli AM, Bisset WM, Smith VV, Lake BD, Milla PJ. Gastric antral dysrhythmias in children with chronic idiopathic intestinal pseudo-obstruction. Gut. 1992;33:1477–81.
37. Reddy SN, DiLorenzo C, Tomomasa T, Snape WJ, Hyman PE. Is electro-gastrography (EGG) a substitute for manometry in the study of gastro-intestinal motility disorders in children. Gastroenterology. 1992;102:A504.
38. Mitros FA, Schuffler MD, Teja K, Anuras S. Pathologic features of familial visceral myopathy. Hum Pathol. 1982;13:825–33.
39. Eltringham WK, Roe AM, Galloway SW, Mountford RA, Espiner HJ. A laparoscopic technique for full thickness intestinal biopsy and feeding jejunostomy. Gut. 1993;34:122–4.
40. Higman D, Peters P, Stewart M. Familial hollow visceral myopathy with varying urological manifestations. Br J Urol. 1992;70:435–8.
41. Puri P, Lake BD, Gorman F, O'Donnell B, Nixon HH. Megacystis-microcolon-intestinal hypoperistalsis syndrome: a visceral myopathy. J Pediatr Surg. 1983;18:64–9.
42. Katz A. Pseudo-Hirschsprung's disease in bantu children. Arch Dis Child. 1966;41:152–4.
43. Singsen BH, Swanson VL, Bernstein BH, Heuser ET, Hanson V, Landing BH. A histologic evaluation of mixed connective tissue disease in childhood. Am J Med. 1980;68:710–7.
44. McDonald GB, Schuffler MD, Kadin ME, Tytgat GNJ. Intestinal pseudo-obstruction caused by diffuse lymphoid infiltration of the small intestine. Gastroenterology. 1985;89:882–9.
45. Jayachandar J, Frank JL, Jonas MM. Isolated intestinal myopathy resembling progressive systemic sclerosis in a child. Gastroenterology. 1988;95:1114–8.
46. Jacobs E, Ardichvili D, Perissino A, Gottignies P, Hanssens JF. A case of familial visceral myopathy with atrophy and fibrosis of the longitudinal muscle layer of the entire small bowel. Gastroenterology. 1979;77:745–50.
47. Brunner HG, Hamel BCJ, Rieu P, Höweler CJ, Peters FTM. Intestinal pseudo-obstruction in myotonic dystrophy. J Med Genet. 1992;29:791–3.
48. Mansell PI, Tattersall RB, Balsitis M, Lowe J, Spiller RC. Megaduodenum due to hollow visceral myopathy successfully managed by duodenoplasty and feeding jejunostomy. Gut. 1991;32:334–7.
49. Smith DS, Williams CS, Ferris CD. Diagnosis and treatment of chronic gastroparesis and chronic intestinal pseudo-obstruction. Gastroenterol Clin N Am. 2003;32:619–58.
50. Chitnis M, Chowdhary S, Lazarus C. Application of the Malone antegrade continence enema principle in degenerative leiomyopathy. Pediatr Surg Int. 2001;17:470–1.
51. Chitnis L, et al. Laparoscopically inserted button colostomy as a venting stoma and access port for the administration of antegrade enemas in African degenerative leiomyopathy. S Afr J Surg. 2011;49(1):44–6.
52. Jena GP. Colonic stricture complicating degenerative leiomyopathy. S Afr J Surg. 1989;27:143–4.
53. Sigurdsson L, Reyes J, Kocoshis SA, Mazeriegos G, Abu-Elmagd KM, Bueno J, Di Lorenzo C. Intestinal transplantation in children with chronic intestinal pseudo-obstruction. Gut. 1999;45:570–4.

Transanal Pull-Through With or Without Laparoscopic Assistance for Rectosigmoid Hirschsprung's Disease

23

Atsuyuki Yamataka, Masahiro Takeda, and Yuta Yazaki

Contents

23.1 Introduction

Surgical cure of Hirschsprung's Disease (HD) involves removing the aganglionic bowel segment and reconstructing the intestinal tract by bringing normally innervated bowel down to the anus while preserving the sphincter mechanism and sensory innervation of the anal transitional zone (ATZ) to ensure good postoperative bowel function (POBF).

In 1995, successful primary laparoscopy-assisted endorectal pull-through with transanal mucosectomy (i.e., L-TAPT) was described by Georgeson et al. [1], and subsequently, in 1998, De La Torre-Mondragon reported a single-stage transanal endorectal pull-through without laparoscopic assistance (pure TAPT) [2], which has been reported to be safe and efficient [3, 4]. Most centers will opt to treat HD using minimally invasive surgery (MIS) using either L-TAPT or pure TAPT.

TAPT is comprised of four key steps that must be performed exactingly for success. They are identification of normoganglionic colon, adequate colorectal dissection, anatomically accurate transanal dissection, and total excision of the posterior aganglionic rectal muscle cuff. Here, the surgical cure of rectal or rectosigmoid type HD using MIS will be described, focusing on a modified L-TAPT procedure developed specifically by the authors that incorporates features of Georgeson's classic

A. Yamataka (✉) · M. Takeda · Y. Yazaki
Department of Pediatric Surgery, Juntendo University School of Medicine, Tokyo, Japan
e-mail: yama@juntendo.ac.jp; mstakeda@juntendo.ac.jp; yyazaki@juntendo.ac.jp

P. Puri (ed.), *Hirschsprung's Disease and Allied Disorders*,
https://doi.org/10.1007/978-3-030-15647-3_23

procedure [1] and De La Torre-Mondragon's procedure [2]. The most distinguishing features are the level at which transanal dissection is commenced, in other words, the anorectal line (ARL), which is the border between the ATZ and colorectal-type mucosa, and is readily visible in viable tissue, and the length of the residual rectal muscle cuff [5].

23.2 Preparing for Surgery

23.2.1 Contraindications to MIS

MIS is generally contraindicated in HD patients if there is a history of previous abdominal surgery (other than stoma surgery), during the acute phase of enterocolitis, or the presence of any coexisting condition that may deteriorate during pneumoperitoneum. When rectosigmoid dilatation is extreme in children older than infants, an ileostomy or colostomy should be considered to reduce risks for complications, such as wound infection and abscess formation or stenosis at the coloanal anastomosis.

23.2.2 Preoperative Patient Preparation

Intensive preoperative bowel preparation is mandatory. Patients without stomas may continue normal oral intake until 2–3 days before surgery. Parents familiar with glycerin enema administration may use daily glycerin enemas with or without bowel irrigation with normal saline to decompress the colorectum. Once admitted to hospital, oral intake is limited to clear fluids only, and intravenous fluid replacement is commenced. Bowel irrigations with normal saline are performed twice daily and magnesium citrate is administered (1 g/kg) until there is no fecal residue forthcoming. An aminoglycoside antibiotic (100 mg/kg/day) is given orally the day before surgery. Broad-spectrum antibiotics such as ceftazidime (120 mg/kg/day) and isepamicin sulfate (8 mg/kg/day) are given intravenously once the patient is fully anesthetized.

Peripheral intravenous nutrition including amino acid and intravenous fat emulsion supplementation is highly recommended because, in total, the period a patient will be nil by mouth both pre- and postoperatively will generally be 4 days. If necessary, more intensively managed nutritional support may be considered using intravenous hyperalimentation through a central venous catheter.

23.3 Surgical Technique

23.3.1 Patient/Surgeon Positioning

After induction of general endotracheal tube anesthesia, the patient is positioned at the end of the operating table in the supine position. The patient's body is disinfected. For infants, the trunk and buttocks are prepared extensively, then the legs circumferentially to the tips of the toes, and sterile stockings are placed on both legs. The legs are raised when transanal dissection is commenced. Children older than infants are positioned in the lithotomy position with their legs in stirrups.

The laparoscopic surgeon and assistant stand on the patient's right side. The transanal pull-through surgeon and an assistant are present, on standby. The scrub nurse stands at the left lower end of the table. A monitor is positioned beyond the patient's feet. The table is placed head-down for laparoscopic colorectal dissection. A urinary catheter is used to decompress the bladder.

23.3.2 Trocar Placement

A 5 mm port is inserted through the umbilicus using an open Hasson technique, and pneumoperitoneum is established with carbon dioxide to a pressure of 8–10 mmHg. Three additional 3 or 5 mm ports are placed in the right upper and lower quadrants and in the left upper quadrant, respectively. A laparoscope is inserted through the 5 mm port in the right upper quadrant. The laparoscopic surgeon's two working ports are the umbilical port for the left hand and the right lower abdominal port for the right hand. The port in the left upper abdomen can be used for either retraction of the colon, or, additionally for the laparoscopic surgeon's left hand.

23.3.3 Laparoscopy-Assisted Colon Suction Biopsy

Laparoscopy-assisted colon suction biopsy can be performed in any infant or child of any size with rectosigmoid type HD, because the sigmoid colon can be mobilized readily to allow the tip of the suction biopsy device to reach the proposed biopsy site. Fortuitously, 80% of HD cases are recto-sigmoid, and laparoscopic-assisted colon suction biopsy is safe, simple, and quick compared with full-thickness biopsy.

After identification of the region of caliber change in the colon laparoscopically by the laparoscopic surgeon, the suction biopsy device is inserted into the anus by the transanal pull-through surgeon (Fig. 23.1) ensuring that the tissue sampling mechanism is orientated correctly to prevent risks for perforation. After the suction biopsy, the laparoscopic surgeon places a metal laparoscopic vessel clip at the biopsy site as a marker. Biopsy specimens are sent for immediate assessment by a pathologist. If the result is aganglionic, the biopsy is repeated more proximally. If ganglion cells are present, the colon is pulled-through to the level of the clip transanally and full-thickness biopsies are taken at 12, 3, 6, and 9 o'clock circumferentially. The coloanal anastomosis is performed only after all biopsies are confirmed to be ganglionic. These extra biopsies are performed to prevent aganglionic transitional zone colon at the level of the clipped biopsy site that has been exposed through the anus from being anastomosed.

23.3.4 Laparoscopic Colorectal Dissection

If the biopsy site is ganglionic, the laparoscopic surgeon starts dissection of the colorectum. A benefit of laparoscopy-assisted procedure, not possible with pure TAPT, is that the mesenteric vessels can be divided distal to the level of the clipped biopsy site, leaving both the marginal artery and vein intact at the level of

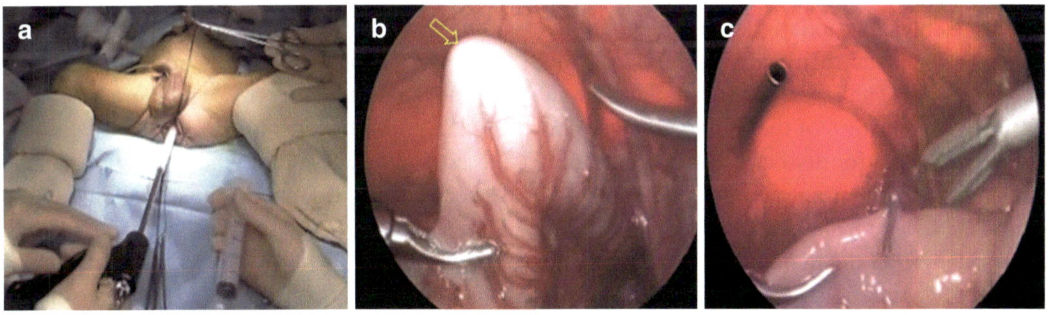

Fig. 23.1 A suction rectal biopsy device is being advanced (**a**) into the colon through the anus by the transanal pull-through surgeon under the supervision of the laparoscopic surgeon until the tip (**b**: open yellow arrow) of the device lies proximal to the region of caliber change. The laparoscopic surgeon places a metal vessel clip at the biopsy site as a marker (**c**)

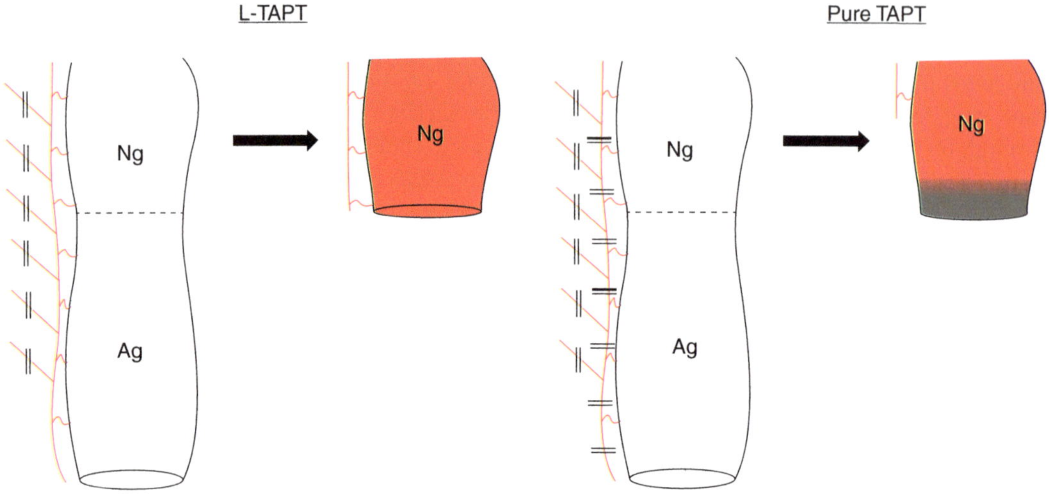

Fig. 23.2 A significant advantage of L-TAPT is the ability to mobilize the colon while keeping marginal arteries intact, unlike during TAPT without laparoscopic coloanal dissection (pure TAPT) where marginal arteries to the pull-through colon must be sacrificed. Short double lines indicate ligation sites. (Ng normoganglionic, Ag aganglionic)

the clipped biopsy site. Then, the mesenteric vascular arcade proximal to the clipped biopsy site is inspected carefully, and vessels divided as required, to enable the pulled-through colon to reach the anus without tension with an intact vascular arcade; that is, intact marginal arteries and veins. Thus, marginal vessels in the pulled-through colon are essentially intact, ensuring good vascular perfusion even in the distal end of the pull-through colon. Further dissection is continued in the rectum distal to the peritoneal reflection circumferentially, which greatly facilitates invagination of the proximal colorectum into the distal rectum during transanal rectal dissection. The laparoscopic surgeon should identify the location of the ureters and vas deferens (in males) for dissection of the distal rectum. Another important point is that dissection of the mesorectum should follow the rectal wall to avoid injuring the hypogastric nerve which is related to ejaculation and the pelvic splanchnic nerve which is related to erection and excretory function.

A significant advantage of L-TAPT is that the colon can be mobilized keeping the marginal arteries at the distal end of the pull-through colon intact to ensure good blood supply to the coloanal anastomosis. In contrast, without laparoscopy, marginal arteries are likely to be injured or need to be sacrificed during dissection (Fig. 23.2).

23.3.5 Transanal Dissection

While awaiting histopathology results, the patient is placed in the lithotomy position by flexing the patient's legs and the transanal pull-through surgeon places 3–0 traction sutures 3–4 cm from the anus at 12, 3, 6, and 9 o'clock to expose the dentate line (DL) and the anal sinuses (Fig. 23.3). The position of the buttocks and these traction sutures are vital for ensuring that a Lone Star Ring Retractor System (LS ring; Lone Star Medical Products, Inc., Stafford, TX) can be attached correctly to expose and confirm the ARL. If positioned and prepared correctly, the LS ring sits snugly and the ARL and entire surgical anal canal prolapses to the anal verge (Fig. 23.4). The anal valves along the DL at the bottom of the anal sinuses are then hooked up using the LS ring allowing the ARL to be identified as a ring at

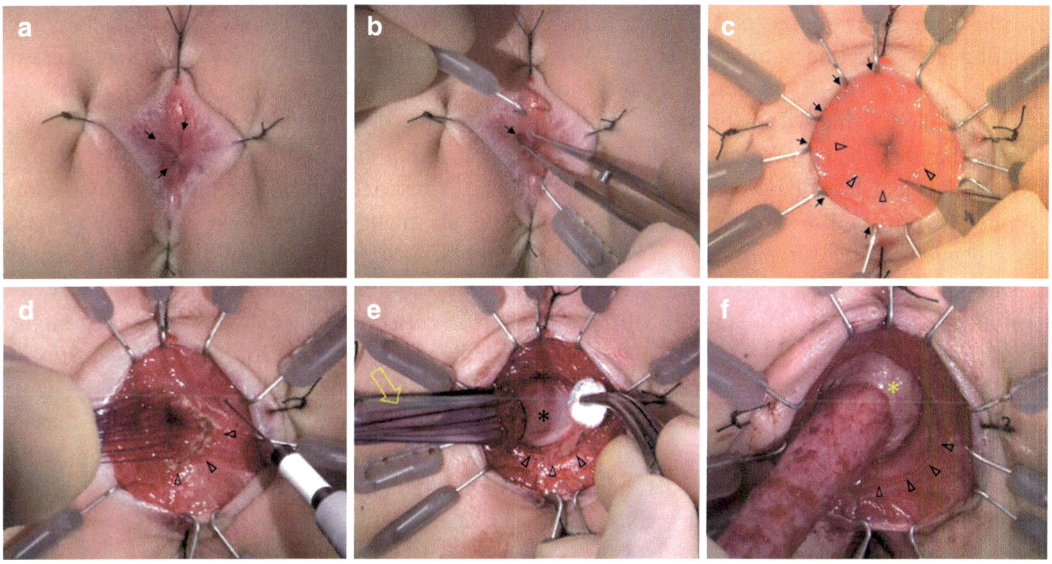

Fig. 23.3 3-0 traction sutures placed circumferentially 3–4 cm from the anus can expose the DL (arrows) (**a**). The ARL (arrowheads) can be identified by hooking the crypts (i.e., anal valves) on the DL to expose the anal transitional zone (between the DL and ARL) with a ring retractor device (**b**, **c**). Note multiple fine traction sutures just proximal to the ARL (arrowheads) and the incision just proximal to the ARL, leaving the ARL intact (**d**). A large bore silicon tube (large open yellow arrow) has been inserted into the rectal lumen (**e**), to facilitate transanal "submucosal" (asterisk) dissection. The rectosigmoid colon begins to invaginate into the rectal muscle cuff (yellow asterisk) and eventually reaches the anus (**f**). When this invagination starts, submucosal dissection is considered to be adequate

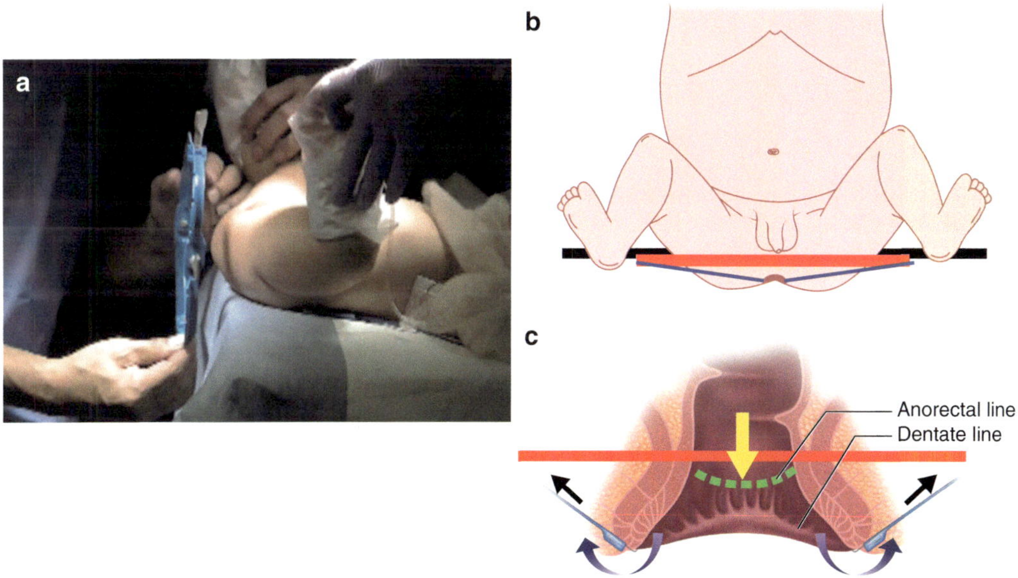

Fig. 23.4 The patient's buttocks should be positioned to hang 3–5 cm over the end of table (**a**) so the ring retractor device sits snugly (**b**) and the ARL and entire surgical anal canal prolapse to the anal verge (**c**)

the top of the anal columns of Morgagni [6]. By omitting these traction sutures or not positioning the patient's buttocks as described, it is most likely that the LS ring will be hooked to the anal verge rather than the DL. When retracted circumferentially, the DL will be spread out roundly and not be retracted toward the anus (i.e., will not prolapse) and the surgeon will not be able to see the ARL under direct vision whatever the surgeon does when the LS ring is in this (incorrect) position (Fig. 23.5).

Multiple fine traction sutures are placed proximal to the ARL and the mucosa incised just proximal to the ARL circumferentially using needle-tipped electrocautery. The ARL and ATZ are left intact (Fig. 23.3). The transanal pull-through surgeon commences near full-thickness rectal dissection transanally progressing cranially for about 10–15 mm in the plane of the rectal muscle layer, taking great care not to injure the external anal sphincter. A large bore silicon tube is inserted into the rectal lumen as a stent, and the plane of dissection is changed to the submucosal plane and continued proximally. As mucosectomy progresses further proximally, the rectosigmoid colon which has already been prepared laparoscopically for pull-through begins to invaginate into the rectal muscle cuff and reaches the anus without any need for dividing the mesenteric vessels transanally. When this invagination starts, submucosal dissection is considered to be adequate and the invaginated muscular wall

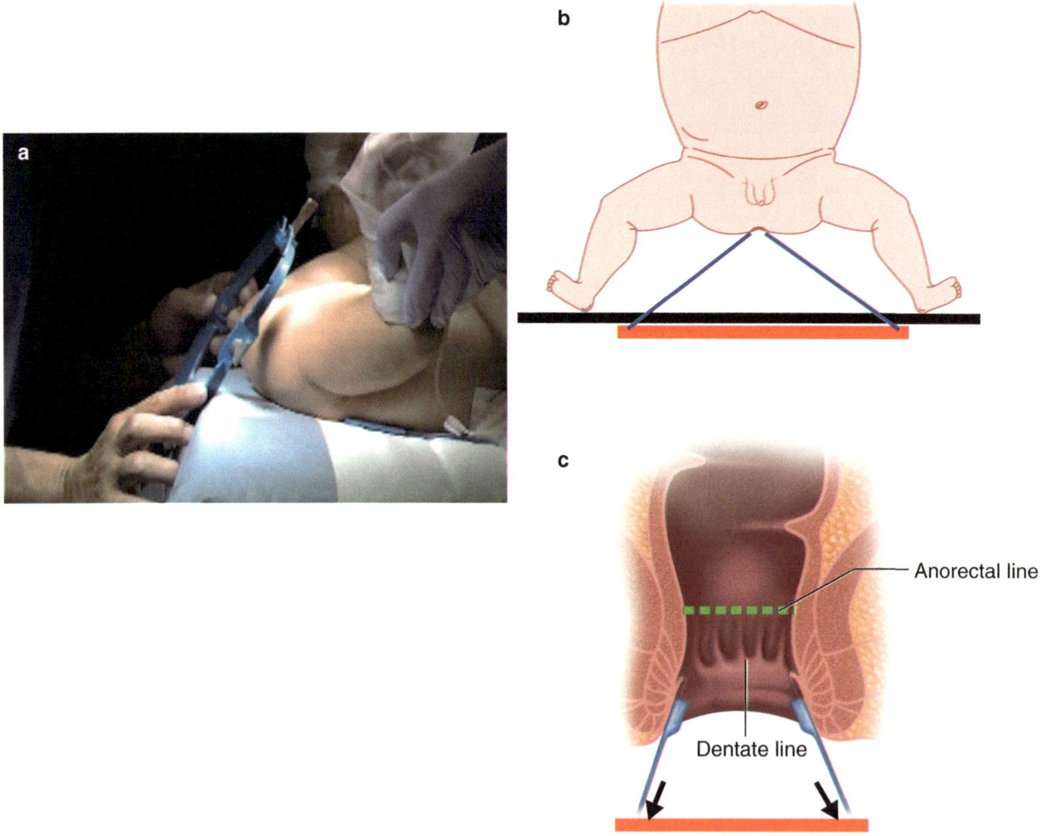

Fig. 23.5 If a patient's buttocks cannot be positioned adequately or the patient is too high on the table (**a**), the ring retractor device will not sit well (**b**), resulting only in dilatation and lengthening of the surgical anal canal without prolapse (**c**). The surgeon will not be able to expose the ARL adequately

of the rectum is divided circumferentially. The proximal rectosigmoid is delivered through the anus externally without applying tension until the proposed site for the coloanal anastomosis marked by the metal clip is identified.

Before the coloanal anastomosis, the pull-through colon is assessed for torsion laparoscopically and tension on both the pull-through colon and vasculature. If there is any tension, further laparoscopic dissection/mobilization is mandatory to prevent retraction of the pull-through colon that may cause leakage at the anastomosis that could lead to pelvic abscess formation.

23.3.6 Total Excision of the Posterior Aganglionic Rectal Muscle Cuff

Before the coloanal anastomosis, the aganglionic rectal cuff should be excised to eliminate any chance for complications caused by the residual cuff to occur. The rectal cuff is divided at the 3 and 9 o'clock positions into anterior and posterior cuffs. The anterior rectal cuff is then divided in the midline (12 o'clock) and then excised till where laparoscopic dissection was performed to, usually slightly distal to the peritoneal reflection (Fig. 23.6). The distal anterior cuff is excised leaving the proximal anterior cuff intact to prevent injury to nerves supplying the urinary tract. The posterior rectal cuff is then divided caudally in the midline (6 o'clock) down to where the mucosectomy was commenced (some 10–15 mm proximal to the ARL) to ensure that achalasia due to aganglionic rectum and structural muscle ring is released completely (Fig. 23.7). In other words, since the first 10–15 mm of rectal dissection from the ARL is nearly full-thickness, the entire posterior aganglionic rectal cuff is removed.

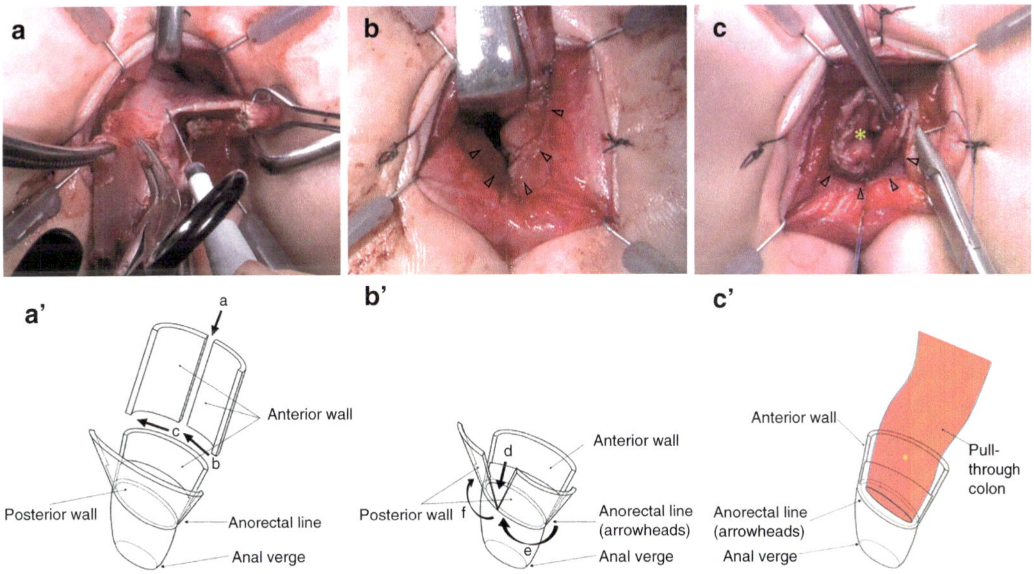

Fig. 23.6 The anterior rectal cuff is divided in the midline (12 o'clock) (**a**) and excised to the point where the laparoscopic dissection was performed (a–c) in **a'**. After "d," "e," and "f" in **b'**, the entire posterior aganglionic rectal cuff is removed while preserving the ARL completely (arrowheads) (**b**). The pull-through colon (yellow asterisk) being anastomosed to the ARL (arrowheads) using interrupted sutures (**c**)

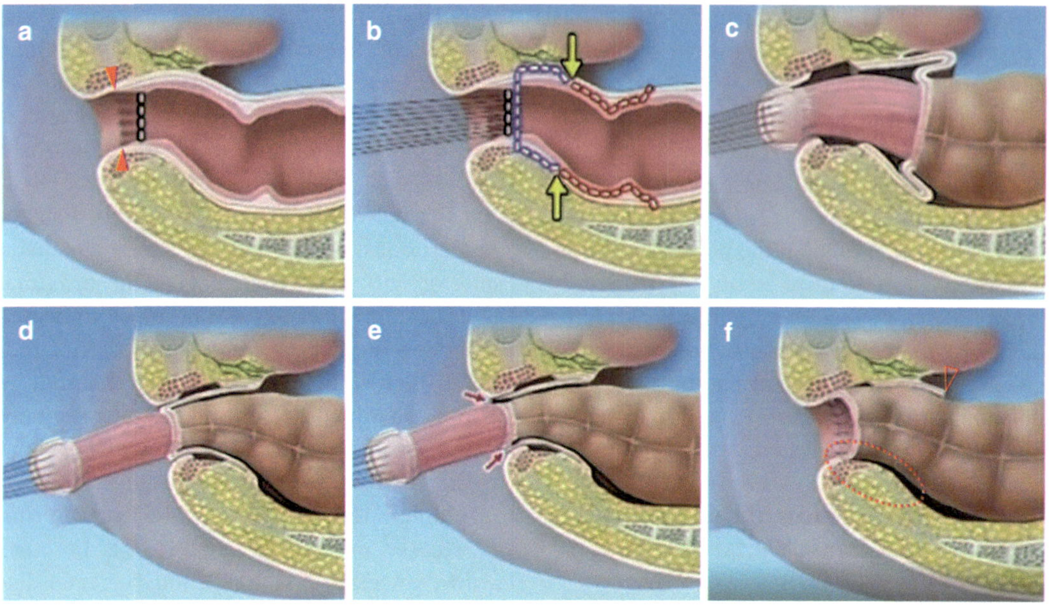

Fig. 23.7 Anatomic relationships in the anal transitional zone. The DL (red arrowheads) is at the bottom of the anal sinuses and the ARL (vertical broken line) is at the top of the anal columns of Morgagni (**a**). The transanal pull-through surgeon commences near full-thickness rectal dissection transanally progressing cranially for 10–15 mm in the plane of the rectal muscle layer (purple broken line; **b**). The yellow arrows indicate where the plane of dissection is changed to submucosal (**b**) and continued proximally between the rectal mucosa and the rectal muscle layers (maroon broken line; **b**), invaginating the proximal colon to the distal colon (**c**) and finally to the anus (**d**). At this time the rectal muscle cuff is divided circumferentially (red arrows; **e**), the posterior rectal cuff is excised totally (red dotted circle; **f**), and the anterior rectal cuff is excised to where the laparoscopic dissection was performed (red open arrowhead)

The pull-through colon is anastomosed just above the ARL using interrupted absorbable sutures.

23.4 Postoperative Care

Provided L-TAPT is performed meticulously without any intra- or postoperative complications, recovery is expected to be unremarkable with routine postoperative care. Intravenous fluids and nasogastric decompression are continued postoperatively until bowel function returns. The urinary catheter is left in place until the next morning. When bowel function returns, oral intake is initiated with tapering of intravenous fluids, typically by 3–4 days postoperatively. Intravenous antibiotics are continued for 3 days postoperatively, and patients can be discharged once a full oral diet is tolerated.

23.5 Complications and Their Management

Complications after L-TAPT can be classified as either early or late. Early serious postoperative complications include anastomotic leakage, retraction of the pull-through colon, abscess formation at the coloanal anastomosis, or consequences of the pull-through of a transitional segment of colon, such as unstable bowel function. Anastomotic leakage, retraction of the pulled-through colon, and abscess formation at the coloanal anastomosis are all secondary to poor perfusion of the distal pulled-through colon. Laparoscopic assistance maintains good blood supply to the entire pulled-through colon because marginal vasculature is never compromised by poor exposure or sacrificing a few vessels as is the case with pure TAPT; marginal vasculature is left intact and ensures successful pull-through. Late complications include intractable constipation, enterocolitis, bowel obstruction, incontinence, and anal stenosis/stricture.

One neonatal case of postoperative obstruction caused by residual rectal cuffs that had only been split in the midline and had folded caudally toward the anus outside the pull-through colon while it was being pulled-through down to the anus [7]. This patient required redo surgery to remove the rectal cuffs using a posterior sagittal approach. After experiencing this case, all posterior rectal cuffs are routinely excised in toto, because splitting the rectal cuff in the midline alone may cause postoperative obstruction.

23.6 Discussion

The DL is the traditional landmark used for the starting point of transanal dissection, with a range of flexibility of 5–20 mm [8, 9] reported as acceptable because the recommendation is "above" the DL. As a consequence, the ATZ may be injured or aganglionic mucosa may be left behind (i.e., if commenced too high, there is a tendency for constipation, and if commenced too low, there is a tendency for staining) (Fig. 23.8). The distance chosen above the DL would appear to be quite subjective, especially when the age and physique of a patient are also taken into account, with the result that postoperative outcome in patients where the DL is used as a landmark can be somewhat unpredictable.

Obviously, a more accurate landmark would be more reliable and the importance of the ARL in HD was actually first suggested by Soave in 1963 [10]. The ARL is a macroscopically observable landmark; synonymous with the suprazonal line and rectal mucosa proximal to the ARL has the texture of pink velvet and distal to the ARL is more whitish [11]. Histologically, the ARL was also considered to be equivalent to the squamous columnar junction, which in mice is the case, with epithelium proximal to the ARL being columnar and distal to the ARL being squamous [12], but in humans, ATZ epithelium is variable

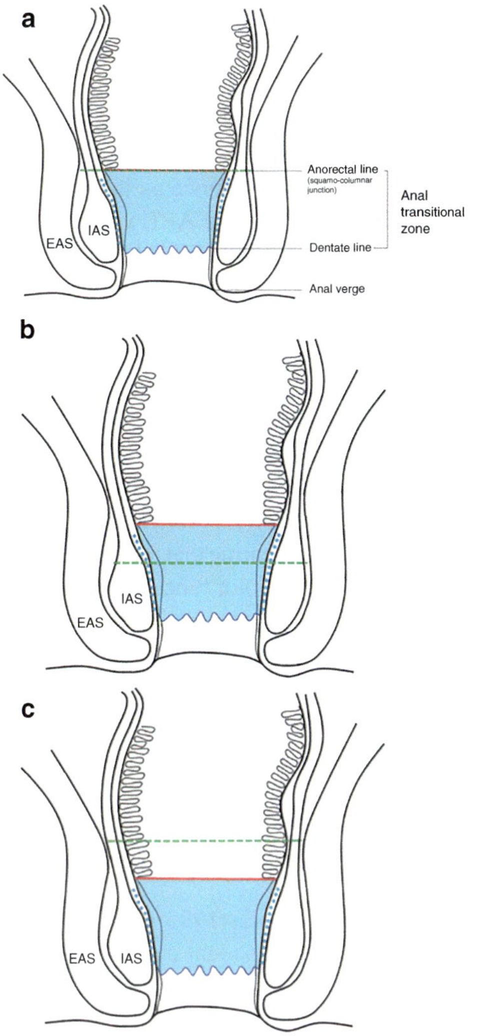

Fig. 23.8 Red solid lines indicate the ARL at the top of the anal columns and blue wavy lines indicate the DL at the bottom of the anal sinuses. The ATZ is the light blue region between the ARL and the DL. The green broken lines indicate where transanal dissection should start. When commenced just above the ARL (**a**), POBF will be more reliable and predictable because the ARL is a fixed landmark. However, if "above" the DL is too low (i.e., below the ARL, (**b**) the ATZ will be injured causing fecal incontinence, and if too high (i.e., above the ARL, (**c**), residual aganglionic rectum will cause constipation. (IAS internal anal sphincter, EAS external anal sphincter)

although epithelium proximal to the ARL is consistently columnar. Thus, the ARL cannot strictly be considered to be equivalent to the squamous columnar junction in humans. Interestingly, the author's most recent research using HD model mice [12], also found that the ARL corresponded with the squamous columnar junction, but that there were no apparent differences in sensory innervation of the ATZ compared with normal mice; proof of the importance an intact ATZ has in HD. In other words, the ARL is synonymous with the top border of the ATZ [11] and this natural demarcation can be located accurately in all patients irrespective of age, size, or build, without any need for subjective interpretation in contrast to "above" the DL.

The author first proposed using the ARL as the landmark for commencing dissection in TAPT in 2006 [6], and by using the modified L-TAPT technique described, the ATZ between the DL and the ARL is preserved, ensuring that the anorectum has normal sensory and motor function, which is crucial for preventing postoperative fecal staining/soiling, while laparoscopic assistance improves mobilization and maintains the blood supply to the pull-through colon. In addition, the posterior rectal cuff should be totally excised. Outcomes should be more reliable if surgeons with a sound knowledge of anatomic relationships in the ATZ commence dissection on the ARL and excise the cuff entirely.

In Georgeson et al.'s 1995 report, they suggested splitting the residual cuff to the level of the proposed anastomosis [1]. There are also reports about short residual cuff remnants being associated with improved short term-results in pure TAPT and L-TAPT cases [13], but from experience, complications related to residual cuffs cannot be resolved by merely leaving some aganglionic cuff behind, no matter how short, or by splitting alone which is inadequate, especially if the residual rectal cuff is longish, because the split may reattach or be retracted/folded as the colon is pulled-through and cause rectal stenosis.

In 2017, Neuvonen et al. reported the long term POBF and quality of life after TAPT (including both pure TAPT and L-TAPT) in relation to controls selected from the general population [14]. In this large series, 75% of patients were socially continent after TAPT. While soiling and fecal accidents experienced during childhood improved with age to be comparable with controls by adulthood, the frequency of stooling remained higher in TAPT cases in adulthood.

Thus, prior to surgery, careful discussion based on the preoperative plan for surgery will ensure parents have realistic expectations and surgeons do not give parents false hope. As with all surgery, experience and confidence will influence operative time but surgeons should not be concerned about time when POBF is concerned. Surgeons must be completely comfortable with the anatomy of the surgical anal canal and be acutely aware that problematic POBF is iatrogenic. There is no excuse for poor outcome due to incomplete knowledge of the SAC [8, 9]. Redo surgery for HD is notoriously difficult and results are not encouraging, especially in cases of postoperative soiling and fecal incontinence caused by ATZ injury [15, 16], because a damaged ATZ will usually only suffer more damage during redo surgery. Surgeons actually have the capacity to seriously disrupt POBF which has the potential to cause lifelong distress.

Outcomes will be more reliable if surgeons with a sound knowledge of anatomic relationships in the ATZ commence dissection on the ARL and excise the cuff entirely.

References

1. Georgeson KE, Fuenfer MM, Hardin WD. Primary laparoscopic pull-through for Hirschsprung's disease in infants and children. J Pediatr Surg. 1995;30:1017–22.
2. De la Torre-Mondragon L, Ortega-Salgado JA. Transanal endorectal pull-through for Hirschsprung's disease. J Pediatr Surg. 1998;33(8):1283–6.
3. Rintala RJ. Transanal coloanal pull-through with a short muscular cuff for classic Hirschsprung's disease. Eur J Pediatr Surg. 2003;13(3):181–6.
4. Langer JC. Laparoscopic and transanal pull-through for Hirschsprung disease. Semin Pediatr Surg. 2012;21(4):283–90.
5. Yamataka A, Miyano G, Takeda M. Minimally invasive neonatal surgery: Hirschsprung disease. Clin Perinatol. 2017;44(4):851–64.
6. Yamataka A, Kaneyama K, Fujiwara N, et al. Rectal mucosal dissection during transanal pull-through for Hirschsprung's disease: the anorectal or the dentate line? J Pediatr Surg. 2009;44(1):266–9.

7. Shimotakahara A, Yamataka A, Kobayashi H, et al. Obstruction due to rectal cuff after laparoscopy-assisted transanal endorectal pull-through for Hirschsprung's disease. J Laparoendosc Adv Surg Tech A. 2006;16(5):540–2.
8. Bischoff A, Frischer J, Knod JL, et al. Damaged anal canal as a cause of fecal incontinence after surgical repair for Hirschsprung disease – a preventable and under-reported complication. J Pediatr Surg. 2017;52(4):549–53.
9. De la Torre L, Cogley K, Santos K, Morales O, Calisto J. The anal canal is the fine line between "fecal incontinence and colitis" after a pull-through for Hirschsprung disease. J Pediatr Surg. 2017;52(12):2011–7.
10. Soave F. A new surgical technique for treatment of Hirschsprung's disease. Surgery. 1964;56:1007–14.
11. Wendell-Smith CP. Anorectal nomenclature: fundamental terminology. Dis Colon Rectum. 2000;43(10):1349–58.
12. Takeda M, Miyahara K, Akazawa C, et al. Sensory innervation of the anal canal and anorectal line in Hirschsprung's disease. Histological evidence from mouse models. Pediatr Surg Int. 2017;33(8):883–6.
13. Nasr A, Langer JC. Evolution of the technique in the transanal pull-through for Hirschsprung's disease: effect on outcome. J Pediatr Surg. 2007;42(1):36–40.
14. Neuvonen MI, Kyrklund K, Rintala RJ, Pakarinen MP. Bowel function and quality of life after transanal endorectal pull-through for Hirschsprung disease: controlled outcomes up to adulthood. Ann Surg. 2017;265(3):622–9.
15. Dingemans A, van der Steeg H, Rassouli-Kirchmeier R, Linssen MW, van Rooij I, de Blaauw I. Redo pull-through surgery in Hirschsprung disease: short-term clinical outcome. J Pediatr Surg. 2017;52(9):1446–50.
16. Pakarinen M. Perioperative complications of transanal pull-through surgery for Hirschsprung's disease. Eur J Pediatr Surg. 2018;28(2):152–5.

Laparoscopically Assisted Pull-Through Operation for Hirschsprung's Disease

24

Jie-xiong Feng, Ting Li, and Ning Li

Contents

Electronic Supplementary Material The online version of this chapter (https://doi.org/10.1007/978-3-030-15647-3_24) contains supplementary material, which is available to authorized users.

J.-x. Feng (✉) · T. Li · N. Li
Department of Pediatric Surgery, Tongji Hospital, Tongji Medical College, Huazhong University of Science and Technology, Wuhan, China

24.1 Introduction

Sixty years ago, the treatment for patients with Hirschsprung's disease (HSCR) was a three-stage approach, namely, colostomy or stoma in the proximal ganglionated intestine followed by pull-through procedures after the infant reached 8–12 months of age, or 10 kg weight, and eventually closure of the colostomy. With the improvement of surgical techniques, one-stage pull-throughs (Soave, Swenson, Duhamel) had been widely performed laparotomically. In recent decades, advanced laparoscopic techniques and instruments have provided a new minimally invasive approach to mobilization and pull-through of the colon [26].

In 1994, Curran et al. reported the feasibility of the Swenson pull-through in 13 mongrel dogs and later applied it on 4 children with HSCR, aging from 10 to 30 months [7]. The first reported successful trial of the laparoscopic Duhamel procedure was carried out on a 2-year-old boy

P. Puri (ed.), *Hirschsprung's Disease and Allied Disorders*, https://doi.org/10.1007/978-3-030-15647-3_24

by Smith BM in 1994 [36]. Later, Georgeson et al. described series of one-stage laparoscopic Soave pull-throughs [10, 11, 28, 44]. In recent years, laparoscopic surgeries have been commonly accepted by most surgeons and a series of modifications have been developed, such as heart-shaped anastomosis (Wang Guo surgery) [15], Z-shaped anastomosis (Ikeda surgery) [40], and ileocolic side-to-side anastomosis (Martin surgery). To achieve better cosmetic results, the conventional laparoscopic procedure (CLP) developed into single-incision laparoscopic procedure (SILP) [28, 45, 48]. Other advances, such as natural orifice transluminal endoscopic surgery (NOTES) [13, 18, 23] and da Vinci robotic laparoscopic-assisted surgery [14, 25], were also reported.

Under the assistance of a laparoscope, patients benefit from the same safety and efficacy as laparotomic procedures, but also gain from better cosmetic results. In addition to the minimized scars, reports showed a more rapid bowel function return, shorter postoperative recovery, better pain control, faster discharge from hospital, and less risk of abdominal contamination and adhesion in laparoscopic procedures compared to laparotomic ones [3, 6, 8, 12, 27, 47]. Laparoscopes also provide clear operative field of view for surgeons. The pulled-through bowel can be visualized to ensure that there is no active bleeding or twisting along the longitudinal axis of the bowel. Moreover, histological determination of the level of transitional zone becomes easier and more convenient with the assistance of a laparoscope [16, 32].

Compared to laparotomic operations, laparoscopic pull-through mainly differs in the procedures in the peritoneal cavity, while the perineal procedures of these two operations are mostly similar.

24.2 Indications

Under the assistance of a laparoscope, the diagnosis of HSCR becomes convenient, and as a result, laparoscopic operations can be used for colonic pathological biopsy in a minimally invasive way. Once diagnosed, most patients are eligible to undergo laparoscopic pull-through, such as patients with common or long-segment HSCR, total colonic aganglionosis (TCA), reoperation, stoma, or allied HSCR disorders. There are also reports on laparoscopic surgery for short-segment HSCR [4, 9, 16, 45] despite the fact that the totally transanal endorectal pull-through procedure is more popular in this situation. The majority of surgeons give preference to one-stage surgery [37–39]. For patients with severe complications, such as severe Hirschsprung's disease-associated enterocolitis (HAEC), malnutrition, huge fecalith, or severe dilation of the proximal bowel, surgery should be staged and a stoma, and an intraoperative biopsy should be performed at first [34].

24.3 Preoperative Preparation

The preoperative preparations for laparoscopic procedures are similar to those for laparotomic ones.

The preoperative work-up includes blood routine, urine routine, stool routine, liver and kidney function, and coagulation function, as well as chest X-ray and ECG. Easily digestible food with high protein is recommended. For patients with malnutrition, enteral and parenteral nutrition should be applied to improve their nutritional condition. Preoperative decompression is usually performed by bowel irrigation with saline or anal dilatation for 6–7 days [24]. For severe and persistent constipation or distension, the bowel preparation may be longer. Oral intake is limited to clear liquids within 14–24 hours before surgery [30]. A nasogastric tube is used for decompression and better exposure just at the beginning of the operation. However, enhanced recovery after surgery (ERAS) studies have shown that [33], prolonged gastrointestinal decompression postoperatively does not promote the recovery of bowel function, nor does it reduce the occurrence of anastomotic leakage, so the nasogastric tube can be removed early after operation. Broad-spectrum intravenous and nonabsorbable enteral antibiotics can be used preoperatively, especially for those with enterocolitis. A Foley tube should be introduced before operation. Blood product should be made available for the patients at high risk of bleeding. Patients suitable for ERAS can be treated by mechanical bowel preparation and oral antibiotics at home on the day before surgery and preoperative antibiotics in the operating room within an hour before incision [35].

24.4 Position of the Patient

Laparoscopic pull-through is usually performed with the patient in the dorsal decubitus position with the legs wrapped. Neonates and infants are placed transversely on the operating table with the legs elevated during the perineal procedures, with the operator standing at the head side. Older patients are placed in a supine lithotomy with the surgeons standing on the right side.

24.5 Port Placement

The ultimate purpose of port placement is to facilitate the surgeons' manipulability, so the placement of the trocars is relatively agile. Different surgeons have their preferred choices, and the position of trocars can vary according to the procedure adopted.

For original laparoscopic Soave procedure [10, 11], three or four 5-mm trocars are placed with the first Hasson's type trocar inserted through the right upper abdomen and two in the left and right abdomen. An extra one if necessary can be placed in the left lower quadrant in some patients to provide retraction of the pelvic structures and to hold the colon in traction during laparoscopic dissection of the rectum (Fig. 24.1). The original Duhamel procedure uses four ports as shown in Fig. 24.2. Three incisions are made separately above the umbilicus and in the left and right upper quadrants, the fourth in the right lower quad-

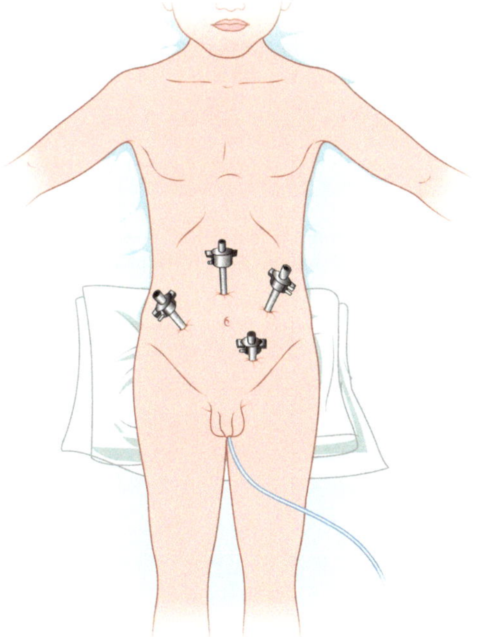

Fig. 24.1 Port placement in the original Soave procedure. The first Hasson's type trocar inserted through the right upper abdomen and the other two in the left and right abdomen. The extra one in the left lower quadrant is introduced in some patients if necessary to facilitate the operation. Currently, the three-incision method is more popular

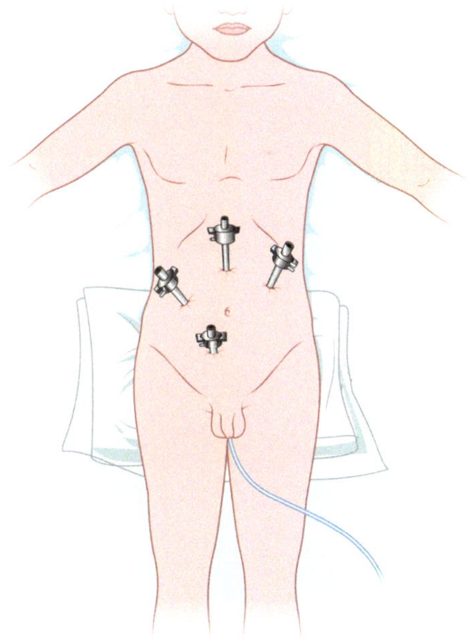

Fig. 24.2 Port placement in the original Duhamel procedure. The three incisions are separate above the umbilicus and in the left and right upper quadrant. The fourth incision is made on the right lower quadrant for the 12-mm port of instruments and endo-cutting stapler. Recently surgeons prefer to make three incisions if manipulation is permitted

rant for the 12 mm port of instruments and endo-cutting stapler [2, 9]. The port placement of Swenson procedure is similar to that in Duhamel with four incisions. Other surgeons prefer three ports, that is, the first port is placed above umbilicus, while the other two ports are inserted in the left and right iliac fossa [17]. The three-incision method has increased in popularity in recent years.

If the patient has a previous colostomy, the stoma can be used for one or two trocar ports [25].

On the basis of these methods mentioned above, port placement has been modified over time. Laparoscopic Soave and Swenson procedures are both suitable for the modified port placement as single-incision laparoscopic procedure (SILP) [28, 45]. Usually, the first port is at the umbilicus while the other two trocars are placed laterally (Fig. 24.3).

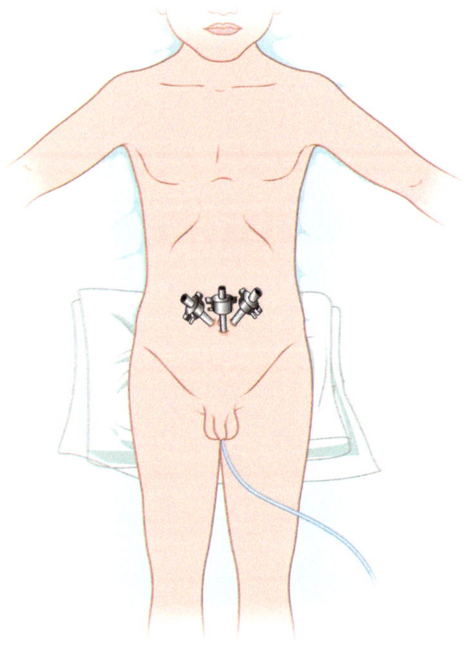

Fig. 24.3 Port placement in single-incision laparoscopic procedure. The first port is at the umbilicus for the laparoscope. The other two ports are placed laterally for the operating instruments. The introduction of a triport is another alternative way

24.6 Laparoscopic Soave Procedure

After anesthesia, the patient is placed in a dorsal position. The lower chest, abdomen, legs, and perineum are cleansed and disinfected. The legs are wrapped with aseptic cloth in advance and elevated during the perineal procedures.

Choose the proper sites to place the trocars and insufflate the abdominal cavity with CO_2. Inspect the abdominal cavity and look for the transitional zone (Fig. 24.4) to identify the site and length of the narrow bowel and the extent of the dilated bowel (Fig. 24.5). Take three or four seromuscular leveling biopsies with the assis-

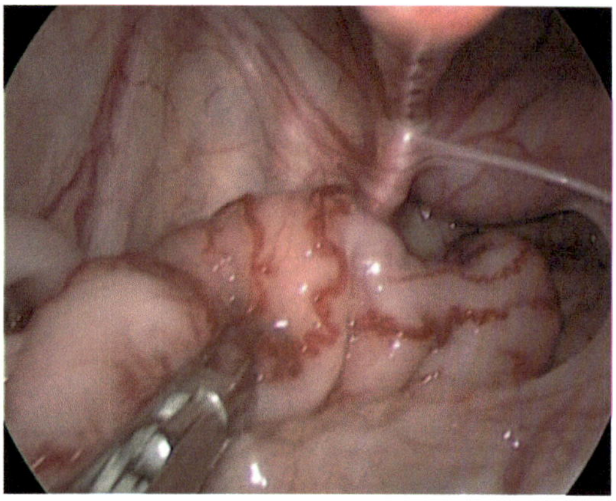

Fig. 24.4 Inspection of the narrow bowel. The narrow bowel is a distinct stricture and stiff without movement

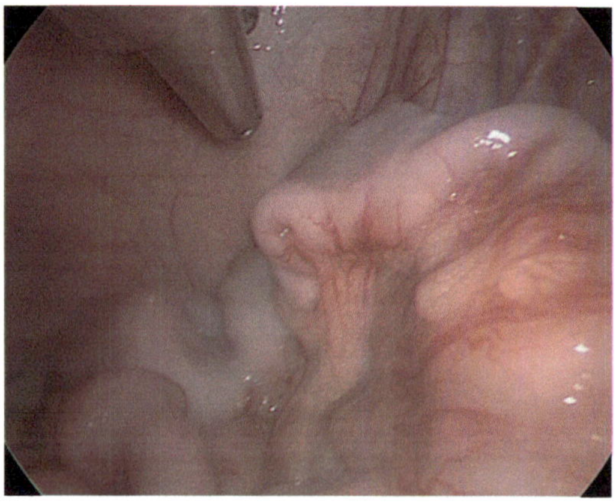

Fig. 24.5 Inspection of the dilated bowel. The dilated bowel is obviously wider with a thicker bowel wall

tance of laparoscopic instruments and send them for rapid frozen section pathological evaluation to determine the normal colon site. Perforation or bleeding of the biopsy site can be closed using figure 8 sutures. If the proximal site still shows abnormal ganglia or nerve fibers, the biopsies should be continued as proximally as possible until the normal colon wall is identified. And then, make a mark on this segment of bowel.

Use an ultrasonic scalpel to mobilize the colon and dissect the colonic mesenteric vessels to approximately 5 cm proximal to the normal colon. Confirm that the normal colon is long enough to reach the deep pelvis without tension. Dissect the sigmoid and descending colon, splenic flexure, gastrocolic omentum, transverse colon, hepatic flexure, and ascending colon if necessary according to the length of the lesion (Figs. 24.6, 24.7, 24.8, 24.9, 24.10, and 24.11). For subtotal resection, the ileocolic vessels should be carefully kept to ensure the blood supply of proximal colon (Fig. 24.12). Surgeons stand on the left side of the patient and accumulate the small intestine from the bottom to the left side of mesentery, then the appendix is grasped, and the ascending colon should be anticlockwisely transpositioned until without torsion followed by concurrent appendectomy (Figs. 24.13 and 24.14). Be aware of protection of ureter when dissecting the sigmoid and descending and ascending colon.

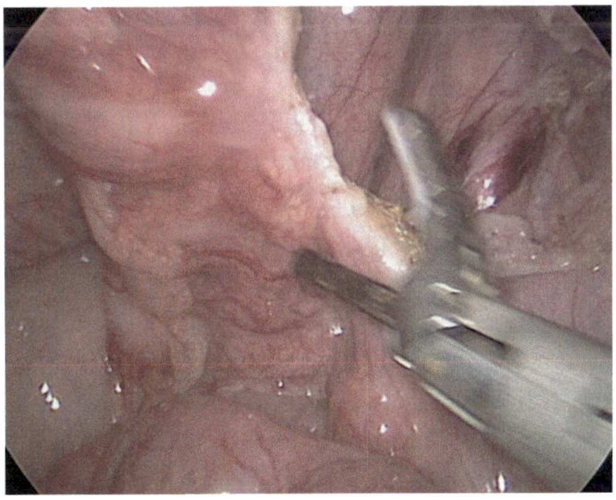

Fig. 24.6 Resection of the sigmoid colon. Open the peritoneum beside the sigmoid colon and dissect the mesentery using an ultrasonic scalpel. Be aware of the protection of surrounding tissues and organs, especially the ureters

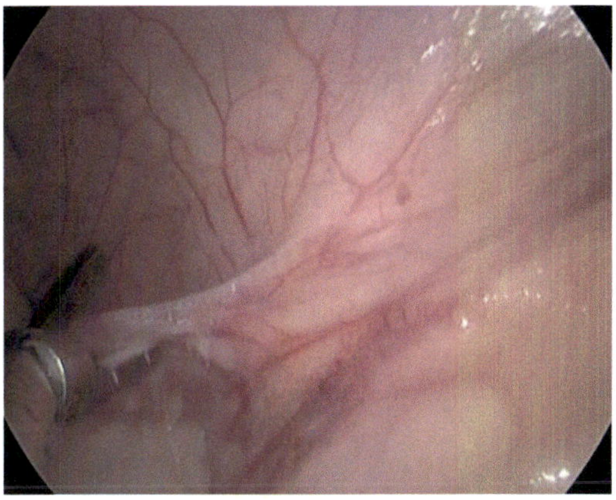

Fig. 24.7 Dissection of the splenic flexure. The splenic flexure is dissected and the surrounding ligaments are dissociated by an ultrasonic scalpel

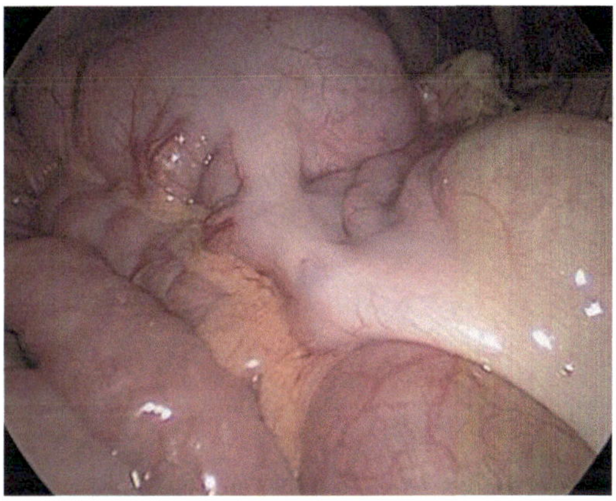

Fig. 24.8 The dilated transverse colon. This indicates that the subtotal resection is needed

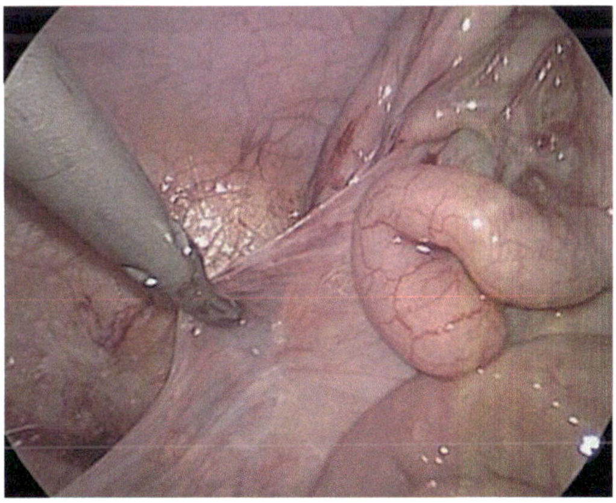

Fig. 24.9 Resection of the peritoneum of ascending colon by ultrasonic scalpel

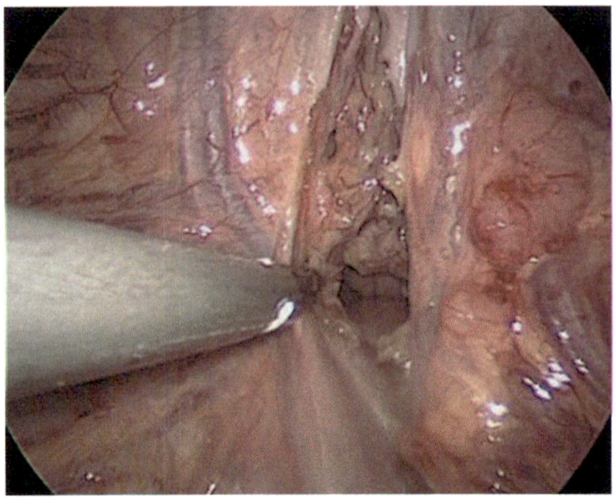

Fig. 24.10 Resection of the middle colic vessels

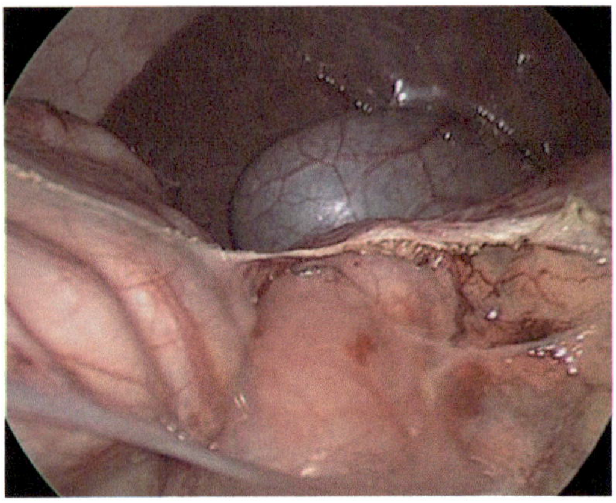

Fig. 24.11 Dissection of the hepatic flexure. Notice the duodenum closely behind the mesentery

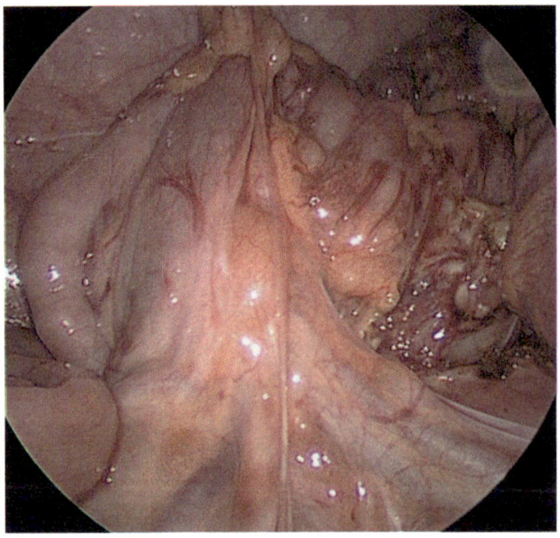

Fig. 24.12 The remaining ileocolic vessels. The ileocolic vessels should be carefully protected to secure the blood supply of the proximal normal bowel

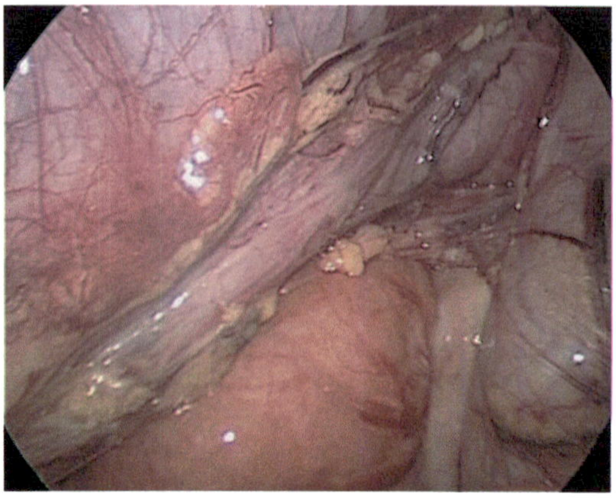

Fig. 24.13 The accumulation of small intestine to the left side of the ascending colon and anticlockwisely transposition of the ascending colon

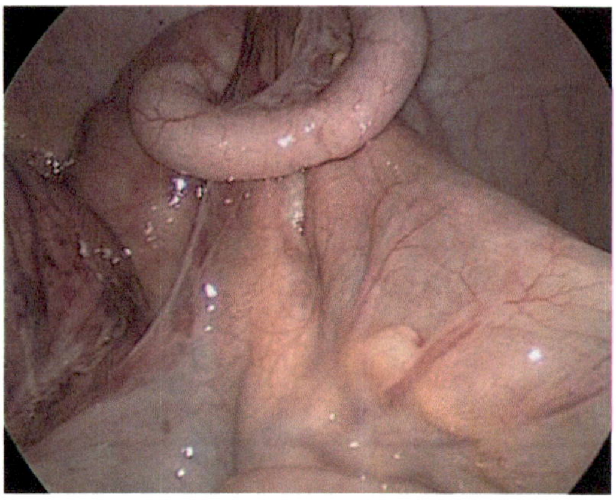

Fig. 24.14 The finish of transposition. There is no torsion of ileocecus

The dissection of distal bowel is performed until the level of peritoneal reflection of the rectum anteriorly and to the level of the coccyx posteriorly. Examine the resected bowel to ensure an adequate dissection and prepare for the perineal procedures (Fig. 24.15).

Anal dilatation is performed to prepare for the following transanal dissection. Six or eight retraction sutures can be placed circumferentially around the anus for better exposure. Circumferentially incise the mucosa 0.5–1 cm above the dentate line and carefully dissect the mucosa from the muscle. The incision of mucosa can also be completed by modified method

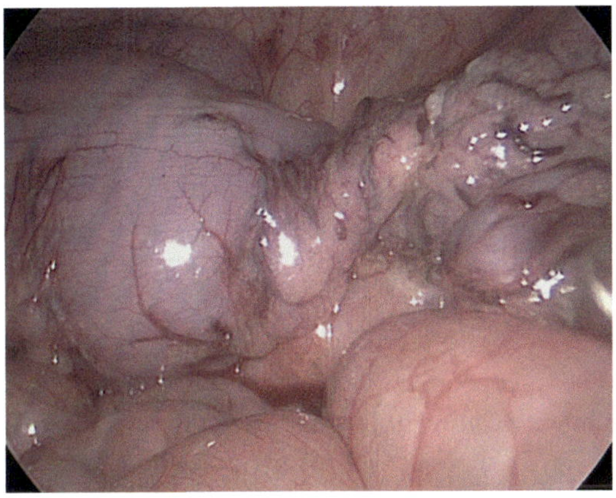

Fig. 24.15 Bowel after dissection. After the dissection of the mesentery, the bowel darkens. The color of the bowel can be helpful for the identification of the blood supply of the remaining colon

with a higher anterior and lower posterior incision. Mucosal stay sutures can be placed either before or after the circumferential incision have been made, which facilitates the traction on the mucosa and provides a more precise endorectal dissection. The submucosa dissection extends cephalad to join the intra-abdominal dissection. An incision is made in the rectal muscle posteriorly, and the muscular cuff is then incised. Shorten the muscular cuff and make an incision in the posterior wall to a V shape. This is important to prevent entrapment of the neorectum by the contracted muscular sleeve, especially after transanal dissection.

Pull down the aganglionic rectum and bowel through the rectal sleeve with the assistance of the laparoscope until the level of identified and marked normal bowel. Pay attention to the direction of the bowel and avoid torsion of the mesentery.

Make sure that the pulled-out bowel is loose enough and is 0.5–1 cm over the anal verge in case of bowel retraction which will lead to anastomotic leakage and pelvic infection. If the retraction looks to carry a high risk, colon exteriorization is suggested. The exteriorized colon is approximately 5–10 cm and should be resected 10–14 days later when the muscular levels of the colon and rectum adhere to each other and the bowel no longer retracts.

Transect the bowel above the normal site and circumferentially and discontinuously suture the anus to the colonic seromuscular level. Finally, circumferentially suture the colonic mucosa to the anal mucosa.

Inspect the abdominal cavity again to secure possible bleeding. For those patients who have the risk of pararectal herniation of the small bowel, reperitonealize the floor of the pelvis laparoscopically.

Remove the laparoscopic instruments and close the incisions. Introduce an anal tube at the end of operation.

Laparoscopic Soave procedure avoids dissection in the pelvic cavity and causes relatively less injuries to the pelvic nerve plexus and organs. With the preservation of the internal sphincter and without the formation of a spur, the risk of soiling and incontinence reduces. However, this procedure can result in internal sphincter syndrome such as recurrent constipation as well. Therefore, the posterior wall of internal sphincter must be split and it is recommended that the patients be treated with anal dilatation for at least 3 months [24]. The muscular sheath should be fixed with the colon which contributes to double levels of muscles surrounding the rectum. The mucosa should be completely desquamated, otherwise, the mucus secreted by the residual mucosa causes interlayer infection, and the pus may extend to the perineum or abdominal cavity, resulting in a fistula or peritonitis.

24.7 Laparoscopic Duhamel Procedure

The preoperative preparation, anesthesia, and position are similar to those of laparoscopic Soave procedure.

After the inspection of the peritoneal cavity and the determination of the transitional zone, seromuscular biopsies for rapid frozen section are performed to identify the normal colonic site. Sometimes the rectum can be suspended by a stay suture placed through the abdominal wall to obtain a better exposure.

Dissection of the colonic mesenteric vessels is similar to that in the Soave procedure to make sure that the normal colon is long enough to reach the deep pelvis. Use one or two endo-cutting staplers to close the colon. After the intra-abdominal transection of the colon, the retrorectal dissection is carried out down to the anus and identified by the laparoscopic light.

Make a full-thickness transverse incision on the posterior rectum at the level of 0.5–1 cm above the dentate line, and pull out the aganglionic colon through the incision using tissue-grasping forceps. The pull-through should be performed under laparoscopic assistance to prevent bowel torsion. To obtain a short rectal stump, perform an extra-anal division of the rectum perpendicular to the anus.

A standard colorectal anastomosis is carried out using interrupted suture followed by resection of the aganglionic bowel. And then introduce a stapler through the anus to divide the posterior rectal wall and the anterior colonic wall.

Although transanal endorectal pull-through has become increasingly popular in these years, Duhamel pull-through, as a traditional and reliable method that helps to decrease recurrent constipation and defecation frequency, is still a good choice, especially for those patients with long-segment HSCR or TCA. This procedure avoids wide dissociation of the pelvic cavity and reduces the risk of damage to the pelvic plexus and postoperative urinary retention. The preservation of the anterior wall of the rectum is beneficial to maintain defecation reflex. However, it is difficult for the transection of the rectum laparoscopically deep enough, leading to a long rectal pouch and colorectal septum. The residual pouch is likely to be infected, and keep coprolite to oppress the bladder and rectum. Moreover, the septum should be divided completely. According to previous research, a short pouch or a completely divided septum contributes to better fecal control, as well as a lower incidence of pouchitis and HAEC [1, 18].

To eliminate the rectal pouch and septum, several modifications have been successfully applied, such as Z-shaped colorectal side-to-side anastomosis [40]. However, laparoscopic Duhamel procedure requires experienced suturing skills and is still challenging for surgeons. Meanwhile, the risk of pelvic infection and soiling still exists.

24.8 Laparoscopic Swenson Procedure

The preoperative preparations, anesthesia, and patient position are similar to Soave procedure.

After the insertion of the ports and insufflation with CO_2, the peritoneal cavity is inspected. Identify the transitional zone under laparoscope and take three or four seromuscular biopsies for rapid frozen sections and make a suture on the bowel as a marker.

Make an incision in the peritoneum around the rectum and dissect the proximal bowel and mesenteric vessels until the ganglionated bowel can reach the pelvic floor without tension. The distal circumferential dissection is then performed to the pelvic floor. The peritoneal reflection from the rectum was dissected on both the left and right sides to 0.5–1.0 cm above the level of the dentate line. To protect the pelvic autonomic nervous system, the upper third of the lateral rectal ligaments was dissected as close as possible to the rectal wall. The ureters and vas deference should be carefully preserved [7].

After adequate proximal dissection is completed, the perineal procedures are performed. Use tissue-grasping forceps to seize the rectum and evert it with the assistance of laparoscopic guidance. Make an incision on the anterior half of the rectal wall proximal to the anocutaneous junction and make interrupted sutures for the anastomosis.

Remove the laparoscopic instruments and close the incisions. Introduce an anal tube.

As the first surgical treatment for HSCR, many operations were developed based on Swenson procedure [7]. However, it lost favor in recent years because of the wider dissection of the pelvic cavity that causes more bleeding and complications, such as anastomotic leakage, urinary retention, pelvic infection, incontinence, and sexual dysfunction [20, 22].

Several modifications improved the dissections to reduce the complications and achieved some good results [21].

24.9 Laparoscopic Heart-Shaped Anastomosis

With the induction of general anesthesia, the patient is placed in a supine position with the legs wrapped like Soave procedure.

Choose the proper positions to place trocars. Conventional three-incision and single-incision methods are both widely used in clinical practice. For a single-incision laparoscopic surgery, make a 0.5 cm skin incision below the umbilicus and place the three trocars, with the first trocar placed in the middle and the other two laterally to form a triangle.

The exploration of the peritoneal cavity and the acquisition of intraoperative biopsies are similar to those performed in the laparoscopic Soave procedure. Make a mark by suture.

Adjust the operating table to lower the head and lean it to the right, to accumulate the intestine in the right upper quadrant. Open the peritoneal reflection closely around the rectum, and dissect the tissues toward the distal direction until the coccyx level via retrorectal approach, and meanwhile pay attention to the ureter protection. Abscise the lateral ligament of the upper third of the rectum (Figs. 24.16 and 24.17).

Resection of the sigmoid colon, descending colon and splenocolic ligament, or the gastrocolic omentum and transverse colon for subtotal resection is similar to those of the laparoscopic Soave procedure.

Operating approach is then changed to the perineum. Dilate the anus to make preparation for the following pull-through of the bowel.

Grasp the upper rectum wall with transanal tissue-grasping forceps, and then the bowel can be pulled out and everted. After incising the rectum, continue to pull out the thick bowel until the marked site appears.

Make a longitudinal split in the posterior wall of the anorectal canal to 0.5 cm above the dentate line, and the incision will show a V shape (Fig. 24.18).

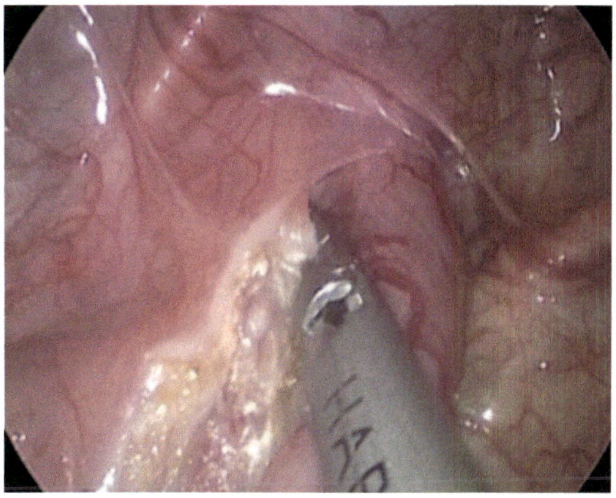

Fig. 24.16 Dissection of the peritoneal reflection closely around the rectum. Pay attention not to damage the nearby ureter and the vas deferens in male patients

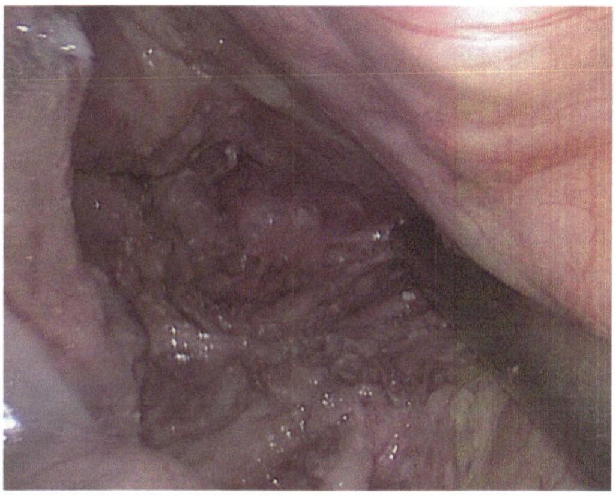

Fig. 24.17 Retrorectal dissection until the coccyx. Avoid the rectal perforation and take care of protection of the surrounding blood vessels and nerves

Carefully clear away the loose connective tissue around the rectum, so that the seromuscular layer of the remaining rectum and colon can be closely sutured. Note that any fat or connective tissue that exists inside the anastomosis will cause malunited stoma and anastomotic leakage.

The first two sutures are located at the tip of the V shape, followed by another three sutures separately at 3, 6, and 12 o'clock as traction stitches. Take notice that the tip of V shape should close to the dentate line, while the 12 o'clock should be approximately 3 cm above the anal verge.

Pull the traction stitches and anastomose the seromuscular layer circumferentially.

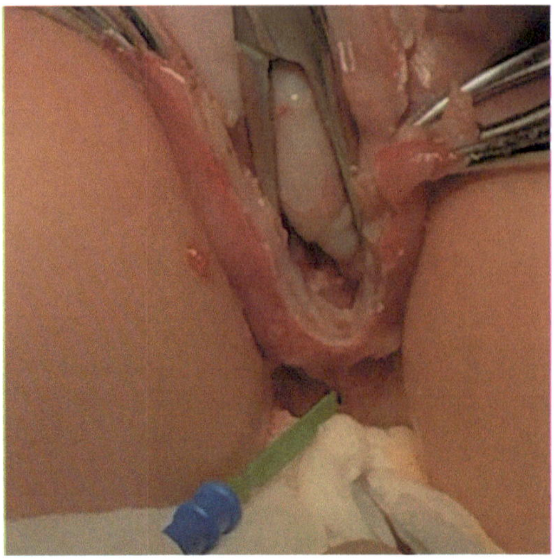

Fig. 24.18 The longitudinal split in the posterior wall of the anorectal canal. The split is approximately 0.5 cm above the dentate line and the incision will show a V shape

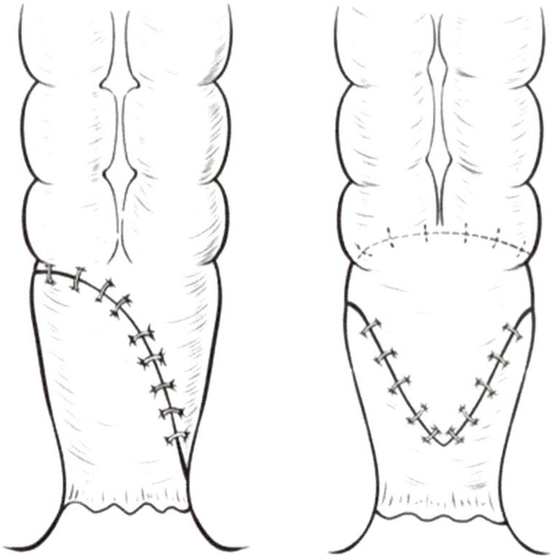

Fig. 24.19 The shape of the anastomosis. The oblique anastomosis is anteriorly high and posteriorly low, like a heart shape

Sutures should be 0.3 cm to the incision verge to make space for the following full-thickness anastomosis.

Resect the extra rectum and colon. Make four full-thickness sutures as traction stitches and subsequent sutures are added to each quadrant to complete the full-thickness anastomosis. After returning the anastomotic stoma, the anterior and posterior anastomoses are, respectively, 3.5–4 and 1.5–2 cm above the anal verge like a heart shape (Figs. 24.19 and 24.20) [43].

Change gloves and inspect the abdomen again to check if there is active bleeding or bowel torsion. In the end, close the incisions on the abdominal wall (Fig. 24.21).

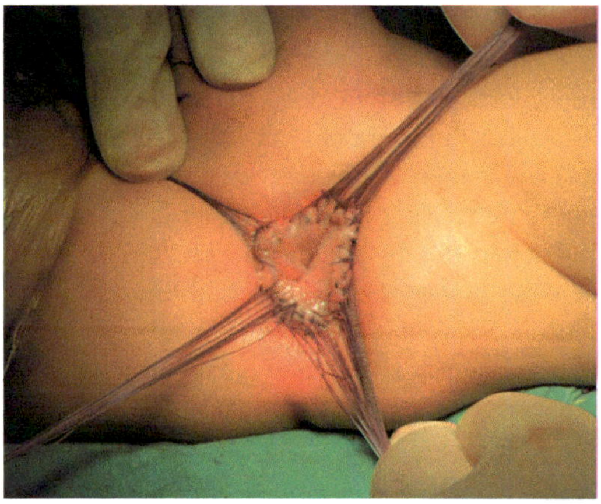

Fig. 24.20 The postoperative anus. The anastomotic stoma is wide enough

With this method, the colon is resected outside the anus and end-to-end obliquely anastomosed to the anorectum, reducing abdominal and pelvic contamination and saving the time of intra-abdominal resection of dilated colon and cuff closure [15, 19]. The Swenson or Duhamel procedures cut away most or at least half of the internal sphincter, causing a higher risk of soiling. Soave procedure preserves almost all the internal sphincter lesion, leading to a higher likelihood of constipation. Laparoscopic heart-shaped anastomosis, on the other hand, prevents too much loss of internal sphincter, as in the Swenson or Duhamel procedure, or too much preservation of internal sphincter, as in the Soave procedure, leading to a lower rate of soiling, constipation, and enterocolitis [19]. Furthermore, the little dissection in the pelvic cavity not only achieves earlier removal of urinary catheter to avoid urocystic infection and painful uroschesis but also reduces secondary damage to the bladder, blood vessels or pelvic nerves, and associated complications.

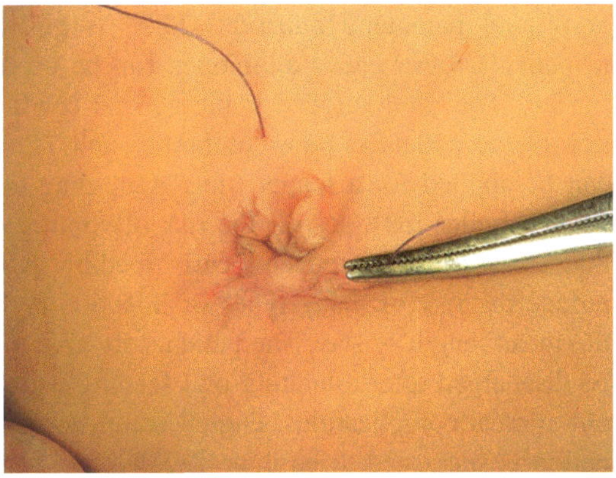

Fig. 24.21 The postoperative abdominal incisions. After intradermic suture, the tiny incisions are beside the umbilicus like the natural umbilical border

24.10 Laparoscopic-Assisted Natural Orifice Transluminal Endoscopic Surgery

As people spend more efforts seeking better cosmetic results these days, a newly developed technique, NOTES, which uses an endoscope inserted through a natural orifice (mouth, urethra, anus, etc.) to avoid external incisions, has been introduced into the treatment of HSCR. This technique can be classified into pure NOTES and hybrid NOTES, with the former allowing for resection of the aganglionic bowel without an abdominal incision while the latter one having an assisted transabdominal incision. Many modifications have been made based on the NOTES concept. A newly developed modification is laparoendoscopic single-site pull-through colectomy (LESS) [41], which combines the minimally invasive laparoendoscopic single-site surgery with the scarless concept of NOTES. Based on the NOTES concept and under the assistance of a laparoscope, a classic endoscope is replaced by a laparoscope, and trocars are inserted transabdominally or transanally. There's a report about transanal laparoscopic procedures that three incisions are all transanal including the gas port using standard laparoscopic instruments [23]. The laparoscopic-assisted NOTES avoid the abdominal incisions with reduced postoperative pain and decreased risk of incision-related complications. But the shortcomings such as clashing and collision of the instruments, poor visualization, possibility of overstretching the anal sphincter, and mesentery of rectosigmoid colon remain to be overcome.

24.11 Laparoscopic-Assisted Pull-Through for Total Colonic Aganglionosis

TCA, which accounts for 3%–15% of HSCR [5], is associated with significantly higher mortality than that of short- or long-segment HSCR.

Laparoscopic-assisted surgeries including the Duhamel and Swenson procedures have been shown to be feasible for patients with TCA in several reports [5], even in neonates with low weight [2]. Besides the cosmetic advantage, the excellent light and magnification provided by laparoscopy facilitate more accurate pelvic dissection. Furthermore, studies show that the laparoscopic approach for TCA patients decreases abdominal trauma and adhesion.

Since most patients with TCA already have a stoma before the pull-through procedures are to be performed, one or two trocars can be introduced through the stoma opening after the dissection of stoma. For TCA patients, the mobilization of the colon, including the descending colon, splenic flexure, transverse colon, hepatic flexure, and ascending colon, becomes convenient under laparoscopic assistance. After the transection of colon transabdominally, the ileum is pulled down and anastomosed to the rectum. The anastomotic procedures can be chosen from Swenson, Duhamel, Soave, or other modifications based on these three methods. One of the successful procedures is the Martin operation, which resects the ascending colon and transverse colon and dissects the pararectal space. The ileum is pulled through the posterior wall of the anus and anastomosed to the descending colon side-to-side. The anterior ileum is anastomosed to the posterior rectum using a stapler as in the Duhamel procedure, or the ileum is anastomosed to the rectum directly as with the Swenson procedure.

Although the operative complications of TCA have decreased significantly in recent years, its mortality is still high. More efforts should be made to decrease the mortality of TCA by modifying laparoscopic procedures.

24.12 Laparoscope-Assisted Reoperation

Although surgical advances achieve better outcomes these days, some patients suffer from persistent complications such as soiling, constipation, and abdominal distention, which may be caused by either pathological or anatomic factors. Residual aganglionic segment or transitional zone is the most common pathological factor, which is the definite indication of reoperation. The anatomic factors include excessive cuff, anastomotic stricture, or gate syndrome [31]. Except for some of the stenosis that can be relieved by regular anal dilatation, the others need a reoperation.

Before reoperation, several factors should be taken into consideration such as what previous procedures have been carried out, the level of anastomosis, blood supply of the rectum, and the pararectal fibrosis or inflammation. Currently, there is no best laparoscopic procedure for reoperation, and the most popular procedures are all feasible. The surgical choice of reoperation depends on the indications for reoperation, the general condition of the patient and the expertise of the surgeons. It has been shown that the laparoscopic-assisted procedure is safe and feasible in HSCR reoperation for constipation recurrences due to residual aganglionosis and transitional zone of the intestine [46]. The Soave procedure is thought to be safer in dissecting the muscular sheath, which reduces pelvic damage.

Although functional outcomes can be improved by reoperation, greater efforts should still be made to decrease complications and avoid reoperation.

24.13 Postoperative Treatment

Routine gastrointestinal decompression is suggested, and oral intake can be started once the bowel function recovers. Before that, intravenous total parenteral nutrition (TPN) is given to patients. Intravenous antibiotics can be used for 2–3 days after surgery. If the general condition of the patient is poor, antibiotics and TPN can be applied for a longer time. According to ERAS studies [33], despite the risk of vomiting that early feeding produces, early feeding can reduce the risk of many types of infection and the mean length of stay. The patients are able to be discharged after tolerating oral feeding without clinical complications. Digital rectal examination is suggested to be done 2–3 weeks after the day of operation during a follow-up visit to inspect the anastomotic width, smoothness, and height [4, 24]. Anal dilatation can be applied if necessary.

24.14 Specific Complications of Laparoscopic Pull-Through Surgeries

Although laparoscopic surgeries have so many attractive advantages, serious problems remain to be solved. Common complications in traditional pull-through surgeries (details in the following chapter) such as constipation, soiling, and enterocolitis still exist with laparoscopic operations, while some laparoscope-specific complications can't be ignored.

24.14.1 Trocar-Associated Complications

The incidence of bleeding at the incision sites or abdominal hematoma is not high, and a small amount of active bleeding can be stopped by electrocoagulation, pressure, or sutures. However, injury to abdominal organs or large blood vessels can cause severe bleeding, fistulas, and even death. To avoid secondary injuries, the dissociation and incision should be gentle and precise. And the position of incision should be carefully chosen. For patients who have had previous abdominal surgery, the first incision should be made using Hasson's method or should be away from the previous incision site.

If a severe injury occurs, the surgeons should assess the severity and the possibility of laparoscopic repair and convert to laparotomy if necessary.

24.14.2 Electric and Ultrasonic-Associated Complications

Improper use of electric and ultrasonic instruments, such as laparoscopic high-frequency electric hook, shear, shovel, or ultrasonic scalpel, may cause severe thermal injuries to the tissues nearby. If the bowel or ureter is injured, complications such as infection or perforation may occur [29]. Most importantly, fatal bleeding may happen unexpectedly if the vessels are injured by the thermal conduct, and it is essential to convert to the laparotomic procedure to control the bleeding as quickly as possible. To avoid thermal injuries, the tissues which are to be resected should be carefully identified, and the tissues nearby should be put away as far as possible.

24.14.3 Pneumoperitoneum-Associated Complications

The most common pneumoperitoneum-associated complication is subcutaneous emphysema [26]. It is usually related to improper puncture, oversize incision, repeated puncture, or overtime operation.

Overpressure in a pneumoperitoneum may be creating a heavy burden on the diaphragm to affect the ventilatory function, leading to hypercapnia and hypoxemia. During the operation, vital signs such as pulse, oxygen saturation, pulmonary ventilation, airway pressure, and arterial blood gas analysis (ABG) should be closely monitored, and pneumoperitoneum pressure should be strictly controlled. Once hypercapnia arises, hyperventilation can be used to eliminate the accumulated CO_2, and if this is ineffective, timely conversion to laparotomy must be undertaken.

Other pneumoperitoneum-associated complications include air embolism, cardiac arrhythmia, and so on.

24.15 Conclusion and Future Directions

Under the assistance of a laparoscope, better cosmetic results, faster return of bowel function, better pain control, and shorter hospital stay can be easily achieved. Newly developed modifications including the laparoscopic-assisted transumbilical procedure, transanal NOTES laparoscopic pull-though, and da Vinci robotic surgery, are potentially promising. However, despite the diversity of surgical choices, there are no significant differences in mortality, recurrence rate of HAEC, and functional outcomes between laparotomic and laparoscopic procedures. Moreover, laparoscopic surgery requires more operating time and a longer learning curve [42]. Although there's still so much to do to improve the postoperative outcomes, the perspective of laparoscopic surgery is full of potential and will likely grow in popularity in the coming decades.

References

1. Antao B, Radhwan T, Samuel M, Kiely E. Short-pouch and low-anastomosis Duhamel procedure results in better fecal control and normal defecation pattern. Dis Colon Rectum. 2005;48(9):1791–6.
2. Bonnard A, de Lagausie P, Leclair MD, Marwan K, Languepin J, Bruneau B, Berribi D, Aigrain Y. Definitive treatment of extended Hirschsprung's disease or total colonic form. Surg Endosc. 2001;15(11):1301–4.
3. Bradnock TJ, Walker GM. Evolution in the management of Hirschsprung's disease in the UK and Ireland: a national survey of practice revisited. Ann R Coll Surg Engl. 2011;93(1):34–8.
4. Carvalho JL, Campos M, Soares-Oliveira M, Estevao-Costa J. Laparoscopic colonic mapping of dysganglionosis. Pediatr Surg Int. 2001;17(5–6):493–5.
5. Cheung ST, Tam YH, Chong HM, Chan KW, Mou WC, Sihoe DY, Lee KH. An 18-year experience in total colonic aganglionosis: from staged operations to primary laparoscopic endorectal pull-through. J Pediatr Surg. 2009;44(12):2352–4.
6. Craigie RJ, Conway SJ, Cooper L, Turnock RR, Lamont GL, Baillie CT, Kenny SE. Primary pull-through for Hirschsprung's disease: comparison of open and laparoscopic-assisted procedures. J Laparoendosc Adv Surg Tech A. 2007;17(6):809–12.

7. Curran TJ, Raffensperger JG. The feasibility of laparoscopic swenson pull-through. J Pediatr Surg. 1994;29(9):1273–5.
8. Curran TJ, Raffensperger JG. Laparoscopic Swenson pull-through: a comparison with the open procedure. J Pediatr Surg. 1996;31(8):1155–6; discussion 1156–1157
9. de Lagausie P, Bruneau B, Besnard M, Jaby O, Aigrain Y. Definitive treatment of Hirschsprung's disease with a laparoscopic Duhamel pull-through procedure in childhood. Surg Laparosc Endosc. 1998;8(1):55–7.
10. Georgeson KE, Cohen RD, Hebra A, Jona JZ, Powell DM, Rothenberg SS, Tagge EP. Primary laparoscopic-assisted endorectal colon pull-through for Hirschsprung's disease: a new gold standard. Ann Surg. 1999;229(5):678–82; discussion 682–683
11. Georgeson KE, Fuenfer MM, Hardin WD. Primary laparoscopic pull-through for Hirschsprung's disease in infants and children. J Pediatr Surg. 1995;30(7):1017–21; discussion 1021–1022
12. Ghirardo V, Betalli P, Mognato G, Gamba P. Laparotomic versus laparoscopic Duhamel pull-through for Hirschsprung disease in infants and children. J Laparoendosc Adv Surg Tech A. 2007;17(1):119–1123.
13. Giuliani S, Betalli P, Narciso A, Grandi F, Midrio P, Mognato G, Gamba P. Outcome comparison among laparoscopic Duhamel, laparotomic Duhamel, and transanal endorectal pull-through: a single-center, 18-year experience. J Laparoendosc Adv Surg Tech A. 2011;21(9):859–63.
14. Hebra A, Smith VA, Lesher AP. Robotic Swenson pull-through for Hirschsprung's disease in infants. Am Surg. 2011;77(7):937–41.
15. Jiao C, Yu D, Li D, Wang G, Feng J. A long-term follow-up of a new surgery method: laparoscope-assisted heart-shaped anastomosis for Hirschsprung's disease. J Laparoendosc Adv Surg Tech A. 2018;28(4):471–5.
16. Kohno M, Ikawa H, Fukumoto H, Okamoto S, Masuyama H, Konuma K. Usefulness of endoscopic marking for determining the location of transanal endorectal pull-through in the treatment of Hirschsprung's disease. Pediatr Surg Int. 2005;21(11):873–7.
17. Kumar R, Mackay A, Borzi P. Laparoscopic Swenson procedure – an optimal approach for both primary and secondary pull-through for Hirschsprung's disease. J Pediatr Surg. 2003;38(10):1440–3.
18. Lamas-Pinheiro R, Henriques-Coelho T, Carvalho JL, Correia-Pinto J. Duhamel pull-through assisted by transrectal port: a hybrid natural orifice transluminal endoscopic surgery approach. J Pediatr Surg. 2012;47(10):1962–5.
19. Langer JC. Persistent obstructive symptoms after surgery for Hirschsprung's disease: development of a diagnostic and therapeutic algorithm. J Pediatr Surg. 2004;39(10):1458–62.
20. Levitt MA, Dickie B, Pena A. Evaluation and treatment of the patient with Hirschsprung disease who is not doing well after a pull-through procedure. Semin Pediatr Surg. 2010;19(2):146–53.
21. Levitt MA, Hamrick MC, Eradi B, Bischoff A, Hall J, Pena A. Transanal, full-thickness, Swenson-like approach for Hirschsprung disease. J Pediatr Surg. 2013;48(11):2289–95.
22. Levitt MA, Martin CA, Olesevich M, Bauer CL, Jackson LE, Pena A. Hirschsprung disease and fecal incontinence: diagnostic and management strategies. J Pediatr Surg. 2009;44(1):271–7; discussion 277
23. Li N, Zhang W, Yu D, Sun X, Wei M, Weng Y, Feng J. NOTES for surgical treatment of long-segment hirschsprung's disease: report of three cases. J Laparoendosc Adv Surg Tech A. 2013;23(12):1020–3.
24. Liem NT, Hau BD. Primary laparoscopic endorectal colon pull-through for Hirschsprung's disease: early results of 61 cases. Asian J Surg. 2006;29(3):173–5.
25. Mattioli G, Pio L, Leonelli L, Razore B, Disma N, Montobbio G, Jasonni V, Petralia P, Pini PA. A provisional experience with robot-assisted Soave procedure for older children with Hirschsprung disease: Back to the future? J Laparoendosc Adv Surg Tech A. 2017;27(5):546–9.
26. Miller SS. Laparoscopic operations in paediatric surgery. Br J Surg. 1992;79(10):986–7.
27. Miyano G, Ochi T, Lane GJ, Okazaki T, Yamataka A. Factors affected by surgical technique when treating total colonic aganglionosis: laparoscopy-assisted versus open surgery. Pediatr Surg Int. 2013;29(4):349–52.
28. Muensterer OJ, Chong A, Hansen EN, Georgeson KE. Single-incision laparoscopic endorectal pull-through (SILEP) for hirschsprung disease. J Gastrointest Surg. 2010;14(12):1950–4.
29. Nah SA, de Coppi P, Kiely EM, Curry JI, Drake DP, Cross K, Spitz L, Eaton S, Pierro A. Duhamel pull-through for Hirschsprung disease: a comparison of open and laparoscopic techniques. J Pediatr Surg. 2012;47(2):308–12.
30. Oancea M, Vatra L, Kadar A, Copaescu C. Laparoscopic approach for rectosigmoidian resection in children. Chirurgia (Bucur). 2014;109(1):117–22.
31. Pena A, Elicevik M, Levitt MA. Reoperations in Hirschsprung disease. J Pediatr Surg. 2007;42(6):1008–13; discussion 1013–1014
32. Ram AD, Scholfield DW, Pimpalwar A. Novel technique of Mapping Biopsies during laparoscopic assisted transanal Soave endorectal pull-through surgery for Hirschsprung's disease's. Ann R Coll Surg Engl. 2017;99(6):504.
33. Rove KO, Edney JC, Brockel MA. Enhanced recovery after surgery in children: Promising, evidence-based multidisciplinary care. Paediatr Anaesth. 2018;28(6):482–92.
34. Shah AA, Shah AV. Staged laparoscopic-assisted pull-through for Hirschsprung's disease. J Pediatr Surg. 2003;38(11):1667–9.
35. Short HL, Heiss KF, Burch K, Travers C, Edney J, Venable C, Raval MV. Implementation of an enhanced

recovery protocol in pediatric colorectal surgery. J Pediatr Surg. 2018;53(4):688–92.
36. Smith BM, Steiner RB, Lobe TE. Laparoscopic Duhamel pullthrough procedure for Hirschsprung's disease in childhood. J Laparoendosc Surg. 1994;4(4):273–6.
37. Teitelbaum DH, Coran AG. Primary pull-through for Hirschsprung's disease. Semin Neonatol. 2003;8(3):233–41.
38. Thomson D, Allin B, Long AM, Bradnock T, Walker G, Knight M. Laparoscopic assistance for primary transanal pull-through in Hirschsprung's disease: a systematic review and meta-analysis. BMJ Open. 2015;5(3):e006063.
39. Tomuschat C, Zimmer J, Puri P. Laparoscopic-assisted pull-through operation for Hirschsprung's disease: a systematic review and meta-analysis. Pediatr Surg Int. 2016;32(8):751–7.
40. Urushihara N, Fukumoto K, Fukuzawa H, Sugiyama A, Watanabe K, Mitsunaga M, Miyake H, Kusafuka J, Aoba T. Outcome of laparoscopic modified Duhamel procedure with Z-shaped anastomosis for Hirschsprung's disease. Surg Endosc. 2012;26(5):1325–31.
41. Vahdad MR, Foroutan A, Najafi SM, Cernaianu G, Trobs RB, Banani SA, Foroutan HR. Totally transanal LESS pull-through colectomy: a novel approach for avoiding abdominal wall incision in children with long-segment intestinal aganglionosis. J Laparoendosc Adv Surg Tech A. 2013;23(3):276–80.
42. van de Ven TJ, Sloots CE, Wijnen MH, Rassouli R, van Rooij I, Wijnen RM, de Blaauw I. Transanal endorectal pull-through for classic segment Hirschsprung's disease: with or without laparoscopic mobilization of the rectosigmoid? J Pediatr Surg. 2013;48(9):1914–8.
43. Wang G, Yuan J, Zhou X, Qi B, Teitelbaum DH. A modified operation for Hirschsprung's disease: Posterior longitudinal anorectal split with a "heart-shaped" anastomosis. Pediatr Surg Int. 1996;11(4):243–5.
44. Wulkan ML, Georgeson KE. Primary laparoscopic endorectal pull-through for Hirschsprung's disease in infants and children. Semin Laparosc Surg. 1998;5(1):9–13.
45. Xia X, Li N, Wei J, Zhang W, Yu D, Zhu T, Feng J. Single-incision laparoscopic versus conventional laparoscopic surgery for Hirschsprung's disease: a comparison of medium-term outcomes. J Pediatr Surg. 2016a;51(3):440–3.
46. Xia X, Li N, Wei J, Zhang W, Yu D, Zhu T, Feng J. Laparoscopy-assisted versus transabdominal reoperation in Hirschprung's disease for residual aganglionosis and transitional zone pathology after transanal pull-through. J Pediatr Surg. 2016b;51(4):577–81.
47. Zhao B, Liu T, Li Q. Comparison of the efficacy and safety of laparoscopic-assisted operations and open operations for Hirschsprung's disease: evidence from a meta-analysis. Int J Clin Exp Med. 2015;8(8):12963–9.
48. Zhu T, Feng J, Zhang W, Wei M, Yu D, Zhang X, Yu K, Kuang H. Subtotal colectomy with a single-incision laparoscopic surgery technique in children with long-segment Hirschsprung disease and allied disorders. Pediatr Surg Int. 2013;29(2):197–201.

Redo Pull Through Operation for Hirschsprung Disease

25

Matthew W. Ralls and Arnold G. Coran

Contents

M. W. Ralls · A. G. Coran (✉)
Pediatric Surgery, University of Michigan, Ann Arbor, MI, USA
e-mail: acoran@med.umich.edu

25.1 Introduction

Congenital aganglionosis was first described by Härold Hirschsprung in 1886, and Orvar Swenson is credited for the first successful treatment of Hirschsprung disease (HD) [1] in 1948. Descriptions of the disease process date back several centuries prior to either of these recognized pioneers of HD [2]. Medical understanding and surgical treatment of HD has changed dramatically over the last 70 years. However, the objective remains the same in that the aganglionic bowel is resected and healthy intestine is anastomosed low in the anal canal above the dentate (or pectinate) line. The most common techniques performed today comprise a laparoscopic-assisted biopsy and mobilization with a transanal approach to an endorectal pull-through (PT). The three commonly used PT techniques include a Swenson or full-thickness resection, a Soave which utilizes a submucosal dissection in the anal canal and rectum to avoid nerve damage, and a Duhamel procedure which involves a posterior side-to-side anastomosis that leaves some diseased rectum in place.

There is no data to suggest that one operative approach is superior to the other [3–5]. Each technique can be associated with its own set of problems. For instance, a Swenson PT can cause pelvic nerve damage if the surgeon deviates from the proper plane. A Soave PT can be complicated by an obstructing muscular cuff if not addressed

P. Puri (ed.), *Hirschsprung's Disease and Allied Disorders*,
https://doi.org/10.1007/978-3-030-15647-3_25

appropriately at the initial surgery and a retained spur after Duhamel PT can be problematic. Regardless of the technique, repair most often leads to satisfactory results in an experienced surgeon's hands. There is a subset of children who will have long-term stooling problems after PT [6]. Patients can present with Hirschsprung-associated enterocolitis (HAEC) which can range from mild cases to life-threatening. Other significant issues comprise intestinal obstruction, severe stool retention, and/or fecal incontinence [7]. Minor postoperative problems may be self-limiting, and many of these stooling disorders can be managed in an outpatient setting through dietary manipulation and a bowel management regimen. On rare occasions (as low as 2% of children from high-volume centers), the child may require a redo PT procedure. These children should be referred to a center with experience in re-operative HD.

25.2 Presentation of Patients After PT

Factors contributing to long-term complications are thought of as either pathologic or anatomic. The leading pathologic cause of complications is residual aganglionosis or transitional zone pathology (RA/TZP). This results from a failure to identify healthy intestine through pathology investigation at the time of initial PT and require redo PT. A meta-analysis of 555 redo PT patients [8] as well as many other large reviews found that RA/TZP [6] were the major causes of failure [9]. These findings highlight the need for experienced pathology support [6, 10]. Even the most experienced surgeons at high-volume centers can experience poor outcomes due to RA/TZP. At the authors' center, a recent review detailed nine patients with RA/TZP as the cause of failed primary PT. The slides from the primary PT were reviewed, and the original PT segment had normal ganglion cells and lacked hypertrophic nerves in eight of nine cases. The ninth was recognized as a pathologic misread and redo PT was performed immediately. The redo PT specimen from each of the remaining eight cases showed findings consistent with RA/TZP discordant from the original pathology interpretation but done by the same pathologist in many cases. This phenomenon supports a concept of an acquired segment of aganglionosis from a variant form of HD [11] and/or secondary aganglionosis due to neuronal cell death from an ischemic insult on the distal PT [12]. Another theory suggests that the aganglionic segment of residual disease normally left behind proximal to the dentate line grows with the child from 0.5 to 1 cm to a segment that is several centimeters in length. Clearly, more data is needed to verify this theory.

The anatomic causes involve stricture, with or without an associated anastomotic leak, retained dilated segment which functions poorly, twisted pull-through segment, or the obstructions specific to the initial operation of retained spur following a Duhamel and Soave (aganglionic) muscular cuff. All of these complications that severely effect HD patients after definitive PT are divided into three groups. These include recurrent HAEC, persistent problems with the passage of stool (e.g., constipation), and soiling/incontinence [13]. Most children with these common presentations will not require a redo PT, and it is up to the surgeon to understand the symptoms and causes to prescribe appropriate definitive management.

Children that eventually go on to require a redo PT are more likely to have suffered an early complication (anastomotic leak, obstruction, twisted-PT, and enterocolitis) and, of course, suffer late complications which require re-evaluation. While inappropriate PT segments have been listed as the leading cause for redo PT, some experts in the field have noted a decline in pathological indications. This may be due to a recent improvement in the education of pathologists and surgeons from international HD interest groups. Leaders in the pediatric colorectal community believe there is a rise in complications due to the muscular Soave cuff and that this is becoming increasingly problematic. The presentations of many of these underlying problems will be similar and are detailed below.

HAEC can be the most serious complication and remains the most common cause of morbidity and death in HD [14]. The exact etiology is unknown [15, 16]. There are no readily available clinical tests or risk factors to predict the development of this disorder. While many centers have their own protocol, there is no single strategy for prophylaxis from this major complication. Logistic regression analysis of risk factors for the HAEC development showed that anastomotic stricture was a significant risk factor in a multi-center review of primary endorectal PT [17]. Therefore, redo PT may be beneficial in controlling recurrent HAEC in patients found to have strictured during their complete workup.

Persistent stooling problems include most commonly constipation, but also recurrent distension and bloating. Constipation can be a common complaint occurring in 9–40% [18, 19] of children after what appears to be a technically excellent operation. The symptoms usually do not develop for weeks to months following the PT. Review of the literature suggests that while obstructive symptoms are common, many patients report improvement with greater follow-up. Stooling has been reported as normal in 58% at less than 5 years of follow-up and 88% of those at greater than 15 years of follow-up [20]. This suggests many children have persistent problems even after a perfect PT. This may be due to continued problems with the internal anal sphincter or the PT segment even after removal of all aganglionic tissue alluding to an incomplete understanding of the pathophysiology of HD.

There are many etiologies of persistent stooling problems and determining the underlying problem for each child may be difficult. One must determine if the issue is caused by a pathological problem. Pathological causes can be described as retained or acquired aganglionosis [21], rarely hypoganglionosis [22], or transition zone pathology which can be associated with either focal or general motility disorders. Less commonly, internal anal sphincter achalasia and "functional megacolon," a chronically dilated distal rectum secondary to chronic difficulty with passing bowel movements, can lead to persistent stooling problems [23]. Some argue that there is a discrepancy in what surgeons and pathologists would call "healthy" colon due to the size of the nerves on pathology report. There is controversy surrounding this topic in the literature [24].

Some children have no identifiable cause for their persistent stooling problems. Many of these children suffer from behavioral stool-holding and are best treated by bowel management regimen consisting of either laxatives or enemas and, perhaps more importantly, behavior modification including support for the child and family [25]. Response to surgical or use of botulinum toxin injections for relaxation of the sphincter is widely variable [26–29]. This is likely due to the differing approaches to indications and to technique of Botox administration [30]. The approach to address all the above causes varies and should be done by one with expertise in order to successfully manage complicated HD cases.

Incontinence should be avoidable with use of proper surgical techniques. However, even in the most experienced hands, some HD patients face this problem. It is important to understand the symptomatology enough to discern true incontinence from overflow or encopresis. Incontinence has been reported in a range from zero in several series [31–33] to as high as 76% in others [34]. Iatrogenic injury can damage anal sphincters. This can be due to performing the anastomosis too low. Soiling may simply be due to a loss of rectal sensation. A very low anastomosis can compromise sensory rectal mucosa. Surgeons must understand the anatomic level of the internal anal sphincters, the major contributor to continence, and their relationship to the dentate line. All dissection and anastomoses must be performed at least 5 mm or more above this level. Damage can also occur when the muscles are overstretched due to the need of increased exposure, and incontinence may also be due to scarring.

By far, the most common cause of soiling after a pull-through is chronic constipation with overflow, or encopresis. For some, a bowel management program is all that is needed. Others fail all management and require a redo PT or a permanent stoma. As previously stated, the critical challenge is for the surgeon to differentiate true incontinence from encopresis or HAEC.

25.3 Workup

Documentation is of utmost importance in any HD case as these records will prove useful for routine follow-up and essential for those requiring reoperation. This should include the signs and symptoms in the neonatal period, associated anomalies, type of presentation, time and method of diagnosis, preoperative course, type of procedure, pathologic material, and detailed postoperative management. Difficult HD cases should be assessed by experienced surgeons at institutions with expertise and infrastructure to evaluate, diagnose, and treat these complex patients.

25.3.1 History and Physical Examination

A complete history should be performed including general condition, developmental milestones, and growth curve, as well as diet and stooling history and the treatments employed to tackle presenting issue. Abdominal exam is important as the examiner can often palpate impacted stool. Rectal examination can help to understand a general sense of the patient's PT as far as level of the anastomosis, signs of stricture, and rectal tone. At times, anal manometry can prove quite useful in distinguishing causes of symptoms. Internal exam with explosive stool implies persistent obstructive symptoms or ongoing HAEC.

25.3.2 Imaging

A plain abdominal film should be done to evaluate the degree of stool burden and evidence of obstruction. A "cut-off sign" is suggestive of active or chronic HAEC [35]. A contrast enema can help identify anastomotic stenosis or stricture, a twist of the pull-through segment, as well as a chronically dilated rectosigmoid segment. One can also evaluate if the colon empties adequately or is hypermotile. Occasionally, irregularities of the mucosal lining can be seen suggesting chronic inflammation after repeated episodes of HAEC.

25.3.3 Diagnostic Evaluation

A rectal biopsy is a necessary step to aid in the diagnosis. This can be done via suction gun or an open technique. In the case of workup after primary PT, the authors prefer open technique. This allows a more thorough rectal evaluation and allows for identification of the dentate line and likely the anastomotic line. Proper identification of these landmarks is crucial for the biopsy to be taken at the appropriate level. Many advocate serial biopsies at 2, 4, and 5–6 cm from the dentate line [36] and review by a pediatric pathologist with experience in this disease process. Anorectal manometry is not widely used in the postoperative evaluation of HD patients, but can provide valuable information. Most patients with defecation disorders after primary PT will have favorable outcomes without the need for an additional operation when following an organized algorithm [37, 38].

25.4 Operative Approach of Redo Pull-Through

Decision that redo PT is necessary can be as challenging as undertaking the operation itself. While general principles apply, patients should be approached as individuals. Redo PT operations carry even higher risk when compared to the primary PT. Operative intervention should be planned according to the child's presentation, initial PT type, specific complication, and underlying pathology. There is an increasing awareness of stooling disorders in HD children who otherwise had a successful PT procedure [39–41]. Stooling outcomes are significantly worse after redo PT compared to those after a primary PT [9]. Importantly, continence is still preserved in the majority of children. No study has found a correlation in outcomes based on the type of PT, either the primary PT or the redo PT [25, 42–44], which again highlights the need for an experienced colorectal team.

25.4.1 Operative Intervention Other than Redo PT

Symptoms may simply be the result of the internal sphincters failure to relax following a technically perfect PT. Spasm of the anal sphincters after a successful pull-through is not uncommon. The diagnosis can be established with anorectal manometry showing high resting pressures [45], but can also be inferred through a good history and physical exam. Typical presentation of such patients includes straining to defecate, occasionally significant constipation, and may present with recurrent HAEC. These children should be initially approached with bowel management regimens including laxatives. With high clinical suspicion and if the child continues to have troubles, botulinum toxin can be used as a temporary sphincter-relaxing measure [26–29, 46–49]. Nitroglycerine paste [50–52] may be successful as well in many children, but the authors do not use this therapy. Broken up into 4–5 equal doses, 40–100 mg of botulinum toxin can be injected between the internal and external anal sphincter using a spinal or micropuncture needle. This can be done with ultrasound to improve efficacy [30] and allow avoidance of injury to the urethra anteriorly. While temporary, many children outgrow their symptoms or learn to overcome their increased sphincter tone making this approach appealing [46]. Botox has been shown to improve difficulty stooling or persistent enterocolitis and decrease hospitalizations [26]. Should these approaches fail to show improvement, an anal sphincterectomy, also referred to as a myectomy, should be strongly considered [53, 54].

Myectomy was first described for the treatment of short-segment HD. The procedure may be indicated in children with persistent stooling problems after a pull-through procedure. Prior to the consideration of myectomy, a biopsy should be done to rule out an aganglionic segment. Myectomy will make a redo PT more difficult due to more scarring in the area. However, a child with persistent enterocolitis who fails to respond to medical treatment may benefit. A second indication for myectomy is for severe constipation symptoms and a severely dilated rectum and sigmoid colon. Caution should be taken as rectal dilation may not resolve even after a correctly performed myectomy and a redo PT with resection of this dilated bowel segment. Controversially, a child with retained or acquired aganglionic bowel less than 3 cm may benefit from a myectomy though many would argue that a redo pull-through may work better in almost all of these patients [52].

25.4.2 Repeat Pull-Through Procedures

The decision to perform a repeat PT represents a challenge for pediatric surgeons. It carries risks far greater than those after the original surgery. It should only be done by a highly experienced surgeon after following a personal or institutional algorithm. However, one should never hesitate to perform a redo pull-through after careful planning by detailed preoperative biopsies, contrast enemas and possibly anal manometry, as detailed above. Each patient should be approached on an individual basis and an operative intervention should be planned according to their presentation, underlying pathology, and previous surgery.

Whether or not the indication for redo is pathologic, confirming the appropriate pull-through segment is of the highest priority. Expertise in frozen section interpretation for the presence of ganglion cells and hypertrophied nerves is required. In the case of a misread frozen section, an inappropriate PT segment will be chosen. If identified on final pathology, it is the author's recommendation to proceed with an immediate redo PT via the same transanal approach. Minimal scarring and adhesions will be present in this time period. Most infants will start to stool spontaneously which may give the surgeon pause based on an initial positive response. Obstructive symptoms will eventually return and one should not be dissuaded from performing the redo.

The appropriate technique for redo PT pull is dependent on what procedure and other interventions have been previously performed on the child and most importantly the contributing factor leading to the need for a redo pull-through. In all cases, laparoscopy can often be useful in exploration, in intra-abdominal and deep pelvic mobilization, and in obtaining leveling biopsies. If laparoscopy is not used, a lower midline incision or extension of a left hockey-stick incision is usually adequate. However, a transverse incision in the lower abdomen may not allow adequate proximal mobilization of the colon which is often needed for a redo PT.

After mobilization of the colon and leveling is confirmed, the PT segment must have adequate length and blood supply. The distal end of the mobilized PT segment should reach to 2 cm below the pubic symphysis without tension. The marginal artery should be preserved to prevent potential devascularization of the distal PT segment. This is less critical if there is a longer time period between the original and redo PT and secondary revascularization has occurred. Damage to the marginal artery can occur at the time of ostomy creation or takedown. A purely transanal dissection is also an option in some children and may prevent inadvertent damage to blood supply. However, in children with a stricture or previous leak, this dissection may be quite difficult and may require intra-abdominal dissection as well.

The ultimate decision for type of redo may not be readily apparent until the time of operation. In general, patients, who have had either a primary Swenson or Soave, do well with a redo endorectal PT. When this fails due to an inability to adequately dissect the submucosal plane, either a full-thickness transanal Swenson or a Duhamel may be utilized; the authors prefer the former. For those patients who underwent a primary Duhamel, a Swenson should be performed. A redo Swenson may be particularly challenging if one attempts to evert the rectum. Scarring may prevent this due to the last 3–4 cm of rectum being densely adherent within the pelvis, and it may be necessary to perform the anal anastomosis within the anal canal without eversion.

For cases in which a stricture is the indication for redo, the choice of a Duhamel or a Swenson is up to the surgeon. It is critical that the surgeon be able to dissect completely below the area of the stricture from the abdomen, or starts below the stricture if performing a transanal Swenson-like redo. Langer has described an interesting approach to handle these strictures [42] using a stapling device to come across the stricture while simultaneously creating a redo Duhamel anastomosis. If this is done, the surgeon will need to account for the thickness involved in the tissue layers to be stapled. If an endorectal PT was the original procedure, the anastomosis would involve the original aganglionic muscularis propria, full-thickness segment of primary PT segment, as well as various amounts of scar tissue. A longer staple height should be considered in this situation. Rarely, one may perform an original Duhamel procedure. In this situation, the anastomosis is created with extra-long Kocher clamps placed in an inverted "V" configuration. These will be left in place until the crushed bowel forms an anastomosis which usually takes 7–10 days.

The surgeon should always be prepared to perform a hand-sewn anastomosis. However, an end-end circular stapled anastomosis is an option. The desired PT segment is stapled at the desired location for the anastomosis. A Swenson dissection is performed within 1–1.5 cm above the dentate line. The neo-rectum can be everted and stapled 1–2 cm above the dentate line to avoid damage to the sphincters. The neo-rectum and staple line is then reinserted into the pelvis which will result in approximately a 2.5 cm length of the anal canal. The staple line of the healthy PT colonic segment is then removed and an anvil of the EEA stapler in sewn in place. A 21–31 mm EEA stapler is then inserted into the rectal remnant and fired creating the anastomosis. The anastomosis should be evaluated with an air bubble leak test after filling the pelvis with saline and by visualizing complete full-thickness donuts on the stapler.

25.4.3 Special Considerations

Primary or redo PT for long-segment HD can be particularly challenging because the use of more proximal segments of bowel can be difficult to manage. Children left with ganglionated colon confined to the cecum would be better served with a completion colectomy and an ileal PT. A cecal PT is concerning due to the risk of twisting the PT as well as size mismatch when the anastomosis is performed.

A protective stoma is always a consideration but the decision should wait until the end of the redo PT. If the surgeon has any reservation about the final anastomosis, a proximal colostomy or ileostomy should be placed. The blood supply is of the utmost importance if a stoma is necessary. The marginal artery is at risk not only at the time during the creation of the stoma but also at the time of ostomy takedown. A safe option is to perform a temporary loop ileostomy, knowing that some small children may need extra attention in dealing with an ileostomy.

There will be a small group of patients that will fail a redo PT. Alternatively, the child's parents and physician may decide that they may not benefit from a redo PT for a myriad of reasons. Children can live a long happy life with a stoma and may have the option for reversal as they age. As with all cases of stomas enlisting assistance from a stomal therapist will help ensure appropriate positioning of the stoma, and also help parents adjust to the changes in stomal care as their child grows.

25.5 Outcomes from Redo Pull-Through

Success rates vary widely after redo PT often due to a wide variability in the definitions of good outcomes [10, 21, 55, 56]. Some report low fecal continence rates (50% range) [57], but this may be due to dissection injury or complications surrounding the primary PT. Others report a 90% cure rate of symptoms after redo PT. However, functional assessment of these patients is not reported [43]. Stooling outcomes are significantly worse in redo PT patients than those in primary PT patients. This emphasizes the fact that this group of children should be approached carefully by an experienced team. Aggressive prevention of functional constipation after anatomic repair is important in avoiding recurrent symptoms of large bowel obstruction.

The authors of this text recently published a large series on redo PT including long-term outcomes [9]. Although complex and difficult, redo PT patients can achieve very good outcomes. There is no correlation with type of initial or redo PT performed and the long-term outcomes. Complications are similar after redo PT compared to primary PT in experienced hands in both types of complications and rates of complication. Early complications include anastomotic breakdown or leaks, abscess, perforation, wound infection, and HAEC. Late complications are also equivalent reported at 30–40%. These late complications consist of constipation, HAEC, stricture, obstruction, and fistula. Only constipation was found to be significantly higher ($p < 0.05$) in the redo PT group. To better understand functional outcomes, a stooling survey [58] was completed through a telephone interview or through scoring based on recent clinic notes with a follow-up averaging 224.5 ± 157.6 months (range 6.3–491.6 months). Scores comprised an evaluation of stooling pattern (e.g., excessively loose or explosive stooling), continence, and/or evidence of enterocolitis. Three categories (continence, stooling pattern, and enterocolitic complaints) were individually scored and a composite score was tallied. Total scores were significantly worse (higher) in the redo PT patients compared to the historically matched group of children undergoing a primary PT for HD (12.2 ± 1.4 vs. 5.5 ± 1.2, $p < 0.05$). Continence scores were not different (2.5 ± 0.7 vs. 3.9 ± 1.0, $p = 0.33$), and the overall total score for the redo PT group was higher in both stooling pattern (1.0 ± 0.2 vs. 4.1 ± 0.4, $p = 0.001$) and enterocolitis scores (2.0 ± 0.4 vs. 4.2 ± 0.4, $p = 0.001$). Daytime continence of the redo PT group was 81%, similar to the rate of daytime continence in the primary PT of 86%. Only a quarter of redo PT patients complained of occasional nighttime soiling.

25.6 Conclusion

Redo PT for Hirschsprung disease requires extensive planning, a thoughtful workup, and experience and expertise from the surgeon and the pathologist. When indicated, however, reasonably good results can be achieved in the majority of cases. No single operative approach is better for redo PT cases; rather, each case should be treated based on the best operative approach for a redo PT, and the decision can be variable with each patient. Lesser procedures may provide relief in a select population, but those with RA/TZP or a mechanical cause of symptoms will likely require a redo PT. The workup, treatment plan, and definitive surgical management should be organized and performed by an experienced, specialized team at a pediatric referral center.

References

1. Swenson O, Bill AH Jr. Resection of rectum and rectosigmoid with preservation of the sphincter for benign spastic lesions producing megacolon; an experimental study. Surgery. 1948;24(2):212–20.
2. Raveenthiran V. Knowledge of ancient Hindu surgeons on Hirschsprung disease: evidence from Sushruta Samhita of circa 1200-600 BC. J Pediatr Surg. 2011;46(11):2204–8.
3. Minford JL, Ram A, Turnock RR, Lamont GL, Kenny SE, Rintala RJ, et al. Comparison of functional outcomes of Duhamel and transanal endorectal coloanal anastomosis for Hirschsprung's disease. J Pediatr Surg. 2004;39(2):161–5. discussion -5
4. Saleh W, Rasheed K, Mohaidly MA, Kfoury H, Tariq M, Rawaf AA. Management of Hirschsprung's disease: a comparison of Soave's and Duhamel's pull-through methods. Pediatr Surg Int. 2004;20(8):590–3.
5. Craigie RJ, Conway SJ, Cooper L, Turnock RR, Lamont GL, Baillie CT, et al. Primary pull-through for Hirschsprung's disease: comparison of open and laparoscopic-assisted procedures. J Laparoendosc Adv Surg Tech A. 2007;17(6):809–12.
6. Coe A, Collins MH, Lawal T, Louden E, Levitt MA, Pena A. Reoperation for Hirschsprung disease: pathology of the resected problematic distal pull-through. Pediatr Develop Pathol: Off J Soc Pediatr Pathol Paediatr Pathol Soc. 2012;15(1):30–8.
7. Levitt MA, Dickie B, Pena A. The Hirschsprungs patient who is soiling after what was considered a "successful" pull-through. Semin Pediatr Surg. 2012;21(4):344–53.
8. Friedmacher F, Puri P. Residual aganglionosis after pull-through operation for Hirschsprung's disease: a systematic review and meta-analysis. Pediatr Surg Int. 2011;27(10):1053–7.
9. Ralls MW, Freeman JJ, Rabah R, Coran AG, Ehrlich PF, Hirschl RB, et al. Redo pullthrough for Hirschsprung disease: a single surgical group's experience. J Pediatr Surg. 2014;49(9):1394–9.
10. Schweizer P, Berger S, Schweizer M, Holschneider AM, Beck O. Repeated pull-through surgery for complicated Hirschsprung's disease--principles derived from clinical experience. J Pediatr Surg. 2007;42(3):536–43.
11. Puri P, Gosemann JH. Variants of Hirschsprung disease. Semin Pediatr Surg. 2012;21(4):310–8.
12. West KW, Grosfeld JL, Rescorla FJ, Vane DW. Acquired aganglionosis: a rare occurrence following pull-through procedures for Hirschsprung's disease. J Pediatr Surg. 1990;25(1):104–8. discussion 8–9
13. Murphy F, Puri P. New insights into the pathogenesis of Hirschsprung's associated enterocolitis. Pediatr Surg Int. 2005;21(10):773–9.
14. Reding R, de Ville de Goyet J, Gosseye S, Clapuyt P, Sokal E, Buts JP, et al. Hirschsprung's disease: a 20-year experience. J Pediatr Surg. 1997;32(8):1221–5.
15. Vieten D, Spicer R. Enterocolitis complicating Hirschsprung's disease. Semin Pediatr Surg. 2004;13(4):263–72.
16. Teitelbaum DH, Caniano DA, Qualman SJ. The pathophysiology of Hirschsprung's-associated enterocolitis: importance of histologic correlates. J Pediatr Surg. 1989;24(12):1271–7.
17. Teitelbaum DH, Cilley RE, Sherman NJ, Bliss D, Uitvlugt ND, Renaud EJ, et al. A decade of experience with the primary pull-through for hirschsprung disease in the newborn period: a multicenter analysis of outcomes. Ann Surg. 2000;232(3):372–80.
18. Gad El-Hak NA, El-Hemaly MM, Negm EH, El-Hanafy EA, Abdel Messeh MH, Abdel Bary HH. Functional outcome after Swenson's operation for Hirshsprung's disease. Saudi J Gastroenterol. 2010;16(1):30–4.
19. Zhang SC, Bai YZ, Wang W, Wang WL. Long-term outcome, colonic motility, and sphincter performance after Swenson's procedure for Hirschsprung's disease: a single-center 2-decade experience with 346 cases. Am J Surg. 2007;194(1):40–7.
20. Yanchar NL, Soucy P. Long-term outcome after Hirschsprung's disease: patients' perspectives. J Pediatr Surg. 1999;34(7):1152–60.
21. van Leeuwen K, Teitelbaum DH, Elhalaby EA, Coran AG. Long-term follow-up of redo pull-through procedures for Hirschsprung's disease: efficacy of the endorectal pull-through. J Pediatr Surg. 2000;35(6):829–33; discussion 33–4.
22. Wei J, Zhang W, Feng JX, Weng YZ, Wei MF, Sun XY, et al. Transumbilical laparoscopic pull-through for children with hypoganglionosis. Zhonghua Wei Chang Wai Ke Za Zhi. 2011;14(10):762–3.

23. Dingemann J, Puri P. Isolated hypoganglionosis: systematic review of a rare intestinal innervation defect. Pediatr Surg Int. 2010;26(11):1111–5.
24. Kapur RP. Submucosal nerve diameter of greater than 40 mum is not a valid diagnostic index of transition zone pull-through. J Pediatr Surg. 2016;51(10):1585–91.
25. Dasgupta R, Langer JC. Evaluation and management of persistent problems after surgery for Hirschsprung disease in a child. J Pediatr Gastroenterol Nutr. 2008;46(1):13–9.
26. Patrus B, Nasr A, Langer JC, Gerstle JT. Intrasphincteric botulinum toxin decreases the rate of hospitalization for postoperative obstructive symptoms in children with Hirschsprung disease. J Pediatr Surg. 2011;46(1):184–7.
27. Koivusalo AI, Pakarinen MP, Rintala RJ. Botox injection treatment for anal outlet obstruction in patients with internal anal sphincter achalasia and Hirschsprung's disease. Pediatr Surg Int. 2009;25(10):873–6.
28. Wildhaber BE, Pakarinen M, Rintala RJ, Coran AG, Teitelbaum DH. Posterior myotomy/myectomy for persistent stooling problems in Hirschsprung's disease. J Pediatr Surg. 2004;39(6):920–6; discussion -6.
29. Jiang d P, Li ZZ, Zhang YB, Jiang ZT. Treatment of anal achalasia after transanal endorectal pull-through for Hirschsprung's disease with topical botulinum toxin. J Trop Pediatr. 2008;54(3):211.
30. Church JT, Gadepalli SK, Talishinsky T, Teitelbaum DH, Jarboe MD. Ultrasound-guided intrasphincteric botulinum toxin injection relieves obstructive defecation due to Hirschsprung's disease and internal anal sphincter achalasia. J Pediatr Surg. 2017;52(1):74–8.
31. Zhang SC, Bai YZ, Wang W, Wang WL. Stooling patterns and colonic motility after transanal one-stage pull-through operation for Hirschsprung's disease in children. J Pediatr Surg. 2005;40(11):1766–72.
32. Teitelbaum DH, Drongowski RA, Chamberlain JN, Coran AG. Long-term stooling patterns in infants undergoing primary endorectal pull-through for Hirschsprung's disease. J Pediatr Surg. 1997;32(7):1049–52; discussion 52-3.
33. Di Lorenzo C, Solzi GF, Flores AF, Schwankovsky L, Hyman PE. Colonic motility after surgery for Hirschsprung's disease. Am J Gastroenterol 2000;95(7):1759–1764.
34. Athanasakos E, Starling J, Ross F, Nunn K, Cass D. An example of psychological adjustment in chronic illness: Hirschsprung's disease. Pediatr Surg Int. 2006;22(4):319–25.
35. Blane CE, Elhalaby E, Coran AG. Enterocolitis following endorectal pull-through procedure in children with Hirschsprung's disease. Pediatr Radiol. 1994;24(3):164–6.
36. Meier-Ruge WA, Bruder E, Holschneider AM, Lochbuhler H, Piket G, Posselt HG, et al. Diagnosis and therapy of ultrashort Hirschsprung's disease. Eur J Pediatr Surg. 2004;14(6):392–7.
37. Chumpitazi BP, Nurko S. Defecation disorders in children after surgery for Hirschsprung disease. J Pediatr Gastroenterol Nutr. 2011;53(1):75–9.
38. Ralls MW, Coran AG, Teitelbaum DH. Reoperative surgery for Hirschsprung disease. Semin Pediatr Surg. 2012;21(4):354–63.
39. Engum SA, Grosfeld JL. Long-term results of treatment of Hirschsprung's disease. Semin Pediatr Surg. 2004;13(4):273–85.
40. Ieiri S, Nakatsuji T, Akiyoshi J, Higashi M, Hashizume M, Suita S, et al. Long-term outcomes and the quality of life of Hirschsprung disease in adolescents who have reached 18 years or older – a 47-year single-institute experience. J Pediatr Surg. 2010;45(12):2398–402.
41. Rintala RJ, Pakarinen MP. Long-term outcomes of Hirschsprung's disease. Semin Pediatr Surg. 2012;21(4):336–43.
42. Langer J. Repeat pull-through surgery for complicated Hirschsprung's disease: indications, techniques, and results. J Pediatr Surg. 1999;34:1136–41.
43. Weber TR, Fortuna RS, Silen ML, Dillon PA. Reoperation for Hirschsprung's disease. J Pediatr Surg. 1999;34(1):153–6. discussion 6-7
44. Moore SW, Albertyn R, Cywes S. Clinical outcome and long-term quality of life after surgical correction of Hirschsprung's disease. J Pediatr Surg. 1996;31(11):1496–502.
45. Dasgupta R, Langer JC. Hirschsprung disease. Curr Probl Surg. 2004;41(12):942–88.
46. Ciamarra P, Nurko S, Barksdale E, Fishman S, Di Lorenzo C. Internal anal sphincter achalasia in children: clinical characteristics and treatment with Clostridium botulinum toxin. J Pediatr Gastroenterol Nutr. 2003;37(3):315–9.
47. Messineo A, Codrich D, Monai M, Martellossi S, Ventura A. The treatment of internal anal sphincter achalasia with botulinum toxin. Pediatr Surg Int. 2001;17(7):521–3.
48. Chumpitazi BP, Fishman SJ, Nurko S. Long-term clinical outcome after botulinum toxin injection in children with nonrelaxing internal anal sphincter. Am J Gastroenterol. 2009;104(4):976–83.
49. Jiang d P, Xu CQ, Wu B, Li ZZ, Zhang YB, Han FY. Effects of botulinum toxin injection on anal achalasia after pull-through operations for Hirschsprung's disease: a 1-year follow-up study. Int J Color Dis. 2009;24(5):597–8.
50. Millar AJ, Steinberg RM, Raad J, Rode H. Anal achalasia after pull-through operations for Hirschsprung's disease – preliminary experience with topical nitric oxide. Eur J Pediatr Surg. 2002;12(3):207–11.
51. Lindsey I, Jones OM, Cunningham C, George BD, Mortensen NJ. Botulinum toxin as second-line therapy for chronic anal fissure failing 0.2 percent glyceryl trinitrate. Dis Colon Rectum. 2003;46(3):361–6.
52. Demirbag S, Tander B, Atabek C, Surer I, Ozturk H, Cetinkursun S. Long-term results of topical glyceryl

trinitrate ointment in children with anal fissure. Ann Trop Paediatr. 2005;25(2):135–7.
53. De Caluwe D, Yoneda A, Akl U, Puri P. Internal anal sphincter achalasia: outcome after internal sphincter myectomy. J Pediatr Surg 2001;36(5):736–738.
54. Heikkinen M, Lindahl H, Rintala RJ. Long-term outcome after internal sphincter myectomy for internal sphincter achalasia. Pediatr Surg Int. 2005;21(2):84–7.
55. Dingemans A, van der Steeg H, Rassouli-Kirchmeier R, Linssen MW, van Rooij I, de Blaauw I. Redo pull-through surgery in Hirschsprung disease: short-term clinical outcome. J Pediatr Surg. 2017;52(9):1446–50.
56. Lawal TA, Chatoorgoon K, Collins MH, Coe A, Pena A, Levitt MA. Redo pull-through in Hirschsprung's [corrected] disease for obstructive symptoms due to residual aganglionosis and transition zone bowel. J Pediatr Surg. 2011;46(2):342–7.
57. Pena A, Elicevik M, Levitt MA. Reoperations in Hirschsprung disease. J Pediatr Surg. 2007;42(6):1008–13. discussion 13–4
58. Kim AC, Langer JC, Pastor AC, Zhang L, Sloots CE, Hamilton NA, et al. Endorectal pull-through for Hirschsprung's disease-a multicenter, long-term comparison of results: transanal vs transabdominal approach. J Pediatr Surg. 2010;45(6):1213–20.

Early and Late Complications Following Pull-Through Operation for Hirschsprung's Disease

26

Rebecca M. Rentea and Charles L. Snyder

Contents

R. M. Rentea (✉) · C. L. Snyder
Department of Surgery, Children's Mercy Hospital, Kansas City, MI, USA
e-mail: rrentea@cmh.edu; csnyder@cmh.edu

26.1 Overview

Since Harald Hirschsprung's classic description in 1886, hundreds of papers have been published on the complications and outcomes following repair of Hirschsprung's disease (HD). Original works by Swenson (1948), Rehbein (1953), Duhamel (1956), and Soave (1964) and their predecessors emphasized large single-institution or even single-surgeon experiences, rendering analysis of comparative outcomes difficult [34]. There has also been an evolution in surgical management from the traditional three-stage approach to minimally invasive laparoscopic techniques and neonatal single-stage reconstruction. Different risks and benefits are ascribed to each operative approach.

As with many conditions, the fact that several different operative approaches are used by different surgeons and institutions is an indication that no one specific approach is best. However, the principles of the operative approach remain the same: removal of aganglionic bowel and advancement of ganglionic bowel to the preserved anal canal, while leaving the surrounding sphincter mechanism and anatomy undisturbed [32].

HD is often viewed by medical professionals, patients, and families as a surgically correctable cause of bowel obstruction. This is only partially true. It is increasingly recognized that many continue to suffer from bowel dysfunction, enterocolitis, soiling or incontinence, and

P. Puri (ed.), *Hirschsprung's Disease and Allied Disorders*,
https://doi.org/10.1007/978-3-030-15647-3_26

decreased quality of life [12]. Complications occurring following the surgical repair of HD can be temporally categorized into early and late complications, with overlap regarding the time they manifest. Some complications (e.g., wound infection, bleeding, stricture, adhesive bowel obstruction, dehiscence, stomal complications) are discussed briefly as they are inherent to any surgical procedure and not unique to HD. Complications can also be categorized as potentially preventable (leak, transition zone pull-through (TZPT), residual aganglionosis, fistulae, damage to the anal canal), partially preventable (constipation, wound complications), and non-preventable (Hirschsprung-associated enterocolitis, HAEC).

The true incidence of each complication is unknown. Operative results often remain limited to single-center or small multicenter series with relatively short-term follow-up. Long-term results (dependent on complications) vary due to differences in the operation performed, surgeon and patient variables, extent of aganglionosis, and the definition of the complications themselves [12, 29, 48].

Evaluation of the child with a suboptimal outcome following pull-through requires a systematic approach aimed at determining the long-term prognosis based on the anatomy following the original surgery, potential need for reoperation, and optimal medical management [31].

26.1.1 Early Complications

Early complications following pull-through manifest within the initial postsurgical period. Early complications often lead to long-term complications (leaks leading to stricture or scarring, damage to the anal canal resulting in permanent incontinence). Between 10% and 15% of children experience at least one early complication after their pull-through procedure [11, 12, 43, 45, 50, 55].

26.2 Wound Infection

Operations for HD are classified as clean-contaminated cases. The risk of wound infection is about 3–4% for primary repairs. Surgical site infections (SSI) have a higher than average incidence (second only to inflammatory bowel disease) after pull-through and stoma creation or closure for children with HD (Fig. 26.1) [13].

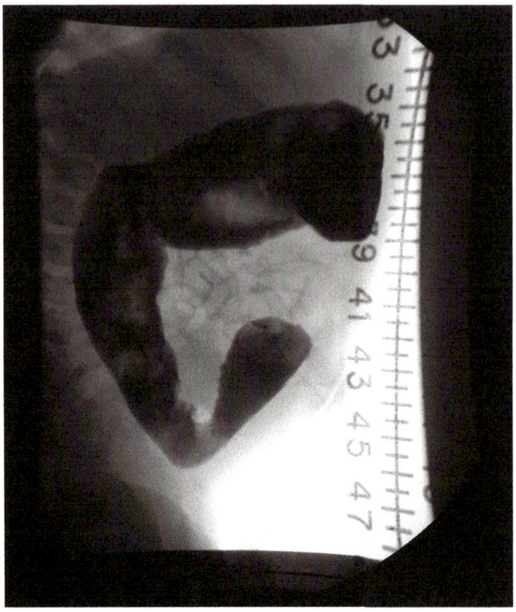

Fig. 26.1 Contrast study through a leveling colostomy demonstrating a stricture (arrow) proximal to the stoma exists

26.2.1 Anastomotic Complications

26.2.1.1 Leak

Anastomotic leaks occur in 1–10% of patients [11, 12, 43, 45, 50, 55]. Factors increasing the risk of leak include tension, ischemia, technical problems, poor nutritional status, general wound-healing problems (immunosuppression and others), residual aganglionosis, and distal obstruction. No specific risk factors have been established for an anastomotic leak in HD [41, 50]. However, postoperative rectal manipulation (temperature, examination, or medications) or in the early postoperative period can potentially damage the repair. A nursing communication prohibiting any rectal temperatures, rectal administration of medications, or procedural manipulations is essential, and a sign should be posted at the bedside.

Suspected leaks are evaluated with water-soluble contrast enemas (Figs. 26.2 and 26.3)

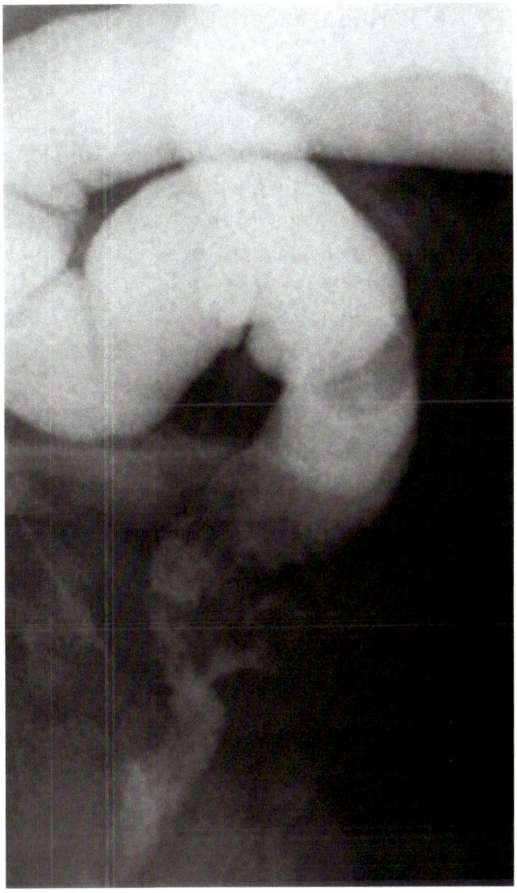

Fig. 26.2 A 1-year-old patient with anastomotic leak following Soave's procedure.

and/or an examination under anesthesia. Minor leaks may be subclinical. Major anastomotic leaks can result in localized abscesses, free peritoneal leakage and sepsis, and may require abdominal washout and diversion. Sequelae such as fluid collections may respond to percutaneous drainage. Studies evaluating indications for redo surgery suggest that a large percentage of strictures (25%) resulted from a clinical history of presumptive anastomotic leaks with recurrent pelvic abscesses or fistulas [31].

26.2.1.2 Cuff/Pelvic Abscess

Cuff abscess is an uncommon complication after the Soave operation, with an estimated incidence of 1–6% [3, 12, 41, 43, 51]. An abscess forms between the rectal muscularis and the colonic pull-through segment. Risk factors include ischemia, retained rectal mucosa, bleeding, pelvic contamination, and anastomotic tension. The treatment varies from broad-spectrum antibiotic coverage (with or without percutaneous drainage) to diversion. Larger or more chronic abscesses or those resulting in fistulas may lead to stricture formation and may eventually result in a late complication of Soave pull-through, such as a Soave cuff (thickened tissue of the rectal muscularis acting as an obstruction from inflammation, discussed later).

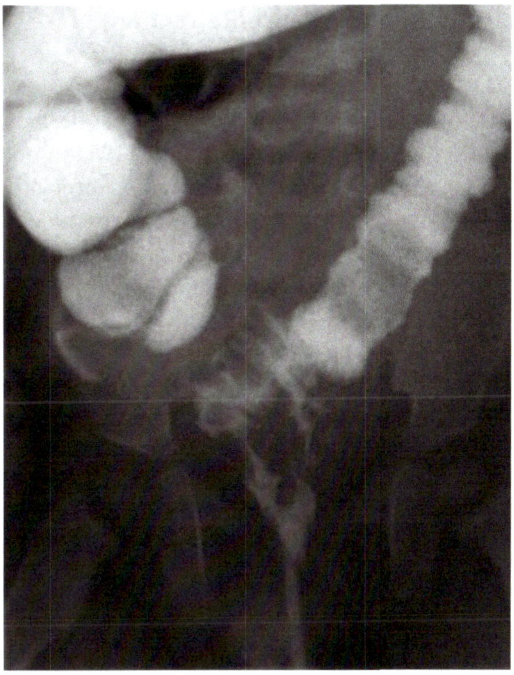

Fig. 26.3 Same patient as in Fig. 26.2, 2 months later. A fistula from the distal to proximal rectum has developed

26.2.1.3 Pelvic Abscess

The incidence of pelvic abscess in HD is approximately 5%. The same factors resulting in leak are also implicated in the formation of pelvic abscesses, with the addition of operative intraabdominal contamination and hematoma formation. CT scans are the diagnostic procedure of choice; the diagnostic accuracy increases if the study is obtained more than 1 week after the procedure. The diagnosis of pelvic abscess requires a high index of suspicion and prompt intervention to avoid further morbidity, such as extension of the infection, systemic sepsis, chronic fistula formation, or necrosis of the pull-through segment. Treatment ranges from percutaneous drainage to washout and stomal diversion.

26.2.1.4 Dehiscence/Retraction of the Pull Through

The incidence of anastomotic dehiscence is about 1–2% in primary pull-throughs [50]. The incidence in redo operations is higher (19% in one recent series) [10] due to the increased difficultly with adequate mobilization, compromised blood supply, and scarring in these cases.

Retraction of the neo-rectum or pull-through segment is rare (less than 1%). Retraction occurs early in the early postoperative period and requires confirmation via examination under anesthesia. It is usually due to tension and inadequate mobilization of the pull-through segment. Transanal repair may be attempted for minimal disruptions. However, depending on the clinical status, retraction may require proximal diverting colostomy and delayed revision in several months.

26.2.2 Fistula

Fistula can be an early or late complication of pull-through for HD. This is usually the result of a leak or perforation. Fistulas can be enterocutaneous, rectourethral, or rectovaginal. Small fistulas or sinus tracts may resolve spontaneously or with local therapy. However, many persist and are one of the most common indications for redo pull-through operation [10, 44].

26.2.3 Stomal Complications

Although rectal washouts are commonly used, a stoma prior to definitive surgery was created in 36% of infants in a national cohort. Delayed diagnosis, enterocolitis, aganglionosis proximal to the splenic flexure, and the presence of other anomalies are associated with stoma complications [4].

Stoma creation and closure has a higher than average risk of infection and other complications in patients with HD [13]. Stoma formation in older children with dilated bowel/megacolon can be technically difficult and is particularly associated with an increased incidence of stomal complications (prolapse, parastomal hernia, skin excoriation, bleeding, retraction, stenosis).

26.2.4 Perineal Excoriation

Perianal excoriation occurs commonly in children undergoing pull-through surgery [11, 29, 43, 51]. It is more common in children with long segment disease and with single-stage transanal pull-throughs in neonates of age under a month [35]. Early involvement of experienced stoma therapists and the use of barrier paste are essential. It is important to prepare the family for this development prior to the operation. The precise cause remains unknown but increased fecal sodium content in loose stools may contribute to the perianal excoriation. The skin irritation usually resolves in 6–8 weeks.

26.3 Late Complications

The incidence of late complications is widely variable but clusters between 15% and 40% [27, 53]. The most common late complications are soiling/incontinence, obstructive symptoms, or enterocolitis (which can also occur prior to diagnosis, preoperatively, or postoperatively). Additional long-term complications due to injuries to the adjacent anatomy (urinary and sexual function) may only manifest long after the original pull-through. Some complications tend to exclude others; for example, fecal incontinence and Hirschsprung-associated enterocolitis (HAEC) are rarely seen together. Long-term bowel function may be poorer in those patients who have experienced enterocolitis [36].

A recent inpatient database analysis found that while the number of operations for HD remained stable, admissions for constipation and enterocolitis have increased over the last decade [23]. Whether this is simply increased recognition or a true change in incidence is unclear.

The (increasing) use of single-stage transanal pull-through, discussed in detail in Chap. 23, in the newborn period initially raised concerns about long-term outcomes compared to the historical staged approach with leveling colostomy, pull-through, and colostomy closure. Although the quality of the evidence in the literature is admittedly poor, several studies identified no major differences in soiling, incontinence, enterocolitis, or constipation [27, 29, 49, 51].

26.3.1 General Approach to Late Complications

A systematic approach to the evaluation of late complications is essential (Fig. 26.4). Excluding enterocolitis, patients generally fall into one of two categories: those that are soiling/incontinent and those that are constipated/obstructed.

The evaluation begins with a detailed history and physical exam. This should include an understanding of the specific operative approach utilized for the pull-through. The technical differences between the different operations is often critical to the accurate assessment of postoperative problems [32]; whether the child had an ostomy created first, any additional interventions that were performed in the perioperative period, and a review of the pathology report and slides (if available) are all important in guiding management [30, 31, 33].

Following a complete history, all patients should undergo an examination under anesthesia (EUA). This includes inspection for [34] integrity of the anal canal (Fig. 26.5a), [1] presence of a stricture, [2] status of the sphincters, [3] presence of a large dilated rectal pouch, or [4] the presence of a palpable Soave cuff. A full-thickness rectal biopsy is also performed for histologic evaluation for patients with obstructive symptoms.

Finally, for all patients with problems following definitive repair of HD, a water-soluble contrast enema is performed to visualize the anatomy after the initial operation. This provides insight into the motility of the colon and any structural anomalies that may account for the patient's symptoms.

26.3.2 Obstruction

The American Pediatric Surgical Association's (APSA) Hirschsprung Disease Interest Group recently published (literature-, evidence-, and expert consensus-based) guidelines to the best approach for common obstructive complications after operation for HD.[30] The incidence of obstructive symptoms was estimated at 10–40%, but rates are higher in patients with long-segment disease or Down syndrome.

26.3.2.1 Etiology

There are five broad causes of obstruction [30]:

- Mechanical (stricture, twisted pull-through, rectal cuff complications, fecaloma or dilated Duhamel, adhesive bowel obstruction)
- Pathologic (transition zone pull-through, residual or secondary aganglionosis)
- Internal sphincter achalasia
- Motility disorders (neuronal dysplasia [IND], global, or focal colonic dysmotility)
- Functional megacolon (stool withholding)

26.3.2.2 Clinical

Constipation is the most common of the obstructive symptoms and some degree of it is extremely common in HD (Fig. 26.6). Its incidence varies widely and may change with time, but rates of approximately 30% are reported, generally unrelated to the type of operation [1, 12, 45, 48]. The literature is rife with retrospective single-institutional studies reporting constipation and other functional outcomes. However, variable definitions of constipation, different operative approaches, patient variables, and other uncontrolled factors limit conclusions and comparisons. Individual or family questionnaires and specialized scoring systems are widely used to assess constipation/obstruction and incontinence, but standardized criteria (such as the Rome III definition and others) are preferable [55]. The evidence suggests that constipation improves over time [25, 48, 55].

Other symptoms vary with the severity of the obstruction and include vomiting, abdominal distension, crampy abdominal pain, recurrent enterocolitis, and failure to thrive. Most children have chronic complications, but an acutely obstructed patient may require admission, cessation of oral intake and or nasogastric suction, and rectal decompression with dilation or irrigations.

Enterocolitis may occur with obstruction and is discussed briefly below, and in detail in Chap. 13.

Mild ongoing obstructive symptoms can be treated symptomatically, but more severe symptoms are approached as outlined below.

26.3.2.3 Evaluation and Treatment

Evaluation of obstructive symptoms begins with a thorough history and physical, including a digital rectal examination [31] (Figs. 26.4 and 26.5). Obstructive symptoms are usually due to either

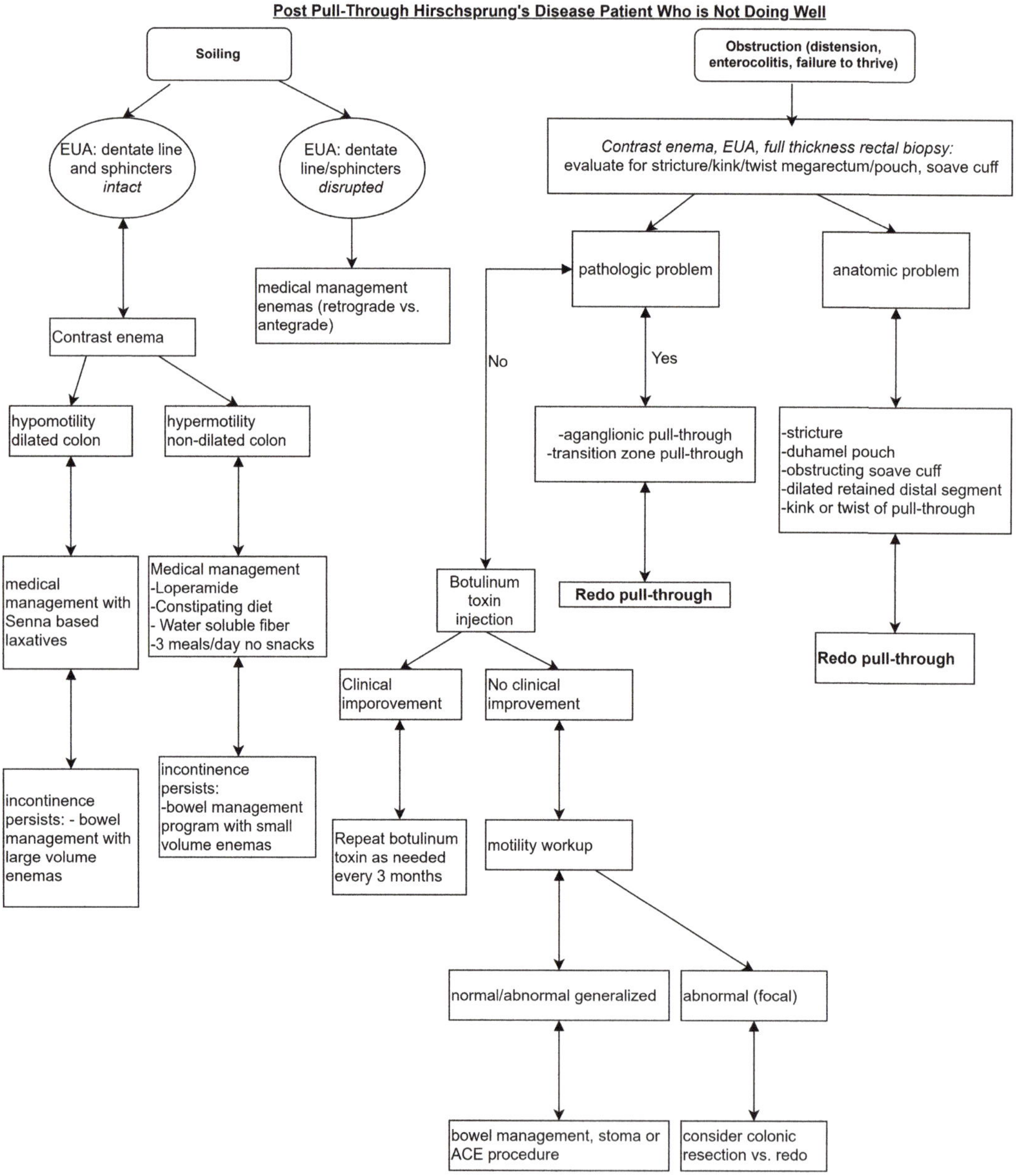

Fig. 26.4 Algorithm for the diagnosis and management of the child with soiling or obstructive symptoms after a pull-through for Hirschsprung's disease. (Modified and reprinted with permission from Langer et al. [30], Levitt et al. [32, 33]. Examination under anesthesia (EUA), antegrade colonic enema (ACE))

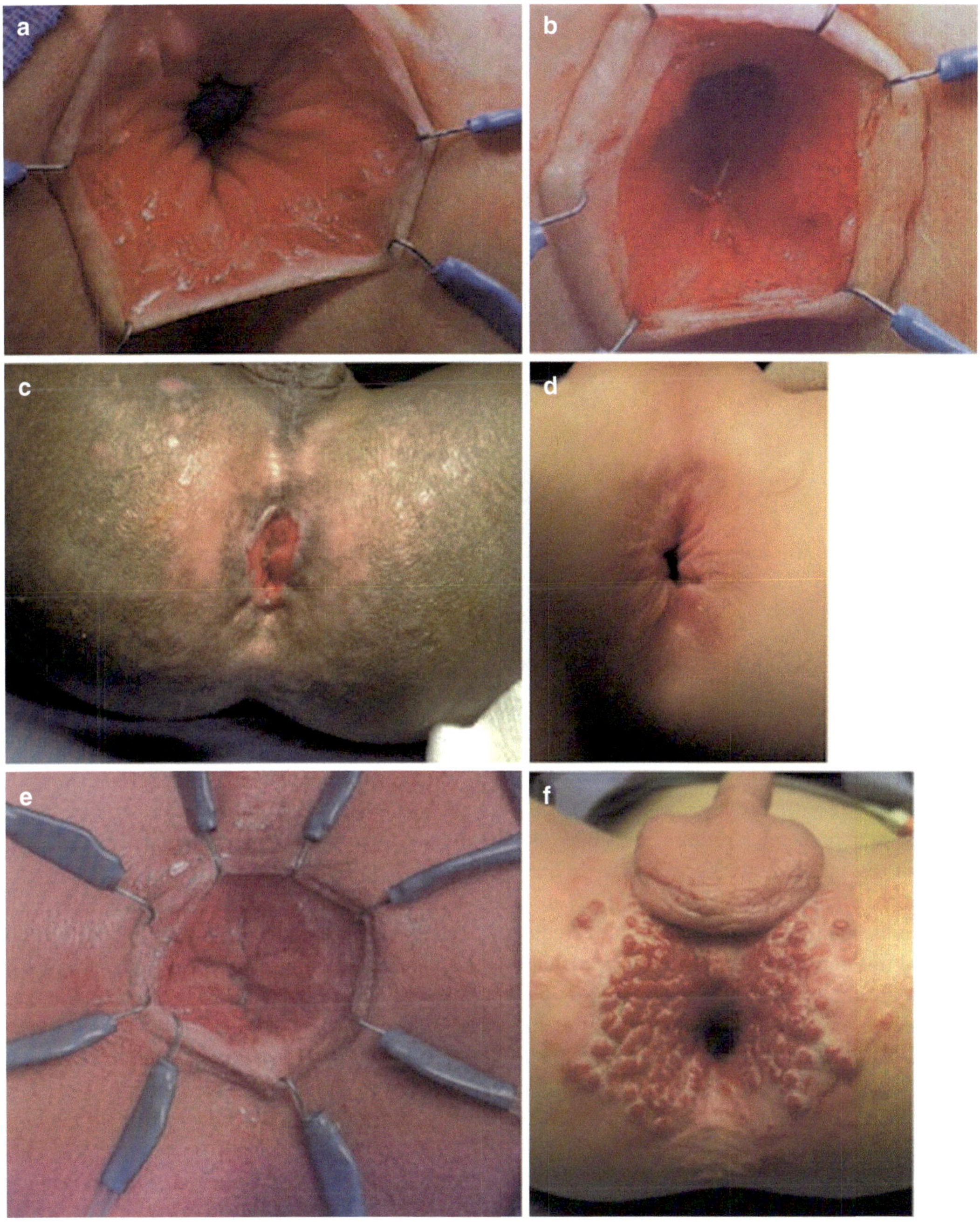

Fig. 26.5 Examination under anesthesia: (**a**) Normal dentate line seen on inspection of the anal canal. (**b**) Loss of the anal canal and the dentate line with the colo-anal anastomosis was sewn to the anal skin. (**c**) An "open anus" likely from excessive stretching of the sphincters during the pull-through and no evidence of a dentate line. (**d**) Patulous anus in an awake patient connoting lax sphincters. (**e**) The right side of the dentate line is missing while the left side is present. (**f**) Severe perineal excoriation from constant soiling related to an open anus with damaged sphincters. (Reprinted with permission (**a**, **c**, **d**, **f**) [32] (**b**) [33])

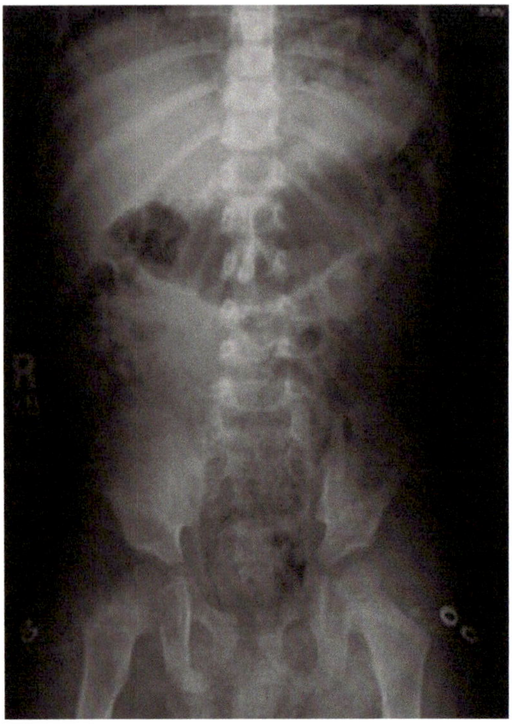

Fig. 26.6 Abdominal plain film demonstrating a large amount of stool in the ascending, descending, and rectosigmoid

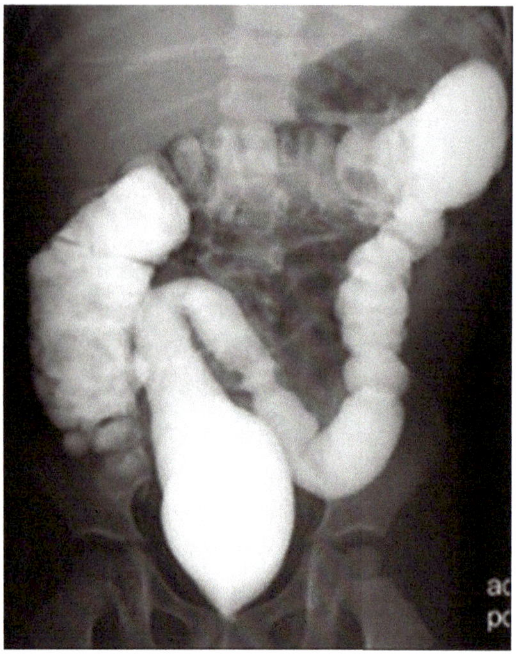

Fig. 26.7 Contrast study of retained dilated segment of colon after a laparoscopic assisted transanal pull-through procedure. The dilated segment led to fecal stasis and enterocolitis. (Reprinted with permission [31])

an anatomic problem (stricture, twisted/kinked anastomosis, megarectum (Fig. 26.7), tight Soave cuff) or a pathologic problem (transition zone or aganglionic pull-through); both usually require surgical revision. Of the two, pathologic complications are the most common [42, 44]. A good water-soluble contrast enema should be obtained for evaluation of the anatomy. To identify pathological causes, a review of the pathology report and slides from prior operations is important, and a full-thickness rectal biopsy should be performed without the use of electrocautery. This allows for evaluation of the submucosa where hypertrophic nerves may be visualized. Specimens are sent fresh to pathology to look for the presence of ganglion cells, absence of hypertrophic nerve fibers and normal acetylcholinesterase staining. Calretinin staining may be helpful as well. It is important to note that a prior successful Duhamel operation will intentionally leave aganglionic bowel around the anterior one-half of the rectum, and a posterior biopsy must be done.

Management following biopsy and contrast enema focuses on known anatomic issues specific to different surgical procedures.

Soave Muscular Cuff The muscular cuff through which the functional ganglionated bowel is passed can cause obstruction, from excessive scarring and fibrosis, if too much muscle was left, if the cuff was not adequately split, or if it rolls down after a Soave procedure [8]. Obstructive symptoms and enterocolitis are the usual presentation. The diagnosis can often be made by palpation of the cuff (band or fibrous thickening around the distal pull-through on digital examination, or on contrast enema (Fig. 26.8). The enema identifies about half the cases [8]. Anorectal manometry provides no additional information that cannot obtained through perineal inspection and radiographs.

This complication can be prevented by leaving only a few centimeters of cuff during the primary operation, with full-thickness splitting of the remainder of the muscle. Definitive treatment requires reoperation, usually via a redo transanal approach.

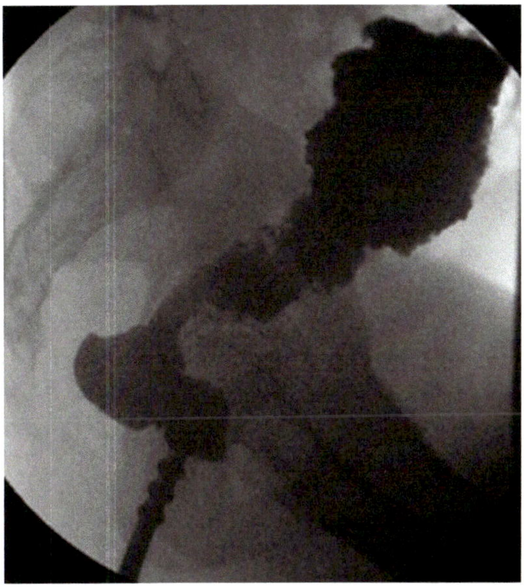

Fig. 26.8 Problematic Soave cuff causing narrowing of the distal pull-through. Note the area of narrowing and the increased distance between sacrum and rectum, consistent with a retained and obstructing Soave cuff. (Reprinted with permission [31])

Twisted Pull- Through A twisted pull-through can be surprisingly difficult to identify. Obstructive symptoms and enterocolitis are the usual nonspecific presentations. Treatment of the enterocolitis with rectal tubes and irrigation proximal to the twist result in improvement while the diagnosis is missed. Digital rectal examination may appear normal. A contrast enema (Fig. 26.9) is often diagnostic, but injection of the contrast above the twist can be misleading. EUA and rectosigmoidoscopy may be helpful. A twisted pull-through is best avoided by careful attention to the pulled-through bowel at the initial procedure (Fig. 26.10), with colored suture to identify the correct orientation, and calibration with a dilator or balloon catheter at the end of the procedure.

Large Duhamel Pouch Obstruction from a Duhamel (where the aganglionic segment of bowel retains stool that becomes impacted and causes obstruction) can lead to a severely dilated rectum refractory to conservative treatment (Fig. 26.11). Care must be taken at the primary operation to avoid leaving an aganglionic spur of bowel anteriorly. One should be alert to the possibility of this

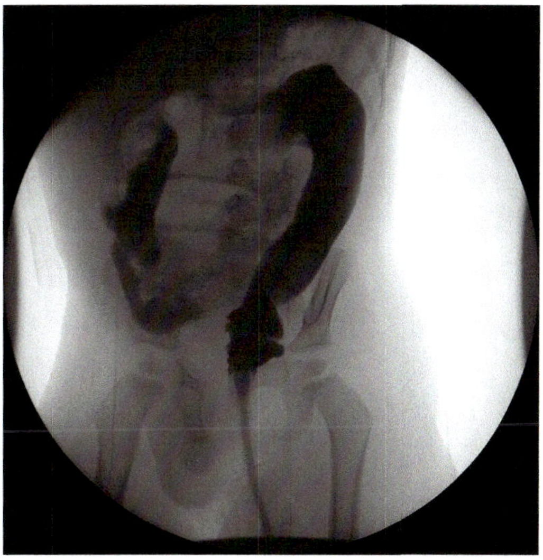

Fig. 26.9 Contrast enema demonstrating a twist of the pull-through

complication in children who have a history of extensive aganglionosis managed with an extended Duhamel or Kimura patches [31]. One treatment option is resection of the Duhamel pouch and conversion to a Swenson procedure.

Strictures Strictures may be due to ischemia, tension, or anastomotic leakage resulting in scarring. Late strictures can be caused by chronic inflammation from stercoral ulceration.

The incidence of anal anastomotic stricture varies from 3% to 35% [11, 12, 50, 51]. Strictures are more common following Soave and Swenson repairs than the Duhamel procedure. Strictures in the intraabdominal colon may occur secondary to ischemia/devascularization.

Dilation is the first line of therapy for early anastomotic strictures. If the obstruction is within reach of a Hegar dilator, then repeated graded dilation is attempted. Mitomycin-C has been reported in limited case series with some benefit. More proximal strictures may require operative stricturoplasty, resection, or redo pull-through.

While early anastomotic strictures may respond to dilation, often they are recalcitrant. It is important to note that strictures do not grow with the child and eventually manifest as worsening obstruction as the child continues to grow

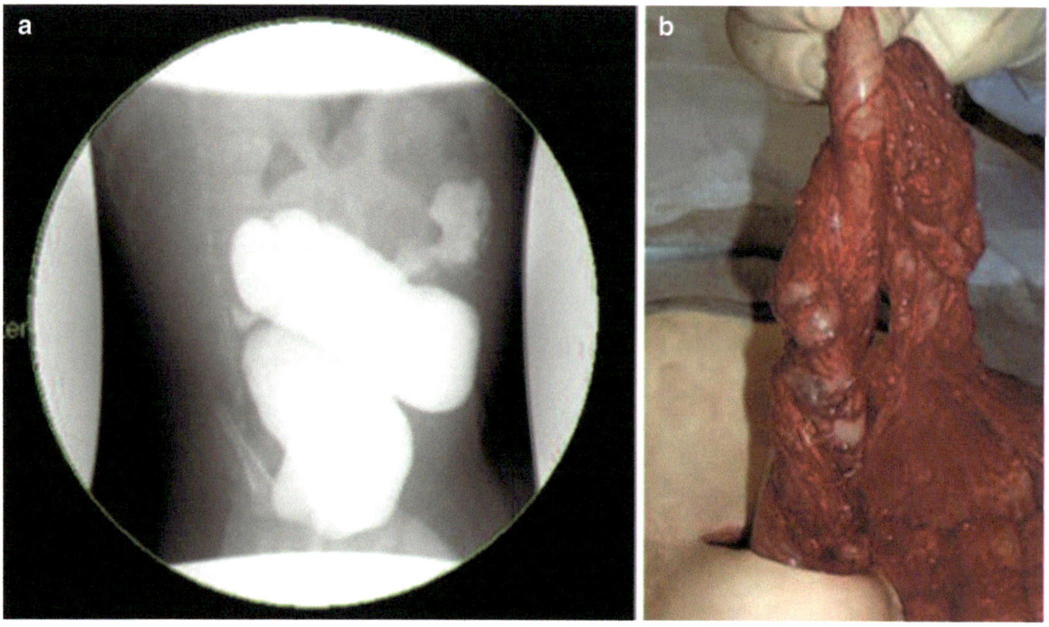

Fig. 26.10 (**a**) Contrast study of a 5-month-old boy after a pull-through procedure showing a bowel obstruction. (**b**) He was found to have an almost 360° twist in his pull-through segment. (Reprinted with permission [31])

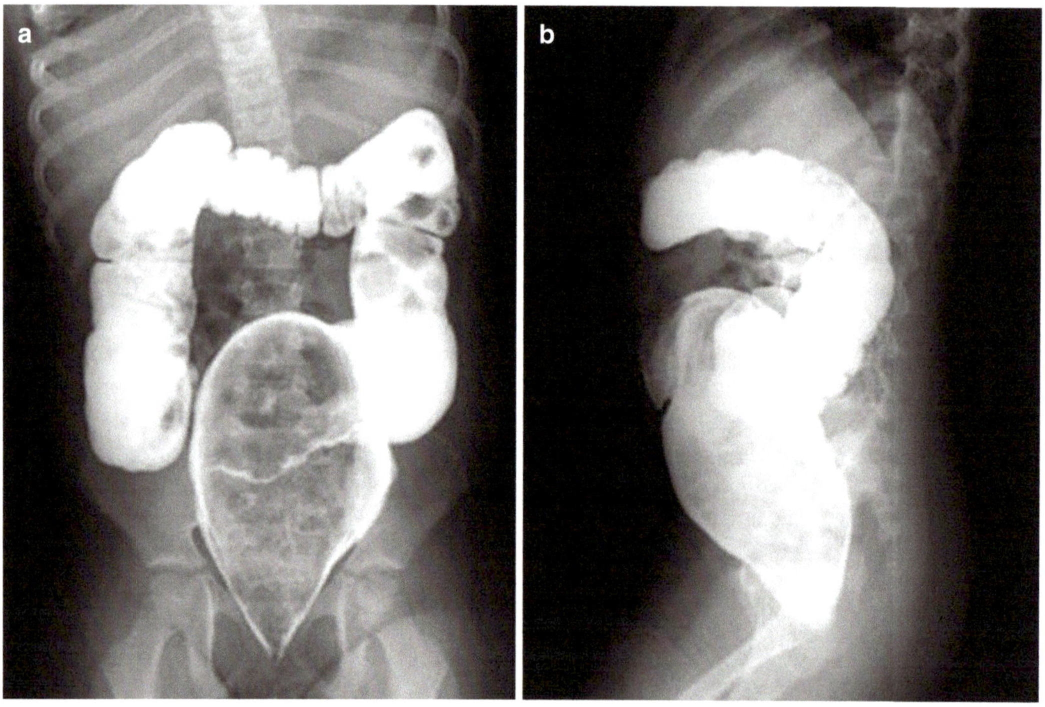

Fig. 26.11 (**a**, **b**) Large Duhamel pouch causing fecal impaction. (Reprinted with permission [31]) Contrast study of retained dilated segment of colon after a laparoscopic assisted transanal pull-through procedure. The dilated segment led to fecal stasis and enterocolitis. (Reprinted with permission [31])

and incorporate more solid food into their diet. As many as one-third to one-half of all clinically significant strictures require surgical intervention. These anatomic complications are often best managed with reoperation (discussed in detail in Chap. 25). In strictures after Soave or Swenson pull-throughs, a Duhamel operation can often be used for salvage.

Adhesive Bowel Obstruction As with any abdominal or pelvic operation, an adhesive bowel obstruction can develop at any time after the definitive repair. Small bowel can also become trapped (internal hernia) underneath the mesentery of the pulled-through bowel.

Pathologic Complications Retained aganglionosis or transition zone pull-through (TZPT) are the most common indications for reoperation (Fig. 26.12) [44]. The timing of the obstructive symptoms may provide a clue as to the cause, with mechanical and anatomic problems usually discovered earlier than pathologic etiologies. It is important to remember that the transition zone is nonuniform; often eccentric and variable from patient to patient. Although the length of the transition zone is usually <5 cm, meticulous histologic examination found a range of 0–12 cm [6, 26]. Circumferential sampling is necessary to clearly identify the TZ, in addition to staying well above the site where ganglionated bowel was found on frozen section [26]. TZPT should be an avoidable complication with careful biopsy and high-quality pathology. Even when this complication occurs, only about one-third of children will need reoperation.

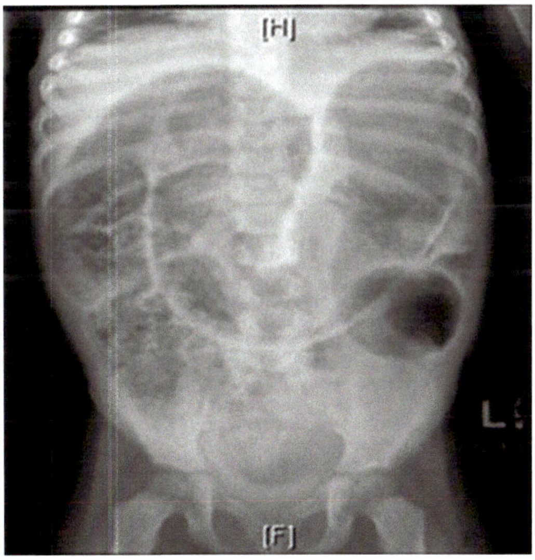

Fig. 26.12 Abdominal radiograph of a 3-year-old child presenting with abdominal distension, fever, and vomiting 1 year after a pull-through procedure. Enterocolitis was treated with irrigations and metronidazole. The patients subsequently underwent a redo pull-through for persistent transition zone bowel. (Reprinted with permission [31])

26.3.2.4 Internal Anal Sphincter Achalasia

One of the hallmarks of HD is failure of the internal anal sphincter to relax in response to distension. Restorative operations to bring ganglionated bowel down to the anorectum do not correct the lack of a rectoanal inhibitory reflex. Persistent obstructive symptoms after otherwise successful pull-through for HD often result from this. The diagnosis is usually made empirically, but manometry is confirmatory. Treatment options include topical nitroglycerin paste or nifedipine cream, intrasphincteric botulinum toxin injection, and internal anal sphincterotomy or myotomy [30].

A trial of injection of botulinum toxin is the initial treatment of choice when normal ganglionated bowel is found on biopsy and no anatomic cause is identified. Variable dosages are reported, but a concentration of 100 U/ml diluted to 10 U/ml with normal saline, injected into four quadrants around the anus with 1 ml of fluid (total of 40 U and 4 ml injected) works well. Ultrasound guidance during the injection of botulinum toxin (the internal anal sphincter is small) may increase the success of the procedure and avoid injection-related complications [5].

If significant clinical improvement occurs after botulinum toxin injection, it can be repeated when symptoms indicate (usually the effects last from 3 to 6 months), or an anorectal myectomy or myotomy can be considered. Repeated botulinum toxin is often preferred to myectomy/myotomy due to concerns about the risk of permanent incontinence with the latter. Nearly three-fourths of HD patients with obstructive symptoms improve with botulinum toxin injection [20]. Adverse reactions are rare, although transient soiling is sometimes seen. Symptoms tend to resolve with time (typically by about 5 years of age), further supporting a nonsurgical approach [30].

26.3.2.5 Motility

Failure to improve with botulinum injection is an indication for manometry and a thorough evaluation of bowel motility, with ingestion of radio-opaque markers or nuclear medicine colonic transit studies. In some centers, specific colonic motility studies are available [30]. If the motility is confined to a segment of colon, a segmental resection may help. Diffuse motility problems and patients with normal motility studies may be treated with bowel management programs (which may include various forms of antegrade colonic enema procedures). Nutritional consultation, high-fiber diets, stool softeners, stimulant laxatives, prokinetic agents, biofeedback training, pelvic physical therapy, and psychological support are all potentially useful adjuncts [30]. A permanent stoma is occasionally needed as a last resort.

26.3.2.6 Stool-Holding Behavior

When normal pathologic findings, absence of anatomic abnormalities, normal motility, and failure to respond to botulinum toxin are present in a child with obstructive symptoms, stool holding behavior is the likely cause. Medical bowel management including a high-fiber diet, stool softeners, laxatives, and prokinetic agents may suffice. Additional treatment options include biofeedback and pelvic physical therapy, and social/psychological support. Anorectal manometry may demonstrate pelvic dyssynergia and may be used as an adjunct to biofeedback and physical therapy. In severe cases, a de-functioning stoma may be necessary [30]. The use of antegrade enemas may be contraindicated (or should be approached with care), since they can worsen the symptoms.

26.3.3 Continence

Postoperative fecal incontinence is a devastating complication following pull-through for HD. The literature regarding postoperative bowel control and fecal continence has not identified a superior initial procedure [1, 38].

26.3.3.1 Incidence

Reported rates of incontinence range widely in various series, with median rates of 20–30% [24, 29, 48]. The incidence of soiling is higher for children with total colonic disease or extensive aganglionosis and in Down syndrome.

26.3.3.2 Evaluation

The evaluation is as previously described (Fig. 26.4). A detailed history and thorough physical examination are followed by a water-soluble contrast enema and examination under anesthesia. The anatomic evaluation is aimed at determining and documenting if the mechanisms for continence are intact through examination and imaging. Normal continence mechanism involves three components: [34] anal canal sensation, [1] an intact sphincter mechanism, and [2] normal colonic motility [32].

26.3.3.3 Evaluation and Treatment

Anal sensation depends on an intact anal canal that allows a child to differentiate between solid, liquid, and gas contents. Anal canal preservation is a key principle of any surgical approach to HD (Fig. 26.5). The Duhamel operation provides less risk of sensory damage but has other complications (e.g., fecaloma) absent from Soave and Swenson procedures.

Damage to the anal canal is an irreversible and avoidable cause of incontinence, highlighting the importance of prevention over treatment [7]. Preservation of 1.5–2.0 cm of the distal rectum is critical. Many experts recommend advancing the hooks of the Lone Star™ above the anal canal [2]. The use of the anorectal line (ARL, the ring at the top of the anal columns) to begin dissection, preserving the surgical anal canal between the anal verge and the ARL, may improve continence.

The sphincter mechanism can be compromised from over-vigorous retraction during primary repair, resulting in lax and/or incompetent sphincters (Fig. 26.5c, d). Gentle graded dilation of the anus only up to a Hegar dilator size two steps greater than the number that corresponds to the age of the patient in months (i.e., 14 Hegar for a 12-month-old), and then placement of the Lone Star™ or other retractor may also limit iatrogenic injury [7].

Sphincter damage has been confirmed in adult studies using anorectal manometry, demonstrating a correlation between functional outcome and anal resting pressures in adults who have repaired HD [21]. Low postoperative resting anal pressures may indicate sphincter damage [2, 55]. Sphincter function can often be indirectly inferred from physical examination (Fig. 26.5) [32].

Factors associated with a damaged anal canal (absent pectinate line, rectal mucosa anastomosed to skin or anoderm) were found to be associated with the need for reoperation compared to symptomatic children with an intact canal in a recent report [2]. Enemas and a coordinated bowel regimen were used in 45/54 patients, with only 2 requiring permanent ileostomy [2]. Even in those children in whom anatomic structures have been damaged, achievement of continence is usually still possible with a daily enema regimen. However, it may be much difficult to obtain in this group. Antegrade enema administration, either through an appendicostomy or cecostomy, may be another option.

Motility is the third factor required for continence. Colonic motility studies are available at some institutions but are not typically part of an initial evaluation. Constipated patients (overflow incontinence) demonstrate an absence of high-magnitude propagating contractions. Colonic motility can be estimated via a contrast enema [33], and categorized as due to hyper- (normal colon caliber on contrast enema; Fig. 26.13) or hypomotile bowel (dilated colon on contrast enema; Fig. 26.14).

Most commonly, incontinence is due to overflow or *pseudo-incontinence* caused by the overflow of liquid fecal material around solid impacted stool in the neo-rectum. Those with intact anatomic structures are treated with laxatives or enemas if they have colonic hypomotility. Pseudo-incontinence will usually respond. High-volume enemas (≥500 mL) are indicated for those who fail a laxative trial. Patients refractory to treatment may also benefit from laparoscopic biopsies, motility, and manometry studies.

Children with hyper-motile, true incontinence are initially managed with loperamide, water-soluble fiber, and dietary modifications. Small-volume enemas (300–500 mL) and a constipating diet are used if needed.

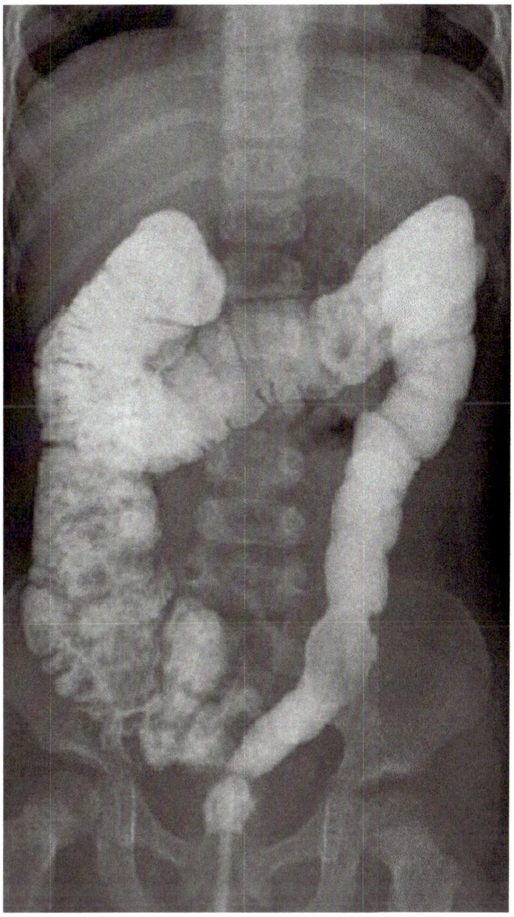

Fig. 26.13 Contrast enema of a patient with a nondilated colon (hypermotile) following Hirschsprung pull-through. (Reprinted with permission [33])

In both hyper- or hypomotile children with intact anatomy, the initial enema regimen can usually be converted to oral laxatives once continence is achieved, assessed at 6–12-month intervals [33].

Most children with HD will achieve satisfactory continence with time. Many studies demonstrate improving incontinence rates with age [12, 24, 38].

26.3.4 Enterocolitis

Hirschsprung-Associated Enterocolitis (HAEC) is the major cause of morbidity and mortality in

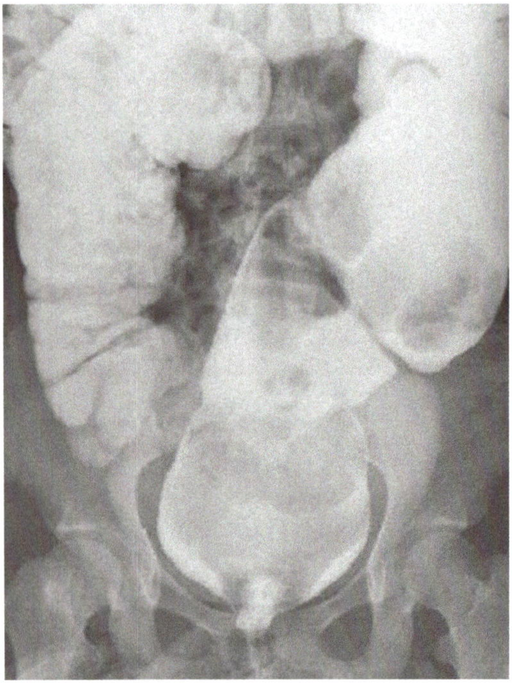

Fig. 26.14 Contrast enema of a patient with a dilated colon (hypomotile) following Hirschsprung pull-through. (Reprinted with permission [33])

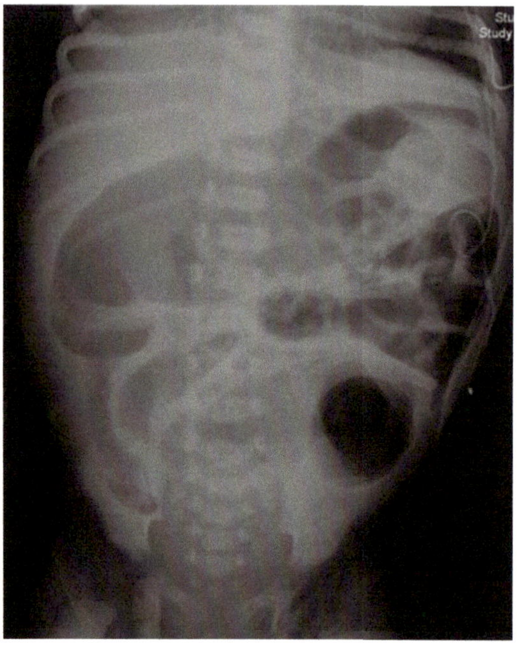

Fig. 26.15 Anteroposterior radiograph demonstrates classic findings of enterocolitis including moderate distension of bowel lumen and edema of bowel wall

HD and is thoroughly discussed in Chap. 13. It is briefly reviewed here due to its interrelation to other early and late complications (Fig. 26.15).

26.3.4.1 Definition

The definition of HAEC has long been problematic, accounting for variations in the reported incidence and results of treatment. The common symptoms – abdominal distension, discomfort, loose foul-smelling stools, fever, decreased appetite, lethargy – are nonspecific and vague (Fig. 26.16). Chronic or recurrent enterocolitis may also lead to failure to thrive.

The simplified classification recently recommended by the APSA HD interest group divides HAEC into possible, definitive, and severe categories, based on clinical history, physical findings, and plain films [19].

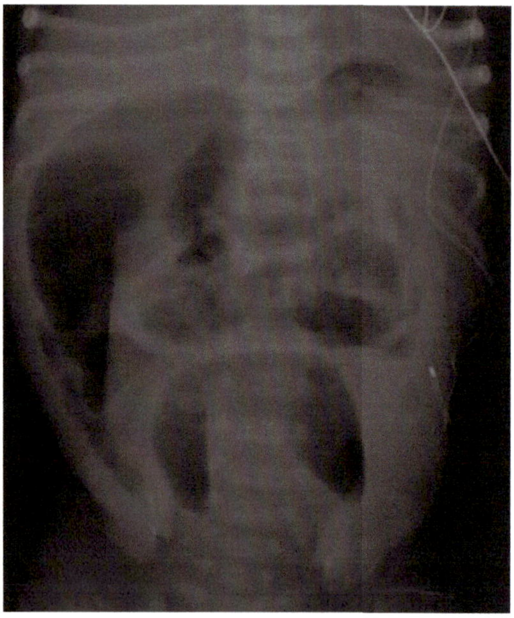

Fig. 26.16 Lateral radiograph demonstrates significant air–fluid levels in a patient with enterocolitis

26.3.4.2 Etiology

Anything that interferes with the normal passage of stool (retained aganglionosis, TZPT, dysmotility, stricture, twist in the pull-through, internal anal sphincter achalasia, or tight muscular cuff following the Soave procedure) can result in stasis and predispose the patient to enterocolitis [31]. However, the etiology of enterocolitis is multivariable and poorly understood, and obstruction alone is likely neither sufficient nor necessary for its development. Abnormalities in the intestinal microbiome (dominance of fungi and bacteria predisposing patients to development of HAEC) [17], impaired intestinal mucosal barrier function (abnormal goblet cells and mucus) [52], altered systemic immune system [18], and bacterial translocation are all possible causative agents [19].

26.3.4.3 Incidence

Enterocolitis has a widely variable incidence of between 15% and 40%, with a mean of about 30% [16, 19, 24, 53, 55]. The incidence of HAEC has no clear relationship with the type of pull-through performed. Wide variation in the postoperative management (postoperative dilations, irrigations, frequency of follow-up, use of botulinum toxin) render comparisons between different operative approaches difficult. Early series noted a higher incidence of HAEC after primary pull-through [12, 51], but increased recognition and more accurate detection in recent years, corresponding with more widespread use of primary pull-through may be the explanation. Down syndrome, long-segment aganglionosis, and prior HAEC are markers for an increased risk of HAEC [19, 21].

26.3.4.4 Prevention

Prevention of enterocolitis is preferable to treatment. Dilations, irrigations, botulinum toxin injections, probiotics, and antibiotic prophylaxis have all been used as preventative measures. Probiotics do not appear to provide a significant reduction in the risk of HAEC, although the quality of the evidence is low [37].

26.3.4.5 Treatment

Due to the potentially life-threatening nature of the disease, erring toward overtreatment of borderline presentations is advisable.

Mild "suspected" HAEC may require only rectal irrigations and oral metronidazole. Definite HAEC may be treated with rectal irrigations, *nil* per os, intravenous hydration, IV metronidazole or broad-spectrum (ampicillin/gentamycin or piperacillin/tazobactam) antibiotics. Severe enterocolitis is life-threatening and may necessitate admission to the PICU as well as the aforementioned, with proximal diversion and/or colectomy [19]. Sepsis, hemodynamic instability, and clinical deterioration indicate the development of toxic megacolon and the need for emergent operation (usually abdominal colectomy and ileostomy). Mortality from fulminant HAEC is considerable.

26.3.4.6 Recurrence

Recurrent HAEC is an indication to search for an underlying late complication, such as mechanical obstruction or a pathologic abnormality. The algorithm is outlined in the obstruction section. If no treatable cause is identified in a child with recurrent HAEC, botulinum toxin injection is recommended, since it may decrease the need for recurrent hospitalization [19].

26.3.5 Voiding and Sexual Dysfunction

There is an increasing recognition that children with HD also have extraintestinal complications. These include impacts on growth and development, urinary and sexual dysfunction, and impaired quality of life into adulthood [12]. These topics are more fully reviewed in Chaps. 31 and 32, and are briefly reviewed here as they relate to complications.

Any operation requiring pelvic dissection risks injury to the nerves controlling bladder and sexual function. The tissue anterolateral to the rectum contains most of the parasympathetic nerve fibers innervating the bladder. Staying very close to the rectal wall during dissection and avoiding blunt dissection in the retrorectal space (which may tear the visceral fascia) may be preventative. Duhamel's and Soave's modifications were designed to reduce the risk of injury to the delicate pelvic structures.

Parasympathetic denervation to the pelvic splanchnic nerves will lead to a flaccid bladder whereas sympathetic denervation to the hypogastric nerves may result in loss of bladder compliance and incompetence of the bladder neck and posterior urethra [12].

Obstructive complications often lead to rectal distension and dilation, a well-recognized cause of urinary symptoms unrelated to any neurogenic operative trauma. Patients with Down syndrome appear to be a unique subset of HD with a higher prevalence of urinary symptoms after surgery [9]. Patients with postoperative urinary complaints should be evaluated with renal and bladder ultrasound and possibly voiding cystourethrography and urodynamic studies. However, long-term voiding dysfunction is uncommon in HD patients [39, 48, 54].

Data regarding sexual dysfunction in adults who have undergone repair of HD is limited due to difficulties in obtaining long-term follow-up. Incontinence and soiling significantly interfere with sexual function. Females may have a higher incidence of sexual dysfunction than males. The incidence of erectile dysfunction is low (1–2%) [48, 54].

26.4 Other

26.4.1 Quality of Life

Long-term outcomes are thoroughly reviewed in Chap. 32. Although urgency, constipation, and more frequent stooling are sources of concern and frustration, frank incontinence with fecal soiling is physically, emotionally, and psychologically disabling. It has a significant impact on patients' social and emotional development and is the primary impact factor determining quality of life [12, 20, 48]. Studies on long-term quality of life (QoL) parameters indicate poorer outcomes for patients with HD compared to controls. The longer the follow-up, the fewer are the number of studies and the poorer the quality of evidence. Improvement in bowel function over time is reported in multiple studies [38, 48].

Importantly, many of the long-term studies find that many adult HD patients report that long-term complications (QoL, sexual and urologic function) were never adequately discussed with them and that their transition from pediatric to adult care providers was difficult or problematic [20].

26.4.2 Down Syndrome

A meta-analysis of Down syndrome and HD found an incidence of Down syndrome in HD patients of 7.3% (based on population prevalence, an incidence of about 0.15% would be expected) [15]. Conversely, less than 3% of those with Down syndrome had HD. Long-segment disease was more common in the Down group. Enterocolitis and soiling were increased, and the mortality for Down patients was higher. Several studies have shown higher rates of HAEC and poorer functional outcomes [12, 48].

26.4.3 Long-Term Cancer Risk

A small percentage (2.5–5%) of HD patients carry MEN2A RET-mutations (discussed in Chap. 12), which are associated with an increased risk of developing of medullary thyroid carcinoma [48]. Limited data suggests the increased risk is small [40].

26.4.4 Total Colonic Aganglionosis

Total colonic aganglionosis (TCA) is defined as aganglionosis affecting the entire colon and less than 50 cm of small bowel and is discussed in Chap. 18. It is uncommon (<10% of HD, or an incidence of about 1 in 50,000) [12]. It is associated with poorer functional outcomes, a higher chance of requiring a permanent stoma, and an increased risk of HAEC [48]. Frank fecal incontinence has been reported in as many as one-third of TCA patients after treatment with a permanent stoma required in 5–18% [48]. Somatic growth impairment is also seen in 1–15% of children. The risk of complications in some reports appears to correlate with the type of pull-through operation, with a higher risk of long-term complications when extensive segments of aganglionic bowel are utilized in the repair [22]. The mortality rate in these children is increased as well [12].

26.4.5 Redo Pull-Through

Early complications from the primary pull-through operation are often the primary cause of the eventual need for reoperation.

Redo pull-through operations (discussed in Chap. 25) are necessary in less than 5% of patients after initial repair [42, 44, 56]. The indications for reoperation can be categorized as [34] anatomic complications (twisted pull-through, stricture or frozen (scarred) pelvis); [1] Histopathologic complications (aganglionosis, transition zone pull-through); and [2] other (rectocutaneous or other fistulas, inflammatory/HAEC).

The most common cause of reoperation is retained aganglionosis or transition zone pull-through, followed by mechanical and anatomic complications [10, 14, 28, 44, 46].

26.4.6 Mortality

The mortality rate from HD is under 2% in most series [15, 50]. A significant reduction in mortality has occurred over the past 40 years. This may be attributed to improved resuscitation and management of comorbidities, use of parenteral nutrition, earlier detection and prevention of enterocolitis, and improved operative and peri-operative care. Long-segment disease and Down syndrome are associated with increased mortality [15]. Apart from children who die of associated cardiac or other major anomalies [47], toxic enterocolitis remains the most common cause of disease-related postoperative death [19]. The mortality of HAEC in previously undiagnosed HD is particularly high.

26.5 Conclusion and Future Directions

HD is a neurogenic intestinal obstruction and should be viewed as a chronic illness. A wide spectrum of complications has been reported following definitive repair of HD. Enterocolitis remains the most serious late complication following primary pull-through. The great majority of children become well-adjusted in adulthood. Early development milestone deficiencies appear to improve over time. The greatest negative impact on quality of life is due to fecal soiling. Rates of fecal incontinence in adolescents and adults have been reported as high as 36–48% with only about half of adults achieving bowel function comparable to controls [48]. Incontinence has been associated in adulthood with lower-emotion quality-of-life scores, limitations on personal and sexual relationships [38], alterations in diet (55.7%), difficulties in peer relationships (15.6%), and school absences (13.3%) and poor academic performance [12].

Continued advances in our understanding of anatomic specific complications and following systematic workup when issues arise will help identify and treat complications. While many patients with HD do well following definitive operation regardless of the technique employed, many are left with significant impacts on their quality of life. Appropriate preoperative conference with family members must include a candid discussion of the importance of realistic expectations and the need for close parental surveillance for late complications. It is important that the family and patient understand that issues with continence may arise so that these issues can be addressed when they occur and minimize the psychosocial impact. Children should be regularly followed post pull-through into young adulthood to assist in identifying issues with soiling and constipation as well as providing anticipatory guidance and transitional care when appropriate.

References

1. Aworanti OM, Mcdowell DT, Martin IM, Hung J, Quinn F. Comparative review of functional outcomes post surgery for Hirschsprung's disease utilizing the paediatric incontinence and constipation scoring system. Pediatr Surg Int. 2012;28(11):1071–8.
2. Bischoff A, Frischer J, Knod JL, Dickie B, Levitt MA, Holder M, et al. Damaged anal canal as a cause of fecal incontinence after surgical repair for Hirschsprung

disease – a preventable and under-reported complication. J Pediatr Surg. 2017;52(4):549–53.
3. Bischoff A, Levitt MA, Peña A. Total colonic aganglionosis: a surgical challenge. How to avoid complications? Pediatr Surg Int. 2011;27(10):1047–52.
4. Bradnock TJ, Knight M, Kenny S, Nair M, Walker GM. The use of stomas in the early management of Hirschsprung's disease: findings of a national, prospective cohort study. J Pediatr Surg. 2017;52(9):1451–7.
5. Church JT, Gadepalli SK, Talishinsky T, Teitelbaum DH, Jarboe MD. Ultrasound-guided intrasphincteric botulinum toxin injection relieves obstructive defecation due to Hirschsprung's disease and internal anal sphincter achalasia. J Pediatr Surg. 2017;52(1):74–8.
6. Collins MH, Reyes-Mugica M. Defining the transition zone of Hirschsprung disease. Pediatr Dev Pathol. 2013;16(4):235–6.
7. De la Torre L, Cogley K, Santos K, Morales O, Calisto J. The anal canal is the fine line between "fecal incontinence and colitis" after a pull-through for Hirschsprung disease. J Pediatr Surg. 2017;52(12):2011–7.
8. Dickie BH, Webb KM, Eradi B, Levitt MA. The problematic soave cuff in Hirschsprung disease: manifestations and treatment. J Pediatr Surg. 2014;49(1):77–80. discussion 80–81
9. Dingemans AJM, Reck-Burneo CA, Fuchs M, Sanchez AV, Lane VA, Hoover E, et al. Urinary outcomes in patients with Down's syndrome and Hirschsprung's disease Eur J Pediatr Surg Off J Austrian Assoc Pediatr Surg Al Z Kinderchir. 2018.
10. Dingemans AJM, van der Steeg HJJ, Rassouli-Kirchmeier R, Linssen MW, van Rooij IALM, de Blaauw I. Redo pull-through surgery in Hirschsprung disease: short-term clinical outcome. J Pediatr Surg. 2017;52(9):1446–50.
11. Elhalaby EA, Hashish A, Elbarbary MM, Soliman HA, Wishahy MK, Elkholy A, et al. Transanal one-stage endorectal pull-through for Hirschsprung's disease: a multicenter study. J Pediatr Surg. 2004;39(3):345–51. discussion 345–51
12. Engum SA, Grosfeld JL. Long-term results of treatment of Hirschsprung's disease. Semin Pediatr Surg. 2004;13(4):273–85.
13. Feng C, Sidhwa F, Cameron DB, Glass C, Rangel SJ. Rates and burden of surgical site infections associated with pediatric colorectal surgery: insight from the National Surgery Quality Improvement Program. J Pediatr Surg. 2016;51(6):970–4.
14. Friedmacher F, Puri P. Residual aganglionosis after pull-through operation for Hirschsprung's disease: a systematic review and meta-analysis. Pediatr Surg Int. 2011;27(10):1053–7.
15. Friedmacher F, Puri P. Hirschsprung's disease associated with down syndrome: a meta-analysis of incidence, functional outcomes and mortality. Pediatr Surg Int. 2013;29(9):937–46.
16. Frykman PK, Kim S, Wester T, Nordenskjöld A, Kawaguchi A, Hui TT, et al. Critical evaluation of the Hirschsprung-associated enterocolitis (HAEC) score: a multicenter study of 116 children with Hirschsprung disease. J Pediatr Surg. 2017.
17. Frykman PK, Nordenskjöld A, Kawaguchi A, Hui TT, Granström AL, Cheng Z, et al. Characterization of bacterial and fungal microbiome in children with Hirschsprung disease with and without a history of enterocolitis: a multicenter study. PLoS One [Internet]. 2015 [cited 2018 Jul 6];10(4). Available from: https://www.ncbi.nlm.nih.gov/pmc/articles/PMC4409062/.
18. Gosain A, Barlow-Anacker AJ, Erickson CS, Pierre JF, Heneghan AF, Epstein ML, et al. Impaired cellular immunity in the murine neural crest conditional deletion of endothelin receptor-B model of Hirschsprung's disease. PLoS One [Internet]. 2015 [cited 2018 Jul 6];10(6). Available from: https://www.ncbi.nlm.nih.gov/pmc/articles/PMC4465674/.
19. Gosain A, Frykman PK, Cowles RA, Horton J, Levitt M, Rothstein DH, et al. Guidelines for the diagnosis and management of Hirschsprung-associated enterocolitis. Pediatr Surg Int. 2017;33(5):517–21.
20. Granström AL, Danielson J, Husberg B, Nordenskjöld A, Wester T. Adult outcomes after surgery for Hirschsprung's disease: evaluation of bowel function and quality of life. J Pediatr Surg. 2015;50(11):1865–9.
21. Heikkinen M, Rintala R, Luukkonen P. Long-term anal sphincter performance after surgery for Hirschsprung's disease. J Pediatr Surg. 1997;32(10):1443–6.
22. Hoehner JC, Ein SH, Shandling B, Kim PC. Long-term morbidity in total colonic aganglionosis. J Pediatr Surg. 1998;33(7):961–6.
23. Huang EY, Tolley EA, Blakely ML, Langham MR. Changes in hospital utilization and management of Hirschsprung disease: analysis using the kids' inpatient database. Ann Surg. 2013;257(2):371–5.
24. Huang W-K, Li X-L, Zhang J, Zhang S-C. Prevalence, risk factors, and prognosis of postoperative complications after surgery for Hirschsprung disease. J Gastrointest Surg. 2017;22(2):335–43.
25. Jarvi K, Laitakari EM, Koivusalo A, Rintala RJ, Pakarinen MP. Bowel function and gastrointestinal quality of life among adults operated for hirschsprung disease during childhood: a population-based study. Ann Surg. 2010;252(6):977–81.
26. Kapur RP, Kennedy AJ. Transitional zone pull through: surgical pathology considerations. Semin Pediatr Surg. 2012;21(4):291–301.
27. Kim AC, Langer JC, Pastor AC, Zhang L, Sloots CEJ, Hamilton NA, et al. Endorectal pull-through for Hirschsprung's disease-a multicenter, long-term comparison of results: transanal vs transabdominal approach. J Pediatr Surg. 2010;45(6):1213–20.
28. Langer JC. Repeat pull-through surgery for complicated Hirschsprung's disease: indications, techniques, and results. J Pediatr Surg. 1999;34(7):1136–41.
29. Langer JC, Durrant AC, de la Torre L, Teitelbaum DH, Minkes RK, Caty MG, et al. One-stage transanal soave pullthrough for Hirschsprung disease: a multicenter experience with 141 children. Ann Surg. 2003;238(4):569–83. discussion 583–5

30. Langer JC, Rollins MD, Levitt M, Gosain A, de la Torre L, Kapur RP, et al. Guidelines for the management of postoperative obstructive symptoms in children with Hirschsprung disease. Pediatr Surg Int. 2017;33(5):1–4.
31. Levitt MA, Dickie B, Peña A. Evaluation and treatment of the patient with Hirschsprung disease who is not doing well after a pull-through procedure. Semin Pediatr Surg. 2010;19(2):146–53.
32. Levitt MA, Dickie B, Peña A. The Hirschsprungs patient who is soiling after what was considered a "successful" pull-through. Semin Pediatr Surg. 2012;21(4):344–53.
33. Levitt MA, Martin CA, Olesevich M, Bauer CL, Jackson LE, Peña A. Hirschsprung disease and fecal incontinence: diagnostic and management strategies. J Pediatr Surg. 2009;44(1):271–7. discussion 277
34. Little DC, Snyder CL. Chapter 29: early and late complications following operative repair of Hirschsprung's disease. In: Hirschsprung's disease and allied disorders. 3rd ed. Berlin, Heidelberg: Springer; 2008. p. 375–7.
35. Lu C, Hou G, Liu C, Geng Q, Xu X, Zhang J, et al. Single-stage transanal endorectal pull-through procedure for correction of Hirschsprung disease in neonates and nonneonates: a multicenter study. J Pediatr Surg. 2017;52(7):1102–7.
36. Menezes M, Puri P. Long-term outcome of patients with enterocolitis complicating Hirschsprung's disease. Pediatr Surg Int. 2006;22(4):316–8.
37. Nakamura H, Lim T, Puri P. Probiotics for the prevention of Hirschsprung-associated enterocolitis: a systematic review and meta-analysis. Pediatr Surg Int. 2017;34(2):189–93.
38. Neuvonen MI, Kyrklund K, Rintala RJ, Pakarinen MP. Bowel function and quality of life after transanal endorectal pull-through for Hirschsprung disease: controlled outcomes up to adulthood. Ann Surg. 2017;265(3):622–9.
39. Onishi S, Nakame K, Kaji T, Kawano M, Moriguchi T, Sugita K, et al. The bowel function and quality of life of Hirschsprung disease patients who have reached 18 years of age or older - the long-term outcomes after undergoing the transabdominal soave procedure. J Pediatr Surg. 2017;52(12):2001–5.
40. Pakarinen MP, Rintala RJ, Koivusalo A, Heikkinen M, Lindahl H, Pukkala E. Increased incidence of medullary thyroid carcinoma in patients treated for Hirschsprung's disease. J Pediatr Surg. 2005;40(10):1532–4.
41. Pini Prato A, Gentilino V, Giunta C, Avanzini S, Mattioli G, Parodi S, et al. Hirschsprung disease: do risk factors of poor surgical outcome exist? J Pediatr Surg. 2008;43(4):612–9.
42. Pini-Prato A, Mattioli G, Giunta C, Avanzini S, Magillo P, Bisio GM, et al. Redo surgery in Hirschsprung disease: what did we learn? Unicentric experience on 70 patients. J Pediatr Surg. 2010;45(4):747–54.
43. Pratap A, Gupta DK, Shakya VC, Adhikary S, Tiwari A, Shrestha P, et al. Analysis of problems, complications, avoidance and management with transanal pull-through for Hirschsprung disease. J Pediatr Surg. 2007;42(11):1869–76.
44. Ralls MW, Coran AG, Teitelbaum DH. Redo pullthrough for Hirschsprung disease. Pediatr Surg Int. 2017;33(4):455–60.
45. Rassouli R, Holschneider AM, Bolkenius M, Menardi G, Becker MR, Schaarschmidt K, et al. Long-term results of Rehbein's procedure: a retrospective study in German-speaking countries. Eur J Pediatr Surg. 2003;13:187–94.
46. Reck-Burneo CA. Interventions for patients with Hirschsprung disease with obstructive symptoms after pull-through: a review of 62 cases: American Pediatric Surgical Association Annual Meeting; 2018.
47. Rescorla FJ, Morrison AM, Engles D, West KW, Grosfeld JL. Hirschsprung's disease. Evaluation of mortality and long-term function in 260 cases. Arch Surg Chic Ill. 1992;127(8):934–41. discussion 941–942
48. Rintala RJ, Pakarinen MP. Long-term outcomes of Hirschsprung's disease. Semin Pediatr Surg. 2012;21(4):336–43.
49. Seo S, Miyake H, Hock A, Koike Y, Yong C, Lee C, et al. Duhamel and transanal endorectal pull-throughs for Hirschsprung' disease: a systematic review and meta-analysis. Eur J Pediatr Surg Off J Austrian Assoc Pediatr Surg Al Z Kinderchir. 2018;28(1):81–8.
50. Sherman JO, Snyder ME, Weitzman JJ, Jona JZ, Gillis DA, O'Donnell B, et al. A 40-year multinational retrospective study of 880 Swenson procedures. J Pediatr Surg. 1989;24(8):833–8.
51. Teitelbaum DH, Cilley RE, Sherman NJ, Bliss D, Uitvlugt ND, Renaud EJ, et al. A decade of experience with the primary pull-through for Hirschsprung disease in the newborn period. Ann Surg. 2000;232(3):372–80.
52. Thiagarajah JR, Yildiz H, Carlson T, Thomas AR, Steiger C, Pieretti A, et al. Altered goblet cell differentiation and surface mucus properties in Hirschsprung disease. PLoS ONE [Internet]. 2014 [cited 2018 Jul 6];9(6). Available from: https://www.ncbi.nlm.nih.gov/pmc/articles/PMC4063789/.
53. Tomuschat C, Zimmer J, Puri P. Laparoscopic-assisted pull-through operation for Hirschsprung's disease: a systematic review and meta-analysis. 2016. Available from: http://www.ncbi.nlm.nih.gov/pubmed/27369964 http://link.springer.com/10.1007/s00383-016-3910-5.
54. Versteegh HP, Johal NS, de Blaauw I, Stanton MP. Urological and sexual outcome in patients with Hirschsprung disease: a systematic review. J Pediatr Urol. 2016;12(6):352–60.
55. Wester T, Granström AL. Hirschsprung disease-bowel function beyond childhood. Semin Pediatr Surg. 2017;26(5):322–7.
56. Zimmer J, Tomuschat C, Puri P. Long-term results of transanal pull-through for Hirschsprung's disease: a meta-analysis. Pediatr Surg Int. 2016;32(8):743–9.

Morphological Basis of Persistent Bowel Problems Following a Properly Performed Pull-Through Operation for Hirschsprung's Disease

27

David Coyle and Prem Puri

Contents

D. Coyle
Temple Street Children's University Hospital, Dublin, Ireland

P. Puri (✉)
National Children's Research Centre, Our Lady's Children's Hospital, Crumlin, Dublin, Ireland
e-mail: prem.puri@ncrc.ie

P. Puri (ed.), *Hirschsprung's Disease and Allied Disorders*,
https://doi.org/10.1007/978-3-030-15647-3_27

27.1 Introduction

Hirschsprung's disease (HSCR) is the most common congenital gut motility disorder and is characterized by the absence of ganglion cells and the presence of hypertrophic nerve trunks affecting the distal bowel (aganglionosis). In the majority of patients (~80%) the extent of aganglionosis is limited to the rectosigmoid region, while a longer segment extending proximally from the internal anal sphincter (IAS) is involved in the remaining ~20% [1]. The gold-standard treatment for this condition is the pull-through (PT) operation. While several variations on this procedure exist, the underlying principle of the PT operation is the transanal resection of the tonically contracted aganglionic segment of bowel with anastomosis of the normally innervated colon to a point just inside the dentate line, preserving the IAS [2].

Despite undergoing a technically well-performed PT operation, many patients experience persistent bowel symptoms at long-term follow-up, including constipation, soiling, and recurrent Hirschsprung-associated enterocolitis (HAEC) [3, 4]. While a demonstrable mechanical cause can be shown in many of these patients, a proportion is experiencing ganglionic bowel dysfunction as the underlying cause. This chapter explores the phenomenon of ganglionic bowel dysfunction in HSCR, including potential mechanisms by which it occurs.

27.2 Causes of Persistent Bowel Symptoms Following Pull-Through Surgery for Hirschsprung's Disease

The range of operations performed to correct HSCR and the varied means of monitoring postoperative outcome (parental questionnaire/validated scoring systems/subjective assessment) make comparison of the outcomes obtained in each study difficult, with the results of each being judged on the merits of the study. For ease, persistent symptoms following PT surgery can be categorized as obstructive symptoms (constipation, recurrent HAEC) and incontinence symptoms [5].

Assessing the prevalence of constipation after PT surgery depends on how it is defined. Studies with statistically meaningful numbers of patients have reported constipation ranging from 9.8% to 55% [3, 6–12]. Postoperative HAEC occurs in 2–35% of patients who have undergone a PT operation [13, 14].

Fecal incontinence and associated soiling is one of the key contributors to the quality of life reported by patients who undergo PT surgery for HSCR. Normal fecal continence is a function of rectal reservoir function, anal canal sensation, and normal anal sphincter function [3]. While loss of rectal reservoir is an inherent side effect of the PT procedure, loss of anal canal sensation may occur due to the commencement of endorectal dissection too close to the dentate line. Interference with the sphincter complex may occur owing to excessive stretching during total transanal endorectal PT or retrorectal dissection during a Duhamel PT [15].

As with constipation, the incidence of post-PT incontinence and soiling may be considerably higher when independently assessed than has been previously thought [3]. Soiling has been reported in various follow-up studies in 12–56% of patients, a small proportion of whom are patients with true incontinence as opposed to overflow soiling [6, 8, 9, 11, 12, 16].

Patients with persistent bowel symptoms may fall into one or more of the following categories of patients: (1) those with mechanical obstruction, due to a stricture or an obstructive cuff of tunica muscularis following a Soave PT procedure; (2) those with recurrent, retained, or acquired aganglionosis; (3) patients with intestinal dysmotility; (4) patients with internal anal achalasia; (5) functional megacolon due to stool holding behaviors [4]. While those with a mechanical obstruction or a retained segment of aganglionic bowel have a demonstrable surgically treatable cause, as is also somewhat the case with internal anal sphincter achalasia, getting control over ongoing bowel symptoms in those with dysmotility or an acquired megacolon can be challenging.

27.3 Investigation of Persistent Bowel Symptoms After the Pull-Through Operation for Hirschsprung's Disease

All patients presenting with persistent bowel symptoms following a pull-through operation should have a detailed clinical assessment, specifically trying to elucidate information about abdominal distension, explosive stools, consistency of stool, vomiting, weight gain, use of any medications that affect gastrointestinal motility, and details about the PT operation and any postoperative complications. A physical examination will also yield information about nutritional status, abdominal distension, and the gross appearance of the anal canal, and whether there are any palpable strictures. A contrast enema is a valuable initial investigation in these individuals as it provides information regarding bowel caliber and motility [4, 5].

An examination of the anal canal under anesthesia is performed to check the integrity of the anal canal, whether the dentate line is intact in its full circumference, and depending on the type of PT operation performed, whether there is an obstructing Soave cuff, or a dilated rectal pouch. Retained aganglionic or transition zone bowel is evaluated by means of a full-thickness rectal biopsy. In the absence of a mechanical obstruction or a damaged anal canal/disrupted dentate line, motility studies including anal manometry and a radio-opaque marker study may provide information about localized or diffuse dysmotility and colonic hyperactivity or atony. Management options depending on the nature of the abnormality found will range from anal dilatations or a redo PT operation, to medical treatment with loperamide, dietary modification, bowel irrigations, or intra-sphincteric botulinum toxin therapy [4, 5].

27.4 The Extent of the Transition Zone in Hirschsprung's Disease

The transition zone (TZ) represents the segment of colon in HSCR at the interface between the tonically contracted aganglionic colon and the "normal" colon, which contains ganglion cells and non-hypertrophied nerve trunks. Characteristically, TZ colon is neuroanatomically abnormal despite ganglion cells being present [17]. Localizing the transition zone prior to curative PT surgery for HSCR is important in operative planning, especially if considering a total transanal approach over a combined transabdominal-transanal approach.

By far the most widely used means of achieving this is the preoperative contrast enema [2]. Radiologically, the TZ typically appears as a site where large caliber dilated colon abruptly funnels into a narrow caliber colon [18, 19]. The presence of irregular contractions, spasm, and mucosal irregularities may also be used as secondary signs indicative of TZ colon [19].

However, concordance between the radiological TZ on contrast enema and the histological TZ varies widely. In neonates and in those with total colonic aganglionosis the colon can appear normal in caliber [20]. Frongia et al. reported 94.4% concordance of contrast enema with the histologically assessed proximal level of aganglionosis in those with RSHD, although it was only 50% accurate in those with LSHD [21]. Muller et al. levelled the TZ according to the corresponding vertebral level and found that, when those with no visible radiological transition zone are excluded, the levels of the radiological and histological TZ were only concordant in 51.9% of children with rectal or rectosigmoid aganglionosis [22]. A striking finding in a study of similar objective by Jamieson et al. was that the radiological TZ was consistently more distal than the histological TZ in those in whom there was discordance (62.5% of cases) [19].

Failure to recognize TZ colon can lead to a retained aganglionic segment following PT surgery, with the potential need for a redo-PT [23]. One retrospective series reported a TZ PT rate of 15% (13 patients), with incorrect interpretation of the intraoperative biopsy being the cause in 7 patients and partial circumference aganglionosis with a ganglionic intraoperative biopsy being the cause in 5 patients [17]. Lawal et al. reported a series of 93 patients referred with persistent obstructive symptoms following PT surgery for HSCR. As part of their workup, a rectal biopsy was performed. Twenty-five patients (26.9%) were found to have retained aganglionic or transition zone bowel, 11 of whom had rectosigmoid disease [23].

There are no agreed criteria defining what constitutes the histological TZ in HSCR. In general, features such as hypoganglionosis, the presence of hypertrophic nerve trunks, and partial circumference aganglionosis are widely quoted characteristics of transition zone colon [17]. Partial circumference abnormalities of innervation pattern have been well described in HSCR. White and Langer (2000) prospectively examined the circumferential distribution of ganglion cells in transition zone colon in 12 patients with HSCR and found a "leading edge" of ganglion cells extending for up to 2.4 cm in the myenteric plexus and 2.1 cm in the submucosal plexus [24]. Das et al. described a series of 20 patients with long-segment aganglionosis, in whom they evaluated the quadrantic innervation of the colon after pull-through surgery. They noted incomplete ganglionation of the full circumference in the transition zone in 8 patients [18].

Only a small number of studies have examined the total extent of the histological TZ in HSCR. A small series by Swaminathan and Kapur measured the gradient change in ganglion cell density in the myenteric plexus moving from aganglionic to ganglionic colon, and estimated the extent of the TZ to be 1–4 cm in length [25]. In a well-designed study examining the resected specimens of 15 individuals with short-segment HSCR (aganglionic segments 1–10 cm in length), Kapur and Kennedy examined several parameters in attempting to delineate the TZ: partial circumference (>1/8) aganglionosis; hypoganglionosis; hypertrophic submucosal nerves; Glut1-positive submucosal innervation; submucosal hyperganglionosis; and the presence of so-called ectopic ganglia in the lamina propria, tunica muscularis, or serosa. They found that the TZ extent was ~5 cm, while the extent of partial circumference aganglionosis is approximately 1–3 cm [26].

A more recent study from the same institution examines the features of the TZ in an expanded cohort of patients, 20% of whom had long-segment disease. In addition to the histological features described earlier, gangliosclerosis (the presence of dense fibrosis usually seen around the myenteric plexus) and eosinophilic periganglioneuritis were also included as criteria in describing the TZ. This study found that although major histological changes such as myenteric hypoganglionosis extended for ~5 cm proximal to the aganglionic segment, subtler histological changes such as eosinophilic periganglioneuritis could extend for up to 15 cm [27].

The use of intraoperative frozen section evaluation of seromuscular colonic biopsies looking for normal ganglionic distribution is a mandatory component of the PT operation for HSCR. Thick sections should be used (14–16 μm) to avoid an erroneous determination of sample aganglionosis [20]. Once a biopsy showing a normal ganglionic pattern is taken, most authors recommend citing the proximal resection margin at a point several centimeters proximal to this biopsy. In his description of the laparoscopic-assisted PT operation in 2002, Georgeson recommended a 10–15 cm margin of ganglionic colon be resected prior to completing the anastomosis [28]. Schäppi et al. recommend that the proximal resection margin be at least 2–3 cm of colon proximal to the first biopsy showing normal ganglion density [20]. Prior to completion of the colo-anal anastomosis it is also highly recommended that a full circumference donut of the proximal resection margin is evaluated by frozen section to allow detection of abnormal distribution of the ganglion cells.

27.5 Abnormalities of Excitatory and Inhibitory Innervation in the Ganglionic Colon in Hirschsprung's Disease

HSCR is one of the most common causes of neonatal intestinal obstruction. Functionally, it is characterized by the presence of a spastic contracted aganglionic segment of bowel causing functional obstruction, which manifests as failure to pass meconium, abdominal distension, bilious vomiting, and enterocolitis [2, 14, 29]. The underlying mechanism giving rise to this contracted segment is thought to concern an imbalance of excitatory and inhibitory neurotransmitters in the aganglionic colon [2].

Enteric smooth muscle cell contractility is modulated by opposing actions of inhibitory and excitatory neurotransmitters and neuropeptides released by the Enteric Nervous System (ENS). The chief excitatory neurotransmitter is acetylcholine (ACh), which acts through nicotinic and muscarinic acetylcholine receptors [30]. Key neuropeptides involved in eliciting an excitatory post-junctional response include substance P (SP), neurokinin A and neurokinin B, which exert their actions through neurokinin receptors NK1, NK2, and NK3, respectively [30]. A range of non-adrenergic non-cholinergic substances act as inhibitory neurotransmitters. Neuronal nitric oxide synthase (nNOS) catalyzes the conversion of L-arginine to nitric oxide in nerve cells. Its activity co-localizes with that of NADPH-diaphorase in nitrergic neurons [31]. Nitric oxide is one of the most important neurotransmitters involved in the relaxation of smooth muscle. It acts by inducing slow hyperpolarization in smooth muscle [30]. Vasoactive intestinal peptide (VIP) causes smooth muscle relaxation by inducing hyperpolarization through a mechanism that is, as of yet, poorly understood. Purinergic neurotransmission largely governs induction of the fast inhibitory junction potential in the smooth muscle syncytium through actions of ATP and β-NAD on purinergic receptors [30].

While data concerning the distribution of excitatory and inhibitory enteric motor neurons in the ganglionic bowel in humans with HSCR are sparse, two studies using a murine model of HSCR have reported abnormal patterns of expression. The earlier of the two studies described a deficiency of nitrergic and peptidergic neurons proximal to the aganglionic segment in lethal spotted mice [32]. More recently, Zaitoun et al. described an inverse relationship between neuronal density and expression of nNOS and choline acetyltransferase, a key enzyme in ACh synthesis, in endothelin B-receptor (EDNRB)-deficient mice, with nNOS expression being reduced in aganglionic bowel and relatively elevated in ganglionated colon, while the converse was true of ChAT [33]. A similar relationship has been reported in a small cohort of children with HSCR. When compared to healthy colon, the imbalance in expression of these two neurotransmitters was not merely due to relative deficiency but rather pathological overexpression of ChAT and nNOS in aganglionic and ganglionic bowel, respectively. Such abnormality may account for the segmental or generalized atony seen in the colons of some patients following a PT operation. This same study found that VIP and Substance P were expressed at normal levels in the ganglionic colon in HSCR [34].

27.6 5-Hydroxytryptamine (Serotonin) and Hirschsprung-Associated Enterocolitis

Hirschsprung-associated enterocolitis (HAEC) is the most serious complication of HSCR, and is the leading cause of disease-related mortality. It occurs in 17–50% of patients with HSCR and may occur before or after a pull through operation [14, 35]. Although a scoring system for HAEC exists, there is no agreed definition of this condition. It is typically described as an inflammatory disease of the colon leading to a spectrum of symptoms ranging from abdominal distension and loose stools to life-threatening toxic megacolon [2, 36]. The etiology and pathogenesis of HAEC are still incompletely understood. It has been proposed that intestinal barrier dysfunction, abnormal innate immunity, and the presence of a disturbed microbiome are all potential contributors to its etiology [14]. However, given that the primary abnormality in HSCR is the absence of enteric ganglia in the distal colon, it follows that the enteric nervous system may have a role in the pathogenesis.

5-Hydroxytryptamine (5-HT), commonly known as serotonin, is a major neuroendocrine signaling molecule. While the gut is the single largest reservoir of 5-HT, the wide range of its functions therein have only been elucidated relatively recently. Most enteric serotonin is stored in the mucosa in the enterochromaffin (EC) cells. Approximately 1–5% of enteric serotonin is stored in the serotonergic enteric nerves, where it acts as a neurotransmitter [37, 38]. The rate limiting step in the synthesis of 5-HT is the conversion of L-tryptophan to 5-hydroxytryptophan by tryptophan hydroxylase (TPH). The conversion of 5-hydroxytryptophan to 5-HT then occurs rapidly through the actions of L-amino acid decarboxylase [39]. However, the synthesis pathway of enteric 5-HT differs depending on whether 5-HT is being synthesized in EC cells, where the TPH1 isozyme of TPH predominates, or in serotonergic neurons, where TPH2 predominates [37, 39].

5-HT has many roles, including activation of intrinsic reflexes such as peristalsis, vasodilation, and secretion. When released from EC cells, mucosal 5-HT has been demonstrated to promote inflammation – an activity that is counterbalanced by its re-uptake via the serotonin transporter (SERT) [37, 40]. Abnormal mucosal 5-HT activity has been demonstrated in inflammatory and functional bowel disorders such as ulcerative colitis and irritable bowel syndrome [41]. Conversely, neuronal 5-HT is anti-inflammatory and neuroprotective, an activity that has obvious importance in the setting of inflammation and enterocolitis, as neuronal damage can frequently result [40]. It has previously been reported that populations of mucosal enterochromaffin cells are deficient in the ganglionic bowel of children with HSCR who have previously had HAEC. It is unclear if this is a facilitator or an effect of HAEC [42].

Serotonergic nerves have previously been shown to make extensive synapses with myenteric ICC – the pacemaker cells of the bowel – as well as nitrergic neurons. This indicates a functional role for serotonergic neurons in modulating nitrergic neurotransmission and pacemaker activity [43]. The intimate spatial arrangement of serotonergic nerves with nNOS-positive nerves is also important as it is thought that, through the intercession of descending inhibitory serotonergic neuronal activity, the release of nitric oxide from nNOS-positive neurons suppresses excitatory cholinergic activity and limits the rate at which high-amplitude peristaltic activity is propagated in mice [44]. Using TPH2 as a surrogate marker for neuronal 5-HT, it has been shown in children with HSCR that serotonergic nerves are reduced in density in the ganglionic colon of children who had experienced HAEC prior to their PT procedure, with the exception of children who had undergone a diverting/levelling colostomy in the neonatal period. The finding of reduced serotonergic neuron density in the aganglionic, transition zone, and ganglionic bowel in these children with HSCR complicated by HAEC is probably reflective of enterocolitis-mediated neuronal damage. The vicious circle of enterocolitis and loss of neuroprotective serotonergic neurons may thus occur [45].

27.7 The S.I.P Syncytium in Hirschsprung's Disease

The movement of intestinal contents in the gut requires coordinated concentric contractions of the smooth muscle layers of the gut wall. The orderly excitatory stimulation of specific smooth muscle cells (SMC) to contract and inhibitory stimulation of others to relax to achieve these peristaltic contractions is conducted by the ENS [46, 47]. Central to the process of peristalsis is the propagation of slow wave electrical activity through the electrical syncytium formed by the SMC, ICC and Platelet-Derived Growth Factor Receptor-α-positive (PDGFRα+) cells, known as the SIP syncytium [48]. ICC have a key role as electrical pacemaker cells in the gut. They are coupled loosely to SMC by gap junction proteins. This loose coupling limits the likelihood of electrical waves dissipating across a large smooth muscle area [46]. The systole-diastole nature of electrical slow wave activity leads to ordered periods of smooth muscle contraction and relaxation, which are essential to propel intestinal contents along the alimentary tract for digestion.

ICC act as intermediaries between enteric motor neurons and SMC, modulating inhibitory and excitatory signals from the enteric nervous system [49]. Abnormalities of ICC distribution have been observed in a range of gastrointestinal disorders including inflammatory bowel disease, idiopathic slow-transit constipation, and necrotizing enterocolitis [50]. At microscopy, these cells can be identified by their immunopositivity for c-kit and anoctamin-1. It has long been recognized that ICC networks are markedly deficient in the aganglionic colon in HSCR. More recently, several studies have demonstrated that ICC networks are less dense in the ganglionic bowel in HSCR [51, 52].

PDGFRα$^+$ cells are fibroblast-like cells that share morphological similarities with ICC but are c-kit negative. They are arranged in discrete networks in the myenteric plexus but also in the tunica muscularis where they form part of the SIP syncytium. They are thought to be involved in smooth muscle relaxation in the bowel and express the small conductance calcium-activated potassium (SK3) channel, which, when activated, facilitates purine-mediated smooth muscle relaxation. The density of both PDGFRα$^+$ cells and SK3 channel expression have both been shown to be reduced in the aganglionic colon in HSCR and, in a proportion of patients, in the ganglionic colon [53, 54].

In addition to these findings indicating abnormalities in the density of cells needed for normal gut motility in the ganglionic colon in HSCR, abnormalities in the expression of functional cellular components in the SIP syncytium have also been described. Gap junctions are channels that couple cells electrically and chemically. They consist of two hemichannels composed of connexin proteins. Several connexins (Cx26, Cx36, Cx43) are involved in mediating the intercellular signaling responsible for colonic motility. Despite being expressed across all the cell types in the SIP syncytium, many of which are reduced in density in the ganglionic bowel of children with HSCR, only Cx26 has been found to be underexpressed in the SIP in HSCR ganglionic colon [55, 56]. Reduced expression of Kv7 channels, which play a role in the membrane excitability of ICCs, and Nav1.9 channels, which play a role in the repolarization cycle of the action potential in specific nerve populations in the colon, have also been described [57, 58].

27.8 Colonic Mucosal Barrier Integrity in Hirschsprung's Disease

Hirschsprung-associated enterocolitis (HAEC) is the most common life-threatening surgical emergency that can affect children with HSCR. Its diagnosis is primarily based on clinical grounds, with abdominal distension, explosive loose stools, fever, and vomiting as some of the key features [13, 14]. A scoring system with 83% sensitivity and 98.7% specificity for diagnosing HAEC has been devised to aid in clinician diagnosis [59]. Its etiology is uncertain and is thought to involve disturbance of the intestinal microbiome, impaired mucosal barrier function, abnormal innate immune response and bacterial translocation, and it affects both the aganglionic and the ganglionic colon [14, 60].

The intestinal microbiome in HSCR has been demonstrated to be less diverse than in healthy individuals, with larger proportions of pathogenic organisms such as Enterobacter and Bacilli [61]. In children with HSCR, Protobacteria and Bacteroidetes are more prevalent in the colons of children with a history of HAEC when compared to those without HAEC. The population of fungal organisms in fecal specimens from children with HAEC has also been shown to be less diverse with an expansion of Candida species [62]. Patients who have previously been treated for HAEC have been shown to have a microbiome more similar to that of children with active enterocolitis than those with HSCR who have never had HAEC [63]. In both cases, it is unclear if these findings are underlying contributors to the development of HAEC or as a result of HAEC. Further prospective studies should be able to elucidate this.

Intestinal mucosal barrier dysfunction is likely be play a strong role in the etiology of HAEC. Numerous components required for normal barrier function have been found to be deficient in the aganglionic and the ganglionic colon of children with HSCR. The potassium channel, TREK-1, is a stretch-mediated channel that is involved in mucosal barrier integrity, as well as mediating the response of gastrointestinal smooth muscle to neural stimulation and mechanical stretch. Its expression is reduced in both aganglionic and ganglionic colon in HSCR compared to controls [64].

Goblet cells in the colon produce a mucus layer that forms a bactericidal and bacteriostatic barrier against bacterial invasion. Nakamura et al. found that populations of goblet cells, as well as a host of factors required for normal goblet cell differentiation and maturation are deficient in both ganglionic and aganglionic colon in HSCR [65]. An abnormal immune response may also partly contribute to the susceptibility to enterocolitis seen both before and after PT surgery. The pro-inflammatory cytokine IL-36γ is overexpressed in the colons of children with HSCR compared to healthy controls [66].

27.9 Conclusions and Future Directions

The proportion of children requiring medical treatment for ongoing problems with constipation, soiling, and recurrent enterocolitis despite having a technically adequate PT operation for HSCR is not trivial. Key to avoiding this problem is the avoidance of retained segments of aganglionic or transition zone colon. This can be best avoided by resecting an adequate margin above the most distal normal intraoperative colonic biopsy and, where possible, doing a frozen section of the proximal resection margin to ensure the absence of partial circumference aganglionosis.

Despite having normal neuroanatomical architecture, the ganglionic colon in HSCR appears to be abnormal in a number of ways. Specifically, there is an imbalance of neurotransmitters, with excessive nitrergic innervation and deficient cholinergic innervation. Important modulators of neurotransmission in the enteric nervous system, such as neuronal serotonin, ICC and PDGFRα$^+$ cells all appear to be deficient in the ganglionic colon in at least some patients with HSCR. The intestinal microbiome is also disrupted in children with HSCR, with those who have experienced HAEC demonstrating the least diversity. It is unclear if this is a cause or an effect as it applies to susceptibility toward HAEC.

Future studies will aim to elucidate if many of the findings described above are primarily abnormalities of the colon or occur as a result of the distension associated with congenital megacolon seen in HSCR. Understanding the basis for these abnormalities is important because even if aganglionosis can be reversed in the future (e.g., stem cell-based therapies), it may not yield a satisfactory result for the patient regarding obstructive symptoms or the occurrence of enterocolitis.

References

1. Haricharan RN, Georgeson KE. Hirschsprung disease. Semin Pediatr Surg. 2008;17(4):266–75. https://doi.org/10.1053/j.sempedsurg.2008.07.005.
2. Dasgupta R, Langer JC. Hirschsprung disease. Curr Probl Surg. 2004;41(12):942–88. https://doi.org/10.1067/j.cpsurg.2004.09.004.
3. Rintala RJ, Pakarinen MP. Long-term outcomes of Hirschsprung disease. Semin Pediatr Surg. 2012;21(4):336–43. https://doi.org/10.1053/j.sempedsurg.2012.07.008.
4. Langer JC. Persistent obstructive symptoms after surgery for Hirschsprung disease: development of a diagnostic and therapeutic algorithm. J Pediatr Surg. 2004;39(10):1458–62.
5. Levitt MA, Dickie B, Pena A. Evaluation and treatment of the patient with Hirschsprung disease who is not doing well after a pull-through procedure. Semin Pediatr Surg. 2010;19(2):146–53. https://doi.org/10.1053/j.sempedsurg.2009.11.013.
6. Chumpitazi BP, Nurko S. Defecation disorders in children after surgery for Hirschsprung disease. J Pediatr Gastroenterol Nutr. 2011;53(1):75–9. https://doi.org/10.1097/MPG.0b013e318212eb53. PubMed PMID: 21694540
7. Zakaria OM. Bowel function and fecal continence after Soave's trans-anal endorectal pull-through for Hirschsprung disease: a local experience. Updat Surg. 2012;64(2):113–8. https://doi.org/10.1007/s13304-012-0140-9. PubMed PMID: 22392576
8. Thomson D, Allin B, Long AM, Bradnock T, Walker G, Knight M. Laparoscopic assistance for primary transanal pull-through in Hirschsprung disease: a systematic review and meta-analysis. BMJ Open. 2015;5(3):e006063. https://doi.org/10.1136/bmjopen-2014-006063. PubMed PMID: 25805527; PubMed Central PMCID: PMCPMC4386272
9. Kim AC, Langer JC, Pastor AC, Zhang L, Sloots CE, Hamilton NA, et al. Endorectal pull-through for Hirschsprung disease-a multicenter, long-term comparison of results: transanal vs transabdominal approach. J Pediatr Surg. 2010;45(6):1213–20. https://doi.org/10.1016/j.jpedsurg.2010.02.087. PubMed PMID: 20620323
10. Nasr A, Haricharan RN, Gamarnik J, Langer JC. Transanal pullthrough for Hirschsprung disease: matched case-control comparison of soave and Swenson techniques. J Pediatr Surg. 2014;49(5):774–6. https://doi.org/10.1016/j.jpedsurg.2014.02.073. PubMed PMID: 24851768
11. Zhang SC, Bai YZ, Wang W, Wang WL. Long-term outcome, colonic motility, and sphincter performance after Swenson's procedure for Hirschsprung disease: a single-center 2-decade experience with 346 cases. Am J Surg. 2007;194(1):40–7. https://doi.org/10.1016/j.amjsurg.2006.10.018. PubMed PMID: 17560907
12. Granstrom AL, Husberg B, Nordenskjold A, Svensson PJ, Wester T. Laparoscopic-assisted pull-through for Hirschsprung disease, a prospective repeated evaluation of functional outcome. J Pediatr Surg. 2013;48(12):2536–9. https://doi.org/10.1016/j.jpedsurg.2013.07.017. PubMed PMID: 24314199
13. Frykman PK, Short SS. Hirschsprung-associated enterocolitis: prevention and therapy. Semin Pediatr Surg. 2012;21(4):328–35. https://doi.org/10.1053/j.sempedsurg.2012.07.007. PubMed PMID: 22985838; PubMed Central PMCID: PMC3462485
14. Austin KM. The pathogenesis of Hirschsprung disease-associated enterocolitis. Semin Pediatr Surg. 2012;21(4):319–27. https://doi.org/10.1053/j.sempedsurg.2012.07.006. PubMed PMID: 22985837
15. Engum SA, Grosfeld JL. Long-term results of treatment of Hirschsprung disease. Semin Pediatr Surg. 2004;13(4):273–85. PubMed PMID: 15660321
16. Mills JL, Konkin DE, Milner R, Penner JG, Langer M, Webber EM. Long-term bowel function and quality of life in children with Hirschsprung disease. J Pediatr Surg. 2008;43(5):899–905. https://doi.org/10.1016/j.jpedsurg.2007.12.038. PubMed PMID: 18485963

17. Kapur RP, Kennedy AJ. Transitional zone pull through: surgical pathology considerations. Semin Pediatr Surg. 2012;21(4):291–301. https://doi.org/10.1053/j.sempedsurg.2012.07.003. PubMed PMID: 22985834
18. Das K, Kini U, Babu MK, Mohanty S, D'Cruz AJ. The distal level of normally innervated bowel in long segment colonic Hirschsprung disease. Pediatr Surg Int. 2010;26(6):593–9. https://doi.org/10.1007/s00383-010-2603-8. PubMed PMID: 20419377
19. Jamieson DH, Dundas SE, Belushi SA, Cooper M, Blair GK. Does the transition zone reliably delineate aganglionic bowel in Hirschsprung disease? Pediatr Radiol. 2004;34(10):811–5. https://doi.org/10.1007/s00247-004-1292-7. PubMed PMID: 15278325
20. Schappi MG, Staiano A, Milla PJ, Smith VV, Dias JA, Heuschkel R, et al. A practical guide for the diagnosis of primary enteric nervous system disorders. J Pediatr Gastroenterol Nutr. 2013;57(5):677–86. https://doi.org/10.1097/MPG.0b013e3182a8bb50. PubMed PMID: 24177787
21. Frongia G, Gunther P, Schenk JP, Strube K, Kessler M, Mehrabi A, et al. Contrast enema for Hirschsprung disease investigation: diagnostic accuracy and validity for subsequent diagnostic and surgical planning. Eur J Pediatr Surg. 2015;26:207. https://doi.org/10.1055/s-0035-1546755. PubMed PMID: 25803244
22. Muller CO, Mignot C, Belarbi N, Berrebi D, Bonnard A. Does the radiographic transition zone correlate with the level of aganglionosis on the specimen in Hirschsprung disease? Pediatr Surg Int. 2012;28(6):597–601. https://doi.org/10.1007/s00383-012-3094-6. PubMed PMID: 22534881
23. Lawal TA, Chatoorgoon K, Collins MH, Coe A, Pena A, Redo LMA. Pull-through in Hirschsprung [corrected] disease for obstructive symptoms due to residual aganglionosis and transition zone bowel. J Pediatr Surg. 2011;46(2):342–7. https://doi.org/10.1016/j.jpedsurg.2010.11.014. PubMed PMID: 21292085
24. White FV, Langer JC. Circumferential distribution of ganglion cells in the transition zone of children with Hirschsprung disease. Pediatr Dev Pathol. 2000;3(3):216–22. PubMed PMID: 10742408
25. Swaminathan M, Kapur RP. Counting myenteric ganglion cells in histologic sections: an empirical approach. Hum Pathol. 2010;41(8):1097–108. https://doi.org/10.1016/j.humpath.2009.12.012. PubMed PMID: 20346481
26. Kapur RP, Kennedy AJ. Histopathologic delineation of the transition zone in short-segment Hirschsprung disease. Pediatr Dev Pathol. 2013;16(4):252–66. https://doi.org/10.2350/12-12-1282-OA.1. PubMed PMID: 23495711
27. Kapur RP. Histology of the transition zone in Hirschsprung disease. Am J Surg Pathol. 2016;40:1637. https://doi.org/10.1097/PAS.0000000000000711. PubMed PMID: 27526297
28. Georgeson KE. Laparoscopic-assisted pull-through for Hirschsprung disease. Semin Pediatr Surg. 2002;11(4):205–10. PubMed PMID: 12407501
29. Kenny SE, Tam PK, Garcia-Barcelo M. Hirschsprung disease. Semin Pediatr Surg. 2010;19(3):194–200. https://doi.org/10.1053/j.sempedsurg.2010.03.004. PubMed PMID: 20610192
30. Koh SD, Rhee PL. Ionic conductance(s) in response to post-junctional potentials. J Neurogastroenterol Motility. 2013;19(4):426–32. https://doi.org/10.5056/jnm.2013.19.4.426. PubMed PMID: 24199003; PubMed Central PMCID: PMC3816177
31. O'Kelly TJ, Davies JR, Tam PK, Brading AF, Mortensen NJ. Abnormalities of nitric-oxide-producing neurons in Hirschsprung disease: morphology and implications. J Pediatr Surg. 1994;29(2):294–9; discussion 9–300 PubMed PMID: 7513759
32. Sandgren K, Larsson LT, Ekblad E. Widespread changes in neurotransmitter expression and number of enteric neurons and interstitial cells of Cajal in lethal spotted mice: an explanation for persisting dysmotility after operation for Hirschsprung disease? Dig Dis Sci. 2002;47(5):1049–64. PubMed PMID: 12018900
33. Zaitoun I, Erickson CS, Barlow AJ, Klein TR, Heneghan AF, Pierre JF, et al. Altered neuronal density and neurotransmitter expression in the ganglionated region of Ednrb null mice: implications for Hirschsprung disease. Neurogastroenterol Motil. 2013;25(3):e233–44. https://doi.org/10.1111/nmo.12083. PubMed PMID: 23360229; PubMed Central PMCID: PMC3578114
34. Coyle D, O'Donnell AM, Gillick J, Puri P. Altered neurotransmitter expression profile in the ganglionic bowel in Hirschsprung disease. J Pediatr Surg. 2016;51(5):762–9. https://doi.org/10.1016/j.jpedsurg.2016.02.018. PubMed PMID: 26951962
35. Menezes M, Puri P. Long-term outcome of patients with enterocolitis complicating Hirschsprung disease. Pediatr Surg Int. 2006;22(4):316–8. https://doi.org/10.1007/s00383-006-1639-2. PubMed PMID: 16463033
36. Pastor AC, Osman F, Teitelbaum DH, Caty MG, Langer JC. Development of a standardized definition for Hirschsprung-associated enterocolitis: a Delphi analysis. J Pediatr Surg. 2009;44(1):251–6. https://doi.org/10.1016/j.jpedsurg.2008.10.052. PubMed PMID: 19159752
37. Gershon MD. 5-Hydroxytryptamine (serotonin) in the gastrointestinal tract. Curr Opin Endocrinol Diabetes Obes. 2013;20(1):14–21. https://doi.org/10.1097/MED.0b013e32835bc703. PubMed PMID: 23222853; PubMed Central PMCID: PMC3708472
38. Gershon MD. Enteric serotonergic neurones ... Finally! J Physiol. 2009;587(Pt 3):507. https://doi.org/10.1113/jphysiol.2008.167676. PubMed PMID: 19182271; PubMed Central PMCID: PMC2670073
39. Gershon MD. Serotonin is a sword and a shield of the bowel: serotonin plays offense and defense. Trans

Am Clin Climatol Assoc. 2012;123:268–80. discussion 80. PubMed PMID: 23303993; PubMed Central PMCID: PMC3540639
40. Mawe GM, Hoffman JM. Serotonin signalling in the gut--functions, dysfunctions and therapeutic targets. Nat Rev Gastroenterol Hepatol. 2013;10(8):473–86. https://doi.org/10.1038/nrgastro.2013.105. PubMed PMID: 23797870; PubMed Central PMCID: PMC4048923
41. Galligan JJ. 5-hydroxytryptamine, ulcerative colitis, and irritable bowel syndrome: molecular connections. Gastroenterology. 2004;126(7):1897–9. PubMed PMID: 15188186
42. Soeda J, O'Briain DS, Puri P. Regional reduction in intestinal neuroendocrine cell populations in enterocolitis complicating Hirschsprung disease. J Pediatr Surg. 1993;28(8):1063–8. PubMed PMID: 7901360
43. Okamoto T, Barton MJ, Hennig GW, Birch GC, Grainger N, Corrigan RD, et al. Extensive projections of myenteric serotonergic neurons suggest they comprise the central processing unit in the colon. Neurogastroenterol Motil. 2014;26(4):556–70. https://doi.org/10.1111/nmo.12302. PubMed PMID: 24460867
44. Smith TK, Park KJ, Hennig GW. Colonic migrating motor complexes, high amplitude propagating contractions, neural reflexes and the importance of neuronal and mucosal serotonin. J Neurogastroenterol Motility. 2014;20(4):423–46. https://doi.org/10.5056/jnm14092. PubMed PMID: 25273115; PubMed Central PMCID: PMC4204412
45. Coyle D, Murphy JM, Doyle B, O'Donnell AM, Gillick J, Puri P. Altered tryptophan hydroxylase 2 expression in enteric serotonergic nerves in Hirschsprung-associated enterocolitis. World J Gastroenterol. 2016;22(19):4662–72. https://doi.org/10.3748/wjg.v22.i19.4662. PubMed PMID: 27217698; PubMed Central PMCID: PMCPMC4870073
46. Sanders KM. Rhythmic electrical activity and regulation of gut motility. Eur Rev Med Pharmacol Sci. 2008;12(Suppl 1):129–31. PubMed PMID: 18924452
47. Baker SA, Mutafova-Yambolieva V, Monaghan K, Horowitz B, Sanders KM, Koh SD. Mechanism of active repolarization of inhibitory junction potential in murine colon. Am J Physiol Gastrointest Liver Physiol. 2003;285(5):G813–21. https://doi.org/10.1152/ajpgi.00115.2003. PubMed PMID: 14561587
48. Peri LE, Sanders KM, Mutafova-Yambolieva VN. Differential expression of genes related to purinergic signaling in smooth muscle cells, PDGFRalpha-positive cells, and interstitial cells of Cajal in the murine colon. Neurogastroenterol Motil. 2013;25(9):e609–20. https://doi.org/10.1111/nmo.12174. PubMed PMID: 23809506; PubMed Central PMCID: PMC3735650
49. Benarroch EE. Enteric nervous system: functional organization and neurologic implications. Neurology. 2007;69(20):1953–7. https://doi.org/10.1212/01.wnl.0000281999.56102.b5. PubMed PMID: 17998487
50. Burns AJ. Disorders of interstitial cells of Cajal. J Pediatr Gastroenterol Nutr. 2007;45(Suppl 2):S103–6. https://doi.org/10.1097/MPG.0b013e31812e65e0. PubMed PMID: 18185068
51. Coyle D, Kelly DA, O'Donnell AM, Gillick J, Puri P. Use of anoctamin 1 (ANO1) to evaluate interstitial cells of Cajal in Hirschsprung disease. Pediatr Surg Int. 2016;32(2):125–33. https://doi.org/10.1007/s00383-015-3822-9. PubMed PMID: 26510736
52. Taguchi T, Suita S, Masumoto K, Nagasaki A. An abnormal distribution of C-kit positive cells in the normoganglionic segment can predict a poor clinical outcome in patients with Hirschsprung disease. Eur J Pediatr Surg. 2005;15(3):153–8. https://doi.org/10.1055/s-2005-837612. PubMed PMID: 15999306
53. O'Donnell AM, Coyle D, Puri P. Deficiency of platelet-derived growth factor receptor-alpha-positive cells in Hirschsprung disease colon. World J Gastroenterol. 2016;22(12):3335–40. https://doi.org/10.3748/wjg.v22.i12.3335. PubMed PMID: 27022215; PubMed Central PMCID: PMCPMC4806191
54. Coyle D, O'Donnell AM, Puri P. Altered distribution of small-conductance calcium-activated potassium channel SK3 in Hirschsprung disease. J Pediatr Surg. 2015;50(10):1659–64. https://doi.org/10.1016/j.jpedsurg.2015.01.013. PubMed PMID: 25783396
55. Coyle D, Doyle B, Murphy JM, O'Donnell AM, Gillick J, Puri P. Expression of connexin 26 and connexin 43 is reduced in Hirschsprung disease. J Surg Res. 2016;206(1):242–51. https://doi.org/10.1016/j.jss.2016.08.010. PubMed PMID: 27916369
56. Nemeth L, Maddur S, Puri P. Immunolocalization of the gap junction protein Connexin43 in the interstitial cells of Cajal in the normal and Hirschsprung disease bowel. J Pediatr Surg. 2000;35(6):823–8. https://doi.org/10.1053/jpsu.2000.6851. PubMed PMID: 10873019
57. O'Donnell AM, Coyle D, Puri P. Decreased expression of Kv7 channels in Hirchsprung's disease. J Pediatr Surg. 2017;52(7):1177–81. https://doi.org/10.1016/j.jpedsurg.2016.12.028. PubMed PMID: 28087137
58. O'Donnell AM, Coyle D, Puri P. Decreased Nav1.9 channel expression in Hirschsprung disease. J Pediatr Surg. 2016;51(9):1458–61. https://doi.org/10.1016/j.jpedsurg.2016.05.007. PubMed PMID: 27297039
59. Frykman PK, Kim S, Wester T, Nordenskjold A, Kawaguchi A, Hui TT, et al. Critical evaluation of the Hirschsprung-associated enterocolitis (HAEC) score: a multicenter study of 116 children with Hirschsprung disease. J Pediatr Surg. 2018;53(4):708–17. https://doi.org/10.1016/j.jpedsurg.2017.07.009. PubMed PMID: 28760457
60. Gosain A, Brinkman AS. Hirschsprung associated enterocolitis. Curr Opin Pediatr. 2015;27(3):364–9. https://doi.org/10.1097/MOP.0000000000000210. PubMed PMID: 25944307; PubMed Central PMCID: PMCPMC4451822

61. Neuvonen MI, Korpela K, Kyrklund K, Rintala RJ, Pakarinen MP. Intestinal microbiota in Hirschsprung disease. J Pediatr Gastroenterol Nutr. 2018;67:594. https://doi.org/10.1097/MPG.0000000000001999. PubMed PMID: 29652728
62. Frykman PK, Nordenskjold A, Kawaguchi A, Hui TT, Granstrom AL, Cheng Z, et al. Characterization of bacterial and fungal microbiome in children with Hirschsprung disease with and without a history of Enterocolitis: a multicenter study. PLoS One. 2015;10(4):e0124172. https://doi.org/10.1371/journal.pone.0124172. PubMed PMID: 25909773; PubMed Central PMCID: PMCPMC4409062
63. Li Y, Poroyko V, Yan Z, Pan L, Feng Y, Zhao P, et al. Characterization of intestinal microbiomes of Hirschsprung disease patients with or without Enterocolitis using Illumina-MiSeq high-throughput sequencing. PLoS One. 2016;11(9):e0162079. https://doi.org/10.1371/journal.pone.0162079. PubMed PMID: 27603009; PubMed Central PMCID: PMCPMC5014423
64. Tomuschat C, O'Donnell AM, Coyle D, Dreher N, Kelly D, Puri P. Altered expression of a two-pore domain (K2P) mechano-gated potassium channel TREK-1 in Hirschsprung disease. Pediatr Res. 2016;80(5):729–33. https://doi.org/10.1038/pr.2016.140. PubMed PMID: 27384506
65. Nakamura H, Tomuschat C, Coyle D, O'Donnel AM, Lim T, Puri P. Altered goblet cell function in Hirschsprung disease. Pediatr Surg Int. 2018;34(2):121–8. https://doi.org/10.1007/s00383-017-4178-0. PubMed PMID: 29383490
66. Tomuschat C, O'Donnell AM, Coyle D, Puri P. Altered expression of IL36gamma and IL36 receptor (IL1RL2) in the colon of patients with Hirschsprung disease. Pediatr Surg Int. 2017;33(2):181–6. https://doi.org/10.1007/s00383-016-4011-1. PubMed PMID: 27853811

28 Bowel Management for the Treatment of Chronic Constipation and Soiling in Patients Operated for Hirschsprung's Disease

Andrea Bischoff and Alberto Peña

Contents

28.1 Introduction

The result of an operation for Hirschsprung's disease (HSCR), performed in a technically correct manner, is frequently a good one; the patients have bowel control, no diarrhea, no constipation, and no enterocolitis. Unfortunately, many times the patients suffer from one of these conditions because of a technically deficient operation; other times, these conditions occur despite a history of a technically impeccable operation, for unknown reasons. Diarrhea after an operation for HSCR may occur because of an extended colonic resection in cases of long-segment aganglionosis. Also, patients who suffer from enterocolitis frequently have very characteristic liquid, fetid stool. This chapter is dedicated to the discussion of constipation and soiling.

A. Bischoff · A. Peña (✉)
International Center for Colorectal and Urogenital Care, Children's Hospital Colorado, Aurora, CO, USA
e-mail: Alberto.Pena@childrenscolorado.org

28.2 Constipation

Constipation following an operation for HSCR may be classified under three categories:

A. Anatomic (mechanical) origin. This includes:
   - Stricture at the anastomosis site
   - Twisting of the pull-through bowel
   - Duhamel operation
B. Histologic error with pull-through of an aganglionic segment
C. Unknown origin

Accordingly, the evaluation of a patient who presents with constipation after an operation for HSCR must be conducted sequentially, trying to rule out the conditions mentioned above.

A. Anatomic origin

Stricture at the anastomosis site – It occurs most likely as a consequence of ischemia of the pull-through colon, and (or) excessive tension at the anastomosis. To prevent that, the anastomosis should never be done in cases with questionable blood supply or duskiness of the ganglionic bowel. In addition, the bowel must descend easily, under no tension.

When performing a trans-anal pull-through for HSCR, the surgeons may find themselves in the situation of being able to reach the normoganglionic bowel, but the bowel looks dusky and (or)

P. Puri (ed.), *Hirschsprung's Disease and Allied Disorders*, https://doi.org/10.1007/978-3-030-15647-3_28

barely reaches the anal canal. Under those circumstances the surgeon should not hesitate to perform a laparotomy or laparoscopy, to be able to visualize clearly the colonic arcades of the blood supply of the colon. If these arcades cannot be seen clearly via laparoscopy, a laparotomy must be done. In order to see clearly the colonic blood supply, it is very helpful to mobilize the splenic flexure.

The diagnosis of a strictured anastomosis can be done by digital rectal exam or, if necessary, under anesthesia. In addition, a contrast enema or a distal colostogram in cases with a colostomy, allows the surgeon to see clearly the location of the stricture.

The management of a stricture will depend on its characteristics. Soft, ring-like strictures deserve a trial of rectal dilatations. These must be performed on daily basis by the parents of the patient. If they declare that it is impossible for them to do it, then the patient will require a surgical resection. Weekly rectal dilatations under anesthesia usually end up provoking a more severe fibrotic process around the rectum and eventually will require an operation. Long, narrow strictures or strictures associated to a history of anastomosis dehiscence, leakage of stool, pelvic abscess, and extensive pelvic fibrosis do not respond to rectal dilatations and must be operated on [1].

The surgical repair of rectal strictures may represent a serious technical challenge. Those procedures must be performed by experienced surgeons hopefully dedicated to the treatment of these problems.

Twisting of the pull-through bowel [2]- This complication occurs at the time of pulling the normoganglionic down to the anal canal. The bowel may be inadvertently twisted. To prevent that complication, there are several intraoperative maneuvers that can be observed, including using a pen to mark all the antimesenteric aspect of the bowel to be pulled down, or else the use of a large rubber tube to be passed through the anus and expected to be palpated through the colon to verify that the bowel was not twisted.

The diagnosis of this condition requires a good index of suspicion and a meticulous contrast enema.

The management of a twisted pulled-through bowel [2] requires surgical intervention, including a resection and re-anastomosis, when the twisted area can be reached easily transabdominally. Sometimes, however, the twisted area is located down into the pelvis and the patient needs a redo pull-through.

Constipation consecutive to a Duhamel pull-through [3] – a widely recognized complication of the Duhamel type of operation is the high frequency of constipation associated to the presence of a giant aganglionic rectal pouch. These patients usually do not respond to the use of laxatives, even if the patients have diarrhea as a consequence of the laxatives, the giant aganglionic segment remains fecally impacted. Therefore, it is generally preferred to resect the aganglionic pouch, which may also be surgically challenging.

B. Histologic error [4, 5] – (pull-through of an aganglionic segment).

In spite of the advances in the histologic diagnosis of HSCR, including sophisticated histologic and immunohistochemically techniques, errors in diagnosis continue to happen, with serious clinical consequences. These errors occur because of one or several of the following events:

Lack of experience of the pathologist. It is not enough to be a board-certified pathologist to be trusted to diagnose HSCR. Some pediatric surgeons are very fortunate to work in an institution with an excellent pathologist with experience in the histologic diagnosis of HSCR. Those pediatric surgeons who do not have that privilege must adopt special routines to ensure they pull down a demonstrated normoganglionic piece of colon. These routines include:

- Not to perform pull-through operations based on frozen sections, unless they have evidence that the pathologist on call has demonstrated experience in the evaluation of frozen sections.
- Take colonic biopsies as a separate procedure; send the specimens to an experienced pathologist and perform the pull-through in another surgical event.

The diagnosis of this condition must be suspected in every patient suffering from constipation, with or without enterocolitis, after an operation for HSCR. A contrast enema may show a characteristic image of a relatively narrow distal colon, followed proximally by a dilated colon, with a "transition" zone in between (Fig. 28.1). The next step in such cases must be a rectal biopsy, taken about 3 cm proximal to the pectinate line.

The treatment for this condition consists in a resection of the aganglionic segment and a pull-through of normoganglionic colon.

There is considerable debate concerning the management of cases in whom the aganglionic segment pulled down is very short (2–4 cms). The question is: How significant is such a short aganglionic segment? Is it capable of producing symptoms of constipation? Perhaps a reasonable approach for those cases could be to manage them medically for a period, and if they do not respond, to proceed with a surgical resection of the aganglionic segment.

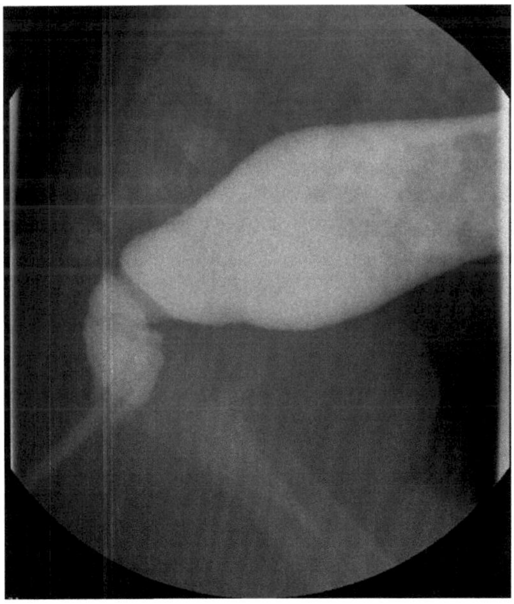

Fig. 28.1 Contrast enema after a pull-through procedure showing residual aganglionic segment with a narrow distal colon followed by a proximal dilated colon

C. Unknown origin

Constipation of unknown origin – It is relatively common to operate two cases suffering from HSCR, using in both cases identical surgical techniques and to observe that the results are different. One patient suffers from constipation and the other does not. Several hypotheses have been postulated to try to explain this.

- A primarily motility disorder of the normoganglionic bowel, without histologic recognizable component
- A lack of relaxation of the "internal sphincter"
- "Pelvic dyssynergia"
- Pull-through of a dilated normoganglionic piece of colon

The proponents of the idea that this problem is a consequence of a "lack of relaxation of the internal sphincter," advocate the use of Botox (botulinum toxin) injected in the area where they supposed is located the evanescent structure known as "internal sphincter." [6] Transient "good results" have been reported with this type of management. There is no evidence of permanent cure.

The proponents of the "pelvic dyssynergia" explanation [7] offer a feedback type of physical therapy.There is evidence indicating that the dilatation of a hollow viscus produces inefficient peristalsis. Therefore, it is generally recommended, during an operation for HSCR, to resect not only the aganglionic segment but also the most dilated portion of the normoganglionic segment.

The treatment of constipation of unknown origin, consecutive to an operation for HSCR, consists in trying to determine the amount of laxative necessary to guarantee the complete emptying of the colon, as radiologically demonstrated [8–10]. In unusual cases, the patients do not tolerate the high dosage of laxative necessary to achieve the goal and the alternative is the use of rectal enemas, per rectum or in an antegrade fashion [11]. When these types of treatment fail to give the patient a good quality of life there is always the possibility of offering a secondary resection.

There is no guarantee that this kind of treatment will solve the problem.

28.3 Soiling (Fecal Incontinence)

Even when in theory, fecal incontinence should not occur in patients operated for HSCR, the fact is that many patients still suffer from this devastating complication [12, 13].

It is important to consider the very significant physiologic changes that are produced in a patient who was subjected to a resection of the rectosigmoid, or even worse, when the resection included longer segments of colon. The rectum, and the sigmoid colon, represent the natural fecal reservoir of humans. The peristalsis of the colon is very active in its most proximal segments (cecum and ascending colon) and becomes less active in the distal portion (descending and sigmoid colon). The rectum has a unique motility pattern. In fact, the rectum remains aperistaltic most of the time, it is very compliant and receives stool, acting as a reservoir until it is full. At some point, an independent mechanism triggers the contraction of the rectum, the person feels the desire to evacuate, holds the bowel movement using the voluntary sphincter until the person reaches the toilet. At that time the rectum expulses all the stool produced during the last 24 h or more. It is that unique motility pattern that allows humans to be social and spend long periods of time without the need to evacuate. The resection of the rectosigmoid leaves the patient without a fecal reservoir. A portion of proximal colon is connected to the lower rectum, very near the pectinate line. That proximal portion of the colon has an active constant peristalsis, which translates in an almost constant passing of stool, similar to what is observed in a colostomy. A good operation for HSCR must preserve the anal canal (area located below the pectinate line), to guarantee the preservation of sensation, which is an essential component of the mechanism of fecal continence. A patient without the rectosigmoid and a well-preserved anal canal will feel the desire to evacuate almost constantly. For that person to avoid episodes of incontinence, he must be paying constant attention to the desire to evacuate and must be using his voluntary sphincter all the time to remain clean in underwear. That may help to understand why some children who were subjected to one of these operations may have problems learning to become toilet trained at the right age, when most children become toilet trained for stool. In other words, it takes a significant effort, cooperation, and attention to become toilet trained after a sigmoid resection.

Let's consider another scenario, which can be the case of a patient without a rectosigmoid and with a destroyed or absent anal canal. This kind of situation will provoke fecal incontinence on a permanent basis. Unfortunately, this scenario is frequently seen in patients who underwent an operation for HSCR.

Based on the explanation above, the routine evaluation of a patient suffering from fecal incontinence after having an operation for HSCR must include an examination under anesthesia to inspect the integrity of the anal canal [14]. This examination is performed with the use of a "Lone Star" * retractor, which is an excellent tool that allows a full inspection of the anal canal, the pectinate line, and the rectal mucosa. Figure 28.2 shows an intact anal canal. Image 3 shows a partially destroyed anal canal and Fig. 28.3 shows a

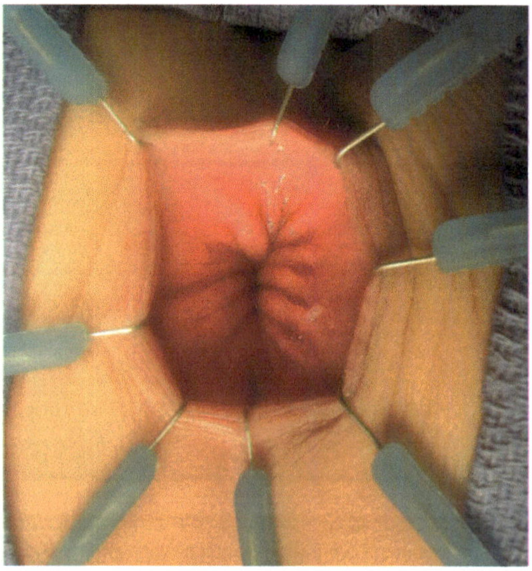

Fig. 28.2 Intact anal canal

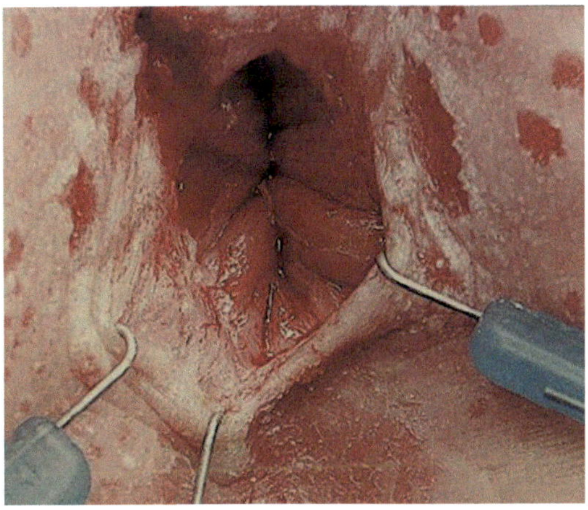

Fig. 28.3 Completely destroyed anal canal

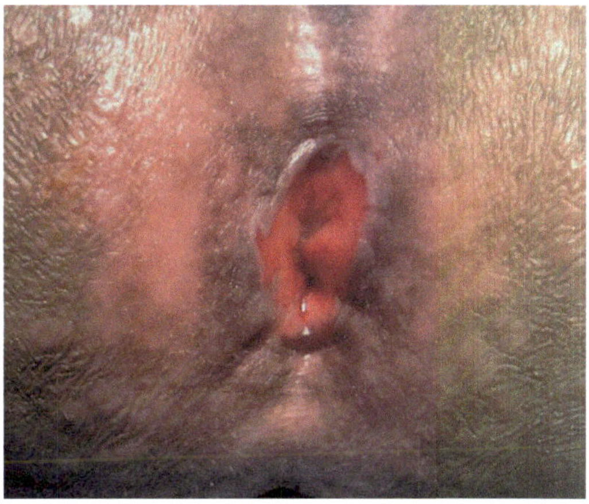

Fig. 28.4 Partially destroyed anal canal

completely destroyed anal canal. The chances of a patient with a destroyed anal canal and resection of the rectosigmoid gaining bowel control are almost nil (Fig. 28.4) [14].

In addition to the examination under anesthesia, the evaluation of fecal-incontinent patients must include a contrast enema, which will provide very valuable information relating to the type of colonic motility of the patient. This information will help us to determine the best type of management that may benefit the patient.

Patients suffering from fecal incontinence and with a destroyed anal canal must be managed with enemas, implementing a "Bowel Management Program," [15–17] which is an excellent way to keep the patients artificially clean in their underwear. If the patient suffers from fecal incontinence, absent or destroyed anal canal and constipation, the bowel management will consist in finding the right type of enema (large volume and concentrated) that will empty the colon daily and will keep the patient clean for 24 h. On the other hand, if the patient suffers from fecal incontinence, absent or destroyed anal canal, and tendency to diarrhea (narrow, short, or spastic colon), the management may be more technically demanding, including finding the right type of enema (small volume of normal saline), but adding medication (Imodium*) and constipating diet to try to paralyze the colon in between enemas to keep the patient clean.

Patients suffering from fecal incontinence and an intact anal canal can be helped by treating the constipation with laxatives or treating the tendency to diarrhea with medication and a constipating diet [13].

When the examination under anesthesia reveals the presence of an intact anal canal, in a patient suffering from fecal incontinence, the management must consist in giving the patient a trial of medical management, administering laxatives if the patient suffers from constipation or medication and constipating diet if the patient suffers from tendency to diarrhea. In addition, it is recommended to give the patient three meals per day, avoiding the snacks in between meals, which may trigger bouts of colonic motility and unexpected episodes of fecal incontinence.

References

1. Peña A, Elicevik M, Levitt MA. Reoperations in Hirschsprung disease. J Pediatr Surg. 2007;42:1008–14.
2. Garrett KM, Levitt MA, Peña A, et al. Contrast enema findings in patients presenting with poor functional outcome after primary repair for Hirschsprung disease. Pediatr Radiol. 2012;42:1099–106.
3. Chatoorgoon K, Peña A, Lawal TA, et al. The problematic Duhamel pouch in Hirschsprung's disease: manifestations and treatment. Eur J Pediatr Surg. 2011;21:366–9.
4. Lawal TA, Chatoorgoon K, Collins MH, et al. Redo pull-through in Hirschsprung's disease for obstructive

symptoms due to residual aganglionosis and transition zone bowel. J Pediatr Surg. 2011;46:342–7.
5. Coe A, Collins MH, Lawal T, Louden E, Levitt MA, Peña A. Reoperation for Hirschsprung disease: pathology of the resected problematic distal pull-through. Pediatr Developl Path. 2012;15:30–8.
6. Koivusalo A, Pakarinen MP, Rintala RJ. Botox injection treatment for anal outlet obstruction n patients with internal anal sphincter achalasia and Hirschsprung's disease. Pediatr Surg Int. 2009;25:873–6.
7. Sun X, Wang R, Zhang L, et al. Efficacy of pelvic floor muscle training for the treatment of fecal incontinence after soave procedure for Hirschsprung disease. Eur J Pediatr Surg. 2012;22:300–4.
8. De La Torre L, Langer JC. Transanal endorectal pull-through for Hirschsprung disease: technique, controversies, pearls, pitfalls, and an organized approach to the management of postoperative obstructive symptoms. Advances in pediatric colorectal surgery, Levitt MA and Peña A. Semin Pediatr Surg. 2010;19(2):96–106.
9. Bischoff A, Brisighelli G, Dickie B et al. Idiopathic constipation: a challenging but manageable problem. J Pediatr Surg 2017 [Epub ahead of print].
10. Levitt MA, Dickie B, Peña A. Evaluation and treatment of the patient with Hirschsprung disease who is not doing well after a pull-through procedure. Semin Pediatr Surg. 2010;19:146–53.
11. Levitt MA, Soffer SZ, Peña A. Continent appendicostomy in the bowel management of fecal incontinent children. J Ped Surg. 1997;32:1630–3.
12. Levitt MA, Dickie B, Peña A. The Hirschsprungs patient who is soiling after what was a considered a "successful" pull-through. Semin Pediatr Surg. 2012;21:344–53.
13. Levitt M, Martin C, Olesevich M, et al. Hirschsprung's disease and fecal incontinence: diagnostic and management strategies. J Pediatr Surg. 2009;44:271–7.
14. Bischoff A, Frischer J, Knod JL, et al. Damaged anal canal as a cause of fecal incontinence after surgical repair for Hirschsprung disease – a preventable and under-reported complication. J Pediatr Surg. 2017;52:549–53.
15. Bischoff A, Levitt MA, Bauer C, et al. Treatment of fecal incontinence with a comprehensive bowel management program. J Pediatr Surg. 2009;44:1278–84.
16. Bischoff A, Levitt MA, Peña A. Bowel management for the treatment of pediatric fecal incontinence. Pediatr Surg Int. 2009;25:1027–42.
17. Bischoff A, Tovilla M. A practical approach to the management of pediatric fecal incontinence. Semin Pediatr Surg. 2010;19:154–9.

Hirschsprung's Disease and Inflammatory Bowel Disease

29

Anna Löf Granström and Tomas Wester

Contents

29.1 Introduction

The first observation suggesting an association between Hirschsprung disease (HSCR) and inflammatory bowel disease (IBD) was reported in a retrospective follow-up of 880 individuals who had undergone Swenson's procedure for HSCR, 9 of whom had developed IBD. No further details were provided [1]. HSCR is a developmental defect of the enteric nervous system caused by incomplete migration, proliferation, differentiation, and survival of enteric nervous system progenitors. Between 5% and 42% of all individuals with HSCR develop an IBD-like acute bowel inflammation, Hirschsprung-associated enterocolitis (HAEC). The risk for HAEC is increased in patients with Down syndrome and total colonic aganglionosis. Some patients have recurrent episodes of HAEC or develop chronic HAEC. The etiology of HAEC is not fully understood, but involves altered intestinal microbiome and immune response. The severity of HAEC varies from mild bouts of explosive, foul-smelling diarrhea and abdominal distension to a severe condition with fever, lethargy, and septicemia. The treatment of mild episodes consists of antibiotics and regular bowel irrigations. IBD arises as a result of the interaction of environmental and genetic factors leading to immunological responses and inflammation in the gastrointestinal tract. IBD usually refers to two disease entities, Crohn's disease and ulcerative colitis, but also includes indeterminate colitis. Crohn's disease is characterized by focal, asymmetric, transmural and occasionally granulomatous inflammation, which can occur in any part of the gastrointestinal tract. Ulcerative colitis is characterized by a continuous mucosal and submucosal inflammation affecting the colon.

A. L. Granström · T. Wester (✉)
Division of Pediatric Surgery, Department of Women's and Children's Health, Karolinska Institutet, Stockholm, Sweden

Pediatric Surgery, Karolinska University Hospital, Stockholm, Sweden
e-mail: tomas.wester@sll.se

P. Puri (ed.), *Hirschsprung's Disease and Allied Disorders*,
https://doi.org/10.1007/978-3-030-15647-3_29

29.2 Epidemiology

Several studies, mainly case series, but also a recent population-based study, have suggested an association between HSCR and IBD (Table 29.1). In a recent systematic review and meta-analysis, Nakamura et al. reported 14 case series including 63 patients with HSCR and IBD, 46 of whom had Crohn's disease. Eighty-six per cent of the patients had total colonic aganglionosis or long segment disease [2]. In a national Swedish population-based cohort study from 1964 to 2013, 20 of 739 individuals with HSCR also had IBD; 15 had Crohn's disease and 5 had ulcerative colitis. Compared with the control group, individuals with HSCR had a five times increased risk of having IBD (odds ratio (OR) 4.99, 95% confidence interval (CI) 2.85–8.45). The patients' age at time of IBD diagnosis was 19 (5–34) years, which did not differ from the control group [3]. In a population-based cohort study from United States, 11 individuals who died of ulcerative colitis from 1991 to1996 also had HSCR [4]. Unfortunately, there is no further information about these individuals. In a combined case series from Canada and Finland, eight patients with HSCR and IBD were reported. The patients presented with IBD 4–21 years after pull-through for HSCR. Three of the patients had trisomy 21 and six patients had chronic or recurrent HAEC [5]. Granström et al. could not show an increased risk for patients with Down syndrome and HSCR to develop IBD [3].

One could speculate whether IBD is detected to the same extent in patients with HSCR as in individuals without HSCR. On the one hand, individuals with HSCR may have easier access to health care and therefore mild forms of IBD are detected. On the other hand, chronic diarrhea is usually a sign of HAEC in young patients with HSCR and also a common symptom in patients with long segment disease, which may cause diagnostic delay with respect to IBD.

29.3 Clinical Presentation

Clinically, patients with HAEC present with distended abdomen, explosive diarrhea with foul-smelling stool, vomiting, fever, and lethargy during the first few years of life [6].

IBD may present in different ways in patients with HSCR. The age at presentation of IBD does not differ between patients with and without HSCR. Patients usually present with IBD as adolescents or adults after surgical treatment for HSCR in the neonatal period. Dray et al. presented a case report of a man who had undergone surgery for total colonic aganglionosis at the age of 18 months who at the age of 34 years presented with chronic rectal bleeding where endoscopy showed ileal Crohn's disease [7]. Kim et al. presented a similar case with a 17-year-old male who underwent surgery for HSCR within the first year of life and who suffered from recurrent HAEC episodes as well as

Table 29.1 Summary of reports on the association between Hirschsprung disease and inflammatory bowel disease

					IBD			HAEC		
Author	Year	Country	Patients number	TCA	UC	Crohn	Unknown	Yes	No	Unknown
Sherman [1]	1989	United States	9				9			9
Cucino [4]	2001	United States	11		11					11
Pena [9]	2007	United States	1			1				1
Dray [7]	2007	France	1	1		1			1	
Pino Prato [10]	2008	Italy	2	1		1	1		2	
Levin [5]	2012	Canada/Finland	8	2		3	5	6	2	
Freeman [13]	2014	Germany	3	1			3	3		
Frémond [12]	2014	France	4	3		4				4
Muller [11]	2016	France	7	6		7			7	
Kim [8]	2017	Korea	1			1		1		
Löf Granström [3]	2018	Sweden	20		5	15				15

Abbreviations: *TCA* total colonic aganlionosis, *IBD* inflammatory bowel disease, *UC* ulcerative colitis, *HAEC* Hirschsprung-associated enterocolitis

uveitis and finally was diagnosed with Crohn's disease [8]. IBD may also present as chronic ulcers after surgery for HSCR. One case report described a patient with a chronic ulcer, where biopsies showed granulomatous IBD. The patient received medical treatment for Crohn's disease and the ulcer healed [9]. In some of the case reports of HSCR and IBD, individuals with HSCR, who initially had recovered from surgery for HSCR, later presented with chronic diarrhea. These symptoms were interpreted as HAEC and treated with metronidazole with insufficient effect. Finally, endoscopy showed IBD and after initiating IBD treatment the symptoms improved significantly [10, 11]. Frémond et al. reported four individuals with HSCR who at an average age of 11.5 years presented with a variant of Crohn's disease called digestive perianastomotic ulceration. One of these four patients had an *NOD2* gene mutation [12]. Freeman et al. discussed that histological findings suggesting IBD in patients with HSCR should not necessarily be considered true IBD, but rather Crohn's disease-like histopathology findings secondary to partial gastrointestinal obstruction after surgery for HSCR [13]. They retrospectively reviewed children with HSCR and identified three individuals who had developed IBD-like findings in intestinal biopsies or resected specimens. Two of the patients had total colonic aganglionosis, one had rectosigmoid HSCR and they did not have trisomy 21. The individual with rectosigmoid HSCR was treated with total colectomy with good result. Of the other two patients, one was treated with steroids, methotrexate and mesalamine, while the other was treated with steroids, mesalamine and azathioprine with good results. Histologically, there was transmural, chronic inflammation, fibrosis, and lymphoid aggregates similar to features seen in Crohn's disease.

29.4 The Link Between HSCR and IBD

HAEC is probably a key factor to explain the association between HSCR and IBD. Recent advances in the understanding of HAEC have focused on mucosal immunity, the role of the intestinal microbiome, and the role of genetics [6]. The pathophysiology of HAEC has similarities with current understanding of IBD, which is thought to result from an aberrant and continuing immune response to the microbes in the gut, in combination with individual genetic susceptibility [14]. Current IBD theories involve an interaction of genetics, host immunity, and environmental factors [15, 16]. There is insufficient evidence to show any environmental factors that explain the association between HSCR and IBD.

29.4.1 Genetics

Approximately 200 genetic variants have been associated with Crohn's disease and, or, ulcerative colitis. These variants explain 20–25% of all IBD cases [17, 18]. Mutations in a number of genes have been associated with HSCR. *RET* gene mutations are encountered in 20–25% of patients with HSCR with a penetrance of 50–70%. Several other genes have been associated with syndromic HSCR, for instance, *SOX10, PHOX2B, KIAA1279, and ZEB2* mutations are seen in Wardenburg syndrome, congenital central hypoventilation syndrome, Goldberg Shprintzen syndrome, and Mowat Wilson syndrome, respectively [19]. There have been a few attempts to show genetic associations between HSCR and IBD. *NOD2* variants, known to be associated with Crohn's disease, did not predispose for HAEC [20]. However, Muller et al. presented an *NOD2* gene mutation in one patient with Crohn's disease and HSCR [11].

29.4.2 Microbiome

Recently, Frykman et al. showed that patients with HAEC had altered bacterial microbiome compared to HSCR patients without HAEC. The bacterial microbiome was particularly characterized by increased Bacteroidetes. Also, the fungal microbiome was altered with increased Candida species, particularly *Candida albicans*, in patients with HAEC [21]. The microbial composition is also altered in patients with IBD with particularly a decreased diversity of bacteria. Bacteroidetes and Firmicutes as well as Clostridia, Ruminococcaceae, Bifidobacterium, Lactobacillus are decreased, whereas Gammaproteobacteriae are increased [22]. Fecal short chain fatty acids are decreased in patients with HAEC, indicating that also the microbiome function is altered [23]. Similar findings have been shown in patients with IBD, who also have decreased short chain fatty acids. Other alterations in microbial function in IBD have been reported such as decreased butanoate and propanoate, decreased amino acid biosynthesis, increased auxotrophy, increased amino acid transport, increased sulfate transport, and increased oxidative stress [22].

29.5 Conclusion

There is evidence that HSCR predisposes for an increased risk of IBD. The pathophysiological link between HAEC and IBD is still unclear, but there are similarities between HSCR and IBD with respect to altered microbiome and inflammatory responses. Probably, HAEC is an important factor. In individuals with HSCR and inflammation affecting the gastrointestinal tract, which is not typical for HAEC, IBD should be considered. This is particularly important in adolescents and young adults with HSCR so as not to delay diagnosis and treatment of IBD.

References

1. Sherman JO, Snyder ME, Weitzman JJ, Jona JZ, Gillis DA, et al. A 40-year multinational retrospective study of 880 Swenson procedures. J Pediatr Surg. 1989;24(8):833.
2. Nakamura H, Lim T, Puri P. Inflammatory bowel disease in patients with Hirschsprung's diasease: a systematic review and meta-analysis. Pediatr Surg Int. 2018;34:149–54.
3. Löf Granström A, Amin L, Arnell H, Wester T. Increased risk of inflammatory bowel disease in a population-based cohort study of patients with Hirschsprung disease. J Pediatr Gastroenterol Nutr. 2018;66:398–401.
4. Cucino C, Sonnenberg A. The comorbid occurrence of other diagnoses in patiens with ulcerative colitis ans Crohn's disease. Am J Gastroenterol. 2001;96:2107–12.
5. Levin DN, Marcon MA, Rintala RJ, Jacobson D, Langer JC. Inflammatory bowel disease manifesting after surgical treatment for Hirschsprung disease. J Pediatr Gastroenterol Nutr. 2012;55:272–7.
6. Gosain A. Established and emerging concepts in Hirschsprung's-associated enterocolitis. Pediatr Surg Int. 2016;32:313–20.
7. Dray X, Sokol H, Vahedi K, Lavergne-Slove A, Marteau P. Pure ileal Crohn's disease without colonic involvement after a long ileo-colonic anastomosis (Lester Martin Procedure) for Hirschsprung's disease: an argument favoring a specific sensitivity of the ileumin a subset of patients with Crohn's disease. Inflamm Bowel Dis. 2007;13:243–4.
8. Kim HY, Kim TW. Crohn's disease with ankylosing spondylitis in an adolescent patient who had undergone long ileo-colonic anastomosis for Hirschsprung's disease as an infant. Intest Res. 2017;15:133–7.
9. Peña A, Elicevik M, Levitt MA. Reoperations in Hirschsprung disease. J Pediatr Surg. 2007;42:1008–13.
10. Pini Prato A, Felici E, Gentilino V, Giunta C, Avanzini S, et al. Uncommon causes of postoperative chronic diarrhoea mimicking enterocolitis in Hirschsprung's disease: is there a role for digestive endoscopy? Pediatr Surg Int. 2008;24:503–7.
11. Muller CO, Rossignol G, Montalva L, Viala J, Martinez-Vinson C, et al. Long-term outcome of laparoscopic Duhamel procedure for extended Hirschsprung's disease. J Laparoendosc Adv Surg Tech A. 2016;26:1032–5.
12. Frémond ML, Viala J, Tréton X, Roy M, Berrebi D, et al. Digestive perianastomotic ulcerations and Crohn's disease. J Crohns Colitis. 2014;8:1624–31.
13. Freeman JJ, Rabah R, Hirschl RB, Maspons A, Meier D, Teitelbaum DH. Anti-TNF-α treatment for post-anastomotic ulcers and inflammatory bowel disease with Crohn's-like pathologic changes following intestinal surgery in pediatric patients. Pediatr Surg Int. 2015;31:77–82.
14. Zhang YZ, Li YY. Inflammatory bowel disease. World J Gastroenterol. 2014;7:91–9.
15. Rabizadeh S, Dubinsky M. Update in pediatric inflammatory bowel disease. Rheum Dis Clin N Am. 2013;39:789–99.
16. Tam PK, Garcia-Barceló M. Genetic basis of Hirschsprung's disease. Pediatr Surg Int. 2009;25:543–58.
17. De Souza HSP, Fiocchi C, Iliopoulos D. The IBD interactome: an integrated view of aetiology, pathogenesis and therapy. Nat Rev Gastroenterol Hepatol. 2017;14:739–49.
18. McGovern DPB, Kugathasan S, Cho JH. Genetics of inflammatory bowel disease. Gastroenterology. 2015;149:1163–76.
19. Mundt E, Bates MD. Genetics of Hirschsprung disease and anorectal malformations. Semin Pediatr Surg. 2010;19:107–17.
20. Lacher M, Fitze G, Helmbrecht J, et al. Hirschsprung-associated enterocolitis develops independently of NOD2 variants. J Pediatr Surg. 2010;45:1826–31.

21. Frykman PK, Nordenskjöld A, Kawaguchi A, Hui TT, Granström AL, Cheng Z, Tang J, Underhill DM, Iliev I, Funari VA, Wester T. Characterization of bacterial and fungal microbiome in children with Hirschsprung disease with and without a history of enterocolitis: a multicenter study. PLoS One. 2015;10(4):e0124172.
22. Kostic AD, Xavier RJ, Gevers D. The microbiome in inflammatory bowel disease: current status and the future ahead. Gastroenterology. 2014;146:1489–99.
23. Demehri FR, Frykman PK, Cheng Z, Ruan C, Wester T, Nordenskjöld A, Kawaguchi A, Hui TT, Granström AL, Funari V, Teitelbaum DH. Altere fecal short chain fatty acid composition in children with a history of Hirschsprung-associated enterocolitis. J Pediatr Surg. 2016;51(1):81–6.

Intestinal Transplantation for Total Intestinal Aganglionosis

30

Joanne Lai and Kishore Iyer

Contents

J. Lai (✉)
Icahn School of Medicine at Mount Sinai, New York, NY, USA
e-mail: Joanne.Lai@mssm.edu

K. Iyer
Recanati/Miller Transplantation Institute, Mount Sinai Medical Center, New York, NY, USA
e-mail: Kishore.Iyer@mountsinai.org

30.1 Introduction

Total intestinal aganglionosis, i.e., involving the entire colon and small intestine, is a rare form of Hirschprung's disease (HD) affecting about 1% of infants with HD. Total colonic aganglionosis with extensive ileal involvement, or near-total intestinal aganglionosis, affects up to 5% of infants with HD [43, 45]. Total aganglionosis was first described in 1951 [6] and was a universally fatal condition due to intestinal obstruction, malnutrition, and infection. Ziegler reported the first long-term survivor in 1987, describing a surgical approach involving myectomy at the transition zone followed by myotomy at the antimesenteric border of the aganglionic small bowel. The myotomized bowel improved absorptive function and motility of the intestine; however, the majority of patients remained dependent on parenteral nutrition (PN) despite this surgical intervention [51, 52]. Postoperative complications and complications from PN resulted in a high morbidity and mortality [44]. Intestinal transplantation is a definitive treatment for patients with total or near-total intestinal aganglionosis who cannot be maintained on PN.

30.2 Intestinal Failure

Intestinal failure is defined as the reduction of functional gut mass below the minimum amount necessary for digestion and absorption adequate

P. Puri (ed.), *Hirschsprung's Disease and Allied Disorders*,
https://doi.org/10.1007/978-3-030-15647-3_30

to satisfy the nutrient and fluid requirements for maintenance in adults or growth in children [18]. Causes of intestinal failure can be subdivided into three categories: short bowel syndrome, disorders of bowel motility, and primary mucosal disease. Intestinal aganglionosis is a motility disorder; however, resection of affected segments of aganglionic intestine results in a foreshortened intestinal length and superimposed short bowel syndrome. The presence of a proximal jejunostomy leads to increased fluid losses and PN is often necessary to fulfill nutrient and fluid demands [43].

30.2.1 Management of Intestinal Failure

PN is a life-sustaining therapy for patients with intestinal failure; however, prolonged use may be limited by its complications. The likelihood of permanent PN dependence is near-certain when the remnant length of normally innervated small intestine is shorter than 50 cm [16, 28]. Children with intestinal failure are at risk for metabolic, infectious, hepatic, and vascular morbidities necessitating multidisciplinary care. A collaborative approach, including nutritional, medical, and surgical management, has improved outcomes for patients who are dependent on PN.

The medical management of intestinal failure is multifaceted. Providing enteral nutrition is fundamental to promote intestinal adaptation. Pharmacologic therapies also play a role in the management of patients with intestinal failure. Proton-pump inhibitors, histamine-2 receptor antagonists, and octreotide are useful during the hypersecretory and hypergastrinemia phase following massive intestinal resection. Anti-diarrheal agents such as loperamide and diphenoxylate-atropine are used to slow intestinal transit. Bile acid sequestrants are used for bile salt malabsorption after terminal ileal resection. Antibiotic agents are helpful in the treatment of small bowel bacterial overgrowth [39]. Administration of growth factors such as teduglutide (Gattex®, Shire-NPS Pharmaceuticals, Lexington, MA, USA), a glucagon-like peptide 2 analogue, are beneficial in intestinal adaptation by increasing villous length and crypt depth, and lowering parenteral nutrition needs [30].

Intestinal failure-associated liver disease is a frequently encountered complication of PN. Optimizing PN, including use of an appropriate type and amount of lipid emulsion, helps to ameliorate intestinal failure-associated liver disease. Traditional lipid emulsions derived from soybean oil are a contributing factor to liver disease in patients receiving PN [12]. Lipid minimization protocols as well as alternative lipid emulsions such as fish oil-based lipid emulsion Omegaven® (Fresenius Kabi, Bad Homburg, Germany), or combination soy, medium-chain triglyceride, olive, and fish oil lipid emulsion SMOFlipid® (Fresenius Kabi, Bad Homberg, Germany), are effective to prevent or treat liver disease due to PN [10, 17, 20, 40].

Meticulous management of the central venous catheter to avoid catheter-related sepsis and loss of vascular access sites is indispensable in the management of intestinal failure. Protocols addressing central venous catheter insertion procedures and exit site care are necessary to prevent infection. Ethanol lock therapy is an intervention shown to prevent central line associated blood stream infection in patients receiving home PN [41].

Surgical interventions have a limited role in intestinal failure due to intestinal aganglionosis. Autologous intestinal reconstruction procedures to taper and/or lengthen remnant intestine may improve tolerance of enteral feeds and promote intestinal adaptation to avoid or, in the least, postpone intestinal transplant for patients with short bowel syndrome. The latter have not been shown to be of sustained benefit in the presence of functional disease such as HD. A high rate of surgical procedures prior to transplant, however, is an independent risk factor for complications after intestinal transplant [19, 42]. Management of intestinal failure due to intestinal aganglionosis is particularly complicated due to the variable length of involved small intestine and the absence of a functional colon. Patients often undergo multiple abdominal operations beginning with removal of the aganglionic bowel. In the situation of total intestinal aganglionosis, it has been suggested that resection of the entire intestine at the time of diagnosis should be avoided. Loss of abdominal domain, or reduced space in the abdominal cavity, becomes a technical challenge at time of transplant. Furthermore, extensive resection of the intestine may be associated with rapid liver deterioration and the need for transplantation early in life. Consideration may be made for creation of a simple stoma to use the proximal jejunum if possible [45]. Conversely, patients may have increased bacterial translocation from the aganglionic segment and often require early enterectomy to prevent sepsis [43]. Another surgical approach recommended for the neonate with total or near-total aganglionosis includes preservation of 40 cm of proximal jejunum to avoid a high output ostomy and to preserve abdominal domain. Most children demonstrated intestinal passage and tolerated enteral feeds either spontaneously or with longitudinal myotomy [28]. Intestinal lengthening procedures may further reduce space in the abdominal cavity and fail to achieve enteral autonomy, causing greater harm than benefit when intestinal transplant is inevitable.

30.2.2 Complications of Intestinal Failure

Complications of intestinal failure (Table 30.1) are frequent and can be grouped into three categories: bowel anatomy-related complications, including malabsorptive diarrhea, fluid and electrolyte disturbances, small bowel bacterial overgrowth, metabolic bone disease, and growth impairment; complications related to the central venous catheter including infection and central vein thrombosis; and, lastly, liver and biliary complications due to parenteral nutrition. These complications, particularly when life-threatening, become indications for intestinal transplantation. It is also important to recognize that patients with very-long-segment HD often have subtle abnormalities in the residual bowel that may have ganglion cells but exhibit poor prograde motility resulting in functional intestinal failure.

Table 30.1 Complications of intestinal failure

Bowel anatomy-related complications	Parenteral nutrition-related complications	Central venous catheter-related complications
Malabsorptive diarrhea Malnutrition Fluid and electrolyte disturbances Micronutrient deficiency Essential fatty acid deficiency Small bowel bacterial overgrowth D-lactic acidosis Oxalate nephropathy Renal dysfunction Metabolic bone disease Acid peptic disease Anastomotic ulceration/stricture Oral aversion Impaired growth	Intestinal failure-associated liver disease Steatosis Cholestasis Fibrosis Cirrhosis Biliary complications	Infection Occlusion Breakage Central vein thrombosis

30.3 Intestinal Transplantation

Intestinal transplantation has become the standard of care for the management of patients with irreversible intestinal failure. Intestinal transplantation was first reported in 1962 by Thomas E Starzl as part of a multivisceral organ transplant. Outcomes following intestinal transplantation remained poor for several decades due to the immunogenicity of the intestine until the development of tacrolimus in the 1990s [48]. With improvements in surgical techniques including procurement and recipient operations, immunosuppression management, and posttransplant monitoring, significant gains in patient survival and outcome have been achieved. Goals of intestinal transplant for intestinal aganglionosis are two-fold: restoration of intestinal absorption and enteral autonomy and also restoration of colonic function with bowel continence if possible [50].

30.3.1 Indications for Intestinal Transplantation

HD is an infrequent indication for intestinal transplantation. Dysmotility syndromes including pseudoobstruction and intestinal aganglionosis account for 18% of pediatric transplants [7, 21, 22]. Based on the international intestinal transplant registry, the common indications for intestinal transplantation are intestinal failure secondary to necrotizing enterocolitis, gastroschisis or volvulus (Table 30.2). As with all causes of intestinal failure, intestinal transplantation must be considered when impending life-threatening complications due to parenteral nutrition arise. The decision regarding timing and appropriateness of intestinal transplantation requires extensive discussion between transplant surgeons, gastroenterologists, social workers, and, most importantly, the family.

Table 30.2 Indications for intestinal transplantation

Indications for pediatric intestinal transplantation
Short bowel syndrome
Gastroschisis
Volvulus
Necrotizing enterocolitis
Atresia
Ischemia
Trauma
Motility disorder
Hirschprung's disease
Chronic intestinal pseudoobstruction
Hollow visceral myopathy
Megacystis-microcolon-hypoperistalsis syndrome
Abnormalities of interstitial cells of Cajal
Idiopathic
Malabsorption
Microvillus inclusion disease
Tufting enteropathy
Tumor
Indications for adult intestinal transplant
Short bowel syndrome
Ischemia
Crohn's disease
Volvulus
Trauma
Motility disorder
Tumor
Gardner's/familial polyposis

The indications for intestinal transplantation as posited by the American Society of Transplantation are irreversible intestinal failure with parenteral nutrition dependence and one or more of the following: liver disease, catheter-related sepsis, impending loss of vascular access, and electrolyte disturbance or dehydration despite parenteral nutrition.

30.3.1.1 Liver Disease

As intestinal failure-associated liver disease progresses, liver fibrosis will persist or worsen. Fibrosis of the liver leads to portal hypertension which manifests with progressive splenomegaly, varices of the esophagus, stomach or stoma, and ascites. These findings may not be apparent in patients who have had extensive small bowel resection. As liver disease progresses, synthetic function of the liver will be affected, seen by prolongation of prothrombin time and hypoalbuminemia. Once liver disease has progressed to bridging fibrosis and cirrhosis or if synthetic function of the liver is affected, the patient must be treated with a combined liver-intestinal transplant. For this reason, early referral to a transplant center prior to the development of irreversible liver injury is imperative as survival outcomes are worse for combined liver-intestine transplantation as compared to isolated intestine transplantation for total intestinal aganglionosis [43].

30.3.1.2 Catheter-Related Sepsis

Sepsis is frequently related to the presence of a central venous catheter which is necessary for the administration of PN. The rate of catheter-related infections itself is not necessarily an indication for transplant. However, if catheter-related sepsis becomes complicated by metastatic infectious loci or if there are recurrent severe life-threatening bacterial or fungal septic episodes, then transplant is indicated.

30.3.1.3 Impending Loss of Vascular Access

Central venous access provides life-sustaining treatment for patients with intestinal failure. When vascular access sites become thrombosed and can no longer be used, patients risk no longer having a means to receive PN. The standard access sites for younger infants are the right and left subclavian and internal jugular veins. The femoral veins can also be considered to be access sites for older children. Referral for intestinal transplantation is indicated upon loss of two of the four available access sites in younger infants, or three of six access sites in older children.

30.3.1.4 Electrolyte Disturbance or Dehydration Despite Parenteral Nutrition

Despite supplementation with parenteral nutrition, electrolyte abnormalities or episodes of dehydration may persist. Extensive intestinal aganglionosis often results in a proximal ostomy with resultant high output. Intestinal transplantation may be essential to maintain fluid and electrolyte balance [33].

30.3.1.5 Expanded Indications

Increasingly, the indications for intestinal transplant have extended beyond these classic indications. Poor quality of life may be taken into account as an indication for transplant. Particularly in the setting of intestinal failure with a known high risk of mortality, early intestinal transplant may be considered before the development of complications associated with PN. These situations include transplant for congenital mucosal disorders such as tufting enteropathy or microvillus inclusion disease which have no effective therapy. Patients with extreme short bowel syndrome defined as less than 10 cm of jejunum are also known to have poor survival due to rapid progression to liver failure. Total intestinal aganglionosis or near-total intestinal aganglionosis with a short functional intestinal length may fall within this category. Referral to a transplant center does not mandate listing for intestinal transplant but does allow physicians specialized in intestinal rehabilitation and transplant to evaluate children at a high risk of morbidity and even death from a rare and complex disease in order to determine optimal timing of transplant [46, 47].

30.3.2 Contraindications to Intestinal Transplant

The decision to list a patient for intestinal transplant is made based on a thorough evaluation by a multidisciplinary team. Contraindications to intestinal transplant exist and are comparable to other solid organ transplants. A comprehensive evaluation of the patient's clinical status must be completed before transplant, allowing transplant candidacy to be considered on an individual basis. Commonly accepted contraindications to intestinal transplant are listed in Table 30.3. Consideration should be made to conditions affecting the quality of life following transplant such as profound neurologic disabilities, life-threatening conditions, or malignancy outside the gastrointestinal tract. The risks of immunosuppression following transplant must also be anticipated. Patients with immunological deficiencies, whether congenital or acquired, are at significantly greater risk due to immunosuppression. Lastly, maintenance of vascular patency for vascular access is essential during transplant and in the early posttransplant period [33].

30.3.3 Allograft Choice

Understanding the extent of affected gastrointestinal tract and associated organs is critical to decide on the appropriate graft for transplantation. The three major types of allografts are (1) isolated intestine; (2) intestine plus liver, which usually includes the duodenum and head of the pancreas to avoid the need for biliary anastomo-

Table 30.3 Contraindications to intestinal transplant

Contraindications to intestinal transplant
Neurologic disabilities
Life-threatening or uncorrectable illness outside gastrointestinal tract
Severe congenital or acquired immunological deficiencies
Nonresectable malignancies
Multisystem autoimmune diseases
Insufficient vascular patency

sis; and (3) multivisceral allograft which contains the stomach, duodenum, liver, pancreas, and intestine.

Studies of the gastrointestinal system including radiologic, endoscopic, histopathologic, and manometric evaluation should be conducted. The presence and extent of liver disease should be determined during the transplant evaluation in order to decide early on whether a liver-inclusive graft is warranted. Laboratory examinations such as transaminases, albumin, and INR are helpful to determine liver function. Platelet count is an indirect marker of hypersplenism and portal hypertension. Abdominal imaging such as an ultrasound, CT with angiography and venography, or MRI and MRI angiography are helpful to determine anatomy, presence of portal hypertension, and patency of abdominal vasculature. Measurement of elevated portal pressures by angiography supports the diagnosis of portal hypertension. The gold standard for assessment of liver fibrosis and cirrhosis is liver biopsy. Following intestinal transplant, cholestasis, steatosis, and, to some degree, fibrosis may be reversible [13]. Irreversible liver disease manifested by hepatic synthetic compromise or clinical sequelae of portal hypertension mandates a combined liver and intestine transplant.

A multivisceral allograft may include any organ along the gastrointestinal tract. A multivisceral transplant may be necessary in extensive motility disorders and widespread abdominal pathology or if vascular complications such as mesenteric thrombosis have occurred. A modified multivisceral transplant excludes the liver and is appropriate for patients with diffuse gastrointestinal disorders involving the stomach or duodenum but preserved hepatic function. Partial intestine and liver grafts can be procured from living donors, but these techniques are not routinely used [4, 35].

Intestinal transplant for total intestinal aganglionosis is unique in that extensive intestinal involvement is present without a functional colon. Transplantation not only allows the reversal of intestinal failure and restoration of intestinal function but also restoration of colonic function including fecal continence. Inclusion of the right colon vascularized by the superior mesenteric artery for patients with total intestinal aganglionosis is recommended. The colon functions to enhance absorption of water and electrolytes. Fermentation of undigested carbohydrates and further absorption also occurs in the colon. Colon graft length is typically 25–45 cm. Early clinical studies suggested an increase in graft loss and sepsis due to an increased bacterial load leading to translocation when the colon is transplanted [49]. Subsequent reports have shown that the inclusion of colon in the graft is not associated with a higher rate of rejection or infection [32]. Inclusion of the right colon improves enteral fluid absorption and allows a permanent colonic pull-through in the future to establish fecal continence without an ostomy [43, 50]. Colonic pull-through prior to ileostomy closure is recommended due to the risk of septic complications due to fecal retention following pull-through [43].

Similar to other etiologies of intestinal failure, the timing of transplant for intestinal failure due to total intestinal aganglionosis is crucial. Patient survival is worse with combined liver-intestinal transplant as compared to isolated intestinal transplant. Inclusion of the liver in the graft may be beneficial for graft survival due to protective effects on the intestinal graft by reducing rejection rates; however, poorer patient survival outcomes may be related to the presence of portal hypertension related to liver cirrhosis [9, 34, 43]. Additionally, the severe shortage of liver-containing grafts globally, due to the direct competition with isolated liver recipients, leads to a significantly higher mortality on the waiting list for patients awaiting liver-inclusive intestinal transplants [26, 27].

30.3.4 Technical Aspects of Intestinal Transplantation

Intestinal grafts are procured from ABO-matched, size-appropriate cadaveric donors. The size of the donor is often a limitation due to the compromised abdominal domain in patients who have had prior abdominal surgery with resulting scarring or a contracted abdominal cavity. For size mismatch, techniques of tissue expansion prior to transplant, graft size reduction, staged abdominal closure, and grafting of abdominal wall or skin onto exposed intestine have all been effective [36].

Allograft procurement begins with careful donor preparation. The administration of systemic and enteral antibiotics for gut decontamination as well as the use of donor lymphocyte depletion with anti-thymocyte globulin (Thymoglobulin®, Sanofi-Genzyme, Cambridge, MA, USA) is not universal, and there is a lack of compelling evidence showing benefit to such practice. During procurement, depending on the need for en bloc inclusion of the liver, preservation of the arterial vessels of the celiac and/or superior mesenteric arteries as well as the venous outflow of the superior mesenteric vein or hepatic veins is vital. After the graft is carefully dissected out, preservation solution, typically University of Wisconsin solution, is infused throughout the graft.

The donor superior mesenteric artery is anastomosed to the recipient's superior mesenteric artery or an infrarenal aortic graft. Venous drainage is directed to the inferior vena cava or into the portal system of the recipient. Portal drainage is preferred if the superior mesenteric vein and venous length are preserved, though no clear immunological or nutritional disadvantage has been demonstrated with systemic venous drainage [5]. For liver-inclusive or multivisceral transplants, the donor aortic conduit is anastomosed to the recipient's infrarenal or supra-celiac aorta, with a single venous outflow through the suprahepatic inferior vena cava.

An isolated intestinal transplant is typically accomplished by end-to-end anastomosis of the recipient remnant proximal jejunum or duodenum with the graft jejunum. The allograft distal ileum is brought out as a stoma allowing access for surveillance biopsies and monitoring of stoma effluent. If the colon is included, a loop ileostomy may still be created to allow surveillance biopsies as the colon may not reflect rejection as sensitively as the ileum [8, 25].

30.4 Post-intestinal Transplant Management

Improvements in graft outcomes have improved in recent decades; however, acute and chronic graft rejection, sepsis, and posttransplant lymphoproliferative disorder remain common causes of posttransplant morbidity and mortality. Intestine graft rejection is more difficult to prevent and treat than rejection of other solid organs, requiring high levels of immunosuppression. Morbidity and mortality following transplant also include potential surgical complications. Long-term complications in survivors, predominantly due to medications, include hypertension, osteoporosis, diabetes and chronic renal failure [2].

30.4.1 Postoperative Complications

Immediate postoperative complications are outlined in Table 30.4. Early postoperative surgical complications include arterial thrombosis, aortic graft pseudoaneurysm, hemorrhage, intra-abdominal infection, and leakage from the gastrointestinal-biliary anastomosis. Acute rejection of the graft may also occur and necessitate an increase in immunosuppression or, in severe cases, graft enterectomy, with return to PN and potential consideration of retransplantation.

Table 30.4 Immediate posttransplant complications

Immediate postoperative complications
Surgical
Abdominal compartment syndrome
Intra-abdominal abscess
Intestinal fistula
Hemorrhage
Intestinal perforation
Intestinal obstruction
Graft thrombosis
Infectious
Bacterial and fungal sepsis
Viral infections – EBV, CMV
Immunological
Acute cellular rejection
Antibody-mediated rejection

30.4.2 Immunosuppression Management

Rejection of the intestine graft is challenging due to the innate immunity of the enterocyte, intestinal leukocytes, mesenteric lymph nodes, and Peyer's patches. The recipient immune system and donor immunocytes brought with the allograft give rise to a two-way interaction of host-versus-graft and graft-versus-host. Intestinal transplantation is also associated with a cascade of inflammatory signals as a result of ischemia reperfusion injury, bacterial signals, and bacterial translocation. Intestine rejection leads to significant morbidity due to the high risk of infection from bacterial translocation which occurs following breakdown of the gut barrier function. The degree of immunosuppression to prevent graft rejection must be weighed against the risks of infection and posttransplant lymphoproliferative disease [26, 27].

Specific immunosuppression protocols vary between centers. Induction protocols typically include anti-thymocyte globulin (Thymoglobulin®, Sanofi-Genzyme, Cambridge, MA, USA) or IL-2 antagonists. Maintenance immunosuppression protocols are based on tacrolimus with occasional additional agents, primarily mycophenolate mofetil and m-TOR inhibitors such as sirolimus. Newer protocols attempt to minimize immunosuppression and promote partial tolerance through the generation of regulatory T-cells [1], though the significant risk of graft loss from severe acute rejection has hindered widespread adoption of such strategies.

Based on the most recent Intestinal Transplant Registry Report in 2015, the majority of recipients are treated with induction therapy using either an IL-2 antagonist, anti-thymocyte globulin, or alemtuzumab (lymphocyte depletion). The majority of survivors are given tacrolimus as maintenance immunosuppression [22].

30.4.3 Surveillance for Graft Rejection

No laboratory marker exists to monitor graft function or graft rejection. Diarrhea or increased stool output, bloody stool output, abdominal pain, fever, weight loss, vomiting, anemia, and hypoalbuminemia are the nonspecific signs and symptoms that suggest rejection. Lymphadenopathy, abdominal distension, ascites, edema, and discoloration of the stoma are physical signs that should trigger evaluation of rejection. Typically, surveillance protocol ileoscopy with intestinal biopsies are carried out to monitor for graft rejection. Zoom endoscopy aids in the endoscopic diagnosis of rejection without the delay of histologic processing. While the optimal frequency of endoscopies is not known, typical surveillance protocols are 1 to 2 per week for the first month after transplant followed by a gradual wean in frequency. Plasma citrulline and fecal calprotectin have been studied as possible screening tests. A cell-based assay using allospecific CD154+ T-cytotoxic memory cells has been shown to predict acute cellular rejection with a high sensitivity and specificity [3].

Endoscopic findings of acute cellular rejection include friable and edematous mucosa, erythema, superficial or deep ulcerations, and, in severe cases, diffuse exfoliation of mucosa. Graft rejection may be patchy. Diagnosis of rejection relies on biopsies taken from multiple locations. Acute cellular rejection can be detected in any organ of the composite graft, even if the intestine remains at greatest risk for acute cellular rejection. Histologic findings in the intestine graft are crypt epithelial cell apoptosis, crypt injury, mixed inflammatory cell infiltrate, villus blunting with architectural distortion, and edema with vascular congestion. Diffuse mucosal ulceration, erosion, and sloughing are seen in exfoliative rejection which has a high risk for graft loss and mortality [25]. Mainstays of treatment for rejection are high doses of corticosteroids, thymoglobulin or alemtuzumab [8].

The role of donor-specific antibodies (DSA) in antibody-mediated rejection and short- and long-term risks of rejection is coming to attention. Presence of preformed DSA has been associated with a higher risk of early graft failure. Development of DSA after transplant, termed de novo DSA, also had an accelerated graft loss of 28% by 2 years after detection of DSA. Mounting evidence suggests a role for immune suppressive regimens to target donor-specific antibodies prior to transplant and de novo DSA after transplant [9].

Chronic rejection is a common cause of late graft dysfunction but is not a mucosal process and hence can be diagnosed only in full-thickness biopsies or following graft enterectomy. Diagnosis is made histopathologically by intimal hyperplasia and obliterative arteriopathy with concentric fibrous intimal thickening of the large- and medium-sized arteries found in submucosal layers of the intestine graft. Recurrent acute cellular rejection may be associated with chronic rejection. No definitive treatment for chronic rejection exists, and retransplantation may be the only solution [38].

30.4.4 Infection

Infection is a common complication following intestinal transplant and is a leading cause of posttransplant mortality. The risk of infection is augmented by high levels of immunosuppression and the potential for bacterial translocation due to breakdown of the gut barrier following ischemia reperfusion injury or episodes of acute rejection. Bacterial infections include bacteremia, sepsis, intra-abdominal abscess, pneumonia, or wound infections.

Common viral infections affecting transplant recipients include cytomegalovirus (CMV), Epstein-Barr virus (EBV), adenovirus, rotavirus, and, rarely, calcivirus. These viral pathogens may cause enteric infection and gastrointestinal symptoms which mimic acute cellular rejection. Strategies for surveillance and prophylaxis of viral infection vary by institution. Routine surveillance of CMV, EBV, and adenovirus in the blood and intestinal biopsies may help in early detection and treatment of infection.

CMV infection develops in 20% of patients, most frequently as enteric infection, but may involve any organ [14]. Ganciclovir, oral valganciclovir and Cytogam® (CSL Behring AG, Bern, Switzerland), a CMV-specific immunoglobulin, are used for prophylaxis and treatment of CMV infection.

Adenovirus also causes enteritis but may also disseminate and infect the brain, liver, lungs, or pancreas. No definitive treatment for adenoviral infection exists. Supportive care and reduction of immunosuppression are the mainstays of treatment. Cidofovir may play a role in the treatment of adenovirus infection, particularly when used preemptively [15].

EBV infects B-cells and can lead to systemic disease in the immunosuppressed patient. EBV infection is often detected as asymptomatic viremia but may lead to invasive EBV disease. The intestinal allograft is the most common location for invasive EBV disease and is visualized endoscopically as mucosal ulcerations of the intestine. Transformation of EBV infection to polyclonal and monoclonal lymphoproliferative diseases and lymphoma is a feared complication. Careful monitoring for EBV viremia and reduction in immunosuppression in the setting of non-malignant EBV disease must be carefully undertaken [23].

30.4.5 Posttransplant Lymphoproliferative Disorder

Posttransplant lymphoproliferative disorder (PTLD) is most commonly an EBV-driven B-cell lymphoproliferation. Non-EBV-related lymphoma such as non-Hodgkin B-cell or T-cell lymphoma may also occur. High levels of immunosuppression and antibody-depleting agents contribute to rates of PTLD which are higher in intestinal transplant as compared to other solid organ transplants. Judicious maintenance of immunosuppression and closer monitoring of EBV have led to improved rates of PTLD, now estimated at less than 10% [22]. Treatment of PTLD includes lowering of immunosuppression and, in advanced cases, use of rituximab, a monoclonal anti-CD20 antibody, and chemotherapy [24]. Lowering or withdrawal of immunosuppression to allow the immune system to develop a cytotoxic T-cell lymphocyte response may lead to rejection, further complicating management of PTLD. The use of cytotoxic T-cell therapy has had promising results [11]. Allograft enterectomy to allow cessation of immunosuppression can also be considered in severe cases.

30.4.6 Graft-Versus-Host Disease

As previously mentioned, the intestine graft carries with it donor lymphoid cells leading to graft-versus-host disease in 5% of intestinal transplant recipients, a rate that is much higher than other solid organs recipients [31]. Donor-derived lymphocytes lead to injury of the skin, native intestine, liver, and bone marrow. Mild cases may resolve without intervention, but severe cases are treated with corticosteroids and carry with it a high risk of mortality.

30.5 Outcomes of Intestinal Transplantation

In the last 30 years, over 2700 intestinal transplants have been performed worldwide. The international experience has reported patient survival as 77%, 58%, and 47% at 1, 5, and 10 years, respectively, with graft survival of 71%, 50%, and 41%, respectively [22]. Specific high-volume centers have reported survival rates at 1, 3, and 5 years of 95%, 84%, and 77%, respectively, and graft survival of 88%, 74%, and 58% [4]. A meta-analysis of intestinal transplantation for total intestinal aganglionosis with 37% isolated intestinal transplants and 63% who underwent multivisceral transplantation, reported an overall survival rate of 66% over a mean follow-up period of 40 months [37].

Of the survivors of intestinal transplant as a whole, the vast majority are able to be fully weaned from PN onto full enteral feeding by either oral route or tube feeding by about 3 months [29]. Most survivors attain significant improvement in quality of life after transplantation and are able to maintain a self-sustained socioeconomic status [2].

30.6 Conclusion

Intestinal transplantation has evolved to be the standard of care for children with intestinal failure and resultant life-threatening complications. Total intestinal aganglionosis or near-total intestinal aganglionosis is a rare but highly fatal form of Hirschprung's disease. Intestinal transplantation offers the potential for enteral autonomy from PN. Early referral to a transplant center allows for optimization of parenteral nutrition and timing of intestinal transplant to enhance outcomes in these patients with irreversible intestinal failure. Following transplant, conscientious management of immunosuppression and vigilance to detect and treat rejection and infectious complications have allowed improvement in patient and graft survival. Intestinal transplantation is a life-saving option for a once universally fatal diagnosis. While short- and medium-term outcomes of intestinal transplant have shown significant recent improvements, long-term survival remains guarded.

References

1. Abu-Elmagd KM, Costa G, Bond GJ, Wu T, Murase N, Zeevi A, Simmons R, Soltys K, Sindhi R, Stein W, Demetris A, Mazariegos G. Evolution of the immunosuppressive strategies for the intestinal and multivisceral recipients with special reference to allograft immunity and achievement of partial tolerance. Transpl Int. 2009;22(1):96–109.
2. Abu-Elmagd KM, Kosmach-Park B, Costa G, Zenati M, Martin L, Koritsky DA, Emerling M, Murase N, Bond GJ, Soltys K, Sogawa H, Lunz J, Al Samman M, Saefer N, Sidhi R, Mazariegos GV. Long-term survival, nutritional autonomy, and quality of life after intestinal and multivisceral transplantation. Ann Surg. 2012;256(3):494–508.
3. Ashokkumar C, Soltys K, Mazariegos G, Bond G, Higgs BW, Ningappa M, Sun Q, Brown A, White J, Levy S, Fazzolare T, Remaley L, Dirling K, Harris P, Hartle T, Kachmar P, Nicely M, O'Toole L, Boehm B, Jativa N, Stanley P, Jaffe R, Ranganathan S, Zeevi A, Sindhi R. Predicting cellular rejection with a cell-based assay: pre-clinical evaluation in children. Transplantation. 2017;101(1):131–40.
4. Avitzur Y, Grant D. Intestine transplantation in children: update 2010. Pediatr Clin North Am. 2010;57(2):415–31.
5. Berney T, Kato T, Nishida S, Tector AJ, Mittal NK, Madariaga J, Nery JR, Cantwell GP, Ruiz P, Tzakis AG. Portal versus systemic drainage of small bowel allografts: comparative assessment of survival, function, rejection, and bacterial translocation. J Am Coll Surg. 2002;195(6):804–13.
6. Bodian M, Carter CO, Ward BC. Hirschprung's disease. Lancet. 1951;1(6650):302–9.

7. Bond GJ, Reyes JD. Intestinal transplantation for total/near-total aganglionosis and intestinal pseudo-obstruction. Semin Pediatr Surg. 2004;13(4):286–92.
8. Celik N, Stanley K, Rudolph J, Al-Issa F, Kosmach B, Ashokkumar C, Sun Q, Brown-Bakewell R, Zecca D, Soltys K, Khanna A, Bond G, Ganoza A, Mazariegos G, Sindhi R. Improvements in intestine transplantation. Semin Pediatr Surg. 2018;27(4)267–72.
9. Cheng EY, Everly MJ, Kaneku H, Banuelos N, Wozniak LJ, Venick RS, Marcus EA, McDiarmid SV, Busuttil RW, Terasaki PI, Farmer DG. Prevalence and clinical impact of donor-specific alloantibody among intestinal transplant recipients. Transplantation. 2017;101(4):873–82.
10. Cober MP, Killu G, Brattain A, Welch KB, Kunisaki SM, Teitelbaum DH. Intravenous fat emulsions reduction for patients with parenteral nutrition-associated liver disease. J Pediatr. 2012;160(3):421–7.
11. DeStefano CB, Desai SH, Shenoy AG, Catlett JP. Management of post-transplant lymphoproliferative disorders. Br J Haematol. 2018;182(3):330–43.
12. El Kasmi KC, Anderson AL, Devereaux MW, Vue PM, Zhang W, Setchell KD, Karpen SJ, Sokol RJ. Phytosterols promote liver injury and Kupffer cell activation in parenteral nutrition-associated liver disease. Sci Transl Med. 2013;5(206):206ra137.
13. Fiel MI, Wu HS, Iyer K, Rodriguez-Laiz G, Schiano TD. Rapid reversal of parenteral-nutrition-associated cirrhosis following isolated intestinal transplantation. J Gastrointest Surg. 2009;13(9):1717–23.
14. Fishman JA, Rubin RH. Infection in organ-transplant recipients. N Engl J Med. 1998;338(24):1741–51.
15. Florescu DF, Islam MK, Mercer DF, Grant W, Langnas AN, Freifeld AG, Sudan D, Basappa R, Dimaio D, Kalil AC. Adenovirus infections in pediatric small bowel transplant recipients. Transplantation. 2010;90(2):198–204.
16. Fouquet V, De Lagausie P, Faure C, Bloch J, Malbezin S, Ferkhadji L, Bauman C, Aigrain Y. Do prognostic factors exist for total colonic aganglionosis with ileal involvement? J Pediatr Surg. 2002;37(1):71–5.
17. Gonzalez-Hernandez J, Prajapati P, Ogoa G, Channabasappa N, Piper HG. A comparison of lipid minimization strategies in children with intestinal failure. J Pediatr Surg. 2018;53:96–100.
18. Goulet O, Ruemmele F, Lacaille F, Colomb V. Irreversible intestinal failure. J Pediatr Gastroenterol Nutr. 2004;38(3):250–69.
19. Goulet O, Sauvat F, Ruemmele F, Caldari D, Damotte D, Cezard JP, Lacaille F, Canioni D, Hugot JP, Berebi D, Sarnacki S, Colomb V, Jan D, Aigrain Y, Revillon Y. Results of the Paris program: ten years of pediatric intestinal transplantation. Transplant Proc. 2005;37(4):1667–70.
20. Goulet O, Antebi H, Wolf C, Talbotec C, Alcindor LG, Corriol O, Lamor M, Colomb-Jung V. A new intravenous fat emulsion containing soybean oil, medium-chain triglyceride, olive oil, and fish oil: a single-center double-blind randomized study on efficacy and safety in pediatric patients receiving home parenteral nutrition. J Parenter Enteral Nutr. 2010;34(5):485–95.
21. Grant D, Abu-Elmagd K, Reyes J, Tzakis A, Langnas A, Fishbein T, Goulet O, Farmer D, on behalf of the Intestine Transplant Registry. 2003 Report of the Intestine Transplant Registry. Ann Surg. 2005;241(2):607–13.
22. Grant D, Abu-Elmagd K, Mazariegos G, Vianna R, Langnas A, Mangus R, Farmer DG, Lacaille F, Iyer K, Fishbein T, Intestinal Transplant Association. Intestinal transplant registry report: global activity and trends. Am J Transplant. 2015;15(1):210–9.
23. Green M, Michaels MG. Epstein-Barr virus infection and posttransplant lymphoproliferative disorder. Am J Transplant. 2013;13(s3):41–54.
24. Gross TG, Orijuela MA, Perkins SL, Park JR, Lynch JC, Cairo MS, Smith LM, Hayashi RJ. Low-dose chemotherapy and rituximab for PTLD: a children's oncology group report. Am J Transplant. 2012;12(11):3069–175.
25. Huard G, Schiano T, Fiel MI, Ward SC, Moon J, Iyer K. Comparative incidence of rejection occurring in small intestinal and colonic mucosal biopsies of patients undergoing intestinal transplantation. Histopathology. 2016;69(4):600–6.
26. Huard G, Schiano T, Moon J, Iyer K. Choice of allograft in patients requiring intestinal transplantation: a critical review. Can J of Gastroenterol and Hepatol. 2017;1–10.
27. Huard G, Schiano TD, Moon J, Iyer K. Severe acute cellular rejection after intestinal transplantation is associated with poor patient and graft survival. Clin Transplant. 2017;31(5):e12956.
28. Hukkinen M, Koivusalo A, Merras-Salmio L, Rintala RJ, Pakarinen MP. Postoperative outcome and survival in relation to small intestinal involvement of total colonic aganglionosis. J Pediatr Surg. 2015;50(11):1859–64.
29. Iyer K, Horslen S, Iverson A, Sudan D, Fox I, Shaw B, Langnas A. Nutritional outcome and growth of children after intestinal transplantation. J Pediatr Surg. 2002;37(3):464–6.
30. Jeppesen PB, Pertkiewicz M, Messing B, Iyer K, Seidner DL, O'keefe SJ, Forbes A, Heinze H, Joelsson B. Gastroenterology. 2012;143(6):1473–81.
31. Kato T, Tzakis AG, Selvaggi G, Gaynor JJ, David AI, Bussotti A, Moon JI, Ueno T, DeFaria W, Santiago S, Levi DM, Nishida S, Velasco ML, McLaughlin G, Hernandez E, Thompson JF, Cantwell P, Holliday N, Livingstone AS, Ruiz P. Intestinal and multivisceral transplantation in children. Ann Surg. 2006;243(6):756–64.
32. Kato T, Selvaggi G, Gaynor JJ, Takahasi H, Nishida S, Moon J, Levi D, Smith L, Hernandez E, Ruiz P, Tzakis A. Inclusion of donor colon and ileocecal valve in intestinal transplantation. Transplantation. 2008;86(2):293–7.
33. Kaufman SS, Atkinson JB, Bianchi A, Goulet OJ, Grant D, Langnas A, SV MD, Mittal N, Reyes J, Tzakis AG, American Society of Transplantation.

Indications for pediatric intestinal transplantation: a position paper of the American Society of Transplantation. Pediatr Transplant. 2001;5(2):80–7.
34. Matsumoto CS, Fishbein TM. Modified multivisceral transplantation with splenopancreatic preservation. Transplantation. 2007;83(2):234–6.
35. Lacaille F, Irtan S, Dupic L, Talbotec C, Lesage F, Colomb V, Salvi N, Moulin F, Sauvat F, Aigrain Y, Revillon Y, Goulet O, Chardot C. Twentyeight years of intestinal transplantation in Paris: experience of the oldest European center. Transpl Int. 2017;30(2):178–86.
36. Millar AJW, Gupte G, Sharif K. Intestinal transplantation for motility disorders. Semin Pediatr Surg. 2009;18:258–62.
37. Nakamura H, Henderson D, Puri P. A meta-analysis of clinical outcome of intestinal transplantation in patients with total intestinal aganglionosis. Pediatr Surg Int. 2017;33:837–41.
38. Parizhskaya M, Redondo C, Demetris A, Jaffe R, Reyes J, Ruppert K, Marin L, Abu-Elmagd K. Chronic rejection of small bowel grafts: pediatric and adult study of risk factors and morphologic progression. Pediatr Dev Pathol. 2003;6(3):240–50.
39. Parrish CR, DiBaise JK. Managing the adult patient with short bowel syndrome. Gastroenterol Hepatol. 2017;13(10):600–8.
40. Premkumar MH, Carter BA, Hawthorne KM, King K, Abrams SA. Fish oil-based emulsions in the treatment of parenteral nutrition-associated liver disease: an ongoing positive experience. Adv Nutr. 2014;5(1):65–70.
41. Rahhal R, Abu-El-Haija MA, Fei L, Ebach D, Orkin S, Kiscaden E, Cole CR. Systemic review and meta-analysis of the utilization of ethanol locks in pediatric patients with intestinal failure. J Parenter Enteral Nutr. 2018;42(4):690–701.
42. Sauvat F, Dupic L, Caldari D, Lesage F, Cezard JP, Lacaille F, Ruemmele F, Hugot JP, Colomb V, Jan D, Hubert P, Revillon Y, Goulet O. Factors influencing outcome after intestinal transplantation in children. Transplant Proc. 2006;38(6):1689–91.
43. Sauvat F, Grimaldi C, Lacaille F, Ruemmele F, Dupic L, Bourdaud N, Fusaro F, Colomb V, Jan D, Cezard J, Aigran Y, Revillon Y, Goulet O. Intestinal transplantation for total intestinal aganglionosis: a series of 12 consecutive children. J Pediatr Surg. 2008;43(10):1833–8.
44. Saxton ML, Ein SH, Hoehner J, Kim PC. Near-total intestinal aganglionosis: long-term following of a morbid condition. J Pediatr Surg. 2000;35(5):669–72.
45. Sharif K, Beath SV, Kelly DA, McKiernan P, van Mourik I, Mirza D, Mayer AD, Buckels JA, de Ville de Govet J. New perspective for the management of near-total or total intestinal aganglionosis in infants. J Pediatr Surg. 2003;38(1):25–8.
46. Soltys KA, Bond G, Sindhi R, Rassmussen SK, Ganoza A, Khanna A, Mazariegos G. Pediatric intestinal transplantation. Semin Pediatr Surg. 2017;26(4):241–9.
47. Squires RH, Duggan C, Teitelbaum DH, Wales PW, Balint J, Venick R, Rhee S, Sudan D, Mercer D, Martinez JA, Carter BA, Soden J, Horslen S, Rudolph JA, Kocoshis S, Superina R, Lawlor S, Haller T, Kurs-Lasky M, Belle SH, Pediatric Intestinal Failure Consortium. Natural history of pediatric intestinal failure: initial report from the Pediatric Intestinal Failure Consortium. J Pediatr. 2012;161(4):723–8.
48. Todo S, Tzakis AG, Abu-Elmagd K, Reyes J, Fung JJ, Casavilla A, Nakamura K, Yagihashi A, Jain A, Murase N, et al. Cadaveric small bowel and small bowel-liver transplantation in humans. Transplantation. 1992;53(2):369–76.
49. Todo S, Reyes J, Furukawa H, Abu-Elmagd K, Lee RG, Tzakis A, Rao AS, Starzl TE. Outcome analysis of 71 clinical intestinal transplantations. Ann Surg. 1995;222(3):270–82.
50. Yann R, Yves A, Jan D, Thierry Y, Goulet O, Lacaille F. Improved quality of life by combined transplantation in Hirschprung's disease with a very long aganglionic segment. J Pediatr Surg. 2003;38(3):422–4.
51. Ziegler MM, Ross AJ 3rd, Bishop HC. Total intestinal aganglionosis: a new technique for prolonged survival. J Pediatr Surg. 1987;22(1):82–3.
52. Ziegler MM, Royal RE, Brandt J, Drasnin J, Martin LW. Extended myectomy-myotomy: a therapeutic alternative for total intestinal aganglionosis. Ann Surg. 1993;218(4):504–11.

Urological and Sexual Outcomes in Patients with Hirschsprung's Disease

31

Kristiina Kyrklund and Mikko P. Pakarinen

Contents

K. Kyrklund · M. P. Pakarinen (✉)
Section of Pediatric Surgery, Pediatric Liver and Gut Research Group, Pediatric Research Center, Children's Hospital, University of Helsinki and Helsinki University Hospital, Helsinki, Finland
e-mail: kristiina.kyrklund@hus.fi; mikko.pakarinen@hus.fi

Synonyms and Abbreviations

CAKUT	Congenital anomalies of the kidney and urinary tract
FMTC	Familial medullary thyroid cancer
GDNF	Glial cell line neurotrophic factor
GFRα1	GDNF family receptor alpha-1
LUTS	Lower urinary tract symptoms
MEN2	Multiple endocrine neoplasia type s2
QoL	Quality of life
RET	REarranged during Transfection
UI	Urinary incontinence

31.1 Introduction

Hirschsprung's disease remains a challenging condition in pediatric surgery. To date, most research has been focused around the postoperative bowel functional outcomes, Hirschsprung's-associated enterocolitis, and the complex genetic basis of this condition. Recent years have also witnessed increasing interest also toward the urological and sexual outcomes, as these are major contributors to individual long-term well-being, comprehensive psychosocial functioning, and quality of life (QoL) [28, 44]. Besides impairments in bowel function and fecal control, the consequences and complications of pelvic surgery and associated genitourinary anomalies may

P. Puri (ed.), *Hirschsprung's Disease and Allied Disorders*,
https://doi.org/10.1007/978-3-030-15647-3_31

have far-reaching effects on urological and sexual outcomes as well as fertility in Hirschsprung's patients. Although the reported incidence of urethral, vasal and ureteric injuries as well as iatrogenic fistulas to surrounding organs during pull-through surgery has been low [44], there is growing evidence from contemporary studies that the incidence of congenital urogenital anomalies, which were also thought to be uncommon, has been underestimated [14]. The significance of postoperative pelvic adhesions on female fertility remains to be elucidated in Hirschsprung's patients, although comparable operative treatment of ulcerative colitis is known to reduce female fecundity [39].

Postoperative impairments in bowel function and fecal incontinence, which variably occur after standard coloanal pull-through operations for rectosigmoid aganglionosis, may have significant negative effects on psychosexual development and social integration. Surgical complications and the need for bowel management or enterostomy may further jeopardize bowel functional outcomes and development of sexual self-esteem [31]. In this chapter, we review the urological and sexual outcome in patients with Hirschsprung's disease and discuss how operative treatment, surgical complications, associated congenital genitourinary anomalies, and the effects of chronic morbidity may modulate them. Increased attention to genitourinary morbidity and strategies to ascertain and support normal psychosexual development in these patients is encouraged.

31.2 Effect of Surgical Treatment on the Genitourinary Tract

The Duhamel procedure and Soave or Swenson type of transanal pull-through are the most commonly used operations to treat Hirschsprung's disease worldwide [49]. Patients usually undergo pull-through surgery in early infancy once the diagnosis has been confirmed. Irrespective of the surgical technique used, low pelvic dissection during rectosigmoidectomy in small infants is associated with a risk of neural damage of pelvic splanchnic nerves (nervi erigentes), which may interfere with genitourinary function including bladder emptying, urinary continence, sexual arousal, and erectile function. The risk for neural damage is higher when dissection is performed outside the rectal wall. In addition, surgical mobilization of the distal colon results in formation of pelvic adhesions, which may reduce female fecundity similar to restorative proctocolectomy in females with ulcerative colitis or adenomatous polyposis [39].

In this respect, endorectal and laparoscopic surgical techniques are theoretically the safest approaches by minimizing dissection outside the rectal wall and associated autonomic nerve injury and by reducing adhesion formation, pelvic scarring, and fallopian tube obstruction. So far, these issues have not been tested in specifically designed and adequately powered clinical follow-up trials in patients with Hirschsprung's disease. However, technically comparable surgery for other pediatric bowel problems has significant consequences on sexual function, especially in females. After childhood restorative proctocolectomy with ileoanal anastomosis for ulcerative colitis, as many as 50% of women report different forms of sexual dysfunction when assessed by validated normative questionnaires [42]. Proctocolectomy complications such as pelvic infection, fistulas, and pouchitis seem to increase the chance of postoperative sexual dysfunction in women. In contrast, erectile dysfunction and retrograde ejaculation in males with ulcerative colitis following childhood proctocolectomy are unusual complications [19, 42].

Direct genitourinary organ injuries are rare but potentially serious complications of pull-through surgery, which may require extensive additional surgery and have significant lifelong consequences.

Recent institutional series suggest an incidence of 1–2% after transanal pull-through, although operative genitourinary complications may have been underreported [44]. In a systematic review of genitourinary complications including 1021 Hirschsprung's patients, the overall incidence of operative ureteric, urethral, vasal, or vaginal injuries after different types of pull-through operations was 0.7% [44]. Most of these were reported after transanal pull-through surgery, which is not surprising due to limited visualization of the intrapelvic space and immediate vicinity of the urethra in males during totally transanal dissection. Iatrogenic fistulas to surrounding organs have developed after both laparoscopic-assisted and open pull-throughs. Two patients with rectourethral and one patient with rectovaginal fistula were identified. Postoperative urinary tract infections and temporary urinary retention may be rarely encountered after pull-through surgery.

31.3 Postoperative Bowel Function

Impairments in bowel function, and especially fecal incontinence, may have important, indirect, and negative consequences on psychosexual outcomes in patients with Hirschsprung's disease. Surgical management of Hirschsprung's disease ranges from simple and uneventful coloanal pull-through in rectosigmoid aganglionosis to permanent high jejunostomy and intestinal transplantation with all associated difficulties and complications [15]. Even following a typical transanal coloanal pull-through for classic rectosigmoid Hirschsprung's disease, a significant proportion of patients suffer from repeated episodes of enterocolitis and outlet obstruction as well as different degrees of fecal incontinence, especially during early childhood. After a Duhamel operation, constipation is a more frequent concern and source of morbidity [5, 24].

Reassuringly, with increasing age, fecal control gradually improves and approaches the level of normal population controls by young adulthood in most, while the reasons for this age-related improvement remains unclear [29]. Operative complications such as residual aganglionosis, transition zone pull-through, twisting of the pulled-through bowel, rolled muscle cuff, misplaced coloanal anastomosis, and stretching-induced sphincter damage further worsen bowel function and fecal control, jeopardizing normal psychosexual development [31]. It should be also borne in mind that although redo pull-through effectively treats recalcitrant obstructive symptoms, bowel functional outcomes remain clearly inferior to those achieved after uncomplicated primary pull-through [10, 37].

A misplaced coloanal anastomosis and stretching-induced sphincter damage represent the most unfortunate complications, because they predispose to permanent fecal incontinence, which is unamenable to redo pull-through and carries significant psychosocial consequences [31]. Performing the coloanal anastomosis at or below the dentate line invariably results in fecal incontinence by removing the transitional epithelium above the dentate line responsible for sensation and ability to differentiate between solid, liquid, and gas. Endosonographic findings of sphincter damage are more common after a totally transanal pull-through with a correlation to decreased anal resting pressure and severity of fecal incontinence [41]. Laparoscopic colonic mobilization may reduce excessive perioperative stretching of sphincters and risk of fecal incontinence. Postponing transanal pull-through beyond neonatal period when patients are physically larger may have a similar positive effect [24]. In general, following a Soave-type transanal pull-through, a coloanal anastomosis that is placed too distally and extensive sphincter injury are the most common reasons for loss of fecal control. Where bowel management or permanent enterostomy is required, social integration and the development of sexual self-esteem may be further affected [4, 9].

True anastomotic strictures requiring extensive dilatations or surgery rarely occur after pull-through. Around 10% of patients require dilatations of the coloanal anastomosis for a few weeks postoperatively [5]. Enterocolitis is an inherent postoperative complication of transanal pull-through surgery and occurs with similar frequency after transanal Soave and Swenson in 10–45% of patients. Most patients experience one or two episodes, and the tendency to enterocolitis episodes decreases over time [29]. Especially when obstructive symptoms are present, recurrent enterocolitis causes significant morbidity akin to that of chronic pouchitis after restorative proctocolectomy for ulcerative colitis, which is known to associate with sexual dysfunction in females [42].

31.4 Associated Urogenital Anomalies in Hirschsprung's Disease

Associated urogenital anomalies in Hirschsprung's patients have, to date, been reported in a relatively low number of series that are mostly retrospective with various methodologies. However, this topic is particularly interesting from a clinical and genetic perspective, as homozygous knockout mice for genes involved in the *Ret* signaling pathway present with renal agenesis or dysplasia in addition to megacolon [1]. The review by Moore [26] examined 4328 patients with Hirschsprung's disease, finding an overall incidence of 21.1% for any types of associated congenital anomalies. A recent analysis found 18 articles published between 1955 and 2014 describing Hirschsprung's patients with either congenital anomalies of the kidney and urinary tract (CAKUT), urological or urogenital anomalies [14]. These yielded an overall prevalence of only 3.6% among 5693 patients. Seven of these studies covering 757 patients were more systematically reported according to the CAKUT criteria established during the late 1990s [35], from which a higher occurrence of CAKUT (9.5%) was proposed [14]. The only two prospective studies to date have suggested the incidence to be even greater, around 20–25% [33, 34], and that earlier estimates have been too conservative.

However, these studies employed systematic renal tract ultrasound screening and clinical evaluation to look for CAKUT, which would have picked up even mild anomalies. As CAKUT encompasses a broad spectrum of clinical and anatomical entities, asymptomatic patients may have avoided detection altogether without routine screening, partially accounting for the low prevalence rates. In order to evaluate the clinical morbidity of CAKUT in Hirschsprung's patients, it is necessary to assess the frequency of individual phenotypes and prevalence of symptoms relating to CAKUT. The occurrence of individual CAKUT phenotypes in the two most recent prospective series, out of a total of 190 patients with Hirschsprung's disease, is presented in Table 31.1. A total of 55 anomalies were found among 43 patients, the most common being renal dysplasia or hypoplasia, vesicoureteric reflux, and hydronephrosis, consistent with historical literature [14]. Of patients with CAKUT, 37% became symptomatic, mainly with urinary tract infections, and 9% required urologic surgery. As shown in Table 31.2, other associated anomalies occurred among 56% of patients with CAKUT,

Table 31.1 Distribution of CAKUT phenotypes among patients with Hirschsprung's disease in recent prospective studies

	N (%)		
CAKUT phenotype	[34] (*n* = 106)	[33] (*n* = 84)	Total (*n* = 190)
Renal dysplasia	9 (9)	7 (8)	17 (9)
Renal asymmetry	1 (1)	0 (0)	1 (0.5)
Renal agenesis	1 (1)	0 (0)	1 (0.5)
Hydronephrosis	5 (5)	7 (8)	12 (6)
Vesicoureteric reflux	6 (6)	3 (4)	9 (5)
Duplex collecting system	2 (2)	3 (4)	5 (3)
Posterior urethral valves	1 (1)	0 (0)	1 (0.5)
Multicystic dysplastic kidney	1 (1)	0 (0)	1 (0.5)
Horseshoe kidney	0 (0)	1 (1)	1 (0.5)

Table 31.2 Other anomalies or syndromes identified among 43 Hirschsprung's patients from recent prospective series

	N (%)		
Other anomalies	[34] (*n* = 22)	[33] (*n* = 21)	Total (*n* = 43)
Isolated CAKUT (no other anomalies)	5 (23)	14 (66)	19 (44)
Cryptorchidism	1 (5)	0 (0)	1 (2)
Ear pit	2 (9)	0 (0)	2 (5)
Hearing impairment	4 (18)	Not assessed	n/a
Mild abnormalities of visual acuity	13 (59)	Not assessed	n/a
Corpus callosum agenesis	1 (5)	0 (0)	1 (2)
Congenital heart disease	2 (9)	2 (10)	4 (9)
Cleft palate	1 (5)	0 (0)	1 (2)
Intestinal atresia	1 (5)	0 (0)	1 (2)
Pigmentation defects	0 (0)	2 (10)	2 (5)
Cat-eye syndrome	1 (5)	0 (0)	1 (2)
Congenital central hypoventilation syndrome	1 (5)	0 (0)	1 (2)
Down syndrome	2 (9)	3 (14)	5 (12)
Familial medullary thyroid cancer	1 (5)	0 (0)	1 (2)

which is more than twice the mean overall prevalence of 21% of associated anomalies among Hirschsprung's patients in general [26]. Down syndrome affects approximately 5% of patients with Hirschsprung's disease and was also the most common syndrome among patients with CAKUT. Urogenital anomalies are known to occur in other syndromes associated with Hirschsprung's disease, including Mowat-Wilson, McKusick-Kaufman, Bardet-Biedl, and Smith-Lemli-Opitz syndromes, but these are in themselves considerably rare. In light of the emerging evidence, routine ultrasound screening of the renal tract in Hirschsprung's patients would permit early identification of CAKUT and potentially better control of CAKUT-related morbidity. To date, no associations have been suggested between the length of segment in Hirschsprung's disease and occurrence of CAKUT in any series.

The prevalence of genital anomalies in males with Hirschsprung's disease, including cryptorchidism, has been consistently reported to be low at around 1–3%. This may relate to these anomalies being outwardly apparent. Recently, two series of adolescent females with bilateral hydrosalpinx and Hirschsprung's disease were described [25, 32]. It remains unclear whether this represented a postsurgical complication or a congenital defect of autonomous innervation. Bilateral hydrosalpinx is extremely rare in sexually inactive adolescents without inflammatory disease, while loss of adrenergic innervation to the fallopian tubes induces hydrosalpinx in the rabbit model.

31.5 Common Genetic Basis of CAKUT and Hirschsprung's Disease

The developments of the enteric nervous system and renal tract share a common genetic background [14]. The major susceptibility gene for Hirschsprung's disease is the tyrosine kinase receptor RET (REarranged during Transfection), with coding sequence mutations being identified in about 30–50% of familial and 15–20% of sporadic cases [2, 46]. Signaling by glial cell line neurotrophic factor (GDNF) through the RET receptor is required for normal growth of the ureteric bud during kidney development in the mouse model [8], being critical for kidney development and ureteric maturation [16]. Outside the kidney, the RET-GDNF signaling pathway has been linked to the pathogenesis of Hirschsprung's disease [14] but also to hereditary cancer syndromes including multiple endocrine neoplasia type 2 (MEN2) and familial medullary thyroid cancer (FMTC) [16]. Mouse models deficient for RET, GDNF, and GFRα1 (GDNF family receptor alpha-1) develop both kidney agenesis and intestinal aganglionosis [33].

In humans, mutations in RET have been found approximately 35% of patients with renal agenesis [40]. Consistent with this, renal dysplasia or agenesis has been the most common variants of CAKUT observed in Hirschsprung's patients [26, 34, 38]. However, a recent mutational analysis of RET, GDNF, and GFRα1 in HSCR patients with CAKUT was unable to identify any clear functional variants in the gene portions assessed to explain the increased occurrence of CAKUT, although the authors concluded that they were also unable to rule out an association [33]. Renal dysplasia or agenesis has been reported as an associated finding in families with both HSCR and FMTC in several reports [13, 23, 34]. This raises the question of whether all individuals with HSCR should be offered routine screening of RET to rule out life-threatening cancer predisposition [2]. Medullary thyroid cancer-associated RET mutations affected approximately 5% of unselected adults with Hirschsprung's disease according to a recent population-based study [45]. Inactivating RET mutations are the most common cause of Hirschsprung's disease and have also been implicated in renal agenesis, whereas activating mutations lead to the familial cancer predisposition syndromes MEN2 and FMTC [17]. Delineating the underlying pathogenetic mechanisms of abnormalities such as CAKUT in Hirschsprung's patients is complicated by variable expressivity and incomplete penetrance, and it remains unclear how RET-mediated signaling cascades lead to these conditions both together and in isolation [17]. To date, two case reports of Wilms' tumor in patients with Hirschsprung's disease have been described [6, 25].

31.6 Urological Outcomes in Hirschsprung's Disease

Unlike in anorectal malformations, spinal or sacral involvement is not a feature of Hirschsprung's disease. Therefore, abnormalities of urological or sexual function would not be expected, except for those arising from iatrogenic trauma during pull-through surgery or congenital anomalies of the urinary tract [44]. The outcomes for urinary continence after surgery for Hirschsprung's disease were recently analyzed from 17 studies from 1972 to 2014, covering 2546 patients [44]. Apart from two, all studies were retrospective.

Good or normal urinary continence outcomes were reported in the vast majority of cases, and the mean prevalence of urinary incontinence (UI) was only 2% over a follow-up period of 17.2 months to 39 years. The overall occurrence of any type of UI ranged from 0% to 10.7%, which is lower than that reported among adults in the general population. From the data, it was not possible to associate the occurrence of UI with any particular type of pull-through [44]. However, in 9/11 of the studies that reported UI, open pull-through procedures had been used and the two studies where mainly minimally invasive techniques were used reported no UI [22, 48]. The prevalence of other lower urinary tract symptoms (LUTS) has also been reported at low rates (1.7–3.8%) following pull-through surgery in past series, as summarized in Table 31.3 [44].

A recent, cross-sectional survey of long-term LUTS among patients who had undergone endorectal pull-through for Hirschsprung's disease found a much higher rate of minor symptoms with active enquiry (Table 31.3) [29]. In comparison to age- and gender-matched controls, there were no significant differences in the prevalence of any type of LUTS apart from mild straining to void, which was reported more often by controls than patients for unknown reasons ($p = 0.008$). Even frequent LUTS was present at entirely comparable levels between patients (14%) and controls (16%; p = NS), supporting the notion of low morbidity attributable to Hirschsprung's or its surgical repair in terms of long-term LUTS. In one older series, where active assessment was used, the rates of UI after surgery for Hirschsprung's disease were also higher than the average of most retrospective studies, around 5–15% [44].

Table 31.3 Comparison of outcomes for lower urinary tract symptoms (LUTS) in HSCR patients from 17 mainly retrospective studies [44] with controlled, patient-reported outcomes from a recent cross-sectional series after a median follow-up of 15 years

	N (%)		
LUTS	[44] (Review, 17 series)	[29] (*N* = 59 patients with HSCR)	[29] (*N* = 177 controls matched to patients)
Urinary frequency	4/106 (3.8)	0 (0)	6 (3)
Urgency	n/a	25 (42)	101(57)
Any UI	52/2546 (2.0)	13 (22)	44 (25)
Dribbling	2/115 (1.7)	n/a	n/a
Straining to void	n/a	6 (10)	48 (27)[a]
Obstructed voiding	4/115 (3.5)	1 (2)[b]	0 (0)
Dysuria	3/106 (2.8)	n/a	n/a
UTIs	1/63 (1.6)	8 (15)	25 (14)
Any LUTS >1/week	n/a	8 (14)	28 (16)

UI urinary incontinence, *UTIs* urinary tract infections

[a] $p = 0.008$ vs patients; p = NS for prevalence of all other symptoms between patients and controls

[b] This patient was found to have a urethral stricture. The patient had undergone an open pull-through operation in the past

Urodynamic function has been uncommonly assessed in patients before and after pull-through surgery. In 1 prospective series of 11 children treated with laparoscopic resection of the aganglionic segment below the cul-de-sac and a Duhamel-type pull-through, an abnormally large cystometric bladder capacity for age was found in 64%, suggestive of partial detrusor denervation [7]. Of these, all but one patient had a significant residual at a mean age of 10 months, but all patients had detrusor contractility and spontaneous voiding. No clinical problems prevailed during the follow-up period, despite the apparent urodynamic changes. Another series examining urodynamics after transanal endorectal pull-through found no disturbances in urodynamic profiles [3]. As laparoscopy-assisted pull-through techniques are a relatively recent addition to the operative repertoire for Hirschsprung's disease, most reports of long-term surgical complications still describe the results of open procedures. More prospective studies are needed to define the prevalence of urologic complications and LUTS following laparoscopy-assisted pull-through, although there are theoretical safety advantages.

31.7 Sexual Functional Outcomes Following Surgery for Hirschsprung's Disease

There is a paucity of literature regarding the sexual functional outcomes among patients with Hirschsprung's disease. The available literature comprises isolated series that describe low rates of erectile dysfunction, ejaculatory abnormalities, and dyspareunia. However, it is likely that many patients have not been systematically followed up during adulthood. A recent analysis [44] largely summarizes the available information regarding sexual functional parameters after pull-through surgery from a total of 10 series identified up to 2014 (Table 31.4). It is possible that issues relating to sexual function were not actively addressed in the past or reported only when patients presented with problems [44]. The controlled sexual functional outcomes among a cohort of 24 patients aged 18–24 years who had undergone endorectal pull-through in childhood for Hirschsprung's disease at a tertiary center were recently surveyed [29]. As shown in Table 31.4, no significant differences were found compared to age- and gender-matched controls in relation to physical sexual functions. Of these parameters, erectile function is the most often

Table 31.4 Sexual functional outcomes among patients with HSCR from 10 studies between 1977 and 2014 [44] and from a recent controlled survey of patient-reported outcomes for sexual function after a median follow-up of 22 years [29]

	N (%)		
Outcome	[44] (10 studies)	[29] (patients with HSCR) *N* = 24 (16 male)	[29] (matched controls) *N* = 72 (48 male)
Erectile dysfunction	5/425 (1)	0 (0)	4 (6)[a]
Absent/retrograde ejaculations	2/84 (2)	0 (0)	0 (0)
Dyspareunia	3/115[b]	n/a	n/a
Infertility (males)	4/115[b]	0/3[c]	n/a
Infertility (females)	2/66 (3)	0/16[c]	n/a
Sexual satisfaction (males)	n/a	13 (79)	32 (67)
Sexual satisfaction (females)	n/a	6 (71)	20 (83)

[a]Erectile hardness score (EHS) <4/4; p = NS between patients and controls for all functional parameters
[b]Number of males and females not specified
[c]Only three males had attempted to become fathers; each had one healthy child and had not required any treatment for infertility. None of the females had attempted to become pregnant

reported in past series, probably as it can be enquired from the parents during childhood when most patients are still under active follow-up. In two studies [22] comprising a total of 145 males and a follow-up period of up to 96 months, the parents had observed spontaneous erections in 98% of patients postoperatively. In the three cases where erections had not been observed, these had not been noted by the parents preoperatively either [22].

The fertility data for patients with Hirschsprung's disease is even more limited. In the two older series of adults, it was noted that 17/53 males (32%) had become fathers [30] and that 56% of patients (34/61), including males and females, had become parents [36]. In the most recent survey of [29], only three patients (all male) had attempted to become parents after a follow-up of up to 24 years, and all had one healthy child each without a need for infertility treatment. There are no studies where systematic assessment of sperm count in males or pelvic ultrasound in females has been performed to answer questions relating to potential fertility after pull-through surgery for Hirschsprung's disease. In females, two patients with scarred fallopian tubes after open Swenson-type pull-through were noted [27], and several cases of bilateral hydrosalpinx have been described [25, 32]. The relationship between bilateral hydrosalpinx and infertility is well established. Further prospective studies are needed to draw definite conclusions regarding the effects of surgery on physical sexual functions and reproductive capacity in Hirschsprung's patients.

31.8 Long-Term Psychosexual Functioning

Hirschsprung's disease is invariably associated with varying degrees of functional bowel symptoms, including deficiencies in fecal continence, enterocolitis, and constipation, particularly during childhood. Patients may need to endure a number of hospital admissions and diagnostic procedures during childhood which, together with fecal control issues, may predispose to impaired emotional psychosocial well-being in the long term [28].

Although fecal control and other symptoms improve over time, impairment of developing self-esteem and perceived self-confidence during childhood can have long-lasting effects that carry over to affect QoL and personal relationships in adulthood. In children, it has been identified that the wider family's perception and the parental response to the child's illness may exert a stronger influence on emotional development and capacity to manage health-related stress than the presence of chronic organic disease [28]. Addressing the emotional domains of social functioning (feelings of embarrassment, feelings of unattractiveness, worries about the future) as well as physical symptoms during medical care, particularly around sensitive times such as adolescence, may serve to alleviate distress and confer wider benefits in terms of improved disease-specific QoL [12].

Psychosexual well-being after childhood surgery for anorectal malformations or Hirschsprung's disease has been assessed in a cohort of young adults using validated methods [43]. Sexual dysfunction was reported by 53% of females with Hirschsprung's disease and sexual distress by 20%. The self-reported psychosexual outcomes were not, however, associated with a reduction in global QoL. A cohort of adult Hirschsprung's disease patients with median age of 43 years operated mainly using Duhamel procedure reported increased harm to sexual life associated with marginally decreased overall QoL [18]. In females with anorectal malformations and Hirschsprung's disease, sexual distress has been associated with perceived self-competence during adolescence [47]. Research has suggested that the majority of both patients with anorectal malformations and Hirschsprung's disease feel that issues relating to sexuality, specifically in relation to their chronic condition, are insufficiently addressed during the course of their medical care [43]. There is currently no guidance regarding the optimal form and timing of discussions around the sensitive issue of sexuality and intimacy in these patients, although such interventions appear to be indicated.

In terms of personal relationships, a survey of young adults with Hirschsprung's disease found no differences in the proportion of patients who were in a sexual relationship (67% of males and 63% of females) compared to matched controls from the general population overall [29]. However, a lower proportion of females were in a stable relationship compared to controls (25% vs 82%, respectively) and male patients (67%; p = NS vs male controls). In this series, no significant differences in physical sexual functions in relation to matched controls and a comparable age of coital debut in both genders were found, encouragingly suggesting willingness to engage in intimate relationships. In patients with anorectal malformations, a later coital debut compared to peers has been reported [20]. Previous work has shown that female patients may experience a negative effect on sexual life from bowel functional issues, with fear of fecal incontinence being perceived as a hindrance for entry into personal relationships [11]. Fortunately, a stoma or antegrade continence enema conduit is only required in a small proportion of patients with Hirschsprung's disease. A stoma, in particular, can significantly impact on self-image, social functioning, and psychosexual well-being of patients, especially if it is permanent. In these cases, appropriate counselling for both patients and families or spouses should be considered to improve coping and adjustment.

31.9 Conclusions and Future Directions

The urological and sexual function outcomes among patients with Hirschsprung's disease represent an important domain in which more in-depth assessment and provision of multidisciplinary care could further improve outcomes. Development of an increased understanding of the disease process from these perspectives, and the implications of Hirschsprung's disease for the genitourinary tract, fertility, and sexual health, necessitates more prospective research. However, the available knowledge suggests that more standardized assessment and follow-up are indicated.

References

1. Amiel J, Lyonnet S. Hirschsprung disease, associated syndromes, and genetics: a review. J Med Genet. 2001;38:729–39.
2. Amiel J, Sproat-Emison E, Garcia-Barcelo M, Lantieri F, Burzynski G, Borrego S, Pelet A, Arnold S, Miao X, Griseri P, Brooks AS, Antinolo G, de Pontual L, Clement-Ziza M, Munnich A, Kashuk C, West K, Wong KK, Lyonnet S, Chakravarti A, Tam PK, Ceccherini I, Hofstra RM, Fernandez R, Hirschsprung Disease Consortium. Hirschsprung disease, associated syndromes and genetics: a review. J Med Genet. 2008;45:1–14.
3. Ates O, Hakguder G, Kart Y, Olguner M, Akgur FM. The effect of dilated ganglionic segment on anorectal and urinary functions during 1-stage transanal endorectal pull through for Hirschsprung's disease. J Pediatr Surg. 2007;42:1271–5.
4. Bischoff A, Frischer J, Knod JL, Dickie B, Levitt MA, Holder M, Jackson L, Peña A. Damaged anal canal as a cause of fecal incontinence after surgical repair for Hirschsprung disease – a preventable and under-reported complication. J Pediatr Surg. 2017;52:549–53.
5. Bjørnland K, Pakarinen MP, Stenstrøm P, Stensrud KJ, Neuvonen M, Granström AL, Graneli C, Pripp AH, Arnbjörnsson E, Emblem R, Wester T, Rintala RJ. A Nordic multicenter survey of long-term bowel function after transanal endorectal pull-through in 200 patients with rectosigmoid Hirschsprung disease. J Pediatr Surg. 2017;52:1458–64.
6. Blatt J, Nakayama D. Wilms tumor associated with Hirschsprung disease. J Pediatr Hematol Oncol. 2007;29:858–9.
7. Boemers TM, Bax TM, van Gool JD. The effect of rectosigmoidectomy and Duhamel-type pull-through procedure on lower urinary tract function in children with Hirschsprung's disease. J Pediatr Surg. 2001;36:453–6.
8. Costantini F, Shakya R. GDNF/Ret signaling and the development of the kidney. Bioessays. 2006;28:117–27.
9. De la Torre L, Cogley K, Santos K, Morales O, Calisto J. The anal canal is the fine line between "fecal incontinence and colitis" after a pull-through for Hirschsprung disease. J Pediatr Surg. 2017;52:2011–7.
10. Dingemans A, van der Steeg H, Rassouli-Kirchmeier R, Linssen MW, van Rooij I, de Blaauw I. Redo pull-through surgery in Hirschsprung disease: short-term clinical outcome. J Pediatr Surg. 2017;52:1446–50.
11. Grano C, Bucci S, Aminoff D, et al. Feelings of depression in people with ARM: the role of critical incidents and perceived difficulties in close and personal relationships. Pediatr Surg Int. 2014;30:823–8.
12. Hartman EE, Oort FJ, Aronson DC, Sprangers MA. Quality of life and disease-specific functioning of patients with anorectal malformations or Hirschsprung's disease: a review. Arch Dis Child. 2011;96:398–406.
13. Hibi Y, Ohye T, Ogawa K, Shimizu Y, Shibata M, Kagawa C, Mizuno Y, Kurahashi H, Iwase K. A MEN2A family with two asymptomatic carriers affected by unilateral renal agenesis. Endocr J. 2014;61:19–23.
14. Hofmann AD, Duess JW, Puri P. Congenital anomalies of the kidney and urinary tract (CAKUT) associated with Hirschsprung's disease: a systematic review. Pediatr Surg Int. 2014;30:757–61.
15. Hukkinen M, Koivusalo A, Merras-Salmio L, Rintala RJ, Pakarinen MP. Postoperative outcome and survival in relation to small intestinal involvement of total colonic aganglionosis. J Pediatr Surg. 2015;50:1859–64.
16. Jain S. The many faces of RET dysfunction in kidney. Organogenesis. 2009;5:177–90.

17. Jain S, Knoten A, Hoshi M, Wang H, Vohra B, Heuckeroth RO, Milbrandt J. Organotypic specificity of key RET adaptor-docking sites in the pathogenesis of neurocristopathies and renal malformations in mice. J Clin Invest. 2010;120:778–90.
18. Jarvi K, Laitakari E, Koivusalo A, Rintala RJ, Pakarinen MP. Bowel function and gastrointestinal quality of life among adults operated for Hirschsprung's disease during childhood. Ann Surg. 2010;252:977–81.
19. Koivusalo A, Pakarinen MP, Natunen J, Ashorn M, Rintala RJ, Sipponen T, Kolho KL. Sexual functions in adulthood after restorative proctocolectomy for paediatric onset ulcerative colitis. Pediatr Surg Int. 2009;25:881–4.
20. Kyrklund K, Taskinen S, Rintala RJ, Pakarinen MP. Sexual function, fertility and quality of life after modern treatment of anorectal malformations. J Urol. 2016;196:1741–6.
21. Levitt MA, Hamrick MC, Eradi B, Bischoff A, Hall J, Peña A. Transanal, full-thickness, Swenson-like approach for Hirschsprung disease. J Pediatr Surg. 2013;48:2289–95.
22. Liem NT, Bui DH, Tran AQ, Vu TH. Early and late outcomes of primary laparoscopic endorectal colon pull-through leaving a short rectal seromuscular sleeve for Hirschsprung disease. J Pediatr Surg. 2009;44:2153–5.
23. Loré F, Talidis F, Di Cairano G, Renieri A. Multiple endocrine neoplasia type 2 syndromes may be associated with renal malformations. J Intern Med. 2001;250:37–42.
24. Lu C, Hou G, Liu C, et al. Single-stage transanal endorectal pull-through procedure for correction of Hirschsprung disease in neonates and nonneonates: a multicenter study. J Pediatr Surg. 2017;52:1102–7.
25. Merlini L, Anooshiravani M, Peiry B, La Scala G, Hanquinet S. Bilateral hydrosalpinx in girls with Hirschsprung's disease: association of two rare conditions. AJR. 2008;190:W278–82.
26. Moore SW. The contribution of associated congenital anomalies in understanding Hirschsprung's disease. Pediatr Surg Int. 2006;22:305–15.
27. Moore SW, Albertyn R, Cywes S. Clinical outcome and long-term quality of life after surgical correction of Hirschsprung's disease. J Pediatr Surg. 1996;31:1496–502.
28. Neuvonen MI, Kyrklund K, Rintala RJ, Pakarinen MP. Bowel function and quality of life after transanal endorectal pull-through for Hirschsprung disease: controlled outcomes up to adulthood. Ann Surg. 2017;265:622–9.
29. Neuvonen MI, Kyrklund K, Rintala RJ, Pakarinen MP. Lower urinary tract symptoms and sexual functions after endorectal pull-through for Hirschsprung disease: controlled long-term outcomes. J Pediatr Surg. 2017;52(8):1296–301.
30. Nielsen OH, Madsen CM. 13–25 years follow-up after Swenson's operation for Hirschsprung's disease. Prog Pediatr Surg. 1977;10:97–102.
31. Pakarinen MP. Perioperative complications of transanal pull-through surgery for Hirschsprung's disease. Eur J Pediatr Surg. 2018;28:152–5.
32. Palazon P, Saura L, de Haro I, Martin Sole O, Albert A, Tarrado X, Julia V. Bilateral hydrosalpinx in patients with Hirschsprung's disease. J Pediatr Surg. 2018. pii: S0022-3468(18)30020-4. https://doi.org/10.1016/j.jpedsurg.2018.01.011. [Epub ahead of print].
33. Pini Prato A, Musso M, Ceccherini I, Mattioli G, Giunta C, Ghiggeri GM, Jasonni V. Hirschsprung disease and congenital anomalies of the urinary tract (CAKUT): a novel syndromic association. Medicine (Baltimore). 2009;88:83–90.
34. Pini Prato A, Rossi V, Mosconi M, Holm C, Lantieri F, Griseri P, Ceccherini I, Mavilio D, Jasonni V, Tuo G, Derchi M, Marasini M, Magnano G, Granata C, Ghiggeri G, Priolo E, Sposetti L, Porcu A, Buffa P, Mattioli G. A prospective observational study of associated anomalies in Hirschsprung's disease. Orphanet J Rare Dis. 2013;8:184.
35. Pope JC, Brock JW, Adams MC, et al. How they begin and how they end: classic and new theories for the development and deterioration of congenital anomalies of the kidney and urinary tract, CAKUT. J Am Soc Nephrol. 1999;10:2018–28.
36. Puri P, Nixon HH. Long-term results of Swenson's operation for Hirschsprung's disease. Prog Pediatr Surg. 1977;10:87–96.
37. Ralls MW, Freeman JJ, Rabah R, et al. Redo pullthrough for Hirschsprung disease: a single surgical group's experience. J Pediatr Surg. 2014;49:1394–9.
38. Sarioglu A, Tanyel FC, Buyukpamukcu N, Hicsonmez A. Hirschsprung-associated congenital anomalies. Eur J Pediatr Surg. 1997;7:331–7.
39. Shannon A, Eng K, Kay M, et al. Long-term follow-up of ileal pouch anal anastomosis in a large cohort of pediatric and young adult patients with ulcerative colitis. J Pediatr Surg. 2016;51:1181–6.
40. Skinner MA, Safford SD, Reeves JG, Jackson ME, Freemerman AJ. Renal aplasia in humans is associated with RET mutations. Am J Hum Genet. 2008;82:344–51.
41. Stensrud KJ, Emblem R, Bjørnland K. Anal endosonography and bowel function in patients undergoing different types of endorectal pull-through procedures for Hirschsprung disease. J Pediatr Surg. 2015;50:1341–6.
42. van Balkom KA, Beld MP, Visschers RG, van Gemert WG, Breukink SO. Long-term results after restorative proctocolectomy with ileal pouch-anal anastomosis at a young age. Dis Colon Rectum. 2012;55(9):939–47.
43. Van den Hondel D, Sloots CE, Bolt JM, Wijnen RM, de Blaaw I, IJsseltijn H. Psychosexual well-being after childhood surgery for anorectal malformation or Hirschsprung's disease. J Sex Med. 2015;12:1616–25.

44. Versteegh HP, Johal NS, de Blaauw I, Stanton MP. Urological and sexual outcome in patients with Hirschsprung disease: a systematic review. J Pediatr Urol. 2016;12:352–60.
45. Virtanen VB, Pukkala E, Kivisaari R, Salo PP, Koivusalo A, Arola J, Miettinen PJ, Rintala RJ, Perola M, Pakarinen MP. Thyroid cancer and co-occurring RET mutations in Hirschsprung disease. Endocr Relat Cancer. 2013;20:595–602.
46. Virtanen VB, Salo PP, Cao J, Löf-Granström A, Milani L, Metspalu A, Rintala RJ, Saarenpää-Heikkilä O, Paunio T, Wester T, Nordenskjöld A, Perola M, Pakarinen MP. Noncoding RET variants explain the strong association with Hirschsprung disease in patients without rare coding sequence variant. Eur J Med Genet. 2018. pii: S1769-7212(18)30076-4. https://doi.org/10.1016/j.ejmg.2018.07.019. [Epub ahead of print].
47. Witvliet MJ, van Gasteren S, van den Hondel D, Hartman E, van Heurn L, van der Steeg A. Predicting sexual problems in young adults with an anorectal malformation or Hirschsprung disease. J Pediatr Surg. 2018;53:1555–9.
48. Yang L, Tang ST, Cao GQ, Yang Y, Li S, Li SW, et al. Transanal endorectal pull-through for Hirschsprung's disease using long cuff dissection and short V-shaped partially resected cuff anastomosis: early and late outcomes. Pediatr Surg Int. 2012;28:515–21.
49. Zani A, Eaton S, Morini F, et al. European Paediatric Surgeons' Association Survey on the management of Hirschsprung disease. Eur J Pediatr Surg. 2017;27:96–101.

32 Long-Term Outcome and Quality of Life After Treatment of Hirschsprung's Disease

Annika Mutanen, Mikko P. Pakarinen, and Risto J. Rintala

Contents

32.1 Introduction

Before the onset of pediatric surgery as an independent specialty and development of modern pediatric surgery, the overall outcome of Hirschsprung's disease was poor as the disease was fatal in most cases. Along with the development of pediatric surgery, the long-term outcomes of Hirschsprung's disease have significantly improved following better understanding of the pathophysiology and pathological anatomy of the disease and development of surgical techniques. While the treatment results have improved, significant attention has been brought to long-term functional, psychosocial, and quality of life issues in children and adults with Hirschsprung's disease. The overall long-term functional outcome expectancy is relatively optimistic; although many patients have some degree of bowel dysfunction and continence defect, they are able to stay socially continent and report a good quality of life [1–3]. In contrast, some patients need special bowel management programs to achieve social continence, or some are even left with persistent incontinence and significant psychosocial problems needing additional medical attention [3, 4].

In this chapter, the long-term outcomes of Hirschsprung's disease regarding bowel function and continence, enterocolitis, and quality of life are discussed. Furthermore, long-term issues related to specific patient groups, such as syndromic patients and total colonic aganglionosis, are reviewed.

A. Mutanen · M. P. Pakarinen · R. J. Rintala (✉)
Section of Pediatric Surgery, Hospital for Children and Adolescents, University of Helsinki, Helsinki, Finland
e-mail: risto.rintala@hus.fi

P. Puri (ed.), *Hirschsprung's Disease and Allied Disorders*,
https://doi.org/10.1007/978-3-030-15647-3_32

32.2 Functional Outcomes

32.2.1 During Childhood

32.2.1.1 Bowel Function

In the majority of studies, the overall bowel function in children with Hirschsprung's disease is reported to be relatively good although a significant number of patients continue to have problems with bowel function (Table 32.1) [1, 4–9]. The bowel function, measured with bowel function score, is clearly worse in children with Hirschsprung's disease than in healthy controls, but it significantly improves with increasing age [1]. In a Nordic multicenter study [4] in children from 4 to 7 years, 8 to 12 years, and 13 to 17 years who underwent transanal endorectal pull-trough for Hirschsprung's disease, problems with ability to hold back stools (69% vs 55% vs 22%) and an urge to defecate (38% vs 24% vs 19%) as well as social problems (28% vs 21% vs 19%) were reported in all age groups [4]. After pull-through operation, stooling frequency is generally higher compared to healthy controls but tends to decrease over time, especially during the first 6 months after surgery [1, 10, 11]. Teitelbaum et al. showed that decreasing stooling pattern with good levels of continence was reached after 3 years of follow-up in patients who underwent a primary endorectal pull-through as infants [10]. Similarly, stooling frequency was shown to decrease after both transabdominal (initial average 5/day vs final 2/day) and transanal (5/day vs 2/day) pull-throughs such that by year 7, there was no difference between the groups [11].

32.2.1.2 Constipation

During childhood, constipation is a relatively common problem after pull-through operation for Hirschsprung's disease as it is reported in 3–36% of patients (Table 32.1) [1, 4–6, 8, 9, 12–15]. Prolonged colonic transition time, abnormal internal sphincter function, or mechanical obstruction such as postoperative stricture or formation of a spur after Duhamel procedure are common causes of constipation [16–18]. Constipation is seen significantly more commonly in patients from 4 to 12 years of age compared to adolescents and adults with Hirschsprung's disease [4]. A significant proportion of children with Hirschsprung's disease, approximately 30% of patients from 4 to 12 years of age, need diet, laxatives, or enemas to treat the constipation after transanal endorectal pull-through operation [4]. In most cases, however, constipation is manageable with diet changes and oral medication.

32.2.1.3 Soiling and Fecal Incontinence

Fecal incontinence and soiling are the major complications after any type of surgery for Hirschsprung's disease. To maintain normal continence, a preserved sphincter function, rectal reservoir, and anal canal sensation are required. In Hirschsprung's disease, several components related to the disease and its repair can interfere with the continence mechanism and cause long-term problems with soiling and incontinence. Patients with Hirschsprung's disease lack normal rectoanal relaxation reflex before and after surgery, consistent with primary defects in the innervation and function of the internal anal sphincter [16, 19]. At pull-through operation, the internal anal sphincter is at least partially interfered, the rectal reservoir is completely or partially lost, and the transitional epithelium responsible for anal sensation may be inadvertently removed. In controlled manometric studies, the resting and maximal anal canal squeeze pressures are significantly lower after Duhamel procedure compared to controls [16, 17]. In Hirschsprung's disease, the fecal continence is largely dependent on sufficient function of the voluntary sphincters because of the impaired function of the internal sphincter [20].

Overall, soiling or incontinence is reported in 4–77% and 1–63% of children with Hirschsprung's disease depending on the study population and the used study methods and definitions of soiling and incontinence (Table 32.1) [1, 4–6, 8, 9, 12–15, 21–23]. Generally, soiling and incontinence problems seem to decrease from childhood toward adolescence [13, 14, 17, 24].

Kim et al. compared the results of transabdominal (mean age 7 years) and transanal pull-through (mean age 11 years) techniques in a

Table 32.1 Summary of studies on incidence of constipation, soiling, and fecal incontinence and quality of life (QoL) after surgical treatment of Hirschsprung's disease

Author	Year	Patients (*n*)	Healthy controls (*n*)	Age (y) at follow-up (median or mean, range)	Main surgical procedure	Rectosigmoid aganglionosis (%)	Used questionnaires	Constipation (%)	Soiling (%)	Fecal incontinence (%)	Quality of life (QoL)
Collins	2017	60	Previously published controls	6 (2–11)	Duhamel, Soave, Swenson	78	BCS, CCSS, VDESS, PedsQL, FICQOL	NR	NR	63	Good overall and physical QoL Reduced psychosocial QoL
Neuvonen	2017	79	171	15 (4–32)	TEPT	86	BFS, GIQLI, SF-36 health survey, PedsQL	3	68	45	QoL comparable to controls in childhood but impaired emotional and sexual domain in adulthood
Bjornland	2017	200	0	10 (4–32)	TEPT	100	BFS	25	77	47	NR
Onishi	2017	16	0	25 (19–37)	Soave	75	ES, QoL questionnaire	31	19	19	Satisfactory social and academic QoL
Tannuri	2017	41	59	8 (7–12)	Duhamel, TEPT	100	FCI, AQLCAFI	NR	NR	37	Impaired QoL compared to controls
Khalil	2015	53	0	6 (5–7)	TEPT	NR	PedsQL	8	NR	10	Good overall QoL Overflow incontinence has significant negative impact on QoL
Granstrom	2015	37	37	28 (20–43)	Soave	95	SF-36 health survey, GIQLI, bowel and urinary function questionnaire	78	NR	19	Good overall QoL but impaired bowel function, and gastrointestinal QoL is common
Yang	2012	167	0	4 (0–5)	TEPT	100	Wingspread scoring system	3	4	1	NR

(continued)

Table 32.1 (continued)

Author	Year	Patients (*n*)	Healthy controls (*n*)	Age (y) at follow-up (median or mean, range)	Main surgical procedure	Rectosigmoid aganglionosis (%)	Used questionnaires	Constipation (%)	Soiling (%)	Fecal incontinence (%)	Quality of life (QoL)
Jarvi	2010	92	53	43 (35–48)	Duhamel	94	BFS, GIQLI	30	48	14	Good overall QoL Slightly decreased gastrointestinal QoL associated with increasing age
Ieiri	2010	43	0	33 (19–55)	Duhamel	79	Bowel function and QoL questionnaire	33	19	17	Good overall QoL Soiling and incontinence clearly impair QoL
Gunnarsdottir	2010	42	0 (age-adjusted reference values)	29 (18–45)	Duhamel	69	SF-36 health survey, GIQLI	12	29	NR	Good overall QoL and comparable to controls Lower scores in young females
Mills	2008	51	0	10 (3–21)	Soave, TEPT, Duhamel	66	Constipation scoring system, PedsQL	8	NR	49	Good overall QoL and comparable to controls
Catto-Smith	2007	84	0	12 (2–42)	Soave		Bowel function and QoL questionnaire	36	NR	17	Good overall QoL Fecal incontinence has significant effect on social activities and QoL
Bai	2002	45	0	11 (8–16)	Swenson	100	Study-specific bowel function questionnaire, QoL scoring criteria	7	38	7	QoL was good in 40%, fair in 47%, and poor in 13% Strong association between fecal soiling/incontinence and decreased QoL

Ludman	2002	30	0	12 (7–18)	NR	50	Kelly score, study-specific interview, CBCL, DSRS, SPP	NR	24	34	Patients with total colonic aganglionosis had more behavioral/ emotional problems compared to patients with rectosigmoid disease No association between fecal incontinence and psychosocial outcome measures
Yanchar	1999	69	0	5 to 15 (<5 to >15)	Soave, Duhamel, Swenson	75	Fecal continence score	13	NR	44	NR
Diseth	1997	19	33	16 (10–20)	Duhamel	64	CBCL, CAS, YSR, CGAS	16	NR	32	Good overall QoL
Moore	1996	178		10 (1–36)	Soave, Duhamel, Swenson	69	Kelly, Wingspread, and Holschneider scoring systems	24	19	7	Good overall QoL Incontinence is associated with long-term psychosocial problems
Heij	1995	63	0	7	Duhamel	65	Bowel function questionnaire	9	35	27	NR
Heikkinen	1995	102	81	31 (15–39)	Duhamel	95	CCS	NR	52	9	NR

AQLCAFI Assessment of Quality of Life in Children and Adolescents with Fecal Incontinence, *BCS* Baylor Continence Scale, *BFS* Bowel Function Score, *CAS* Child Assessment Schedule, *CBCL* Child Behavior Checklist, *CCS* Clinical Continence Scoring, *CCSS* Cleveland Clinic Constipation Scoring System, *CGAS* Children's Global Assessment Scale, *DSRS* Depression Self-Rating Scale, *ES* evacuation score of the Japan Society of Anorectal Malformation Study Group, *FCI* Fecal Continence Index, *FICQOL* Fecal Incontinence and Constipation Quality of Life, *FOS* Rintala functional outcome score, *NR* not reported, *GIQLI* Gastrointestinal Quality of Life Index, *PedsQL* Pediatric Quality of Life Inventory, *SPP* Self-Perception Profile for Children-Adolescents, *TEPT* transanal endorectal pull-through, *VDESS* Vancouver Dysfunctional Elimination Syndrome Survey, *YSR* Youth Self-Report, * > 1/week

multicenter study, and they found no significant differences in continence scores between the two groups, and the scores did not significantly change with increasing time [11]. Similarly, Neuvonen et al. reported that the type of transanal pull-through (totally transanal or combined) did not significantly influence overall outcome by means of bowel function score [1]. Tannuri et al. compared children who underwent the Duhamel operation to patients with transanal pull-through technique and found similar outcomes according to the fecal continence index [22]. On the other hand, the findings in the large Nordic multicenter study suggested that totally transanal approach is associated with worse outcome than transabdominally or laparoscopically assisted transanal pull-through [4].

32.2.2 Beyond Childhood

32.2.2.1 Bowel Function

Overall, bowel function seems to improve over time when looking at studies showing results 20 years and more after pull-through (Table 32.1) [1, 4, 25]. Neuvonen et al. showed that bowel function score was significantly better after transanal endorectal pull-through in patients more than 18 years of age compared to younger patients [1]. Similar results were reported by Bjornland et al. in a multicenter study after transanal endorectal pull-through, including no social problems related to bowel function in 74%, normal ability to hold back stools in 77%, and mostly or always feeling an urge to defecate in 100% of patients [4]. In contrast, Conway and Granstrom both reported impaired bowel function in adults after Duhamel or Soave pull-through [2, 26]. Although the stooling frequency has been reported to decrease over time during childhood, abnormal stooling frequency persisted in 50% of patients to adulthood [1, 10]. At older age, bowel function seems to be deteriorating as older age predicts poor bowel function [25].

32.2.2.2 Soiling and Fecal Incontinence

Although it is unlikely that surgery-related anatomical defects of anal function that are the cause of fecal incontinence in Hirschsprung's disease significantly improve over time, the fecal incontinence rate reported by patients seems to diminish after puberty [4, 13, 14, 24]. Several studies have reported that fecal incontinence rate improves with age as problems with fecal continence were more common among toddlers and children and less common in teenagers and adults [1, 13, 14, 17, 24]. In more detail, all aspects of fecal control, including urgency, rectal sensation, ability to hold back defecation, fecal soiling, and fecal accidents, improved to levels that no longer significant differences were detected beyond the age of 18 years compared to healthy controls [1]. Overall, socially disturbing incontinence seems to be relatively uncommon in adults, and it has minor impact on the psychosocial functioning which is likely reflecting the advanced coping and adapting capabilities of adults [2, 15, 25].

32.3 Enterocolitis

Hirschsprung's disease-related enterocolitis is a fairly frequent complication that may affect the outcome of patients before and after pull-though procedure. Enterocolitis is reported to occur in 6–50% and 2–35% of Hirschsprung's disease patients in the pre- and postoperative period [27]. Enterocolitis is a potentially life-threatening complication and late mortalities after pull-through operation are reported to relate to enterocolitis in up to 50% of cases [28, 29]. While any patient with Hirschsprung's disease is at risk of enterocolitis, there are certain patient groups with significantly increased risk, including patients with Down syndrome, long-segment disease, prior episodes of enterocolitis, and familial history of Hirschsprung's [30–33].

Enterocolitis is closely related to overall bowel function. In a recent multicenter study, the history of frequent episodes of enterocolitis was significantly higher in patients who reported soiling often or always compared to those who had soiling never or rarely [4]. In contrast, the overall rates of any soiling or fecal accidents (which included infrequent symptoms) did not differ significantly between patients with persistent enterocolitis compared to enterocolitis-free patients [1].

Hirschsprung's-related enterocolitis and inflammatory bowel disease have similar clinical symptoms, including diarrhea, hematochezia, and colicky abdominal pain, and both conditions are characterized by an abnormal intestinal mucosal barrier function and alterations in intestinal microbiota [34–38]. Although it still remains unclear whether inflammatory bowel disease and Hirschsprung's disease have a common etiology, inflammatory bowel disease has been reported to relate to Hirschsprung's disease [39–41]. Both Crohn's disease and ulcerative colitis are seen in patients with Hirschsprung's disease, but Crohn's disease is reported to be more common [40]. Lof Granstrom et al. showed in a nationwide population-based register cohort that the risk for inflammatory bowel disease is significantly increased (OR 4.99) among patients with Hirschsprung's disease compared to sex- and age-adjusted healthy controls [40]. In a meta-analysis by Nakamura et al., patients with extensive colonic aganglionosis who continued to suffer from enterocolitis after pull-through operation were more susceptible to develop inflammatory bowel disease [34]. In the long-term follow-up, it is important for clinicians to keep in mind that chronic enterocolitis-type symptoms may as well be a sign of inflammatory bowel disease in patients with Hirschsprung's disease.

32.4 Total Colonic Aganglionosis

Total colonic aganglionosis is a severe form of Hirschsprung's disease with related significant short- and long-term morbidity, including enterocolitis, perianal excoriation, frequent bowel movements, constipation, soiling, fecal incontinence, metabolic complications, and failure to thrive. Overall, no superior operative approach for total colonic aganglionosis has been confirmed with respect to postoperative morbidity, occurrence of enterocolitis, functional outcome, or mortality [20, 42]. Enterocolitis is a common complication and often a chronic problem in patients with total colonic aganglionosis. The incidence of enterocolitis is significantly higher in patients with total colonic aganglionosis, ranging from 20% to 55%, compared to patients with a rectosigmoid disease [31, 32, 42]. In a recent meta-analysis by Laughlin et al., enterocolitis was the most frequent complication after pull-through arising in 42% of patients with total colonic aganglionosis [43].

Soiling and fecal incontinence are common during childhood and in adults in patients with total colonic aganglionosis. Overall, at least 30–50% of the patients with total colonic aganglionosis suffer from fecal incontinence later in childhood or adolescence [31, 32, 44, 45]. In a meta-analysis by Laughlin et al. with a mean follow-up time of 9.6 years, satisfactory or normal bowel control was reported in 60% of patients with total colonic aganglionosis, while soiling, fecal incontinence, or another poor outcome was found in 34% and 7% requiring a permanent stoma [43]. Surprisingly, in a study by Ludman in patients with total colonic aganglionosis, the continence score was not affected by the length of the aganglionosis or the length of the small bowel resection [23]. The overall mortality rate is reported as high as 20%, with pre-pull-through mortality of 16% and post-pull-through mortality of 6% [43]. Metabolic complications, nutritional deficiencies, growth retardation, and failure to thrive are well-described complications in patients with total colonic aganglionosis, which highlights the need for close multidisciplinary long-term follow-up [45–47].

32.5 Syndromic Hirschsprung's Disease

Hirschsprung's disease has been associated with numerous relatively rare syndromes which further influence the long-term outcome of these patients. Down syndrome, being the most common syndrome related to Hirschsprung's disease, is found in 2–16% of all patients with Hirschsprung's disease [30]. Mortality and morbidity rates are higher in Down syndrome patients with Hirschsprung's compared to non-syndromic patients. The increased mortality rate in Down syndrome patients with Hirschsprung's is mostly related to the frequent comorbidities, including cardiac anomalies [30, 48]. Postoperative complications, such as enterocolitis, constipation, soiling, and incontinence, are more common in Down patients with Hirschsprung's compared to non-syndromic patients [30]. Furthermore, the overall functional prognosis is significantly inferior in Down syndrome patients than in non-syndromic Hirschsprung's disease patients [4, 20, 30]. Down syndrome patients tend to resume bowel control much slower, and many of them, especially those with chronic enterocolitis, suffer from fecal incontinence as adolescents and adults [20]. Catto-Smith et al. reported 87% incidence of fecal incontinence among Down syndrome patients at mean age of 12 years [6].

Hirschsprung's disease is also known to be associated with more uncommon syndromes such as Shah-Waardenburg syndrome, Mowat-Wilson syndrome, cartilage-hair hypoplasia, and hypoplastic left heart syndrome [20, 49]. Patients with Shah-Waardenburg and Mowat-Wilson syndrome are prone to enterocolitis and develop postoperative bowel control very slowly [20]. Cartilage-hair hypoplasia is a metaphyseal chondrodysplasia with growth failure, impaired immunity, and high incidence of associated Hirschsprung's disease. Cartilage-hair hypoplasia patients with Hirschsprung's disease have worse outcome compared to other Hirschsprung's disease patients, including very high incidence of severe pre- and postoperative enterocolitis and increased mortality rate [50].

32.6 Hirschsprung's Disease and Cancer

Besides causing Hirschsprung's disease, the *RET* proto-oncogene germ line mutations are responsible for the development of multiple endocrine neoplasia type 2 (MEN2A) and familial medullary thyroid carcinoma [51]. The *RET* mutations are found in up to 50% of the familial and in 15–30% of the sporadic Hirschsprung's disease cases [52]. On a population-based cohort study from Finland, the risk of medullary thyroid carcinoma, but no other cancers, was found to be increased in patients with Hirschsprung's disease after mean follow-up of 30 years [53]. Virtanen et al. reported that the medullary thyroid carcinoma-associated *RET* mutations are restricted to exons 10 and 13 affecting ~5% of unselected adult patients with Hirschsprung's disease [54]. Based on the known increased risk for medullary thyroid carcinoma, mutation screening for *RET* exons 10 and 13 may be advisable in patients with Hirschsprung's disease, not only limited to familial or long-segment diseases [54].

32.7 Quality of Life

Quality of life can be measured in general health-related or symptom-specific measures; both are useful in assessing quality of life of Hirschsprung's disease patients. Generic quality of life questionnaires, such as PedsQL and SF-36 health survey, help to understand general health and well-being independent of the disease and simultaneously making it possible to compare quality of life between different diseases or to healthy control subjects (Table 32.1). The symptom-specific questionnaires, such as GIQLI and FICQOL, have the advantage of focusing on specific issues relevant to a specific disease (Table 32.1). Assessing the overall quality of life is complex as the relationship between disease-specific functioning and quality of life remains unclear [55]. This highlights the need for longitudinal studies assessing the disease-specific functioning with validated age-specific quality of life questionnaires.

32.7.1 Quality of Life in Children

In contrast to earlier reports that show little or no limitations in quality of life, the recent detailed studies show on average more physical, psychosocial, and overall quality of life problems in children with Hirschsprung's disease compared to controls, although the effects are small (Table 32.1). Collins et al. reported a good overall quality of life in children with Hirschsprung's disease at a median age of 6 years but a reduced psychosocial quality of life compared to reference subjects [21]. In contrast, Tannuri et al. reported impaired overall quality of life in children with Hirschsprung's disease at a median age of 8 years compared to healthy controls [22]. The effect of disease-specific symptoms, such as incontinence, soiling, and constipation, on quality of life varies between different study populations as most studies indicate a significantly reduced quality of life related to these symptoms in comparison to few studies with very little or no association [5, 6, 55, 56]. Interestingly, impaired psychosocial functioning appears to have a stronger effect on quality of life than the disease-specific symptoms [55, 56].

When comparing children and adolescents, children with Hirschsprung's disease report better quality of life than adolescents. In contrast, adolescents reported less bowel functional problems than children. It seems, that despite less continence problems in adolescents, they are more prone to quality of life problems compared to children [55].

In a study comparing outcomes of children and adolescents with Hirschsprung's disease or anorectal malformation, the overall quality of life was comparable between the groups [56]. In the same study, both patient groups reported more psychosocial problems in all domains compared to healthy controls [56].

32.7.2 Quality of Life in Adults

In general, adult patients with Hirschsprung's disease report a good overall quality of life with no significant difference to healthy age-matched reference subjects [2, 25, 57, 58]. However, some patients are left with persistent impaired bowel function, such as soiling and incontinence, significantly impacting their overall and gastrointestinal quality of life [6, 59]. Gunnarsdottir et al. reported a good overall quality of life in adult patients after a Duhamel procedure [60]. In this study young females had lower overall quality of life scores compared to males or older patients [60]. Jarvi and Granstrom both reported a good overall quality of life in adults after Duhamel or Soave procedure, while impaired gastrointestinal function and gastrointestinal quality of life were more common in patients compared to controls [2, 25]. A worrying finding was that in some studies, the degree of impairment of bowel function and symptom-specific quality of life is shown to be associated with increasing age [25, 61]. This is notable as it may have a significant impact on quality of life of older patients with Hirschsprung's disease and might impact follow-up strategies.

32.7.3 Quality of Life and the Effect of the Extent of Aganglionosis

Overall, patients with more severe forms of Hirschsprung's disease are more prone to have reduced quality of life compared to patients with shorter segment aganglionosis [44, 60]. A significant number of patients with total colonic aganglionosis have fecal soiling, incontinence, and frequent episodes of enterocolitis extending to adulthood which may have significant psychosocial implications [23, 31, 32, 45, 46]. Gunnarsdottir et al. showed that patients with aganglionosis extending to the right colon had lower overall quality of life than patients with aganglionosis limited to the left colon [60]. Patients with more severe forms of the disease reported lower levels of perceived self-competence and global disease-specific functioning, which in turn predicted overall quality of life, in a study by Hartman et al. [56] Similarly, Ludman et al. showed that patients with total colonic aganglionosis with or without small bowel involvement have more often behavioral and emotional problems compared to patients with rectosigmoid aganglionosis [23].

32.8 Summary

The long-term outcomes of Hirschsprung's disease have significantly improved following a better understanding of the pathophysiology and pathological anatomy of the disease and development of surgical techniques. While the treatment results have improved, it has become clear that the functional, psychosocial, and quality of life issues in children and adults with Hirschsprung's disease need specific attention in the long term. Patients with Hirschsprung's disease are at risk for several complications, including functional and psychosocial issues that are often passed on from childhood to adulthood and may have a significant effect on long-term quality of life. Although symptoms such as constipation, soiling, and fecal incontinence often have a tendency of improving over time, these still are commonly seen in adolescents and adults with Hirschsprung's disease. All patients with Hirschsprung's disease need close follow-up during childhood as well as during adulthood.

References

1. Neuvonen MI, Kyrklund K, Rintala RJ, Pakarinen MP. Bowel function and quality of life after transanal endorectal pull-through for hirschsprung disease: controlled outcomes up to adulthood. Ann Surg. 2017;265(3):622–9.
2. Granstrom AL, Danielson J, Husberg B, Nordenskjold A, Wester T. Adult outcomes after surgery for hirschsprung's disease: evaluation of bowel function and quality of life. J Pediatr Surg. 2015;50(11):1865–9.
3. Wester T, Granstrom AL. Hirschsprung disease-bowel function beyond childhood. Semin Pediatr Surg. 2017;26(5):322–7.
4. Bjørnland K, Pakarinen M, Stenstrøm P, et al. A nordic multicenter survey of long-term bowel function after transanal endorectal pull-through in 200 patients with rectosigmoid hirschsprung disease. J Pediatr Surg. 2017;52(9):1458–64.
5. Khalil M. Long-term health-related quality of life for patients with hirschsprung's disease at 5 years after transanal endorectal pull-through operation. Qual Life Res. 2015;24(11):2733–8.
6. Catto-Smith AG, Trajanovska M, Taylor RG. Long-term continence after surgery for hirschsprung's disease. J Gastroenterol Hepatol. 2007;22(12):2273–82.
7. Bai Y, Chen H, Hao J, Huang Y, Wang W. Long-term outcome and quality of life after the swenson procedure for hirschsprung's disease. J Pediatr Surg. 2002;37(4):639–42.
8. Moore SW, Albertyn R, Cywes S. Clinical outcome and long-term quality of life after surgical correction of hirschsprung's disease. J Pediatr Surg. 1996;31(11):1496–502.
9. Heij HA, de Vries X, Bremer I, Ekkelkamp S, Vos A. Long-term anorectal function after duhamel operation for hirschsprung's disease. J Pediatr Surg. 1995;30(3):430–2.
10. Teitelbaum D, Drongowski R, Chamberlain J, Coran A. Long-term stooling patterns in infants undergoing primary endorectal pull-through for hirschsprung's disease. J Pediatr Surg. 1997;32(7):1049–52.
11. Kim AC, Langer JC, Pastor AC, et al. Endorectal pull-through for hirschsprung's disease-a multicenter, long-term comparison of results: transanal vs transabdominal approach. J Pediatr Surg. 2010;45(6):1213–20.
12. Yang L, Tang S, Cao G, et al. Transanal endorectal pull-through for hirschsprung's disease using long cuff dissection and short V-shaped partially resected cuff anastomosis: early and late outcomes. Pediatr Surg Int. 2012;28(5):515–21.
13. Mills JL, Konkin DE, Milner R, Penner JG, Langer M, Webber EM. Long-term bowel function and quality of life in children with hirschsprung's disease. J Pediatr Surg. 2008;43(5):899–905.
14. Yanchar NL, Soucy P. Long-term outcome after hirschsprung's disease: patients' perspectives. J Pediatr Surg. 1999;34(7):1152–60.
15. Diseth TH, Bjornland K, Novik TS, Emblem R. Bowel function, mental health, and psychosocial function in adolescents with hirschsprung's disease. Arch Dis Child. 1997;76(2):100–6.
16. Heikkinen M, Rintala R, Luukkonen P. Long-term anal sphincter performance after surgery for hirschsprung's disease. J Pediatr Surg. 1997;32(10):1443–6.
17. Bjornland K, Diseth TH, Emblem R. Long-term functional, manometric, and endosonographic evaluation of patients operated upon with the duhamel technique. Pediatr Surg Int. 1998;13(1):24–8.
18. Baillie CT, Kenny SE, Rintala RJ, Booth JM, Lloyd DA. Long-term outcome and colonic motility after the duhamel procedure for hirschsprung's disease. J Pediatr Surg. 1999;34(2):325–9.
19. Jarvi K, Koivusalo A, Rintala RJ, Pakarinen MP. Anorectal manometry with reference to operative rectal biopsy for the diagnosis/exclusion of hirschsprung's disease in children under 1 year of age. Int J Colorectal Dis. 2009;24(4):451–4.
20. Rintala RJ, Pakarinen MP. Long-term outcomes of hirschsprung's disease. Semin Pediatr Surg. 2012;21(4):336–43.
21. Collins L, Collis B, Trajanovska M, et al. Quality of life outcomes in children with hirschsprung disease. J Pediatr Surg. 2017;52(12):2006–10.
22. Tannuri AC, Ferreira MA, Mathias AL, Tannuri U. Long-term results of the duhamel technique are superior to those of the transanal pullthrough: a study of fecal continence and quality of life. J Pediatr Surg. 2017;52(3):449–53.
23. Ludman L, Spitz L, Tsuji H, Pierro A. Hirschsprung's disease: functional and psychological follow up comparing total colonic and rectosigmoid aganglionosis. Arch Dis Child. 2002;86(5):348–51.
24. Reding R, de Ville de Goyet J, Gosseye S, et al. Hirschsprung's disease: a 20-year experience. J Pediatr Surg. 1997;32(8):1221–5.
25. Jarvi K, Laitakari EM, Koivusalo A, Rintala RJ, Pakarinen MP. Bowel function and gastrointestinal quality of life among adults operated for hirschsprung

disease during childhood: a population-based study. Ann Surg. 2010;252(6):977–81.
26. Conway SJ, Craigie RJ, Cooper LH, et al. Early adult outcome of the duhamel procedure for left-sided hirschsprung disease – a prospective serial assessment study. J Pediatr Surg. 2007;42(8):1429–32.
27. Frykman PK, Short SS. Hirschsprung-associated enterocolitis: prevention and therapy. Semin Pediatr Surg. 2012;21(4):328–35.
28. Swenson O, Sherman JO, Fisher JH, Cohen E. The treatment and postoperative complications of congenital megacolon: a 25 year followup. Ann Surg. 1975;182(3):266–73.
29. Pini Prato A, Rossi V, Avanzini S, Mattioli G, Disma N, Jasonni V. Hirschsprung's disease: what about mortality? Pediatr Surg Int. 2011;27(5):473–8.
30. Friedmacher F, Puri P. Hirschsprung's disease associated with down syndrome: a meta-analysis of incidence, functional outcomes and mortality. Pediatr Surg Int. 2013;29(9):937–46.
31. Wildhaber BE, Teitelbaum DH, Coran AG. Total colonic hirschsprung's disease: a 28-year experience. J Pediatr Surg. 2005;40(1):203–6; discussion 206.
32. Menezes M, Pini Prato A, Jasonni V, Puri P. Long-term clinical outcome in patients with total colonic aganglionosis: a 31-year review. J Pediatr Surg. 2008;43(9):1696–9.
33. Dong Q, Li G, Dong J. Identification of risk factors for postoperative recurrent hirschsprung associated enterocolitis. J Pediatr Surg. 2018.
34. Nakamura H, Lim T, Puri P. Inflammatory bowel disease in patients with hirschsprung's disease: a systematic review and meta-analysis. Pediatr Surg Int. 2018;34(2):149–54.
35. Nakamura H, Tomuschat C, Coyle D, O'Donnel A, Lim T, Puri P. Altered goblet cell function in hirschsprung's disease. Pediatr Surg Int. 2018;34(2):121–8.
36. Prideaux L, Kang S, Wagner J, et al. Impact of ethnicity, geography, and disease on the microbiota in health and inflammatory bowel disease. Inflamm Bowel Dis. 2013;19(13):2906–18.
37. Frykman P, Nordenskjöld A, Kawaguchi A, et al. Characterization of bacterial and fungal microbiome in children with hirschsprung disease with and without a history of enterocolitis: a multicenter study. PLoS One. 2014;10(4):e0124172.
38. Neuvonen MI, Korpela K, Kyrklund K, Rintala RJ, Pakarinen MP. Intestinal microbiota in hirschsprung disease. J Pediatr Gastroenterol Nutr. 2018; epub ahead of print.
39. Sherman JO, Snyder ME, Weitzman JJ, et al. A 40-year multinational retrospective study of 880 swenson procedures. J Pediatr Surg. 1989;24(8):833–8.
40. Lof Granstrom A, Amin L, Arnell H, Wester T. Increased risk of inflammatory bowel disease in a population-based cohort study of patients with hirschsprung disease. J Pediatr Gastroenterol Nutr. 2018;66(3):398–401.
41. Levin DN, Marcon MA, Rintala RJ, Jacobson D, Langer JC. Inflammatory bowel disease manifesting after surgical treatment for hirschsprung disease. J Pediatr Gastroenterol Nutr. 2012;55(3):272–7.
42. Marquez TT, Acton RD, Hess DJ, Duval S, Saltzman DA. Comprehensive review of procedures for total colonic aganglionosis. J Pediatr Surg. 2009;44(1):257–65; discussion 265.
43. Laughlin DM, Friedmacher F, Puri P. Total colonic aganglionosis: a systematic review and meta-analysis of long-term clinical outcome. Pediatr Surg Int. 2012;28(8):773–9.
44. Roorda D, Witvliet MJ, Wellens LM, et al. Long-term outcome and quality of life in patients with total colonic aganglionosis in the Netherlands. Colorectal Dis. 2018;20(8):719–26.
45. Escobar MA, Grosfeld JL, West KW, et al. Long-term outcomes in total colonic aganglionosis: a 32-year experience. J Pediatr Surg. 2005;40(6):955–61.
46. Hoehner JC, Ein SH, Shandling B, Kim PC. Long-term morbidity in total colonic aganglionosis. J Pediatr Surg. 1998;33(7):961–5; discussion 965.
47. Urla C, Lieber J, Obermayr F, et al. Surgical treatment of children with total colonic aganglionosis: functional and metabolic long-term outcome. BMC Surg. 2018;18(1):58–018.
48. Quinn FM, Surana R, Puri P. The influence of trisomy 21 on outcome in children with hirschsprung's disease. J Pediatr Surg. 1994;29(6):781–3.
49. Ahola JA, Koivusalo A, Sairanen H, Jokinen E, Rintala RJ, Pakarinen MP. Increased incidence of hirschsprung's disease in patients with hypoplastic left heart syndrome – a common neural crest-derived etiology? J Pediatr Surg. 2009;44(7):1396–400.
50. Makitie O, Heikkinen M, Kaitila I, Rintala R. Hirschsprung's disease in cartilage-hair hypoplasia has poor prognosis. J Pediatr Surg. 2002;37(11):1585–8.
51. Asai N, Jijiwa M, Enomoto A, et al. RET receptor signaling: dysfunction in thyroid cancer and hirschsprung's disease. Pathol Int. 2006;56(4):164–72.
52. Amiel J, Lyonnet S. Hirschsprung disease, associated syndromes, and genetics: a review. J Med Genet. 2001;38(11):729–39.
53. Pakarinen MP, Rintala RJ, Koivusalo A, Heikkinen M, Lindahl H, Pukkala E. Increased incidence of medullary thyroid carcinoma in patients treated for hirschsprung's disease. J Pediatr Surg. 2005;40(10):1532–4.
54. Virtanen VB, Pukkala E, Kivisaari R, et al. Thyroid cancer and co-occurring RET mutations in hirschsprung disease. Endocr Relat Cancer. 2013;20(4):595–602.
55. Hartman EE, Oort FJ, Aronson DC, Sprangers MA. Quality of life and disease-specific functioning of patients with anorectal malformations or hirschsprung's disease: a review. Arch Dis Child. 2011;96(4):398–406.
56. Hartman EE, Oort FJ, Sprangers MA, et al. Factors affecting quality of life of children and adolescents with anorectal malformations or hirschsprung disease. J Pediatr Gastroenterol Nutr. 2008;47(4):463–71.

57. Onishi S, Nakame K, Kaji T, et al. The bowel function and quality of life of hirschsprung disease patients who have reached 18 years of age or older - the long-term outcomes after un... - PubMed - NCBI J Pediatr Surg. 2017;52(12):2001–5.
58. Heikkinen M, Rintala R, Louhimo I. Bowel function and quality of life in adult patients with operated hirschsprung's disease. Pediatr Surg Int. 1995;10:342–4.
59. Ieiri S, Nakatsuji T, Akiyoshi J, et al. Long-term outcomes and the quality of life of hirschsprung disease in adolescents who have reached 18 years or older – a 47-year single-institute experience. J Pediatr Surg. 2010;45(12):2398–402.
60. Gunnarsdottir A, Sandblom G, Arnbjornsson E, Larsson LT. Quality of life in adults operated on for hirschsprung disease in childhood. J Pediatr Gastroenterol Nutr. 2010;51(2):160–6.
61. Hartman EE, Oort FJ, Visser MR, et al. Explaining change over time in quality of life of adult patients with anorectal malformations or hirschsprung's disease. Dis Colon Rectum. 2006;49(1):96–103.

9783030156466